Understanding
Nursing Care

For Churchill Livingstone:

Commissioning editor: Ellen Green
Project manager: Valerie Burgess
Project development editor: Mairi McCubbin
Design direction: Judith Wright
Copy editor: Pat Croucher
Indexer: Lisa Weinkove
Sales promotion executive: Maria O'Connor

Understanding Nursing Care

Edited by

Patricia I. Peattie BSc (SocSc) CertEd MHSM RGN RSCN RNT
Principal, Lothian College of Health Studies, Edinburgh

Stanley Walker STD RGN RCT RNT
Formerly Vice-Principal, Lothian College of Health Studies, Edinburgh

FOURTH EDITION

CHURCHILL LIVINGSTONE
EDINBURGH HONG KONG LONDON MADRID MELBOURNE NEW YORK AND TOKYO 1995

CHURCHILL LIVINGSTONE
Medical Division of Pearson Professional Limited

Distributed in the United States of America by Churchill
Livingstone Inc., 650 Avenue of the Americas, New York,
N.Y. 10011, and by associated companies, branches and
representatives throughout the world.

First published 1978
Second edition 1981
Third edition 1987
Fourth edition 1995

ISBN 0 443 046360

British Library of Cataloguing in Publication Data
A catalogue record for this book is available from the
British Library.

Library of Congress Cataloging in Publication Data
A catalogue record for this book is available from the
Library of Congress

Produced by Longman Singapore Publishers (Pte) Ltd.
Printed in Singapore

Contents

Contributors

Mary Bronte DipCNE RGN CritCareNursing Cert RCNT RNT
Heartstart Co-ordinator (Scotland), British Heart Foundation
12 Care implications of disorders of the cardiovascular system

John Davidson BEd CertEd RMN RNMH RCNT
Senior Nurse Teacher, Lothian College of Health Studies
7 Care implications of disorders of learning

Christine Donnelly BA RGN ONC DipHV RNT
Nurse Teacher, Lothian College of Health Studies
11 Care implications of disorders of the locomotor system

Helen A. S. Dougan BEd DipCNE RGN RCNT RNT
Nurse Teacher, St Columba's Hospice, Edinburgh
3 The role of the nurse

Isobel M. Gibson BSc DipEd RGN SCM RCNT RNT NeuroCert
Nurse Teacher, Lothian College of Health Studies
5 Care implications of disorders of the nervous system

Patricia M C Gillies RGN RNT
Nurse Teacher, Lothian College of Health Studies
6 Care implications of disorders of the sensory organs

Morag A. Gray DipCNE CertNursTeaching MN RGN RCNT RNT
Senior Nurse Teacher, Lothian College of Health Studies
12 Care implications of disorders of the cardiovascular system
13 Care implications of disorders of the respiratory system

Shirley Gregor BSc DipEd RGN SCM RCNT RNT
Nephro-urological Nursing Dip
Nurse Teacher, Lothian College of Health Studies
17 Care implications of disorders of the genito-urinary and reproductive system

Janis Greig BSc DipLSN RGN RMN RNT
Nurse Teacher, Lothian College of Health Studies
8 Care implications of disorders of mood

Dorothy Horsburgh BA(Hons) MEd RGN RCNT RNT
Nurse Teacher, Lothian College of Health Studies
15 Care implications of disorders of the gastrointestinal system

Doreen MacLean BA RGN RSCN RM HV RNT
Senior Nurse Teacher, Lothian College of Health Studies
1 Health and society

Robert G. Mitchell BA MSc RMN RGN RNT
Senior Nurse Teacher, Lothian College of Health Studies
10 Care implications of disorders of personality

Patricia J. Steele MEd RGN SCM HVCert RNT
Nurse Teacher, Lothian College of Health Studies
2 People and health

Marylyn Stewart BSc RGN RCT RNT
Nurse Teacher, Lothian College of Health Studies
14 Care implications of disorders of the blood and immune system

David J. Tait BSc(Hons) MSc RMN RGN RNT
Nurse Teacher, Lothian College of Health Studies
9 Care implications of disorders of thought and perception

Margaret B. Thomson BA RN RM RCNT RNT
Former Senior Nurse Teacher, Lothian College of Health Studies
Tutor Counsellor, Diploma and Degree Courses in Nursing, Distance Learning Centre, South Bank University, London
16 Care implications of disorders of the endocrine system

Anne Waugh BSc(Hons) MSc CertEd SRN RNT
Nurse Teacher, Lothian College of Health Studies
4 Science and the art of nursing

Preface

There have been many changes in health care in the eight years that have passed since the publication of the third edition of *Understanding Nursing Care*. There is now an increased emphasis on health education, health promotion and preventative medicine. The delivery of health care services has changed, with a greater emphasis than ever before on value for money, efficiency gains and care in the community. The role of nurses in the management of care has never been more vital, and the need for a flexible adaptable practitioner is even more crucial.

To meet these challenges, the preparation of nurses and midwives is now achieved through an educational programme which is more student centred, requiring the learner to become an informed doer, and a thinking, accountable, autonomous practitioner on registration. In addition, direct entry courses leading to registration as a midwife make this text relevant to these students also.

The new format of this edition of the book underlines the changes and contributes to the development of appropriate intellectual skills which underpin all practice.

The first four chapters now provide the generic framework within which all nursing practice takes place. Chapters 1 and 2 are concerned with broad social aspects of health and illness, and the individual within his own context. Chapter 3 explores the role of the nurse, care planning strategies and research issues, whilst Chapter 4 considers the scientific issues which underpin the diagnostic and therapeutic practice of medicine and nursing, explaining the mutual dependence of the one upon the other.

The changing pattern of disease, and increased emphasis on common care strategies, have led to a review of the remaining chapters. There is more emphasis on the care of people with a mental illness, reflecting the increase in mental health problems and learning disability. Some chapters in previous editions relating to specialist areas of care have been put together to create one chapter on care of people with disorders of the sensory organs, and one chapter on care implications of disorders of the genitourinary and reproductive systems.

While this fourth edition looks somewhat different from its predecessors, we would nevertheless like to acknowledge our indebtedness to the original editors, Anne Chilman and Margaret Thomas, without whose foresight and hard work the book would never have been developed, and also to the original contributors, upon whose work much of this edition is based. For our part as Book Editors, we would like to thank our own team of contributors, who have been drawn from the wider resource of the whole Lothian College, which was created in 1989 and operates on several sites throughout the Lothian Region. The many changes and developments in nursing and midwifery education in recent years have informed the development of this work as well as placed additional burdens upon the authors.

We have assumed that the reader has some knowledge of the sciences, and included only that which aids an understanding of the accompanying text. We have directed readers, through suggestions for further reading and assignments, which may be study topics, written activities or discussion, to deepen their understanding of the role of the nurse in particular care settings and for specific care needs.

Despite all the changes in the text, and a new layout to make it user friendly, the purpose of the book remains unchanged: to foster an *understanding* of why certain care strategies are appropriate; to encourage an informed, perceptive, sympathetic and empathetic approach to each patient and his carers; and to enable the nurse, as an equal member of the caring team, to promote the best interests of those in her care.

As had our predecessors, we have had much help from the publishers, without whose guidance and encouragement, in the midst of all the other pressures, this edition might never have been completed.

Individual authors have sought help from many varied sources, and we are grateful to all those colleagues for giving their time and expertise to the development of various aspects of the text.

Edinburgh
1995

Patricia I. Peattie
Stanley Walker

Fundamentals of health, illness and professional nursing practice

Fundamentals of health, illness and professional nursing practice

SECTION CONTENTS

This section provides the framework within which nursing practice takes place. The first two chapters look at the social context of health and illness, and at the individual in a personal context. Chapter 3 considers the role of the nurse, care strategies and research issues. Chapter 4 considers the scientific areas that underpin both medical and nursing practice, and explains their mutual interdependence.

1

Health and society

Doreen MacLean

INTRODUCTION

In many countries health has become a major social and political issue. This is due in part to the World Health Organizations' strategy for attaining health for all by the year 2000. The strategy was adopted by the 33 members of the European region, and Britain as a member state is therefore committed to achieving the 38 targets which have been set. Some of these targets will be referred to later in this chapter.

In addition, the costs of providing health care within the National Health Service (NHS) are escalating at an alarming rate. In the year ending 31 March 1993, the total cost of the Health Service in the UK was £34 912 million. Health care must not only be effective, it must also provide value for money.

The importance of health to and within society is further emphasized by the amount of attention given to health issues by the media, especially television and the press. Even a cursory study of most daily newspapers will reveal at least one article relating to health.

In July 1992, the Government published a strategy for improving the health of England – 'The Health of The Nation' – in which they detailed five key areas for action: coronary artery disease and stroke, cancers, mental illness, HIV / AIDS and sexual health and accidents. Objectives and targets were set for each key area. Scotland has also identified five key areas on which to focus attention but in recognition of the poorer dental health of the Scottish people, has chosen to replace mental health with dental and oral health (Scottish Office 1992). In setting out these priority areas, the Government hopes to shift the focus of the Health Service from that of sickness to health and sees the setting of these targets as one way of improving the nation's health.

The emphasis on health is reflected in *The Role and Function of the Professional Nurse* (1992), which states:

The National Nursing and Midwifery Consultative Committee is strongly of the view that professional nursing practice must be grounded in health rather than illness, though it acknowledges that this may represent a major shift in concept among non-nurses, where the prevailing image of the professional nurse is often associated with the nurse's work in acute sectors.

Nurses, then, as health professionals must be concerned with the health of patients and clients throughout the life-span and should be able to assess the health status of those with whom they come into contact either in the community or in hospital.

THE VALUE OF HEALTH

A wise man ought to realize that his health is his most valuable possession

Hippocrates 460–377 BC (Strauss 1968a)

All health is better than wealth

Sir Walter Scott 1771–1832 (Strauss 1968b)

Health-care professions may find it surprising that the above statements were made so many years ago. They could just have easily come from more recent health education material. Man's preoccupation with health has a very long history and is not just the product of our present-day 'health conscious' society.

Increased knowledge of the causative factors of disease and technological advance has meant that many of the health problems of previous decades, such as infectious disease, have been all but eliminated. Immunization against smallpox is no longer necessary in Britain because the disease has virtually been eradicated on a worldwide scale. People are living longer and the Nation's children are undoubtedly healthier than they have ever been. It is however important to stress that despite the obvious improvements in health status, many members of society adopt and continue to pursue health behaviours which are not conducive to health and which may, and often do, prove to be life threatening. The value placed on health and the priority accorded to it by lay members of society is often at variance with what health professionals believe it to be. Indeed many people probably see health as the opposite of illness and only consider it when in fact they become ill.

Peter O'Neill (1983) suggests that health should be promoted as a 'way of life' and that 'illness is often caused by neglecting those factors in our daily lives over which we could have complete control if we chose to exercise it'.

This may well be true, but the situation is not as straightforward as the aforegoing suggests, since many groups in society chose to ignore the many public exhortations to lead healthier lifestyles. The World Health Organisation has described tobacco smoking as an 'epidemic' and as the most important cause of preventable disease and premature death, yet as one smoker stops, another young person usually takes his place by beginning to smoke.

It is clear that some members of the general public do not see health as their most valuable possession. This seems to be a somewhat neglected area of research, but Calman (1987) describes a study involving 20 women who were asked if there were things more important to them than health. The majority (18) said that their health was not their most important concern. Concerns about the family, and children in particular, were mentioned along with the threat of nuclear war and employment prospects. This was a very small study and as such not statistically significant. It would also have been interesting to find out what values and priorities men and people in different age groups would have reported. The study does however serve to illustrate that to presume health is valued above all other aspects of daily life is somewhat misguided and likely to lead to inappropriate health care.

Paradoxically, too much concern and value placed on health is frequently seen as socially unacceptable. A frequent greeting in Britain is 'How are you?', but do we really want to know in explicit detail exactly how that person is? Even health professionals may find this somewhat daunting! The state of hypochondria is well illustrated in the following:

The surest road to health, say what they will,
– Is never to suppose we shall be ill
– Most of these evils we poor mortals know,
– From doctors and imagination flow

Charles Churchill 1731–1746 (Strauss 1968c)

CONCEPTS OF HEALTH

The word health has been variously defined, interpreted and explained. It has been the subject of much debate, discussion and controversy in recent years but there is as yet, no universally agreed definition of what health actually is. This is largely because health means different things to different people and is likely to vary with age, sex, socioeconomic group and culture.

It is then perhaps misguided to attempt to define health by attaching a specific fixed label such as might be found in a dictionary. In this respect, dictionary definitions are not helpful, as they usually equate health with wholeness. This in turn is likely to fuel debate as to what is meant by 'whole'. Seedhouse

(1986a), recognizing the difficulties inherent in defining health, states that: 'What has emerged from the volumes of writing on health is an indigestible spaghetti of confusion'.

Much of this confusion arises undoubtedly because health is a word which is frequently in use. It has become fashionable to prefix many other words with it. We have health foods, health farms and health centres to name but a few. Familiarity leads us to believe that we understand its meaning, that is until we begin to question what it means. This point is well illustrated in the words of Saint Augustine: 'What, then, is time? If no one asks me I know; if I wish to explain it to someone that asks, I do not.' Seedhouse (1986b).

Aggleton (1990) suggests that definitions of health fall into two main categories:

1. *Official definitions* – the views of doctors and other health professionals.
2. *Lay beliefs* – the views of those not involved professionally with health issues or what might be called the more popular perceptions of health. Such beliefs, according to Aggleton, 'co-exist along with official views about health and they even inform the actions of doctors, nurses, health visitors and health education officers'.

Official definitions of health may be set out in negative terms, as in the absence of disease or illness or more positively in terms of physical and mental fitness or personal strength and ability. To consider health merely as the obvious absence of disease or illness poses immediate problems. It is possible for disease to exist without the individual being aware of it, while on the other hand, a person may feel ill despite a lack of obvious features of the disease. Furthermore, there are many individuals for whom disease has meant permanent disability, such as amputation of a limb or paralysis, but who nevertheless lead happy and productive lives. Indeed, those people affected by the drug thalidomide, who were born with missing or rudimentary arms, would undoubtedly claim to be healthy.

Positive definitions of health include the well-known and much quoted World Health Organization (WHO) statement (1946) which regards health as: 'A state of complete physical, mental and social well-being and not merely the absence of disease or infirmity'.

While it is important to consider the relationship between physical, social and psychological influences in health, there will be few who are capable of achieving such an idealistic state. This definition would exclude a great many people who consider themselves to be healthy, yet have minor anxieties or stresses that are part of everyday living.

The ability to utilize personal strengths and energies to adapt to one's environment and adjust to changing situations is believed by some theorists to be indicative of health. Dubos (1959) states that: 'Health and happiness are expressions of the manner in which the individual responds and adapts to the challenges that he meets in everyday life.' This view of health is attractive since much of nursing practice is concerned with enabling people to adjust to changed circumstances brought about by illness and disease. It is important, however, to stress that some forms of adaptation may be somewhat negative. Passive acceptance of circumstances may inhibit recovery and suicide would not be considered to be an appropriate form of adaption to the pressures of life.

Despite high levels of unemployment in recent years, society still places a great deal of emphasis on the importance of work. For some, to return to work after sickness signifies a return to health. Parsons (1981) supports his concept and defines health as: 'the state of optimum capacity of the individual for the performance of the roles and tasks for which he has been socialized'.

Thus, health is essential for the smooth running of society and, by implication, low levels of health should be discouraged.

Parsons (1981) is quite clear about the 'sick role' which brings rights and obligations for the incapacitated person – the right to be legitimately excused work and the obligation to cooperate with the prescribed care. This approach to health, though useful in some respects, fails to take account of anything but physical health. No consideration is given to other aspects of health such as psychological and social factors, without which no assessment of health would be complete. In addition, Parson's approach to health makes no mention of the fact that some types of work may, by their very nature, prove to be damaging to health. Policemen, firemen, miners and those in the armed forces face situations which are likely to be hazardous to both their physical and psychological health. Nurses too may find some aspect of their work emotionally as well as physically demanding, with some seeking to counteract the stress by smoking.

In recent years, health has come to be regarded as a commodity, something which can be obtained or lost, even bought and sold if one subscribes to private health care. Health is frequently 'advertised' on television and magazines alongside exhortations to buy particular brands of soap powder – an attempt to harness the power of the media for health education purposes. Modern medicine, according to Seedhouse (1986c), supports the image of health as a commodity: 'Health appears to be a thing which exists apart from people, which may be captured if the right procedure is followed. This sort of health can be lost if a person has a diseased organ, but with appropriate treatment can be restored.'

This view of health is somewhat dehumanizing and simplistic and it does not take account of the complexities inherent in human interactions. There is however some merit in the idea of 'marketing' health. Health visitors, whose main concern is to improve and maintain the health of the community, have for many years recognized the value of moving out of health centres and clinics to provide health education and information in shopping centres and similar places (Quickfall 1992). The increasing use of the word client rather than patient emphasizes the notion of individuals being consumers of health care.

Initiatives such as the 'Patient's Charter' are encouraging people to develop a more active role in the provision of health services and they are being asked to share in the responsibility for their own health. This being so, it is important to consider what the lay person believes about health.

Lay beliefs are many and varied and depend on culture, socioeconomic status, age and sex. However, at this point, a few examples will serve as illustration.

Many women see health as their ability to perform tasks in the household and believe they have to look after the family even when they are ill. Indeed, some women believe that by carrying on instead of going to bed they are likely to recover more quickly. To give in to the illness is to admit weakness and indeed lay beliefs frequently have moral overtones. There is still a great deal of anxiety generated by the HIV virus and AIDS despite widespread health education campaigns. Some of those infected are considered to be innocent: babies and those who contracted the disease by being given infected blood. On the other hand there are those who are thought to be guilty: the drug abusers and homosexual men. These latter groups are already being seen by members of society as deviant and the development of AIDS is seen as just retribution.

Colds and chills figure largely among lay beliefs, especially in relation to causative factors. Sitting in a draught, failing to wear a hat while exposed to the night air or getting one's feet wet, are all thought of as causes of colds.

DIMENSIONS OF HEALTH

In recent years there has been increasing interest in the concept of holistic health. The patient is a unique individual whose physical needs may well be influenced by social, emotional or spiritual factors and nurses have been encouraged to consider not only the patient's physical needs but also the social, emotional and spiritual needs. In this way, patients can receive care that is planned, with the knowledge that all the dimensions of health are interrelated and interdependent (Fig. 1.1).

All the theories and approaches to health stated above serve to illustrate that to look for one all-embracing definition of health is inadvisable if not impossible. Nurses and their patients may look at health from differing perspectives but what is important is that the nurse recognizes and takes account of this when planning care.

MEASUREMENT OF HEALTH

Health, as we have seen, is an extremely difficult concept to define. This being so, it follows that the measurement of health will likewise be fraught with problems. Most measures of health are in reality measures of disease and illness, although attempts have been made to focus attention on more positive measures of health. Bowling (1991) describes the measurements of subjective health states and details a large number of studies which examine components of positive health, including social well-being, psychological well-being and quality of life. She argues that although it is easier to measure departures from health, reliance on such negative definitions of health will provide little information on the 80–90% of the population who do not experience chronic physical limitation or substantial psychiatric impairment. Health may be seen as a continuum ranging from positive health and well-being to negative health states and ultimate death (Fig. 1.2). Individuals may be at different points on the continuum on any given occasion.

The promotion of positive health by focusing on measures such as nutrition, physical activity and dental health, as well as environmental factors such as housing and recreation, does however provide a useful supplement to the more traditional negative methods of measuring health.

This view is supported by WHO (1983) who believe there is a need to strengthen health, with one of the main aims being to reduce disease and its consequences. In this respect, the emphasis should be on:

1. Adding life to years by ensuring the full development and use of an individual's total or residual

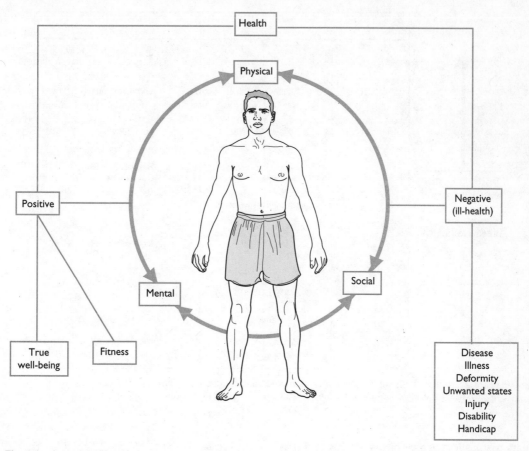

Fig. 1.1 A model of health.

physical and mental capacity to derive full benefit from and to cope with life in a healthy way.

2. Adding health to life by preventing and reducing disease and disability.

3. Adding years to life by reducing premature deaths and therefore increasing life expectancy.

The health of the community is routinely measured using information obtained from a variety of sources. The task of collating, analysing and publishing much of this data is the responsibility of the Office of Population Censuses and Surveys (OPCS). This information includes mortality statistics, births, abortions, congenital malformations and incidence of communicable diseases and cancers.

It is a statutory requirement that all births and deaths be notified, therefore few, if any, will be missed. It is however only necessary to inform the health authorities of certain notifiable communicable diseases, e.g. dysentery, cholera, tuberculosis, measles and sexually transmitted diseases. This system is designed to assist in the control of disease. Registers are also kept of people with congenital malformations, cancers and industrial disease. In addition, information is also obtained by routine collection of hospital inpatient and outpatient statistics. This, however, will exclude those conditions not requiring hospital attendance.

The General Household Survey has been conducted annually since 1971 using a random sample of some 12 500 households in England and Wales. The health section includes questions on chronic and acute illness, general practice consultations and many other variables related to health. However, since this information is self-reported, it may not be entirely accurate.

There have also been three National Morbidity Surveys since the Health Service began, the most recent being in 1981–82. In these, selected general practitioners recorded details of consultations, diagnoses and referrals, as well as age and sex of the patients.

In Scotland the Registrar General is responsible for

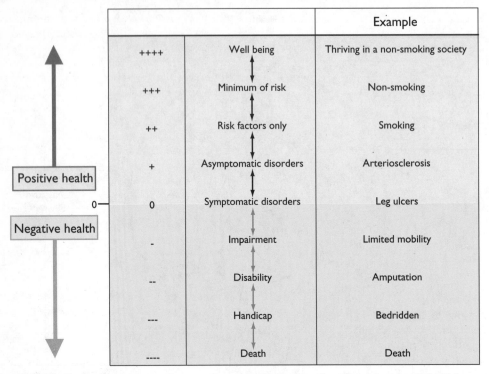

Fig. 1.2 Health status as a continuum – demonstrating ranges of positive (+) and negative (–) health, using the effects of smoking as an example. (Adapted from Catford 1983, figure 1)

population statistics such as births, deaths and marriages while Scottish health statistics are published by the information and statistics divison of the Common Services Agency.

Despite the fact that the above measures are far from ideal, they do provide information on the distribution of disease and disability within the community. Indices of death and disease, despite being in direct contrast to health, can prove useful in assessing needs and in planning health services. In addition, official health statistics can be used to make international comparisons. These statistics, however, are likely to prove more valuable if supported by appropriate information from the many social surveys conducted each year which look at health from a much broader perspective.

GENDER AND HEALTH

For most of the last decade, mortality rates for both sexes have declined – the chances of living longer have improved for both men and women. Until 1989 males had consistently higher mortality rates in every age group from birth to old age, but in 1991 and 1992

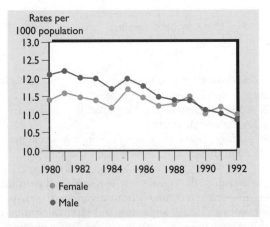

Fig. 1.3 Male and female death rates in the UK. (Source: Central Statistical Office, 1994 Annual Abstract of Statistics)

mortality rates for women were higher than those for men (Fig. 1.3). The expectation of life for women is greater than that for men by 5–6 years. This means that in the 75+ age group the numbers of women in the population greatly outnumber men by a ratio of 2 : 1 (Fig. 1.4). This may be one of the factors influ-

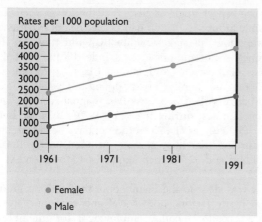

Rates per 1000 population

Fig. 1.4 Population of males and females aged 75+ in the UK. (Source: Central Statistical Office 1994 Annual Abstract of Statistics Table 2.3, pp 6–7)

encing the changing death rates, since death is more common in this age group.

It is interesting to look at gender differences in causes of death. In 1992 in Britain, 3467 males died from suicide and self-inflicted injury, whereas the figure for women was 1054.

One matter of concern is the rising number of deaths due to accidents and violence. Males still outnumber females in this regard, but the gap is narrowing (Fig. 1.5).

It is worth noting that in Scotland the number of women dying from lung cancer has increased in recent years and has now overtaken the number of deaths due to cancer of the breast. This however is not so in England and Wales where in 1992 13 663 women died of breast cancer and 10 994 died from lung cancer.

A study of morbidity patterns reveals that women

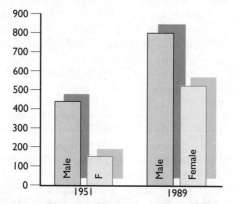

Fig. 1.5 Accident and violence as cause of death in the UK. (Source: Central Statistical Office 1991 Social Trends 21, Table 7.5 p. 116)

consistently record higher rates of chronic and acute sickness. Mental illness is consistently present in much higher levels in women with one woman in four being likely to suffer from serious depression at some time in her life (Wood 1989). In addition, anorexia, anxiety and deliberate self-harm are more commonly diagnosed in women. Women are twice as likely to attempt suicide as men but most successful suicides are committed by men. This may indicate that attempted suicide in women is a cry for help, whereas men may suppress depression until self-destructive impulses reach a lethal level (Briscoe 1989).

More women than men are diagnosed as being mentally ill. The number of admissions to psychiatric hospitals in Scotland in 1991 was 14 202 males and 16 054 females. Various suggestions have been offered to account for this difference. It is felt that socialization factors are important (Briscoe 1989) – girls are socialized to express their feelings to a greater extent than boys and need more emotional support. Women who have a close confiding relationship are less likely to suffer depression. The increased incidence of the nuclear family may well have removed some of the traditional support networks which were previously available to young families and to women in particular.

Women are believed to exhibit more health-seeking behaviour then men and consequently make more use of the health-care services. Women are said to report more symptoms because it is more acceptable to do so. It may also be easier for a housewife or woman in part-time employment to get to the surgery. Illness is seen to be stigmatizing in men but much less so in women. The 'stiff upper lip', which is very much a part of British culture, is considered to be a factor in the identification and treatment of mental health problems in males.

Life circumstances are known to influence the mental health of women, in particular variables such as poverty, employment status, marital status and motherhood. Frequently some, if not all, of the above combine to create an atmosphere of stress. Solberg (1989) states that women 'are more vulnerable to becoming poor and as a group are more likely than men to live in poverty. In addition, once a woman becomes poor, she will remain in poverty for a longer period than a man would.'

A consequence of the high levels of marriage breakdown in recent years is the increase in single-parent families, with women frequently being responsible for the home and child care. Though some of those women will be in employment, circumstances usr dictate that they will be in poorly paid jobs.

The lack of free or cheap child-care provision for the preschool child leads to the stresses of role conflict for the mother. Housing may well be substandard and the mother's ability to provide a well-balanced diet for herself and her children will be compromised.

It is never easy and may be impossible to relieve stress and anxiety by changing an individual's circumstances. This being so, it is perhaps not surprising that in the 1980s, general practitioners frequently prescribed drugs to relieve symptoms if not the cause of stress-related illness. In 1983, general practitioners issued 23 million prescriptions for benzodiazepines, better known to the lay population as valium, and up to half of these were repeat prescriptions. The cost of these prescriptions to the NHS was £37.5 million. The cost to many individuals was the experience of withdrawal symptoms when trying to stop taking the drug (Smith & Jacobson 1988). The vast majority of these prescriptions were for women. The 'valium experience', however, was not all negative – many women set up or joined self-help groups to ease the withdrawal process, and a number of these groups have continued with the aim of providing support and practical help to women who require it.

SOCIOECONOMIC FACTORS INFLUENCING HEALTH

In March 1977, David Ennals, who was at that time Secretary of State for Social Services, made the following statement:

The crude differences in mortality rates between the various social classes are worrying. To take the extreme example, in 1971 the death rate for adult men in Social Class V (unskilled workers) was nearly twice that of adult men in Social Class I (professional workers). When you look at death rates for specific diseases the gap is even wider. The first step towards remedial action is to put together what is already known about the problem. It is a major challenge for the next ten or more years to try to narrow the gap in health standards between different social classes   (Townsend et al 1992)

Consequently, a research working group was appointed under the Chairmanship of Sir Douglas Black, then President of the College of Physicians. The remit of the group was: 'to assess the national and international evidence and draw some of the implications for policy from the evidence on inequalities in health'.

This task was completed in 1980 and the report of the working group, subsequently known as the 'Black Report', was released by the Department of Health and Social Security at the beginning of the August Bank Holiday in the same year.

The report made it clear that the lower socioeconomic groups in Britain had poorer health experience throughout all stages of life than did those in the highest socioeconomic groups. Indeed if the mortality rates of those in Occupational Class I (professional workers and families) had applied to Classes IV and V (partly skilled and unskilled manual workers and their families) during the years 1970–72, 74 000 lives of people under age 75 would not have been lost. It is disturbing that this estimate included nearly 10 000 children and 32 000 men aged 15–64 (Townsend et al 1992).

It was clear to the members of the working group that many factors, both social and economic, influenced health. Income, employment (or unemployment), housing, education, access to transport and individual life-styles were seen to be important determinants of health, with members of the higher socioeconomic groups being able to exert more control over these aspects of their lives than is possible for members of the manual classes. In addition poorer health status experienced by the lower socioeconomic groups did not appear to result in the increased use of health services, indeed the reverse was true.

Despite the importance of Black's findings and the implications they contained for the health of Britain, it was made quite clear by the Secretary of State for Health and Social Security in the foreword to the report that 'additional expenditure on the scale which could result from the report's recommendations is quite unrealistic in present or any foreseeable economic circumstances. I cannot therefore endorse the group's recommendations'. (Department of Health and Social Security 1980).

Despite these comments, the Black Report stimulated a great deal of interest both in this country and in Europe. Researchers continued to collect evidence of inequalities, and in March 1987 the Health Education Council published an update by Margaret Whitehead called 'The Health Divide'. This received a great deal of media coverage despite the cancellation of the expected press conference, which was seen by many as 'an attempt to cover up vital information about the nation's health'. It is interesting to know that this sentiment was also expressed in the House of Lords when members could not obtain copies of the report for a debate on the NHS, because all copies had been distributed by the end of the month in which it had been published.

In the years since the publication of the above reports, their findings have been re-examined (Smith et al 1990) and the information updated (Townsend et al 1992). There is no evidence to suggest that inequalities have lessened. In some respects, notably social class differences in mortality, the gap may have become even greater.

The use of socioeconomic status alone as a determinant of health does however pose problems in that not everyone can be allocated to a social class, as it is dependent on occupation. In addition, the social class of a married woman is based on the occupation of her husband. In an attempt to overcome some of the difficulties inherent in measures of social class, Carstairs and Morris (1990) have devised 'an area measure of deprivation which reflects the socioeconomic characteristics of the population and which permits most of the records, routinely collected in the Health Service to be analysed, using the post code of the areas of residence'. Their four variables used to generate deprivation scores were:

1. *Overcrowding:* persons in private households where there is more than one person per room as a proportion of all persons in private households.
2. *Male unemployment:* proportion of economically active males who are seeking work.
3. *Low social class:* proportion of all persons in private households with head of households in Social Class IV or V.
4. *No car:* proportion of all persons in private households with no car.

These variables were combined to give a single score for each post code area in Scotland. The resultant scores ranged from 1 to 7, or most affluent to most materially deprived. The collection of data in this way has provided confirmation that inequalities do exist and that both morbidity and mortality rates vary dependent on the socioeconomic status of the area in which an individual lives.

The same measure of deprivation has also been used to explain differences in mortality rates between Scotland and England. The greater deprivation experienced in Scotland may well result in excess mortality, particularly in young adults. The links between wealth and the nation's health are well documented and it is a matter of some concern to health professionals that the numbers and proportions of individuals in poverty in Britain continues to rise. The poverty line is derived from Households Below Average income, based on 50% of average income after housing costs. This shows that in 1988/89 nearly 12 million people were living in poverty. Of these, 3.1 million were children, which represents 25% of all children, compared with 1.4 million (10% of all children) in 1979.

The first target of the World Health Organization's European Strategy for Health for All by the Year 2000 concerns inequality. Britain is committed to reducing inequalities by 25% by the year 2000. If this is to be achieved, steps must be taken to reduce poverty and improve the social circumstances of those members of society who are most materially disadvantaged.

CULTURE, LANGUAGE AND HEALTH

Britain has become a multicultural and multiracial society. This means that most of us will have some contact with people from other nations and cultures many of whom will have different traditions, language and religions.

Nurses are not expected to be fluent in foreign languages or conversant with the customs and religions of all ethnic groups. The nurse is however expected to: 'recognise and respect the uniqueness and dignity of each patient and client and respond to their need for care irrespective of their ethnic origin, religious beliefs, personal attributes, the nature of their health problem or any other factor' (United Kingdom Central Council for Nursing, Midwifery and Health Visiting (UKCC) 1992). The nurse then must learn to be sensitive to the cultural needs of patients. Some of these needs will be similar to those of the native population but there are also likely to be differences in attitude to and expectations of health care. There may also be differences in the use which is made of health services.

The best source of information on ethnic issues is the patient and his family and care should always be taken to ensure that they are actively involved in planning care. Nevertheless, consideration of some of the customs and practices of the main ethnic minority groups in Britain will enable the nurse to be more confident in delivering care.

It is important to note that most of those labelled as belonging to other cultures are in fact British by birth, having parents or grandparents who came into this country, often many years ago. In addition, not all of these people will be practising members of their culture. Thus assumption and stereotyping should be avoided.

Consideration should be given to the following areas detailed below.

Language

Differences in language may create barriers to effective communication. Many people, especially those who are older, have only a very basic knowledge of English and will readily become confused, therefore nurses should be prepared to use simple English and speak slowly and distinctly.

Younger members of the family may have greater command of English but difficulties can arise, especially in situations where matters of an intimate or confidential nature are to be discussed. Friends and family members should therefore only be used as interpreters in emergency situations. Most hospitals and health centres will have information and contact numbers where advice and/or interpreters can be obtained. Where verbal communication is difficult, non-verbal communication becomes an important aspect of interaction – a warm smile can relieve anxiety and convey a caring attitude.

Diet

In many cultures religious beliefs put limitations on diet and food preparation. Some foods may be prohibited.

Hindus do not eat meat. Some, but not all will eat eggs. Dairy produce is usually acceptable but only if it is free of animal fat. Indeed strict vegetarians will be unwilling to eat even vegetarian items served from the same plate or with utensils which have been used for meat.

Jews and Muslims will only eat meat which has been killed in a specific way, which ensures that as much blood as possible is drained from the meat before cooking. The pig is a totally forbidden animal and it would be most unusual for a Jewish or Muslim person to eat pork in any form.

The Chinese, especially the older generation, believe that rice is the only food which will provide them with energy. For this reason they may request, if hospitalized, that food be brought in by their relatives.

The increasing number of vegetarians in Britain means that many hospitals and institutions now have vegetarian dishes on the menu each day. This is likely to be useful in meeting the dietary needs of many cultures. In addition it may be possible to obtain special diets, e.g. kosher meals for Jews, if requested.

In some cultures there is a requirement to fast at certain times of the year. Buddhists may not eat after 12 noon on Buddha's birthday. Most Jews will observe Yom-Kippur, the day of atonement, which is a 25-hour fast taking place in the autumn. During Ramadan, a Muslim will fast between sunrise and sunset. In most cultures however exceptions to fasting will be allowed for the pregnant woman or if the health of the individual requires it.

Hygiene/client care

Asian people prefer to wash in running water, therefore a shower is preferable to a bath. The provision of a jug of water to wash the genitals after using the toilet is appreciated. Many Asians observe the right hand/left hand rule of hygiene where the right hand is used for eating and the left hand is for washing. This may present problems if one or other hand cannot be used. In many cultures the individual is required to wash thoroughly before prayer. Privacy for prayer would also be appreciated. In many circumstances, female patients will not wish to be examined by a male doctor. Where this is necessary in an emergency, a female member of staff should always be present.

All individuals have feelings of modesty and these should be respected. Some ethnic minority groups will however be extremely loath to remove clothing in the presence of others and there may be some articles of clothing which have particular significance to the faith of the individual, such as the 'Kaccha' or undershorts won by Sikh women (McCall 1991). Equally, a request for the removal of a turban in public would cause a Sikh male acute embarrassment. In this context the necessity to wear a short hospital gown for surgery and X-ray would be unacceptable in some cultures.

Death/bereavement

In every society death and dying are associated with specific customs and practices. Indeed, there will be some individuals who although not previously practising their cultural traditions wish to do so when death is imminent. The Muslim may wish to lie facing Mecca with members of his/her family reciting prayers at the bedside, whereas the Sikh will gain comfort by reciting hymns from the Sikh Holy Book. The Hindu may wish to lie on the floor to be near to Mother Earth and would be more comfortable dying at home since to do so has religious significance. The advice of the family should always be sought. This is specially important in relation to what should be done when the person is dead, since some cultures, e.g. Muslims, do not allow a person who is not of their faith to touch the body. In addition, strict Muslims consider the body to belong to God and therefore no part of it can be removed. Thus post-mortems and organ donation would be forbidden. The Coroner, or the Procurator Fiscal in Scotland, may in certain circumstances however order a post-mortem to be carried out.

The health status of ethnic minority groups has been highlighted recently by the Chief Medical Officer (Doult 1992). He emphasized the differences in health patterns among the various groups. These include an increased incidence of congenital malformations among all Asian groups, higher numbers of deaths from heart disease in people born in the Indian subcontinent and a higher incidence of death from strokes among people born in the Carribean, the Indian subcontinent and Africa. Why this should be so is not clear but being non-white, unemployed or an unskilled worker in over-crowded and substandard housing are all factors which are likely to contribute to the poorer health experienced by many members of immigrant groups in Britain.

The above is intended to serve only as a guide. Nurses should take every opportunity to learn from and about each individual they care for, whether in hospital or within the community.

Greater understanding of the cultural aspects of difficulties that the person may be facing should increase --- our ability to plan appropriate care.
Being able to discuss problems with cultural understanding can help in itself to put a distressed mind more at ease.
(Dobson 1983)

BEHAVIOUR AND HEALTH

The European Regional Strategy for attaining Health For All by the Year 2000 states: 'it is becoming more and more apparent in all countries of Europe regardless of their stage of development, that the prevailing lifestyles are often the major cause of ill health, while alternative lifestyles would be strongly promotive of health and well being'.

In the nineteenth century, efforts to improve and maintain health were based largely on changes in the environment such as improved housing and sanitation. In twentieth-century society, most infectious diseases have been controlled only to be replaced by diseases which are caused by unhealthy attitudes and habits – smoking, overeating, drug and alcohol abuse and lack of exercise are all major contributions to mortality and morbidity.

Smoking

It is estimated that 1500 deaths or one in six deaths in the Lothian Region in Scotland are directly attributable to smoking. In the UK, cigarette smoking is considered to be responsible for more than 100 000 deaths per year. Added to this is the considerable impairment to quality of life for those suffering from smoking-related diseases.

The Royal College of Physicians of London argues that cigarette smoking is 'as important a cause of death as were the great epidemic diseases that affected previous generations in this country', and believes that 'action to protect the public against the damage done to so many of them by cigarette smoking would have more effect upon the public health in this country than anything else that could now be done in the whole field of preventative medicine'.

The extent of risk involved in smoking is estimated as follows: 'among 1000 young male adult smokers in England and Wales, 1 will be murdered, 6 will be killed in the road and 250 will be killed prematurely by tobacco' (Royal College of Physicians 1983).

The cost of smoking to society is high, with an estimated loss to industry of 50 million working days per year. In addition, the cost to the NHS of caring for patients with smoking-related diseases is substantial, prompting some people to suggest that since this harm is self-inflicted, treatment should not be accorded priority within the Health Service. This is not a view shared by the majority of health professionals.

The harmful effects of smoking extend beyond the individual himself and the dangers of 'side-stream' or passive smoking are being increasingly identified (see Ch. 7). Mortality from all causes including lung cancer is considered to be higher among passive smokers. One study (Wald et al 1986) suggests that non-smokers who live with smokers face a 35% higher risk of developing lung cancer than those who do not. Children are at risk before and after birth. Smoking is associated with low-birth-weight babies and a higher risk of miscarriage and pregnancy complications, while children of parents who smoke are more likely to be admitted to hospital with respiratory infections.

Despite this evidence, Government strategies to control smoking have been very limited. They have set targets to reduce by the year 2000 the proportion of men smoking to 22% and women to 21%. Frequent requests however for a complete ban on the advertising of cigarettes have as yet gone unheeded. Paradoxically many sports are dependent on sponsorship from tobacco companies and although cigarette advertising on television is banned, brand names frequently appear. A regular increase in tax revenue on cigarettes does lead to reduced consumption, but evidence from countries where there is already a complete ban on advertising suggests that this is much more successful in reducing the numbers of people who smoke. The Government however, have increased funding to the

Health Education Board for Scotland to enable them to address smoking as a major priority with emphasis on women and young people. Efforts are also being made to create a smoke-free health service as soon as possible.

Alcohol

Most people in Britain drink alcohol and taken in moderation, this is an enjoyable experience. Unfortunately, drinking too much or drinking even a small amount at the wrong time, e.g. when driving a car, can lead to tragedy and ill health.

In recent years emphasis has been placed on the amount people drink and the pattern of consumption. However, it matters very little whether alcohol is consumed as wine, spirits or beer – from the perspective of damage to health and intoxication, the important factor is the level of alcohol consumption. The metabolism of alcohol takes place in the liver and consequently the risk of irreversible liver damage is increased in relation to the amount drunk.

It is important to note that the breakdown of alcohol may take several hours. Therefore after moderate drinking late in the evening and even a good night's sleep, the blood alcohol level may still be above the legal limit for driving well into the next morning. Unfortunately, there is no satisfactory means of speeding up the metabolism of alcohol, thus drinking black coffee or having cold showers makes little or no difference.

Alcohol taken in excess leads to impairment of physical, psychological and social functioning.

It is estimated that between 15% and 40% of patients in hospital wards, outpatient and accident and emergency department drink too much alcohol. In one emergency department (Robertson 1989), 40% of evening attenders had recently consumed alcohol while after midnight very few patients admitted for whatever reasons were sober. In addition patients who had consumed alcohol and sustained injury fared worse than their sober counterparts.

The links between alcohol consumption and violence are well recognized and the Criminal Justice Act 1990 banned the consumption of alcohol on the way to and during sports events in the hope of reducing violence such as football hooliganism. Much alcohol-related violence takes place in the home and women and children are especially vulnerable in this respect.

While it is not possible to state precisely what levels of alcohol consumption are sensible or dangerous, The Royal Colleges of Psychiatrists, General Practitioners and Physicians have suggested the following (Hartz et al 1990):

Low risk	14 units for women	
	21 units for men	per week
High risk	35 units for women	
	50 units for men	

One unit of alcohol is approximately equivalent to half a pint of beer or one standard single measure of spirit or one glass of wine (Fig. 1.6).

Alcohol-free and low-alcohol wines and beers have become popular among those who intend to drive, but the amount of alcohol may vary and it is wise to refer to the individual label where the alcoholic content must by law be clearly stated.

Many groups exist within the community to help those with alcohol dependence and support is available for spouses and other family members; Alcoholics Anonymous, Al-Anon, Al-Ateen are examples. Community alcohol teams and alcohol treatment centres also exist, but education aimed at reducing alcohol consumption would in part, at least, obviate the need for these services.

One of the most effective ways of reducing supply and demand is to increase the price of alcohol. Alcohol consumption has risen in the last 20 years as the price in terms of disposable income has decreased. Increased taxation on alcohol is possible, though not popular, and would go some way towards reducing demand and consequently limiting the harmful effects of what is still seen as 'our safest, most useful recreational drug' (Robertson 1989).

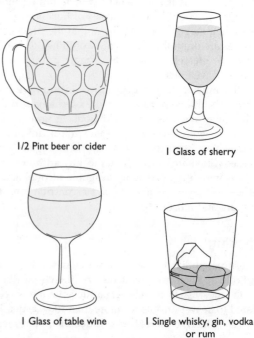

1/2 Pint beer or cider

1 Glass of sherry

1 Glass of table wine

1 Single whisky, gin, vodka or rum

Fig. 1.6 Drinks containing one unit of alcohol

Diet

Another hazard to health is obesity. A few years ago, a product which promised an easy way to lose weight hit the headlines. All the individual had to do was drink a cup of special tea three times a day. Not surprisingly the product failed, although initially there was so much interest that some stockists sold out. Unfortunately, losing weight requires more effort. If this were not so the proportion of the population who are overweight would be greatly reduced. It is estimated that 31% of male adults and 32% of females are overweight and that at any given time, 65% of women and 30% of men are trying to reduce their weight.

Excess weight is associated with several health problems including coronary heart disease, cancers and gall bladder disease, although the relationship is more complex than straightforward cause and effect.

Sugar is not only unnecessary for health, it is a major factor in both obesity and dental decay. Sugar does provide energy, but this can be obtained from other healthier sources. A diet which is high in fat, especially animal fat, will lead to the accumulation of fat on the walls of the arteries and by reducing blood flow lead to clotting which is especially serious in the vessels of the heart. A significant reduction in the incidence of coronary heart disease could be achieved by reducing substantially the amount of fat in the diet. Too much salt may lead to high blood pressure which is a high risk factor for heart disease and strokes. Fibre or roughage on the other hand is beneficial to health by controlling blood sugar levels and keeping the bowel healthy. Fibre also creates a feeling of fullness yet is low in calories. Whole grain cereals are useful sources of fibre, but one would do well to examine the ingredients in proprietary breakfast cereals. A recent survey by 'Which Way to Health 1992' revealed that some cereals have as much fat as two fried eggs and more sugar than a tube of fruit gums in each 'average' helping. In addition the 'average' helping quoted on the packet was less than most people actually ate.

It is encouraging to note however that changes in diet have taken place in the last 50 years (Wells 1992). Bread consumption has declined but white bread is still the most popular. Butter consumption has also declined to half of the amount consumed in 1980 and a quarter of that in 1970. Margarine consumption has also fallen while in contrast that of low-fat spreads has increased. The consumption of whole milk has declined as has the consumption of sugar.

The relationship between behaviour, life-style and health is not simple. Many factors influence health, some of which are very powerful, but outwith individual control. It is easy to blame the victim and in doing so obscure the social, economic and environmental factors which force people into unhealthy lifestyles. Health doesn't just happen, it is a continuously developing process which must be viewed in the context of society.

EMPLOYMENT, UNEMPLOYMENT AND LEISURE

It has been argued that 'a man's closest link to his society is his job or profession. The health of the individual in a society and the health of the society depend on how they are linked to each other and the most significant link is in the work relationship' (Levenstein 1964).

Paid employment is for most people a vital and significant part of their everyday lives. This work is likely to have both personal and social meanings but it is difficult to separate the two, since each is very much a product of the other.

Personal meanings of work are largely shaped in the process of socialization and social communication. To be an adult is synonymous with being in work. Life becomes serious and it is assumed that someone who is not working is 'playing'. Thus for the adult, life consists of alternating periods of work and play, a pattern which has changed very little over the years. A shorter working week and increased levels of unemployment have however altered the balance somewhat by increasing the amount of leisure time available.

This emphasis has been brought to bear upon work design by dominant groups in most countries of the modern world and can be described as 'instrumental' – the emphasis is on the practical outcome of work as opposed to the value of the work experience itself for those involved in it. Work is designed exclusively around such criteria as profits, output production norms and effective worker performance rather than aiming to provide a humane and fulfilling life for those engaged in it.

Many workers have been socialized into accepting that it is reasonable and only to be expected that work should be organized in this way. In addition, many workers so internalize this meaning of work that they themselves take an instrumental view by valuing it largely for it's outcome in terms of the weekly wage or the monthly salary. Work has no real significance for their personal life, development and growth. The effects of socialization are not however exerted uniformly and with equal effect upon all members of society. Factors such as family, social class and educational background mediate between the individual and the means of employment and serve to reinforce or mitigate the effects of socialization. Some individuals do have low expectations and aspirations with respect to the intrinsic rewards and are prepared to forgo a measure of intrinsic satisfaction for the sake of greater extrinsic rewards. Others however learn a more complex set of orientations to work which include not only the achieving of (usually greater) extrinsic rewards but also intrinsic satisfaction thus allowing for psychological growth and self-fulfilment. Most professions would be included in this category. Educational attainment is normally a prerequisite for entry into such occupations, thus excluding some members of society.

In the light of the aforegoing it could be argued that work for the majority of people has little or no meaning other than in terms of its cash rewards. This form of reasoning however would be failing to take account of the various meanings work has for the individual on a personal level. Work provides an opportunity for the individual to relate himself to society and view himself as making a useful contribution to that society by the provision of goods and services. This is explained by Sofer (1970) as follows:

> The operator assembles cars or machines, the farmer grows food, the physician reduces pain, the teacher broadens the intellectual horizons of his students, the policeman protects citizens against law breakers. The unemployed man by contrast has seen the clock go round but he has nothing to show for the hours that have passed.

Employment provides the individual with status and self-respect. Occupation indicates man's place in society. Words like miner, doctor, shopkeeper, solicitor are more than convenient labels, they indicate and illustrate aspects of a whole way of life. This is perhaps more obvious in the negative sense as when someone is described as unemployed or retired, the inference being that the person is in some way out of step with mainstream society.

In addition, work provides a meaningful activity which helps the individual to structure his time and discipline himself to perform a particular activity at a given time. This activity may even provide distraction from private worries, emotional problems and domestic crises. The 'workaholic' may be reacting to as well as causing marital disharmony and breakdown.

The workplace has always been for some a place to meet people, converse and perhaps form friendships outwith the immediate family. A woman who has previously been tied to the home because of child rearing may welcome the chance to regain employment outside the home and so extend her range of social contacts.

Work is also significant in terms of personal identity. An occupational role allows an individual (in this instance male) to define himself both to himself and others and to explain his place in the world. Indeed man's work is one of the things by which he is judged and certainly one of the more significant things by which he judges himself. 'A man's work is one of the more important parts of his social identity, of his self; indeed of his fate in the one life he has to live, for there is something almost as irrevocable about choice of occupation as there is about choice of a mate' (Hughes 1951).

Since work is such an important part of societal life, it follows that it can exert a powerful influence on health. Occupational health services are now an important part of most organizations and legislation exists to ensure the health and safety of the work force (Health and Safety at Work Act 1974).

Many nurses now specialize in occupational health nursing, which includes health surveillance of the workforce, pre-employment health screening and health promotion. The occupational health nurse will also be involved in the management of illness and injury at work.

Some occupations are by their very nature hazardous. Coal miners not only risk injury at or near the coal face but also risk developing lung diseases such as pneumoconiosis which result from the regular inhalation of coal dust. Diseases due to the inhalation of mineral dusts can also occur in those whose work entails contact with iron, steel and asbestos. The inhalation of cotton flax or hemp dust may prove injurious to textile workers and fungal spores from mouldy hay, straw or grain may cause damage in agricultural workers, the so-called 'farmers lung'. Irritant gases and fumes if inhaled can precipitate bronchial asthma. Some occupations are known to be associated with the development of cancers – those working with rubber or some dyes risk bladder cancer and leukemia while those in the plastics industry may develop tumours of the liver. Exposure to insecticides either in production or use is known to be associated with skin, liver and lung cancers.

The above risks can however be minimized or even eliminated by improvements in industrial practice. Measures such as wearing respirators, damping of dust and efficient ventilation systems have been shown to be effective. In this context, the Control of Substances Hazardous to Health (COSHH) Regulations 1988 aim to protect those workers who are exposed to irritant or toxic substances, pesticides, dust and fumes, micro-organisms and cancer-causing agents by ensuring that employers and employees cooperate in the provision and maintenance of safe work habits.

Accidents at work may result in loss of life and are responsible for a significant number of lost days to industry. Most could be prevented. Some accidents occur in much the same way as those outside the work environment simply because people are there and are moving about. Others are linked to the production process and involve machinery and tools as well as human error. It is encouraging to note that the number of deaths from accidents at work has been reduced to the lowest on record but there is no improvement in the non-fatal injury rate which has remained at around the same level since 1986/87. Work however, influences not only the physical health of the individual but also his mental health. Work-related stress is frequently referred to as a cause of ill health. This may be caused by the pressure of work itself or by attempting to balance the demands of both work and family life. The current high rates of unemployment may threaten job security with older people feeling more vulnerable. Indeed stress may be increased by failing to delegate work to a younger person. Those in professional or managerial positions may be able to exert some control over working conditions but may suffer from a very heavy workload.

Melhuish (1982) describes pressures intrinsic to work itself as being:

1. Qualitative, when the skills of the individual are not matched to the requirements of the job and consequently the work is too difficult to do, or
2. Quantitative, where there is quite simply too much work to do.

Work underload however or work which is repetitive or boring may prove to be just as stressful.

Many people respond to stress by increasing their alcohol intake and by increased tobacco smoking. It is interesting to note that a recent study of stress among nurses in Scotland confirmed that stress was associated with the use of alcohol but not with smoking (Plant et al 1992).

The last 20–30 years have seen rising unemployment, a reduction in working hours and longer paid holidays for those in work. This has resulted in more time being available for leisure pursuits. Unfortunately, increased leisure does not necessarily equate with good health. Watching television and entertaining friends and relatives have remained the most popular home-based leisure activities for the past 15 years (Central Statistical Office 1993a). The former activity discourages exercise and the latter may result in excess of alcohol and calories.

It is somewhat disturbing to note that teenagers are less active than they were 50 years ago, indeed physical activity has 'radically decreased' (Durnin 1993). This is a great pity because exercise is known to promote good health and physical fitness and 'is emerging as a key element in most national health promotion recommendations and strategies' (Dargie & Grant 1991). Regular exercise reduces the incidence of coronary heart disease and other vascular disorders. For those who are overweight, exercise, especially when combined with a low-calorie diet, will produce weight loss. Exercise is beneficial to health in every age group. In middle age, activity may decrease as the demands of child rearing and household tasks become less and in the elderly inactivity may even be mistakenly encouraged in an attempt prevent injury and falls. Indeed exercise reduces the likelihood of falling (Fiastarone et al 1990). It is also suggested that regular exercise would reduce the risk of hip fractures by half and thus prevent some 20 000 such fractures each year (Law et al 1991). This would not only enhance the well-being of the elderly person but would also reduce the significant costs of these injuries to the Health Service.

Exercise can be taken in various forms and need not necessitate a major change in life-style. Walking short distances instead of taking the car or climbing stairs rather than using a lift can easily become a way of life. Activities such as swimming can be enjoyable as well as being an excellent form of exercise.

Despite the beneficial effects of exercise, care needs to be taken to increase activity gradually and stop if there is any distress. Exercise should be taken on a regular basis and not in sporadic bursts. Any pain experienced should be taken seriously and medical advice sought if necessary.

Too much exercise can in fact damage one's health. Athletes who overtrain risk developing 'athletes disease', the symptoms of which are 'under performance, fatigue, depression and vulnerability to disease' (Vines 1993). British physiologists are currently researching the link between exercise and its effects on the immune system of athletes. It is possible that exercise makes the individual succumb more readily to infection but leisure-time exercise, if carried out sensibly, is unlikely to have this effect.

In recent years the motor car has become an important part of most people's lives, allowing them to seek leisure pursuits some distance from home. However, it has also produced congestion in the more popular parts of the country, especially at weekends. There is increasing concern by both local and central government agencies at the increased volume of traffic passing over roads which were never designed to cope with the load. At the time of writing there is even a proposal to build a second road bridge over the River

Forth. At the same time, many local authorities have attempted to ban the motor car from the centre of towns, making it easier for public transport to pass along as well as reducing levels of air pollution.

Adequate time for leisure and recreational activities is an important determinant of health, but problems can and do arise if an individual has too much unstructured time at his disposal. The unemployed can find themselves in just such a situation.

Involuntary unemployment is a very real threat to health for both the unemployed person and his family. Indeed the threat of redundancy has been found to have an adverse effect on health (Mattiasson et al 1990).

Reference has already been made to the meanings associated with work. It follows then that loss of a job is a major life crisis which is likely to lead to other losses such as loss of income, loss of home because of inability to make mortgage or rent payments and loss of a car. Increasing family tensions as a result of unemployment may also lead to family break up and loss of a spouse. In addition, unemployment brings with it a loss of identity which employment provides. It is then not surprising that for many, life loses its meaning and purpose.

Many writers have referred to a series of psychological phases in unemployment, similar to those associated with bereavement (Fagin & Little 1984). The first phase is one of shock and disbelief. The individual has difficulty in accepting that 'it could happen to me'. There is a sense of disorientation and confusion and an inability to plan for the future. This gives way to a period of denial and unrealistic optimism.

A holiday feeling prevails and various overdue tasks around the house are attended to. Job loss is considered to be temporary and there is little concern about the future. This phase will last for a few weeks at most, to be followed by increasing anxiety and distress. The holiday feeling is over and money may be running out. All the jobs about the house have been done. The first attempts to find work are likely to be unsuccessful. Job seeking begins in earnest. Numerous letters of application will be written, most of which remain unanswered. Even where a job interview is granted the applicant is unsuccessful. Hopes of finding a job fade and the 'unemployed identity' is gradually assumed. At this point a change in personality may be noticed, the individual becomes moody and irritable, has difficulty sleeping and major rows erupt within the family over trivial incidents. Eventually, a feeling of resignation is experienced. Job seeking becomes haphazard and a large part of the day is spent sleeping or daydreaming.

Fagin (1993) suggests that

there is a tendency to withdraw from social life and even from family activities. The television often becomes the main source of interest and distraction and there is no discrimination over the programmes which are watched. One individual is reported to have said "I know all the children's and women's afternoon programmes even when I'm not interested in them"

More than 10 years later, while children's television programmes can be easily identified in the *Radio Times*, this is not the case for programmes likely to appeal to women viewers. Afternoon programmes seem to be suitable for both sexes, which may be a reflection of the fact that more women are in employment and thus not at home in the afternoon, or an indication that television programmes are responding to the fact that in 1992, 1 846 000 men in Britain were unemployed (Central Statistical Office 1993b).

There is now little doubt that long-term unemployment has an adverse effect on both mental and physical health. Sadly, there is often a great deal of stigma associated with unemployment, the victim being treated as if he was solely to blame for his situation. It is presumed that a job could be found if the individual tried harder. In common with other forms of stigma the victim is labelled as 'feckless and work-shy', a social security 'scrounger' because he/she is dependent on state benefits. Consequently depression is a common feature of unemployment (Case History 1.1).

The unemployed are in the majority among those who commit suicide or deliberately injure themselves (Platt & Kreitman 1984). This would seem to be so not only in Britain but in most other countries' studies. Studies consistently support the fact that suicide and parasuicide rates increase with rising unemployment. A high proportion of those who take overdoses are found to be unemployed. This is confirmed by a study

---

Case History 1.1

Hutchings & Gower (1993) tell the story of Michael who had been unemployed for 6 years. He had tried to find employment and had even moved to another part of the country seeking work.

During a visit to the Department of Employment, he felt that it was implied that he was not trying hard enough to find work and there was a threat to stop his benefit. Michael said: "Something went inside me and I felt like that ever since. I went outside and sat in the car and cried" Michael did go back inside the Department and saw a different person who suggested he see a doctor.

of men in Edinburgh which found that the para-suicide rate among the unemployed was 10 times greater than among the employed (Platt & Kreitman 1984).

The effect of unemployment on physical health is less clear cut. Poor health and illness may well lead to job loss. On the other hand associations have been found between unemployment and ill health. Hospital admission rates and outpatient referrals may be higher in the unemployed but this may reflect a greater willingness to attend or be admitted to hospital because the threat of losing one's job by taking time off no longer exists. Stress is considered to be a factor in many illnesses and there is little doubt that for most people unemployment is stressful. This may result in increased smoking and consumption of alcohol, which in turn predisposes to cardiovascular disease, lung cancer and cirrhosis of the liver.

The effects of unemployment are not only personal however, the family must cope with the painful move from prosperity to poverty. Husband and wife may face reversal of roles if the wife finds employment or is already employed. The husband ceases to be the main breadwinner and this reinforces his feelings of worthlessness and rejection. Some marriages, especially if previously unstable, will end up in divorce. Children in the family may develop sleeping problems and feeding difficulties as well as behaviour disorders. Given the stressful environment, the possibility of non-accidental injury may also be increased.

In circumstances where unemployment is due to closure of what is the main source of jobs in a town, whole communities will be affected.

Unemployment is a social problem which shows no sign of diminishing to any great extent, at least not in the foreseeable future. Nurses therefore are likely to care for many people without employment and should do so with the knowledge that unemployment is a health risk for both the patient and his family and needs to be taken into account when care is planned.

MAN'S ENVIRONMENT – FRIEND OR FOE?

The house a person lives in has an important influence on his health. People who can afford to purchase a house will have some degree of choice, not only of the house itself but also the locality in which it is situated. Those unable to contemplate purchase are dependent on renting from the local authority or a private landlord. In the UK local authority housing has never been able to meet demand, a problem intensified in recent years by the sale of large numbers of houses at greatly discounted prices to those who had been tenants for 2 years or more.

Local authorities are obliged to deal with housing which falls below the 'tolerable standard' or lacks one or more of the standard amenities. The main requirements of the 'tolerable standard' are that a house should:

1. Be structurally stable
2. Be free from dampness
3. Have a toilet available for the exclusive use of the occupants of the house and be located within the house
4. Have a sink with a satisfactory supply of hot and cold water
5. Have satisfactory provision for heating, lighting and ventilation.

Unfortunately cuts in public expenditure may make it difficult for local authorities to meet their obligations in this respect.

Several studies have explored the effects of damp housing on health, but it is difficult to prove cause and effect since other factors influencing health may coexist such as smoking, low income and overcrowding. In addition, dampness has often been described by local authorities as condensation and blamed on the tenant not heating the house properly.

Hunt (1988) explored the links between damp housing and ill health. This was a 'double blind' study in which information on dampness was collected by environmental health officers and interviews on health were conducted by a separate group of researchers.

Their separate findings were not put together until the whole study was complete, thereby minimizing bias and subjectivity. The findings revealed that 'the presence of damp was associated with particular streets and building types' which meant that the inhabitants were unlikely to be responsible for the damp. Women living in damp houses do experience more emotional distress in terms of anxiety and depression, which is not surprising if one considers how unpleasant it must be to live with mould, peeling wallpaper and unpleasant smells.

Housing conditions were found to be positively associated with physical ill health in children. Symptoms included aches and pains, diarrhoea, anxiety and headache. Respiratory problems, especially wheeze and coughs, were also more frequently reported in children from damp houses. Children living in houses where there was obvious mould were in addition more likely to suffer from vomiting and sore throats.

Cold houses are also hazardous to health, especially

for the elderly. The elderly and the chronically sick spend most of each day at home and consequently need to heat their houses for longer periods each day. Unfortunately many elderly people live in houses which have no central heating and which cost a great deal to heat adequately, especially on a limited income. The imposition of value added tax on gas and electricity in the UK is unlikely to improve this state of affairs. As room temperature falls, the risk of hypothermia increases and the possibility of literally freezing to death may become a reality.

A common sight in most large cities today is of someone begging and holding up a card stating that he/she is homeless. In addition many people spend the night in underground stations, shop doorways and other uncomfortable locations, only protected from the elements by means of cardboard boxes. Homeless groups also include families in bed and breakfast accommodation, women and children in refuges, people living in squats, hostel inhabitants, many of whom are mentally ill, alcoholics or drug abusers. There are also people who live with friends and family (sometimes causing overcrowding) because they have no home of their own.

In times of recession, the homeless total rises due to repossessions caused by an inability to make mortgage repayments. The effects of homelessness on health include: mental health problems – depression, isolation and suicide; development delay and behaviour problems in children – aggression, bed wetting and poor sleep. There is also an increased incidence of infectious diseases such as tuberculosis, dysentery and hepatitis A. Poor safety standards are likely to be a feature of temporary accommodation, thus increasing the risk of accidents especially to children (Pritchard 1990). The term 'temporary accommodation' may well be something of a misnomer since some families are placed in this accommodation for months or even years. What it means to bring up children in bed and breakfast accommodation is summed up in the following statement from a single parent living in one room with two children aged 15 months and 5 years:

It is damp. I've got no gas due to leaks. I've got no hot water. I can't cook without gas and it is detrimental to my children's health. Both my daughters have been ill, the eldest never had asthma until I moved here and the youngest is in hospital due to a bad chest

(Heyden 1992)

The infamous London smog of December 1952, caused by a build up of smoke and sulphur dioxide in stagnant foggy air, killed 4000 people from heart and lung disease and almost certainly gave impetus to the British Government to legislate. The 1956 Clean Air Act established Smoke Control Areas, within which the emission of domestic smoke is prohibited. The legislation also controls smoke, dust and fume emissions from industrial premises.

An article in *The Times* (Davie 1994) highlighted the dangers to health from vehicle pollution and stated that more than 7 billion tonnes of carbon monoxide are pumped into the atmosphere of Britain every year, 90% of it from vehicle exhausts. This is likely to cause drowsiness and headaches and may result in exacerbation of bronchial asthma. Small children on foot or in push-chairs are particularly at risk because they are at exhaust height where the levels of carbon monoxide are higher. Since carbon monoxide reduces the oxygen-carrying power of the blood, this poses a serious health problem.

In recent years, there has been growing concern about environmental issues. The greenhouse effect, acid rain and damage to the ozone layer are frequently cited as causes for concern. Some gases, especially carbon dioxide, behave like the glass in a greenhouse, trapping heat so that the temperature of the earth rises. Greenhouse gases are produced by burning fossil fuels, deforestation and by industrial activity. To prevent this global warming, energy needs to be used more efficiently and alternative sources of energy utilized.

The ozone layer protects the earth from harmful ultraviolet radiation which can cause skin cancer. This protective layer is destroyed by increased concentration of man-made gases, the most significant of which are chlorofluorocarbons (CFCS) used mainly in aerosols. The use of CFCS has fallen markedly in recent years.

Two main gases contribute to acid rain, sulphur dioxide and oxides of nitrogen. These are produced by burning fossil and other fuels, the main sources being power stations, industrial output and cars. The amount of acid reaching the ground is dependent on the concentration of acid in the rain and the amount of rain falling. Acid rain causes damage to plants and animals as well as to buildings.

Water is essential to life and health and in 1990 the average domestic water consumption was around 140 litres per person per day. More than 60% of this was used in toilet flushing, baths and showers and washing machines, the latter using 100 litres of water per load (Central Statistical Office 1993c). Tap water is treated to make it suitable for drinking and must conform to the EC Drinking Water Directive. Water can become contaminated by pesticides and fertilizers from agriculture, discharges from industry and microorganisms from sewage. Fortunately, such contamination is rare. In older houses, the presence of lead piping may result in tap water containing toxic levels of lead, the effects of which may be abdominal pain, headache, irritability and eventual coma and death. There is also some evidence of a link between exposure to lead and behaviour and learning difficulties in children (Walker 1992). The Environmental Health Department is responsible for taking routine samples of water for chemical and microbiological examination.

The privatization of the water industry in England and Wales has resulted in escalating costs for the consumers. People on low incomes and on benefits who find difficulty in paying high water bills risk water disconnection with obvious implications for health since it is not possible to boil a kettle, wash or flush the toilet.

Each year, environmental health officers receive thousands of complaints about noise. This noise emanates from a variety of sources and while for many it is unpleasant, for others it is actually damaging to health. Noise at work is a major cause of hearing loss and the Health and Safety Executive estimates that 1.7 million people are deaf due to occupational exposure to noise (Goodlee 1992). Much of this could be prevented by the use of personal ear protection if exposure is unavoidable. Ear protection although provided is not always worn by the employee and although legislation exists, this is not always enforced.

Leisure activities such as going to discos are important sources of noise and are potentially damaging to hearing. The use of personal stereos has also caused some concern, especially when being used in noisy situations where the volume is increased to compete with the background noise.

Noise produced by traffic such as cars, lorries and aeroplanes while not causing deafness may nevertheless damage health by causing lack of sleep. Sleep loss is likely to result in reduced efficiency during the day. Noise has also been found to have an adverse effect on the performance of intellectual skills. In addition, fewer accidents occur when noise levels are reduced (Goodlee 1992).

In 1991 in Britain 4868 people died as a result of road traffic accidents. During the same period, 4455 people died as a result of accidents in the home or other communal establishment (OPCS 1991). Accidents are also a major cause of ill health and disability. Prevention would therefore reduce premature death and disability. Furthermore, the prevention of accidents would reduce the considerable demands made on the Health Services. Accidents in the home are common in the young and in the elderly, largely

because our homes are designed by able-bodied adults for able-bodied adults. This very often means that children, the elderly, the disabled and the handicapped are seriously disadvantaged. In children, the type of injury sustained is closely related to their stage of development. Infants under 1 year are especially liable to choking and suffocation on food or secretions in the early weeks and inhaled toys or sweets or other small objects such as peanuts later on. Children aged 1–2 years are at risk because of their newly acquired mobility, often surprising their parents by their speed and agility. Their precarious balance renders them liable to accidents such as scalds from pans pulled off the cooker and drowning by overbalancing into a bath of water. By the age of 3–4 years, overbalancing and falls are less common but at this stage the child is likely to be venturing outside and the hazards of ornamental pools and garden implements are obvious. At this stage the child can also gain access to road traffic with possibly serious consequences.

The garden can be a hazardous place for adults too. Good weather is very often the stimulus to rush into the garden and do everything before it rains, which may lead to a back injury that then prevents the individual enjoying the garden for some time to come. In this respect, increasing age does not necessarily make the individual more sensible. It is not uncommon for elderly people to sustain fractures by overexertion and strain, especially when degeneration makes bones more likely to break. The use of electrical equipment such as lawn-mowers increases the risk of serious injury, especially if the individual is distracted by someone else in the garden, or by a neighbour. Even tools like forks, spades and rakes if not used carefully can cause serious injury. Putting the fork through one's foot or standing on a rake, which then hits one on the face, is not uncommon.

Sensory deprivation in the elderly renders them more susceptible to accidents, where failing sight or impaired hearing may be a fact in the accident aetiology. These very same factors also make the elderly more vulnerable to road traffic accidents.

The reduction in the numbers of accidents which occur both in the home and on the roads is both an individual and a collective responsibility. It is important to recognize that an accident is possible, not inevitable.

Accident prevention should be considered under the headings:

1. Education This increases awareness of the factors predisposing to accidents in all age groups and encourages foresight rather than the hindsight of tragedy. The Royal Society for the Prevention of Accidents (ROSPA) and the Child Accident Prevention Trust (CAPT) are active in education, but also seek to influence safety standards and legislation.

2. Engineering This encompasses design and construction – the manufacture of fire-retardant furniture, the design of houses to include smoke detectors and safety glass and the design of roads with minimization of accident potential in mind.

3. Enforcement This is used where standards are set, e.g. the Lion Mark indicates that toys meet current safety standards and legislation exists as in the use of seat belts in cars. At the present time pressure is being put on the Government to legislate for the provision of seat belts in coaches, especially when transporting children.

The one constant however in all accidents is human behaviour. Safety is not someone else's responsibility but is the responsibility of each and every individual.

HEALTH AND THE FAMILY

The year 1994 has been designated the Year of the Family, but what does it mean to be a family in the 1990s?

Although there has been a reduction in the number of households containing a married couple with children, more than eight out of ten dependent children still live in this type of family (Central Statistical Office 1993c). Many of the traditional features of family life have however been challenged in recent years. Thirty per cent of live births are to parents who are not married, although the majority are registered by both parents indicating a stable relationship. The number of pregnancies where the parents marry before the birth of the child has fallen significantly. This is an indication of changing attitudes and is perhaps to be welcomed since the imminent arrival of a baby is not the best foundation on which to base a marriage. The UK has one of the highest marriage rates in the European Community but it also has one of the highest divorce rates.

Marital status does influence health. Research has found that mortality rates are lowest for the married, higher for the single and higher still for those widowed or divorced. Morbidity patterns indicate that the widowed and divorced appear to experience most illness. Single people however suffer less morbidity than those who are married (Open University 1985).

Lone parenthood is very much a feature of the 1990s either because of divorce, separation or death of a partner. There are also a substantial number of one-parent families where the parent, usually the mother, is single.

Despite the rise in the divorce rates, most divorcees, especially men, remarry. Thus many children will grow up in families where one partner is a step-parent. In many instances the child will continue to have contact with the natural parent, a situation which may prove difficult for the child and result in a conflict of loyalties.

In recent years the family has been the focus of marked social change, a situation which many people will find difficult to accept. The assumption that couples should marry for life, should want to have children and that the woman will want to stay at home to care for those children, is no longer valid. Some couples will choose not to have children and those who do may well seek alternative child-care provision outwith the home. Rapidly changing technology and high levels of unemployment makes some mothers fear that a return to the work force at a later date will be difficult, if not impossible. It was thought for many years that a child was deprived if his/her mother could not provide the loving care a child needs. Indeed this ideology may have been responsible for keeping a child with parents who were incapable of caring adequately for the child.

Evidence now suggests that there are suitable substitutes for maternal care and that having paid employment outside the home may have a beneficial effect on a mother's well-being. Rutter (1981) found that working mothers were less anxious about separation generally and fathers took a more active interest in family life. The effects of day care on children's development is obviously dependent on the quality of the substitute care and there is a substantial body of research that indicates that day care is not harmful and may even be beneficial to development, especially in the preschool age group (Moss & Melhuish 1991).

Adequate child-care facilities are however not available for all children. Much of the available provision is in the private sector and thus expensive, and state provision is insufficient to meet the demand.

There are then many different types of families, from the single parent to the extended family. Where the extended family exists, grandparents may provide help and support and may also be available to care for children. It is important to recognize that there is not one ideal 'traditional' family, nor is it helpful to suggest 'cause and effect' solutions to social problems. It is often claimed that children from broken homes are insecure and emotionally deprived. This is just as likely to be true for children brought up in stable family settings.

VIOLENCE IN THE FAMILY

Most individuals have deeply held beliefs about family life in terms of the roles and relationships which exist therein. It is however a painful reality that: 'statistically it is safer to be on the streets after dark with a stranger than at home in the bosom of one's family, for it is there that accident, murder and violence are likely to occur' (Brandon 1976). In 1991 four-fifths of female homicide victims were related to or knew their attacker. Sixty-two percent of such homicides were committed by husbands or other family members (Central Statistical Office 1993d).

In 1974, Erin Pizzey provided one of the most vivid accounts of violence directed towards wives or female partners. *Scream Quietly or the Neighbours will Hear* contained personal stories from women who had suffered such violence and gave the impetus for setting up Women's Aid. This is a voluntary organization whose aims include the provision of a temporary refuge for battered women and their children. They also offer support, advice and help to any woman who asks for it, regardless of whether she is a resident.

It is estimated that one in four women in Britain are hit by their partner (Horley 1991) but the true extent of the problem is difficult to determine since domestic violence takes place behind closed doors, away from the public eye. The women themselves may find it difficult to ask for help and have often suffered abuse for many years before finally leaving a violent husband. The woman may be financially dependent on the husband to support her and her children. There is also a belief by some members of society that a woman is in some way to blame because she must have provoked the attack.

The family has been described as a 'conflict prone situation' because 'the members spend considerable amounts of time together, often confined in a relatively small space. It follows that the greater amount of time spent together by family members, the more frequent are the events and issues around which disputes and disagreements may arise' (Okell-Jones 1982). Sadly some of these disputes result in violence.

The most vulnerable member of the family is the young child. Each year many children are killed or injured by the deliberate actions of those charged with their care. Fractures, burns, lacerations, bites, bruising and damage to the central nervous system are common injuries. It may be difficult to understand why these injuries occur but the parents may have suffered violence themselves or have grown up with little experience of love. Poor housing and lack of money may also precipitate child abuse. Sometimes parents make unreasonable demands for perfection and obedience in the child because of lack of knowledge or understanding of the developmental needs of young children.

Abuse may be emotional, the child being rejected and treated with indifference, or may take the form of neglect.

In recent years, child sexual abuse has been increasingly identified. The events of Cleveland and Orkney with their subsequent enquiries will be familiar to many. The idea that any adult could abuse a child in this way is abhorrent to society. It is unthinkable, yet professionals believe that one in four female and one in ten male children have suffered some kind of sexual abuse and some would put the figure even higher (Bagley & King 1990). More than one child in a family may be at risk and the abuse may have continued for many years before detection.

Sexual abuse prompts the largest single group of calls to Childline Scotland, the telephone help-line. Public outrage demands that such children be protected and much of the responsibility for this rests with the Social Work Department. The dilemma for social work that this presents is aptly described by Asquith (1993):

in cases of alleged abuse of children, precipitate intervention is seen as unwarranted and as an invasion of the rights, autonomy and privacy of the family, whereas the failure to intervene in certain cases is also seen as reprehensible because of the direct consequences for the children involved.

The elderly are also at risk of abuse. Those most vulnerable are 'over the age of 75, female, roleless, functionally impaired, lonely, fearful and living at home with an adult child' (Sadler 1989). People are living longer in Britain, which means that the numbers of people aged over 75 are increasing. Increasing age is likely to result in impaired physical and mental functioning with consequent loss of independence. Only a small proportion of these people will be cared for in hospital or some other institution. The burden of care will therefore fall to an informal carer, usually a family member but sometimes a friend or neighbour. In many circumstances, these carers will receive minimal, if any, support from statutory agencies. It is not difficult to understand why the carer sometimes resorts to verbal, emotional and even physical abuse.

It is estimated that informal carers number more than 1.7 million; this rises to 6 million if those providing care, but not living in the same household, are included (Garrett 1989).

A substantial number of elderly people are cared for by a spouse of the same age who may find it difficult to cope with the physical demands of providing care but a sense of duty makes them reluctant to admit this. Younger carers may have had to leave paid employment, which reduces their income substantially. This results in feelings of resentment and guilt.

Not everyone being cared for at home is elderly. Some are handicapped or chronically ill. In this context an important group of carers are schoolchildren who look after a disabled parent. Child carers frequently remain hidden in the community, because to alert social services to their predicament is likely to result in the child being taken into care.

The family has an important role both in health and illness, but most families will require help to avoid the effects of stress and exhaustion. Respite care is available to give families a rest from caring but nurses and other professionals working in the community must be alert to the needs of the carer as well as those of the person being cared for.

Collaboration in protecting or restoring health between the patient, the family and the health care system has been described as a therapeutic triangle – an expression which clearly reflects the reciprocal influence of all three parties   (Cigoli & Binda 1993).

THE NATIONAL HEALTH SERVICE

The National Health Service (NHS) has been in existence since July 1948. At its inception, it was assumed that there was a fixed amount of illness in the community which would be reduced by providing health care which was free at the point of need. It was anticipated that the population would become healthier and consequently demand for the service would decrease. Thus in due course, less money would require to be spent. More than 45 years later, this assumption seems naive to say the least.

For the first 25 years of its life, the NHS comprised three sections:

1. General practitioners, dentists, opticians and pharmacists were administered by Executive Councils.

2. Social Health Authorities were responsible for environmental health and services such as maternity and child welfare clinics, health visitors, community midwives, health education, immunisation and ambulances.

3. Hospital services – The Ministry of Health (now the Department of Health) was responsible for funding.

During the 1960s, the concept of the District General Hospital was born. This hospital would provide facilities for all but the rarest illnesses and would serve a population of more than 100 000. Several new hospitals were built and many more were upgraded to District General Hospital standards.

In 1974, the first NHS reorganization took place and the tripartite structure was modified. Local authorities were no longer responsible for Community Health Services. These and the hospitals became the responsibility of Area Health Authorities which in turn were accountable to Regional Health Authorities. District management teams were responsible for the day to day running of the health services. In Scotland there were no regional authorities, only areas and district levels. Scotland was divided administratively into 15 Area Health Boards.

A feature of this reorganization was the establishment of Local Health Councils to represent the views of the public. Local Health Councils also inform the public about NHS developments.

In 1982, Regional Health Authorities were removed in England and in 1984 the districts were abolished in Scotland, the aim being to delegate power to the local level.

At the same time, concern was growing about the efficiency and effectiveness of Health Service management. The government was advised that there was a lack of individual responsibility and accountability (Department of Health 1983). A stronger, clearer management system was required. General managers were appointed on fixed-term contracts and paid by results. The most significant effect of this reform was that functional management where each profession managed its own affairs was no longer thought to be necessary.

Further changes in the organization of the NHS were announced in the Government's white paper 'Working for Patients' published in 1989. The main proposals were:

1. Purchaser/provider market   A separation of roles of purchaser and provider. Health Boards would be free to purchase services from the public, private or voluntary sector including their own units or NHS 'trusts'. Major hospitals were encouraged to apply for trust status and thus be free from Health Board control. Hospital funding would be dependent on the ability to gain contracts for services. General practitioners would be allowed to control their own budgets as fund holders.

2. Professional accountability Doctors and nurses would become more accountable to managers for their performance. Medical and nursing audit systems would control quality and standards of care.

3. General practice Patients were to have greater choice of general practitioner, who in turn would be allowed to advertise. Greater emphasis was to be placed on prevention of disease.

The last few years have also seen changes in priority needs of particular patient groups for health services and in the provision of community care. The policy of community care aims to enable more vulnerable people to live in the community and thus reduce the number of people living in long-stay hospitals and institutions. This would include the elderly, the mentally ill and people with learning difficulties. There is however some concern that the necessary funding for this initiative will fall short of what is required and may lead to increased pressure on informal carers.

In July 1991 the Citizen's Charter was published. This committed those working in public services to improve standards and seek to meet the needs of those who use the services. Later that year (September 1991) the Patient's Charter, based on the same principles, set national targets for improving health.

The Patient's Charter commits the NHS to minimum standards of health care, including guaranteed waiting times for outpatient consultation and hospital treatment. In addition, information about the Health Service will be provided with an invitation for individuals to give NHS management their opinions on the service. In Scotland, individual Health Boards have been charged with implementing the Patient's Charter at local level both within the community and hospital settings.

What has been described above is the professional or formal health-care system in Britain and as such is the legitimizer of illness. Most health care, however is self care, dealt with without professional intervention, by the use of over-the-counter medicines or advice from friends and family. Self-help groups are a common feature of British society and exist to provide help and support to individuals who have health problems in common. Many members of self-help groups will however, have had contact with the professional sector at some point in their illness.

COMPLEMENTARY THERAPIES

Complementary therapies such as acupuncture, herbalism, aromatherapy and reflexology have become increasingly popular in recent years, in fact some therapies are now being offered by medical practitioners. A survey conducted among 100 general practice trainees indicated that 80% wished to train in at least one method and 21% had already used one (Reilly 1983).

People may seek complementary therapies for a variety of reasons which may include:

1. Failure of orthodox medicine.
2. Differing beliefs about health and illness.
3. Holistic approach of many complementary therapies.
4. Complementary therapists spend more time with patients.
5. Patient may feel comforted by the use of touch in many therapies including aromatherapy and reflexology.

This is confirmed by Trevelyan (1993), who suggests that: 'To those seeking a supplement or an alternative to orthodox medicine, the complementary therapies appear to offer a gentle, personalised form of treatment based on "holistic principles".'

The British Medical Association is somewhat cautious in its support of complementary therapies, largely because of a lack of scientific evidence to support their effectiveness, but concedes, 'The development of medicine has been assisted in the past by concepts and techniques originating from unorthodox sources. For such ideas to be accepted they should be evaluated by methods based on sympathetic scientific observation. Thereafter, they may well be incorporated into main stream medicine' (British Medical Association 1986).

Thus complementary therapies should not be rejected but rather evidence should be found to support the efficacy of such treatments. In addition, at a time of financial stringency, evidence of cost-effectiveness would do much to encourage the use of complementary therapies within the NHS.

HEALTH PROMOTION

This chapter began by looking at the targets set for improving the health of the nation by the year 2000. It is, in fact, the stated purpose of the Health Service in Scotland to promote health and individual health boards have been charged with improving the health of their local population. Many have already published local versions of the Patient's Charter. The Health Service is a major employer; one in 15 of the employed population in Scotland works in the NHS. NHS staff as a group have obvious potential for health promotion, a fact recognized in the Patient's Charter:

'NHS staff will be expected to promote good health personally – and all NHS premises should reflect this'. It follows then that nurses have an important part to play in health promotion both on a personal and a professional level. Much has been written concerning the nurse as a role model for health and nurses teaching by example. It has been suggested that 'smoking and overeating should always be avoided by nurses in uniform. While they are best avoided altogether, if they must be indulged in, – – best done in private' (Smith 1984). While the above philosophy will result in nurses who smoke being hidden from public view, recent policy decisions by many health boards have perhaps encouraged the opposite. In making health board premises and their grounds smoke-free zones, smokers who are unable to give up the habit are likely to congregate outside where they are very much in the public view! On a more positive role, however, many nurses have used the opportunity to give up the habit. Nurses do need to consider their own health – not many will be perfect examples of positive health.

The overweight nurse who smokes may be seen to lack credibility. She may nevertheless be an effective communicator and possess personal qualities such as warmth and empathy. Falling short of perfection may enable her to be more understanding of patients who are also less than perfect.

The reader may well be asking at this point 'What is health promotion?' Downie et al (1991) provide an excellent definition in the following: 'Health promotion comprises efforts to enhance positive health and prevent ill health through the overlapping spheres of health education, prevention and health protection.'

Health education

Health education includes activities which enhance well-being and diminish ill health as well as those which influence the knowledge of policy makers and health professionals. It is important that health education should involve two-way communication. Many successful initiatives are the result of listening to what the consumer needs and wants rather than imposing services based on professional perceptions of need.

Prevention

The aim of preventative activity is to reduce the risk of disease by removing the cause. An individual who stops smoking will reduce the risk of developing lung cancer and coronary artery disease, although the best form of prevention would be to have never smoked.

Prevention also includes the early detection of disease before symptoms of disordered function appear. The taking of cervical smears will identify precancerous cells and thus prevent the development of cancer of the cervix in women. The management of established disease to avoid or limit handicap or disability is also preventive – a patient with diabetes whose condition is well controlled is less likely to suffer from the various complications of the disease.

Patient education designed to facilitate recovery, assist adaptation and prevent complications is an important component of this form of prevention.

Health protection

Health protection includes measures taken to ensure a healthy environment and protection from accidents or disease. Measures such as seat-belt legislation, control of communicable diseases and the addition of fluoride to water supplies to prevent dental decay are all examples of health protection.

Downie et al (1991) believe that 'the cardinal principle of health promotion is empowerment'. Health education seeks to empower by providing necessary information and helping people to develop skills and a healthy level of self-esteem. The provision of good preventative services and the shaping of a healthful environment through health protection also contribute to this process of empowerment.

Nurses have the potential to be in the forefront of health promotion. No other professional group has as much contact with patients. A positive approach to health is everybody's business but nurses should see this as an area of high priority.

This chapter has provided an overview of health and its links with society. Nurses are the largest single group employed in the Health Service and work both in hospital and in the community. They are therefore ideally placed to play an important part in improving the health of the Nation and achieving the targets of Health For All by the Year 2000.

Suggested assignments

Discussion topics
1. Much ill health could be said to be self-inflicted since it relates to unhealthy life-styles.

   Why do many people choose to ignore advice aimed at helping them to lead healthier lives?

(cont'd)

2. Many members of society are opposed to the addition of fluoride to the public water supply, yet this is an effective and inexpensive method of reducing dental decay in the community.

   Is it ethical to deny people, especially young children, the benefits this would provide?

3. Limiting the numbers of motor cars in city centres would reduce noise and air pollution and result in decreased traffic congestion. Deaths from road accidents would also be reduced.

   Discuss the feasibility of implementing such a policy in Britain's city centres.

4. The numbers of elderly people in Britain are steadily increasing.

   What implications does this have for the provision of health and social services?

REFERENCES AND FURTHER READING

Aggleton P 1990 Health. Routledge, London, p 4

Asquith S 1993 Protecting children Cleveland to Orkney: more lessons to learn. HMSO, London, p 2

Bagley C, King K 1990 Child Sexual Abuse. Tavistock/ Routledge, London, p 75

Bowling A 1991 Measuring health. Biddles, Guildford, p 6

Brandon 1976 Physical violence in the family – an overview in Borland M Ed. Violence in the family

Briscoe M 1989 Sex differences in mental health. Update 39(9): 834–839

British Medical Association 1986 Alternative therapy. Chameleon, London, p 78

Calman M 1987 Health and illness – the lay perspective. Tavistock, London, p 25

Carstairs V, Morris R 1990 Deprivation and health in Scotland. Health Bulletin 8(4): 162

Catford J C 1983 Community Medicine: Positive health indicators 5(2) p 125

Central Statistical Office 1993a, Social trends 23. HMSO, London, p 141

Central Statistical Office 1993b Social trends 23. HMSO, London, p 62

Central Statistical Office 1993c Social trends 23. HMSO, London, p 32

Central Statistical Office 1993d Social trends 23. HMSO, London, p 167

Cigoli V, Binda W 1993 Health and the family world health, 46th year, no 6, November/December, p 7

Dargie H, Grant S 1991 Exercise. British Medical Journal 303: 910

Davie T 1994 Children at exhaust height are hit by traffic fumes. *The Times* 18 February, p 8

Department of Health and Social Security 1980 Inequalities in health. Department of Health and Social Security, London

Department of Health and Social Security 1983 National Health Service management enquiry. Department of Health and Social Security, London

Dobson S 1983 Bringing culture into care. Nursing Times 79(6): 57

Doult B 1992 Don't ignore the needs of ethnic minorities. Nursing Standard Vol. No. 3 November 3rd p 12

Downie R S, Fyfe C, Tannahill A 1990 Health promotion models and values. Oxford Medical Publications, Oxford, p 59

Dubos R 1959 The Mirage of Health. Harper Dow, New York p 23

Durnin J 1993 Teenage TV couch potatoes. New Scientific Supplement 140(1894): 15

Eyles J, Donovan J 1990 The social effects of health policy. Avebury, Aldershot

Fagin L 1993 Physical and psychological aspects of unemployment. Update 26(8): 1356

Fagin S, Little M 1984 The forsaken families. Penguin Books, Harmondsworth, p 40

Fiastarone M A, Marks E C, Ryan N D et al 1990 High density training in nonagenarians. Effects on skeletal muscle. Journal of American Medical Association 263: 3029

Garrett G 1989 Caring in Great Britain today, Professional Nurse Vol 4 Issue 10 p 485

Goodlee F 1992 Noise: breaking the silence. British Medical Journal 304: 110

Hartz C, Plant M, Watts M 1990 Alcohol and health. The Medical Council on Alcoholism, London, p 3

Heyden C 1992 Bed and breakfast blues. Health Service Journal 102(5323): 22

Horley S 1991 Positive health indicators. Paper at Families of the 90s Conference, London (cited in Tattam M 1991 Nursing Times 87(46): 7)

Hughes E 1951 In: Esland G, Salaman G, Speakman M(eds) People and Work. Holmes McDougall, Edinburgh; Open University Press, Milton Keynes, p 158

Hunt S 1988 Housing can damage your health. Edinburgh Council Social Services, No 35, Link Up, pp 10–15

Hutchings J, Gower K 1993 Unemployment and mental health. Community Psychiatric Nursing Journal 13(5): 17

Kendall S 1993 Inequalities in health and the provision of care. South Bank University, London

Law M R, Wald N J, Meade T W 1991 Strategies for prevention of osteoporosis and hip fracture. British Medical Journal 303: 456

Levenstein A 1964 Why people work. Collier Books, New York, p 20

McCall J 1991 Ethnic minorities – meeting cultural needs. Surgical Nurse 4(4): 22

Mattiasson L, Lingarde F, Nilsson J A, Theorell T 1990 Threat of unemployment and cardiovascular risk factors. British Medical Journal 301: 465

Melhuish A 1982 Work and health. Penguin Books, Harmondsworth, Middlesex, p 113

Moss P, Melhuish E 1991 Current issues in day care for young children, Department of Health. HMSO, London, p 49

National Nursing and Midwifery Consultative Committee 1992 The role and function of the professional nurse. Scottish Office, Home and Health Department, Edinburgh

Okell-Jones C 1982 In: Scottish Education Department(ed) Violence in the family. HMSO, London, p 12

O'Neill P 1983 Health crisis 2000. Heinemann Medical Books for World Health Organisation, London, p x

OPCS 1991 Mortality statistics – injury and poisoning, Series DH4, No 17. HMSO, London

Open University 1985 The health of nations. The Open University, Milton Keynes, p 80

Parsons T 1981, Definitions of health and illness in the light of American values and social structure. In: Caplan A L, Englehardt H T and M'Cartney J J (eds) Concepts of health and disease – interdisciplinary perspectives. Addison-Wesley, Wokingham, Berks, p 69

Pizzey E 1974 Scream Quietly or the Neighbours will hear. Harmondsworth, Penguin

Plant M L, Plant M A, Foster J 1991 Stress, Alcohol, Tobacco and illicit drug use amongst Nurses. Journal of Advanced Nursing 17: 1057–1067

Platt S, Kreitman N 1984 Trends in parasuicide and unemployment among men in Edinburgh, 1968–1982. British Medical Journal 289: 1032

Pritchard S 1990 Safety of children in temporary accommodation. Health Visitor 63(6): 194

Quickfall J 1992 Selling health in the market, professional care of mother and child. 2(4): 116

Reilly D 1983 Young doctors' views on alternative medicine. British Medical Journal 287: 338

Robertson C 1989 Alcohol, trauma and the emergency department, Edinburgh Medicine (54): 7–9

Royal College of Physicians 1983 Health or smoking. Pitman, London, p 2

Rutter M 1981 Maternal deprivation reassessed, 2nd edn. Penguin Books, Harmondsworth, Middlesex, p 173

Sadler C 1989 Driven to desperation. Nursing Times 85(27): 18

Secretary of State 1992 The health of the nation – a strategy for health in England. HMSO, London

Seedhouse D 1986a Health, the foundations for achievement. John Wiley, Chichester, p i

Seedhouse D 1986b Health, the foundations for achievement. John Wiley, Chichester, Frontispiece

Seedhouse D 1986c Health, the foundations for achievement. John Wiley, Chichester, p 34

Smith A, Jacobson B 1988 The Nation's Health. King Edward's Hospital Fund, Kings Fund Publishing Office, London; Health Education Council, London, p 139

Smith G, Bartley M, Blane D 1990 The Black Report on socioeconomic inequalities in health, 10 years on. British Medical Journal 301: 373

Smith J 1984 Prevention by example. Nursing Mirror 139(13): 18

Sofer C 1970 Men in mid career: a study of British managers and specialists. Cambridge University Press, Cambridge, p 86

Solberg S 1989 Women and mental health. In: Hardy L (ed) Issues in women's health. Churchill Livingstone, Edinburgh, pp 97–98

Strauss M B (ed) 1968a Familiar medical quotations. JA Churchill, London, p 201

Strauss M B (ed) 1968b Familiar medical quotations. JA Churchill, London p 204

Strauss M B (ed) 1968c Familiar medical quotations. JA Churchill, London, p 204

Tattam A 1991 Challenge to protect women victims of violence in the home. Nursing Times 87(46): 7

Trevelyan J 1993 Fringe benefits. Nursing Times 89(7): 32

Townsend P, Davidson N, Whitehead M 1992 Inequalities in health, the Black Report and the health divide. Penguin Books, Harmondsworth, Middlesex, p 1

United Kingdom Central Council for Nursing, Midwifery and Health Visiting 1992 Code of Professional Conduct Clause 7

Vines G 1993 Overdosing on exercise. New Scientist 140 (suppl): 9 October, 13

Wald N, Wanchahal K, Thomson S, Cuckle H 1986 Does breathing other peoples tobacco smoking cause lung cancer. British Medical Journal 293: 1221

Walker A 1992 Drinking water – doubts about quality. British Medical Journal 304: 177

Wells D 1992 Nutrition, social status and health. Nutrition and Food science (2): 16

WHO 1946 The Constitution. WHO, Geneva

WHO 1983 Targets in Support of the Regional Strategy for Health For All By 2000, EUR/RC 33/9, Rev 1, October 28th, p 1. WHO, Geneva

WHO 1993 Health for all targets: the health policy for Europe, revised edn. Regional Office for Europe WHO Copenhagen

Wood C 1989 The reality of women's health. Nursing Times 85(48): 54

2

People and health

Patricia J. Steele

In this chapter the aim is to provide an understanding of how individuals make decisions about their health status and identify how individual health care needs may be meet through nursing practice.

To promote this understanding it is necessary to explore the relevance of 'the study of behaviour' to nursing. The 'systematic study of behaviour of people and animals' is known as **psychology** (Hall 1982). Generally speaking behaviour refers to activities that can be observed, such as socializing, playing games or going to work. However, Hall suggests behaviour should be interpreted in a much wider sense to cover 'thoughts, emotions and utterances as well as acts'. Hall's definition of behaviour in this wide sense can therefore include anything a person may do. This is the definition of behaviour that will be used throughout the discussion on people and health.

Health as discussed in Chapter 1 is a complex concept. However through this discussion it should now be possible to appreciate the interrelationship and interdependence which exist between all of the aspects of health. For example, admission to hospital affects the patient's physical, psychological, emotional, social and spiritual health. It is upon this holistic view of health that the discussion in this chapter will be based.

The definition of nursing which is used is that formulated by Virginia Henderson (1966). For a more detailed discussion of nursing see Chapter 3 on the role of the nurse. Henderson's definition of nursing highlights the health promotional role of the nurse in her care of both the sick and well in society. It also identifies the importance of health care and rehabilitation within the nurse–patient/client relationship.

Nursing is a complex business, therefore the more that is understood about human behaviour the greater the likelihood that nursing care relevant to the health care needs of the individual will be provided. This chapter is divided into the following five sections:

Understanding behaviour

Two areas are covered: (1) the relationship between the study of behaviour and nursing is examined; (2) the paradox of formulating general rules to explore behaviour whilst emphasizing the uniqueness of the individual is analysed.

The individual's view of the world and self

The complexity of the dynamic process of interpreting and interacting with the world by the individual is considered, and the development of attitudes and values and how they may be amenable to change.

The right to choose

This section consists of three parts, which examine:

- how individuals make decisions and relate this to health choices.
- the concept of risk, and how it may be estimated differently by individuals. This discussion also addresses how conflicts may arise between individuals who hold differing views about health issues.
- individual rights – moral, ethical and legal issues. This discussion considers the power differential between professionals and client; parents and children, and poses the question, to what degree should professionals or carers act for those whose ability to act for themselves is diminished? The rights of the individual in relation to euthanasia, living wills, and participation in research are also explored.

Life transitions

This section is composed of five parts:

Human development and discusses the concept of life transitions and how individuals may be affected by them in terms of adaptability, coping and vulnerability to illness.

Ageing provides a brief review of the ageing process and makes reference to other texts to enhance understanding of the continuing individual differences and rights of the elderly in society.

Acute illness considers the effect in relation to self

and significant others, for example, spouse, parents or children, the individual's perception of the threat of illness and how it may alter his view of the world. How illness may affect attitudes and health-related behaviour is also addressed.

Chronic illness and disability discusses the effects in relation to self and significant others. Issues discussed include self-image, quality of life and adaptation skills.

Dying and bereavement is discussed, with particular reference to the issue of loss and the many responses which exist.

Individual uniqueness

This section concludes the chapter by exploring issues of individual uniqueness of:

- clients
- significant others
- nurses.

in relation to effective functioning in the provision of health care.

UNDERSTANDING BEHAVIOUR

Nursing as we have indicated in the introduction has become a complex business. It has developed from an activity which concentrated primarily on the provision of care and comfort to the sick to one which involves a holistic approach to health care and the utilization of current research in nursing practice. (A detailed account of the development of the nursing profession is to be found in Kenworthy et al 1992, ch. 10.)

Holistic health care is described by Redman (1988) as embodying a number of the precepts of the consumer ethic. These include:

1. The provision of comprehensive health care programmes that address the physical, psychological and spiritual needs of those who need help.

2. Programmes that should meet the unique needs of the individual.

3. Remedies that promote further dependence should be exchanged for therapeutic approaches which mobilize the individual's capacity for self healing and independence.

4. An emphasis on education and self care rather than treatment and dependence.

5. Health care settings should be used for education, volunteer work and socializing as well as for care in health and illness.

Therefore individualized care involves coping with the needs of the whole person. It includes the 'promotion of health' which incorporates 'health education, prevention and health protection' as well as tending to physical needs (Downie et al 1990).

In order to integrate the theory (nursing knowledge) and practice of nursing (practical skills) a 'process of nursing' has evolved. The 'nursing process' as it is termed describes a four-stage cycle of assessment, planning, implementation and evaluation. This process is initiated whenever a patient or client presents with an illness or an interest in health promotional or health maintenance issues.

Carrying out the nursing process requires a wide range of professional skills. These include gathering and providing information, clarifying thinking, reflecting feelings or teaching a skill.

For example a young mother may be admitted to the ward for an appendicectomy. Although initially her immediate needs may be physical, careful nursing assessment may reveal she is a very heavy smoker. Using a caring and sensitive approach the nurse may elicit her reasons for smoking. Through an understanding of the patient's behaviour and her concerns about smoking, the nurse will be able to provide information on the dangers of smoking and the help available should the patient wish to stop which will lead to long-term health benefits for the patient and her family.

In providing nursing care, we need to remember there is a person at the centre of every illness and health issue (Hall 1988). An appreciation of the uniqueness of each individual relative to his current health status, age, sexuality, abilities, attainments and social background is important if a good personal relationship between the nurse and patient/client is to be established. This relationship should result in a willingness from both nurse and patient to co-operate to aid recovery and/or achieve one's health potential.

In the discussion so far the term behaviour and its relationship to nursing has been identified. In doing so the importance of caring for the patient/client as an individual has been highlighted.

In general, however, the understanding of how individuals behave results not from the scientific study of individuals but from the study of groups of people (Carlson 1990). It is therefore important to develop the understanding of behaviour by consideration of the paradox of formulating general rules to explain behaviour whilst emphasizing individual uniqueness.

Psychology is the scientific study of behaviour. Its purpose is to explain behaviour and to understand its causes. In general, explaining behaviour means discovering its causes, i.e. the events that are responsible for its occurrence. Therefore, according to Carlson, if the events that cause behaviour to occur can be described, it has been explained.

Generally when research is carried out, the researcher has no particular interest in the individual subjects whose behaviour is being observed. Instead there is an assumption that the subjects are representative of the larger population being studied. This representative group of subjects is usually referred to as a **sample** of the larger population. Because of factors such as time, expense and accessibility it would not be possible nor practical to observe the behaviour of the whole of the adolescent population. Therefore, the researcher would collect such information from a subset or smaller group, a **sample** of the adolescent population. In this way the knowledge gained would be representative of the total adolescent population being studied.

The researcher would then be able to generalize the results from this specific study to the adolescent population as a whole.

In conclusion the findings from the study would provide information on the behaviour of adolescents in general, not simply about the specific subjects who participated in the study. (See Ch. 3 for further comment on research in nursing. A more detailed account of the research process in nursing is to be found in Cormack 1991.)

Certain types of behaviour have been associated with health and disease, and these will be discussed below.

Favourable health behaviours and practices

A Californian study which involved a general community population over a 10-year period showed seven favourable health practices:

- never smoking cigarettes
- limiting alcohol consumption
- controlling weight
- sleeping 7–8 hours daily
- eating breakfast almost every day
- never or rarely eating between meals
- regular physical activity.

The behaviours were proved to be highly correlated with physical health. The more practices followed, the healthier the individual (Breslow & Enstrom 1980). Further research in the USA demonstrated that the results of the Californian study were applicable to the general population.

Unfavourable health behaviours and practices

Relationships between life-style and disease have also been documented. Cancers are the second leading cause of death in the UK. Although there is still insufficient knowledge about the causes of cancer, a causal link has been found between smoking and lung cancer; the risk of death from lung cancer increases with the number of cigarettes smoked and decreases when the number of cigarettes is reduced or stopped altogether.

Cardiovascular disease also provides an example of the synergistic effect of risk factors, that is when several risk factors are present the probability of the disease developing is greater than the sum of the individual probabilities associated with each risk. However, in discussing risk factors it must be remembered that there is no absolute link between a risk factor and the development of a disease. The association between lung cancer and smoking is well established. Ninety per cent of lung cancer deaths are attributable to cigarette smoking, yet only a small proportion of heavy smokers develop lung cancer – a fact many smokers employ to resist changes in their unfavourable health behaviour. Although personal behaviour contributes to the health status of the individual, it is not the only or main influence on the health of the population (Whitehead 1989).

Wider socioeconomic and environmental circumstances also influence health, and some of these are outwith the individual's control. These influences and their effects in determining the health status of the individual will be discussed in more detail.

THE INDIVIDUAL'S VIEW OF THE WORLD AND SELF

As a result of experiences, individuals develop a set of assumptions to help them make sense of the world in which they live (Kneisl & Ames 1989). These assumptions provide a basis for predicting the behaviour of others and the effect of behaviour on others. For example, 'families are responsible for the care of family members; the way to get ahead in this world is to work hard at academic studies'.

These assumptions form the individuals 'world view' and help to guide their perceptions, behaviour, emotional state and well-being. This assumptive world view is a perspective that develops during childhood and is taken for granted. Attitudes and values of the culture are passed on during the early years from parents, other family members, neighbours and church,

at a later date school and workplace transmit similar ideas. Therefore, within a close knit community one's world view is likely to be shared by other community members.

When others share one's world view a greater sense of interpersonal harmony is likely. However when world views are mismatched, frustrations and interpersonal conflicts become inevitable.

An understanding of a person's world view is of importance in the provision of health care. As Kneisl and Ames suggest, mismatched world views frequently account for dissatisfaction from clients about health care providers and health care providers' dissatisfaction with clients.

For example in Hindu or Sikh communities, relatives will be anxious that a mother has complete rest after the birth of a baby. This attitude is based on the belief that the mother is at her weakest at this time and therefore susceptible to infection and injury (Lothian Community Relations Council 1988). This period of 40 days' confinement may be at variance with western views. If the health visitor is unaware of the mother's world views she will be concerned at her lack of activity and attendance at the well baby clinic. In voicing these concerns the health visitor may unwittingly cause distress to the mother, affecting future relationships with health care providers resulting in an unwillingness to seek further health care.

Attitudes, beliefs and values

Attitudes

Attitudes play an important part in how an individual views the world and behaves towards it. Redman (1988) defines an attitude as, 'a learned emotionally toned predisposition to react in a particular way towards an object, idea or person', or as Atkinson and colleagues suggest, attitudes may be described as 'likes and dislikes', affinities for, and aversions to, certain objects, persons, groups or situations (Atkinson et al 1987).

Therefore a person's taste in music, clothes, sports and leisure pursuits all reflect his/her attitudes, as do the people chosen as friends. Attitudes are affected by the individual's beliefs and values and are reflected in both his/her feelings and behaviour.

Beliefs

Beliefs tend to be cognitive in nature, that is, they involve 'thinking, knowing and understanding'. They are created by the acquisition of knowledge and result in acceptance of a statement, fact or an idea as being true.

Certain factors have been identified as influencing the strength of a belief (Downie et al 1990). These include the credibility of the source of the message or information. This may be in the form of the written or spoken word, such as in books or on the radio. Or it may be in the form of a visual presentation, for example a lecture or television performance.

The relevance of the information and the extent to which it fits in or clashes with existing beliefs is also considered to be an important factor, as is the quality and appropriateness of the method of communication.

Values

Whereas a person's beliefs provide an indication of what he believes to be true, a person's values are expressions of how he believes an object or relationship affects him. Values therefore pertain to feelings and emotions. Examples of personal values include self-determination, self-government, sense of development and sense of responsibility (Downie et al 1990). In general, ones values tend to be of a permanent nature.

It has become generally accepted that attitudes consist of three different aspects or components: affective, behavioural and cognitive (Carlson 1990). The affective component is limited to a person's values and consists of the kinds of feelings a particular topic may arouse. The cognitive component is limited to a person's beliefs, beliefs which according to Carlson may be expressed in words. The behavioural component consists of a tendency to behave in a particular way with regard to a particular topic.

Carlson suggests the way attitudes are formed is similar to the way in which an individual can be persuaded to change them. However he does make the point that whereas peoples' attitudes are normally formed by implicit processes, attempts to change peoples' attitudes are usually explicit and deliberate.

Attitude formation

Affective components of attitude

The affective component, the emotional aspect of an attitude, is primarily formed through direct or vicarious classical conditioning (Carlson 1990).

Direct classical conditioning This involves direct contact with the attitude object, for example children may not show any fear of a nurse until they experi-

ence an injection. As the nurse is associated with a painful injection, many children may become upset at the sight of the nurse. The attitude of the child towards the nurse will be negative.

Vicarious classical conditioning This mechanism involves the observation of the emotional reactions of particularly significant others to the attitude object (conditional stimulus). For example, the way children see their parents react towards members of ethnic communities will influence the direction of their reactions. Therefore if the parent reacts in a positive way the child is more likely to develop a positive attitude towards ethnic groups and conversely a negative attitude if the reaction is a negative one.

The affective component of attitudes has been found to be resistant to changes even after an individual has changed his opinion on a particular subject. For example, a nurse may have overcome a childhood racial prejudice to enable her to provide a high standard of nursing care for people of other races but may experience unpleasant emotional feelings at the sight of a mixed racial couple.

As Carlson suggests, such a discrepancy between belief and feelings frequently results in people feeling guilty.

Cognitive components of attitudes

Most beliefs about particular issues are acquired in a direct manner. This may occur through reading, or hearing a fact or statement. Other people may reinforce attitudes by expressing particular opinions.

As children, attitudes are formed through imitating or modelling the behaviour of people who play an important role in the child's life. (Hetherington & Parke 1986). This influence frequently occurs without the model's awareness.

The family is an important source of learning in a child's early years, and its members are important examples for him. Parents therefore have a significant role to play in the development of their children's health attitudes by setting a good example themselves. Children whose parents smoke are, for example, much more likely to take up smoking. As the child develops the peer groups and media influences are also very powerful in the formation of attitudes.

Behavioural components of attitudes

The term behaviour has already been identified as encompassing a range of phenomena involving our thoughts, emotions, words and actions.

The behavioural component is interesting because

people do not always behave as their expressed beliefs and attitudes would lead one to assume. For example a nurse may counsel patients or clients on the health benefits of giving up smoking but continue to smoke the dreaded weed herself when she is stressed. Whilst a teenager may hold an anti-drug attitude he may smoke marijuana when with friends to avoid being ostracized by the group.

Therefore, as suggested by Downie et al, difficulties arise when it is assumed that what a person says or does is a true reflection of his/her attitude (1990). Nevertheless a relationship between attitudes and behaviour has been shown to exist but this relationship is influenced by many factors (Carlson 1990) including:

1. the degree of specificity
2. the motivational relevance
3. self-attribution
4. general constraints on behaviour.

The degree of specificity is an important variable that affects the relationships between a person's attitude and his behaviour. Specific attitudes tend to predict the behaviour better than general attitudes towards behaviour.

Atkinson et al (1987) cites a study by Davidson & Jacques (1979) which demonstrated that women's attitudes toward birth control correlated (0.08) with a woman's use of oral contraceptives over a 2-year period but attitudes towards the pill specifically correlated (0.07) with that behaviour.

Motivational relevance in general, expressing attitudes verbally towards particular topics or issues, is less time consuming than having to put words into actions. Even when a person feels strongly about a particular issue research shows that he is unlikely to behave positively towards it unless it has some personal significance.

For example the membership of a pressure group to bring about changes in the law regarding drinking and driving is most likely to be composed of persons who have had a relative killed or maimed by the actions of a drunk driver.

Self-attribution the way a person forms his/her attitude affects the relationship between attitude and behaviour. Attitudes which are based on direct experience are shown to predict behaviour better than attitudes formed from just reading or hearing about an issue. Thus, attitudes that are based on people's prior behaviour are a good indicator of future behaviour. In conclusion, personal experience appears to form the most consistent attitude–behaviour relationship.

Other constraints on behaviour may result from a lack of knowledge to connect attitudes to the relevant behaviours or the relevant behaviour may be considered very unpleasant and therefore avoided. Also the effects of other attitudes, motives and circumstances may not be known, producing discrepancies between attitude and behaviour (Redman 1988).

Attitude change

Attitudes may be changed in two main ways (Downie et al 1990):

1. By the provision of information which is inconsistent with current beliefs, i.e the information may conflict with the person's existing beliefs. The aim is to provide the information in an attractive and pleasing manner to aid both its acceptance and retention by the individual. This may be achieved by the use of newspapers, books, leaflets, radio, leaflets and television or by the lecture method.

2. By making people behave in a manner which is inconsistent with their current beliefs. This may be achieved by direct exposure to the attitude object, by the use of role play or by direct observations: or by changing the rewards and costs of different courses of behaviour, for example by legislation. Therefore role play may be used in schools to teach about drug abuse, whilst direct observation may be an appropriate way of enabling a patient with a colostomy to cope with his/her new situation by providing him/her with the opportunity to meet a 'model' patient who copes well with a colostomy. Using legislation to ensure motorbike riders wear crash helmets to reduce the risk of head injuries if in an accident provides a further example of how attitudes change can occur.

However even when information is provided, attitude change may not occur.

Studies have shown that four main factors are involved in the provision of information for attitude change to occur:

- the communicator
- the communication
- the recipient
- the medium of communication.

Characteristics of the communicator

Three important factors have been identified as influencing change in people's opinions (Carlson 1990).

The first factor is **expertise or credibility**. This refers to the amount of knowledge the communicator appears to have about the subject of the message. In general people are more likely to be persuaded by someone they believe to be an expert in his/her particular field. This individual may be a professional, for example a nurse specialist in stoma care or a lay person, such as an ex patient who is coping well with the care of his stoma.

Secondly the communicator's **motives and intentions** are of importance. If people think the communicator is likely to benefit (particularly financially) by his/her message then they are less likely to conform to his/her wishes. They are also unlikely to do as the communicator says if the message is directed at them personally. Studies have shown that if the communicator is perceived as unconcerned about convincing his/her audience, the message is more likely to persuade listeners to change their attitudes.

Finally **attractiveness, likeability and similarity**. It has been shown that people are more likely to be persuaded to change their attitude if the message is presented by an attractive person than an unattractive person. Likewise similarity of the communicator to the recipient has also been found to be effective.

It is suggested that by presenting an attractive role model image, the recipient is more likely to strive to become like the role model and assume similar attitudes. If the model is too different then the gap between the two may be seen as being too wide and no change will be attempted.

A method currently being used which utilizes this information is peer group education amongst teenagers to encourage them to make positive choices in sexual relationships, protecting themselves and partners from unwanted pregnancy and HIV infections.

Characteristics of communication

Both the characteristics of the communicator and the context of the communication are important if a change of attitude is to take place.

Three main characteristics that affect the persuasiveness of messages have been identified: argumentation, repetition and fear.

Argumentation This means that when attempting to persuade a change in attitude, whether the communicator should present one side or both sides of an argument to his/her audience. Studies show both can be effective but the choice is dependent on the predisposition of the recipient.

Carlson (1990) suggests if the audience is sympathetic to the communicator's viewpoint, then only one side of the argument is necessary. However if initially the audience is predisposed towards the opposing viewpoint then both points of the argument should be presented. The opposing view being presented first and then discredited by the opposite argument. For most situations, presenting both sides of the argument is more effective. The communicator appears better informed, less biased and less interested in influencing the audience, and is therefore more convincing.

Repetition The more a person is exposed to a stimulus the more he/she will learn to like it or at least tolerate it. By repeating the same message over and over again a positive attitude can be obtained.

However two other factors have been shown to interact with the frequency of exposure effect. First stimuli are required to be of a relatively complex nature otherwise people become bored. Secondly indefinite exposure to even complex stimuli eventually begins to lose its effectiveness. Nurses and health educators need to bear this information in mind in the development and presentation of health promotional material.

Fear or threat Fear or the use of threat can be used not only to induce compliance but to bring about a change in attitude. Health threats or fears have frequently been incorporated into health messages to dissuade people from indulging in health risk behaviours. Messages aimed at persuading people to stop smoking, use a condom or tan safely, are all based on fear. Disregarding these messages, it is argued, will result in lung cancer, AIDS or skin cancer.

Although fear-producing methods of persuasion have been found to be effective, this is only so under certain circumstances.

Three factors that make fear-inducing messages effective in changing attitudes have been identified as:

1. the perceived harmfulness of the event
2. the perceived likelihood the event will take place
3. the perceived effectiveness of avoiding risk-taking behaviour (Rogers 1975).

However, current thinking suggests fear appeals have a limited value as their effects are sometimes short lived (Taylor 1991). Where behaviour change requires to be maintained, or where the individual is repeatedly exposed to temptation, other attitude change techniques which provide information linked to a positive health message are more likely to be effective in motivating behaviour change.

Other communication factors which have been shown to influence change include:

1. The relevance the information has to the recipient at a particular moment in time.
2. Simplicity in transmitting the message.

3. Use of alternative methods of communication such as music, drama or comedy to convey the message.

4. If the message includes specific action recommendations which are easily carried out, then a change in attitude and behaviour is more likely to occur. (Downie et al 1990, Taylor 1991).

The recipient

Characteristics of the recipient play an important part in influencing change.

Personality factors have been identified as contributing to differing levels of persuadability. Individuals who have a low self-esteem appear to be more easily influenced than those who have a high level of self-esteem, as the former are less likely to be confident in their own opinions and therefore seek acceptance by the communicator.

Self-esteem can also be related to intelligence. Intelligent individuals tend to be persuaded by complex messages rather than simple messages that are unsupported by facts. It is suggested this occurs because they are confident enough to resist messages that contain no supporting evidence (Carlson 1990). Also people who are able to present a range of counter-arguments to the message are less likely to be influenced to change their mind (Niven 1989). Individuals may also resist attitude change if they believe their right to make up their own mind is being denied.

Interestingly, men have been found to be less open to persuasion than women (Downie et al 1990).

Cognitive dissonance

So far the discussion has considered how attitudes affect behaviour, but it is also possible for behaviour to affect attitudes. This situation occurs when a person's behaviour is inconsistent with the attitude he holds. For example a person may believe that smoking can seriously damage health but continue to smoke 40 cigarettes a day. This inconsistency between attitude and behaviour causes him/her to experience discomfort or dissonance.

To resolve this discomfort the person may stop smoking, that is, change his/her behaviour, or he/she may change his/her attitude by developing justifications or excuses to resolve the inconsistency, such as, 'my grandfather lived till he was 93 and he smoked all his life' and 'anyway I enjoy my cigarettes, they are the only pleasures left in life'. Studies show that in general, people are more likely to change their attitude than their behaviour (Festinger 1957).

This finding has implications for health educators – it is frequently difficult to understand why some people, despite professional advice, continue to practice negative health behaviours undeterred by the likelihood of endangering their health.

For a more detailed account of attitudes and persuasion see Brigham (1991), Chapter 4.

THE RIGHT TO CHOOSE

Decision making and health choices

Everyday life involves making decisions. According to Tschudin (1992) before any decision can be made there has to be a choice. She suggests that it is necessary to have at least two alternatives to choose from and that all the possibilities and alternatives require to be 'seen and recognised' before a decision can be made. To reach a stable decision, five crucial steps have been identified (Niven 1989). These include:

1. Appraising the challenge – are the risks serious if no change is made?

2. Survey alternatives – searching for an acceptable alternative to resolve the problem.

3. Weighing alternatives – which alternative is best. Identifying the best alternative and based upon this identification a decision is made to follow a specific course of action.

4. Deliberating about commitment – developing a plan – providing interested others with information about the person's commitment.

5. Adhering despite negative feedback – staying with the plan to implement the decision despite the emergence of new thoughts or opportunities.

It is argued that if any of the five stages is omitted or carried out without conviction then the decision may be reversed when difficulties arise (Redman 1989). Redman proposes that major errors may result if decisional conflict is not resolved. The individual applies defective coping mechanisms in an effort to avoid conflict by the use of procrastination, absolving themselves from responsibility or using rationalizations that minimize expected unfavourable outcomes. The individual may also try desperately to find a way out of the dilemma by jumping from one alternative to another, seeking short-term solutions to the problem. Unfortunately this method of coping does not deal with the full range of consequences nor resolve the initial conflict in the long term.

Several factors have been found to influence decision making. The influence of other people is identified as being of major importance in decision making (Sutherland 1978). This influence may extend from the 'general effect of norms' that is, what people believe is expected of them, to the very powerful effect of the influence of significant others such as, parents, spouses and, as Sutherland suggests, 'some other local source of wisdom'.

What influences an individual's decisions about health choices is very important. As has already been discussed, parents play an important role in influencing children's beliefs. Health beliefs appear to develop relatively early in life. By the age of 11 or 12 years of age most children will have developed stable health beliefs that resemble those of adults. The home is therefore a very powerful learning environment. Studies show that in homes where parents do not teach positive health habits other educational efforts to do so are frequently found to be ineffective (Taylor 1991).

Individuals also make decisions about what is appropriate health behaviour as a result of information gained through 'mass health education campaigns'. The current National Health promotion to use a condom to prevent contracting HIV provides a useful example of how people may be encouraged to make a positive health choice related to their sexual behaviour.

Other health topics used in mass health education campaigns to promote positive health choices include childhood immunization programmes, healthy eating, exercise, relaxation and the benefits of stopping smoking and reducing alcohol consumption.

As Downie (1990) suggests, to choose health means the individual must choose the 'goods' and 'life-style' which are likely to lead to and enhance health. Unfortunately at the time when initial health habits are developing during childhood and adolescence, there is little incentive to practice good health behaviours because most individuals are 'healthy'.

Unhealthy behaviours such as heavy smoking, drinking, eating to excess and avoiding exercise appear to carry no apparent health risks. Because the cumulative effects of these negative health habits may not become evident for several years, many young people show little concern for their eventual health status at the age of 40 or 50 years. Also at the same time that individuals may be making decisions about their health behaviours, pressures from the tobacco, alcohol and confectionery manufacturers may influence them into making unhealthy behaviour choices (Sutherland 1979).

For other individuals, we find their health choices are limited by their socioeconomic circumstances.

In 1988–89 one-fifth of the population of the UK, between 11 and 12 million people, were found to be living in poverty (Oppenheim 1993).

As discussed in Chapter 1, the major advances in health status are associated more often with improvements in social circumstances than with medical advances. Therefore where people are able to exercise greater choice related to the factors that affect health, such as housing, the environment, employment, leisure activities and consumption, this generally results in an improvement in their health status (Smith & Jacobson 1988).

These factors are important to the consideration of the concept of risk and how it may be estimated differently by individuals. Throughout life people may take risks either by proceeding in a particular way without regard to the possibility of the dangers involved, or despite knowing the dangers involved.

Epidemiology, the study of the distribution and determinants of disease in communities, provides data on the health of populations and the causes and risk factors related to ill health. Consequently such information also provides the potential basis for health promotion and disease prevention within populations. The major risk factors related to premature death and ill health in the UK have been identified as smoking, an unhealthy diet, alcohol, low physical activity, high blood pressure and obesity.

In the promotion of health and the prevention of disease it is of importance to be able to identify clients who are perceived to be at risk of developing a particular disease or health problem. However despite identifying clients 'at risk' and informing them of the health risks they are taking, some people continue to practise negative health behaviours. Health professionals may find it very difficult to understand why, in spite of all the medical evidence available, individuals continue to practise unhealthy behaviours – why do individuals continue to behave in this 'risky' fashion throughout life?

Ewles & Simnett (1992) suggest that much health behaviour appears to develop without decision making. It often just happens in response to individual group circumstances and external events. This may be particularly true in adolescence when taking risks appear to be the norm. Risks may be taken out of simple curiosity or occur as a response to peer pressure. Most adults are also able to recount dares or taking risks to demonstrate their rebellion against their parents or other authority during their own youth.

People have also been found to hold an unrealistic optimism about the likelihood they will develop major health problems (Taylor 1991). Taylor considers this is true for several reasons:

1. People exaggerate their ability to control their health. Consequently they may ignore health threats, believing the threat does not exist or that if it does develop they will be able to deal with it.

2. Individuals may have little experience of health threats and they will underestimate their vulnerability. Individuals who have never experienced a serious illness may find it difficult to imagine what it would be like. This may be particularly true for young people who are often at their peak of physical fitness and typically view themselves as invulnerable (Plant & Plant 1992). When tragedies do occur, to others, they rationalize that it will never happen to them, appearing somehow to believe that they are protected by some invisible shield.

3. People may believe that if they have had a healthy childhood without evidence of disease then they are unlikely to succumb to ill health during adult life.

Taylor suggests this unrealistic optimism undermines legitimate worry about risk. This may reduce the likelihood that such people will engage in positive health behaviour or accept health habit interventions.

Other reasons why people may take risks by making unhealthy behaviour choices are that they may not perceive their behaviour to be unhealthy or that they are placing themselves at risk. Where they consider there is one element of risk involved they may then assess that the benefits of their actions outweigh the risks and the negative health choice is made. For example, a mother may argue that the alleviation of stress by smoking outweighs the dangers of smoking. It is also worth noting that her alleviation of stress will be attained at least in the short term, whilst the risk of contracting any of the smoking-related diseases is a risk she is prepared to take and deal with should it occur at some time in the future. Others may be aware of the risks associated with unhealthy behaviour but because of other constraints be unable to practise healthy choices. For example if there is insufficient money to feed the family, choice of food is limited. Therefore a mother may choose foods that are cheap and filling but not necessarily nutritious. Thus, what may be seen as irresponsibility by professionals may be seen by the client as the most responsible action that could be taken under the circumstances.

In general most people see health as an important value. However they appear unable to see a relationship between their actions and the risk of poor health (Taylor 1991). In other words, people do not seem to

be very good at assessing their health risks. Thus, as suggested by Niven (1989), the role of prevention is to convince people that they are at risk of poor health. He proposes that by highlighting the similarities between those who are affected by disease and those who are not is a necessary step to encourage a change in negative health behaviours and thereby reduce health risks. Where negative health behaviours are unable to be eradicated, it is suggested that the risks can be reduced using preventative health strategies (Plant & Plant 1992). Using this minimization technique includes providing clean needles to intravenous drug users, promoting the use of condoms to encourage safe sex and ensuring safety equipment is used when indulging in dangerous sports. In general this provides people with the knowledge and skills to enable them to take control over certain aspects of their lives and reduce health risks even if the risks cannot be completely eliminated. These practices have been found to be more effective than the use of fear tactics. However, not everyone agrees with such practices, considering them to be too permissive and a soft option in dealing with major health issues.

The right of choice to practice 'risky' health behaviours also requires to be balanced against the effect of such behaviours on others. Examples of such behaviours include the effects of passive smoking, drinking and driving, and having unprotected sexual intercourse.

Health professionals have to respect the right of individuals to their own point of view and their right to choose, but health professionals also have a responsibility to help people become more self-aware, to gain a greater understanding of themselves, their attitude and their feelings and help them to clarify their values and attitudes (Ewles & Simnett 1992).

Two different categories of rights have been identified, option rights and welfare rights (Fromer 1981). Option rights are concerned with personal freedom; they do not entitle a person to total freedom but allow behaviour within certain limits. Sometimes the limits are clearly defined, as in setting certain standards of dress for particular occasions, or less clearly defined, when one claims the right to play loud music however, wherever and whenever one pleases (Rumbold 1993). As a result, the rights of individuals may overlap and conflict.

Welfare rights on the other hand are rights decreed by law. Legislation ensures the provision of resources to meet such basic needs as clean water, food and shelter. Other rights such as the right to vote, be protected and defended (Tschudin 1992) can also be claimed.

It is important that individuals are aware of and can recognize their rights. In doing so an individual becomes more aware of the rights of others and less likely to violate their rights. This is particularly important in nursing. The United Nations Declaration of Human Rights (1948) reflects basic human needs and includes the right to health via an adequate standard of living and to medical care.

Nevertheless, the right to health care and the concept of patient's rights is relatively new. The rights of patients and clients to either consent to or refuse the treatment or even choose an alternative method of treatment may result in conflict between the patient/client and the health professional (Rumbold 1993). This conflict is likely to arise, according to Rumbold, due to the health professionals 'perceived duty' to always act in such a way that will benefit the patient. This conflict may extend from the beginning to the end of life.

In this chapter it is not intended to discuss in detail the pros and cons of abortion or euthanasia but to consider briefly the rights of those involved. Despite the Abortion Act (1967) legalizing abortion, abortion remains a highly emotive topic touching the lives of all those involved. The rights of the fetus, the mother, the father and the nursing staff all need to be considered.

The fundamental ethical issue in abortion is at what point does a fetus become a person and at what point does that person have the rights to an existence (Mason & McCall Smith 1991). At one extreme there is the strict legal principle which states that 'no rights are vested in a human being until it has achieved a separate existence from its mother'. At the other there is a religious viewpoint that the fetus has and should be regarded as having its own life from the moment of conception.

The argument against abortion is based on two moral assumptions. First that it is wrong to kill a human being and secondly that the unborn child is a human being and therefore has the right to life of any human being. However, several arguments have been put forward to justify abortion in particular circumstances (Rumbold 1993).

First there are those who consider abortion should be available on demand. They argue that a woman has rights over her own body and therefore has the right to an abortion if she does not wish to proceed with the pregnancy. This may be of particular importance when the pregnancy has arisen as the result of rape or incest, where the quality of life of the mother is weighed against the quality of life of the unwanted infant.

The issue of comparing the value of the developing human life with another value is reflected in the 1967 Abortion Act, which gives grounds for abortion as follows:

1. The continuance of the pregnancy would either involve risk to the life of the pregnant woman or risk injury to the physical or mental health of any existing children of her family, greater than if the pregnancy was terminated.
2. There is substantial risk that if the child is born it will suffer such physical and mental abnormalities as to be severely handicapped.

Therefore as Rumbold argues, the values with which the life of the fetus is being compared are the life of the mother, the quality of life of siblings and the potential quality of life for the fetus. These, as Rumbold suggests, apart from the life of the mother, are somewhat unequal values, and pose the question, 'how realistic is it, to equate the value of life to the quality of life?'

The underlying ethical issue relating to abortion is when the unborn child becomes a person. Since 1992 (Still birth (Definition) Act) the 24th week of the pregnancy has been identified as the point at which the fetus can be presumed capable of an existence separate from the mother. Prior to this time the fetus may be legally destroyed or as in the case of abnormal fetuses, where the mother is at risk, until birth.

In so far as abortion is concerned, the father has no rights (Mason & McCall Smith 1991). This is the case irrespective of the reasons for the abortion and applies even in cases which do not relate to the mother's health. However once the child is born, it would appear, according to current practice, that the father would have a voice equal to that of the mother as to the future care of an abnormal infant. This care includes staying with the parents, foster care, or adoption. Theoretically the father could override the mother's objections despite the burden of caring. In practice, the future care of abnormal infants is based on the wishes of the parents in the assumption that marital harmony exists. However, Mason & McCall Smith argue that any possible clashes of interest would be minimized if the absolute importance of the infant's rights were defined by law.

Before considering the rights of the nurse and abortion, it may be helpful to consider the rights of the nurse in more general terms.

As has already been discussed, two different types of rights exist, option rights and welfare rights. As members of society, nurses are entitled to these same rights as everyone else. However these rights are not unlimited. Certain constraints exist which prevent individuals exercising personal rights because they impinge on the rights of others or because there is a duty to act in a particular way.

When one becomes a nurse, one also accepts the duties associated with being a nurse (Rumbold 1993). These duties include ensuring patients exercise their rights to health care and that the patient comes to no harm. These two duties may limit the rights of the nurse as an individual.

However, there may be occasions when in order to carry out these 'nursing duties' the nurse will be justified in exercising her personal rights, such as the right to act in accordance with her conscience. In doing so, this may conflict with her duty to her employer. Tschudin (1992) defines conscience 'as a state of moral awareness, a compass directing ones behaviour according to the moral fitness of things'.

As discussed in an earlier section, values and beliefs are influenced by several factors, a sense of what is right and wrong being instilled by parental, cultural and religious influences. Therefore in developing a conscience an individual is aware of behaviours which are either acceptable or unacceptable according to his/her own values and beliefs. In making an appeal to conscience, the individual claims that to behave in a particular way would be a betrayal of his/her personal values and beliefs (Rumbold 1993).

Freedom of thought, conscience and religion and the freedom of opinion and expression are, according to the Universal Declaration of Human Rights (1948), rights to which all people have an entitlement. Therefore, nurses have the right to 'appeal to conscience', to refuse to behave in any way that may infringe their personal freedom of belief and expression.

The right to make a conscientious objection is also recognized in clause eight of the UKCC Code of Professional Conduct (UKCC 1992). This states: 'as a registered nurse, midwife or health visitor, you must report to an appropriate person or authority, at the earliest possible time, any conscientious objections which may be relevant to your professional practice'.

Having discussed the rights of the nurse in general terms let us now consider how they may be applied to the practice of abortion.

Research shows that many nurses due to their religious beliefs hold a conscientious objection towards abortion. The 1967 Abortion Act allows nurses to be excused from participation in abortion procedures if they hold such an objection. However, it is worth noting that the 'conscientious clause' cannot be invoked if the treatment is directed towards the saving of life or of preventing grave permanent injury to the life of the mother (Mason & McCall Smith 1991).

Nurses also have a duty to care for a woman prior to and after the abortion procedures. There are many reasons why a woman decides to have an abortion, therefore nurses have to be particularly sensitive to the feelings of the patient during this time. Good psychological care of the patient before, during and after the procedure cannot be overemphasized as it plays an important part in the patient's recovery.

Nurses may also be called upon to counsel patients and help them decide whether to continue with the pregnancy or have an abortion. It is important that the nurse does not present a biased point of view, but presents information in such a way that she helps the woman understand the implications of abortion and the varying options open to her. In doing so the nurse enables the patient to make the decision that is right for her.

The two most important events in life are birth and death. In the western world death is frequently portrayed by the media as either a dramatic interruption of life or as a lengthy battle fought and lost. Occasionally death may be regarded as appropriate, for example when the person is elderly and has led a full and happy life, but for many, death is perceived as an unnatural intrusion into life rather than a stage along the 'life–death continuum' (Hinchliff 1989). Hinchliff suggests that for some the continuum may be short, for others long, encompassing every stage of man's development from childhood through to old age.

Medical technology has played a major part in influencing the current concept of death. Ludovic Kennedy (1990) argues that whilst modern medicine has prolonged life resulting in a lengthy and satisfying life for some, it has also led to prolonged and miserable dying for others. This is considered to be one of the main factors behind the hospice movement, where one of the aims is to achieve effective control over physical and mental pain to enable the patient to die a dignified death. Others attempt to control their dying by seeking legislation which allows them the right to choose freely and lawfully the time, the method and place of death. However, although suicide has been legal in Scotland for some considerable time (in England since 1961), helping someone to end his life is not.

Given the choice most people would choose to die peacefully with dignity in preference to dying suddenly or suffering a lingering painful death. This easy or gentle death is the literal meaning of **euthanasia**. The word **euthanasia** being derived from the Greek words *eu* and *thanatos* meaning a 'good death'.

Today, euthanasia is more likely to be understood to mean 'the bringing about of a good death', where

Box 2.1   Text of the Voluntary Euthanasia Society of Scotland Living Will (Advance Directive)

TO MY FAMILY, MY PHYSICIAN AND MY SOLICITOR

This declaration is made by me ....
(Full name and address)

at a time when I am of sound mind and after careful consideration

I, the said .... in the event of my being unable to take part in decisions concerning my medical care due to my physical or mental incapacity, and in the event that I develop one or more of the medical conditions listed in clause (3) below and in the event that two independent physicians conclude that there is no reasonable prospect of my making a substantial recovery, do hereby DECLARE that my wishes are as follows, VIZ:-

(1) I request that my life should not be sustained by artificial means such as: life support systems, intravenous fluids and/or drugs, tube feeding.

(2) I request that distressing symptoms caused either by illness or by lack of food or fluid should be controlled by appropriate sedatative treatment, even though such treatment may have incidental and secondary effect of shortening my life.

(3) The said medical conditions are:-
1. Severe and lasting brain damage sustained as a result of an accident or injury.
2. Advanced disseminated malignant disease.
3. Advanced degenerative disease of the nervous and/or muscular systems with severe limitations of independent mobility, and no satisfactory response to treatment.
4. Stroke with extensive persisting paralysis.
5. Pre-senile, senile or Alzheimer type dementia.
6. Other conditions of comparable gravity.

(4) I request that, in the event of my becoming incapable of giving or withholding consent to any medical treatment or procedures proposed to me, the Court of Session to be petitioned to appoint as my tutor the following person:-

\ ....
whom failing:-

: ....

Whom failing: such other person may be deemed by the court to be a fit person. It is my specific request that in exercising his or her powers to consent or withhold consent on my behalf to any medical treatment or procedures, my tutor shall take into account, in any determination of what is in my best interests, the requests which I solemnly make in clauses (1) and (2) of this document.

And I declare that I hereby absolve my medical attendants of all real liability arising from action taken in response to and in terms of this declaration.

I reserve the right to revoke this determination at any time, before witnesses, in writing or orally.

: ....
(Signature)   (Town/Place)   (Day/Month/Year)

(If you write above this signature "adopted as holograph" this under Scottish Law authenticates this document without the necessity of witnesses to your signature.)

NB: This document has been devised in accordance with the Law of Scotland.
Those resident in England can obtain a form from the V.E.S London.
Those resident elsewhere should seek local advice.

Issued by: Voluntary Euthanasia Society of Scotland
17, Hart Street
Edinburgh
EH1 3RN.

one person brings about the death of another who wishes to die. This is often referred to as mercy killing, an illegal act. Four types of euthanasia have been identified. Passive, active, voluntary and involuntary:

- *Passive euthanasia* is allowing someone to die by passive means, either by withholding or withdrawing life-sustaining treatment.
- *Active euthanasia* actively causes death through a direct action such as administering a lethal injection to end a person's life.
- *Voluntary euthanasia* is when an individual freely gives consent to his death and decides when and how to end life. It is worth noting that the person does not have to be competent to assert the wish to die.
- *Involuntary euthanasia* occurs when the individual is incompetent to make this decision and others make it for him. It is argued that certain medical practices such as giving large doses of pain-killing drugs which eventually cause the patient's death or the withholding of life-sustaining treatments to comatosed patients could come into this category.

As discussed earlier, for most people the preference would be to die with dignity rather than suffer a lingering death. However difficulties may arise due to a conflict of values and rights between those of the patient and doctor. Whereas the patient may not wish life to be prolonged under certain circumstances, for example, severe and lasting brain damage as the result of an accident, the doctor may feel bound by his professional code to preserve life and this may take precedence over the rights and values of the patient.

In an attempt to counteract this situation, many people, whilst in good health and spirits, have provided written instructions in the form of a **living will** or **advance declaration** (Box 2.1) which reflects their certain wishes regarding treatment choices if and when they become incapable of making or communicating a decision (VESS 1993).

The living will does not provide authorization for active euthanasia, which is a criminal offence, but clear guidelines regarding treatment should the person develop certain irreversible conditions from which no recovery would be expected. It does not cover circumstances other than those described. The text of the Voluntary Euthanasia Society of Scotland (VESS) Living Will (Advance Directive) is given in Box 2.1.

On completion of the document persons are advised to place a copy with someone whom they trust. This may be a solicitor, GP, medical consultant, friend or relative. They are further advised to carry a Living Will Alert Card, to inform the person finding it that a living will has been signed and where it may be found (Fig. 2.1). To alert medical and nursing personnel that a patient's medical notes/records contain a living will document, a living will sticker is available which can be attached to the patient's notes/records (Fig. 2.2).

Provision has also been made under both Scottish and English Law that if a person is incapable of making his/her wishes known, for example, if the patient is comatosed or mentally incapacitated, then a proxy, usually a friend, relative or lawyer, will bring notice of the document to the attention of the doctor concerned. This action should result in treatment being carried out in accordance with the wishes expressed in the advance directive. If this does not occur then legal proceedings on behalf of the patient can be implemented. The British Medical Association (1993) has said that a valid advance directive should be accorded the same weight as any other valid expression of a competent patient's wishes. However, it is worth noting, that under the present law, although living wills are legal there is no penalty for ignoring them.

VESS suggests that advance directives should be updated at 5-year intervals to verify that no change of mind has taken place since the initial completion of the document. However, should the person change his mind then the declaration can be revoked at any time. This can be done by destroying the document or by stating orally or in writing that the document no longer represents the persons wishes.

Allowing someone to die does not mean that the patient is abandoned without care. Rather as Henderson (1966) suggests where recovery is not possible then the function of the nurse is to assist the patient towards a peaceful death.

Individual rights have been further identified in the Patient's Charter (DOH 1991), in particular these rights as they apply to children and persons suffering from mental handicap (learning difficulties).

As a general rule, medical treatment, even that of a minor nature, should not be carried out unless the doctor has received the patient's consent. However, when a patient attends his GP or hospital doctor it is assumed the patient is giving his/her consent to examination and treatment. Nevertheless the patient is entitled to be given an accurate and understandable explanation of the diagnosis, its implications, what treatment is available and what it may involve.

The patient is also entitled, as far as it is practical, to be involved in making decisions about his/her care

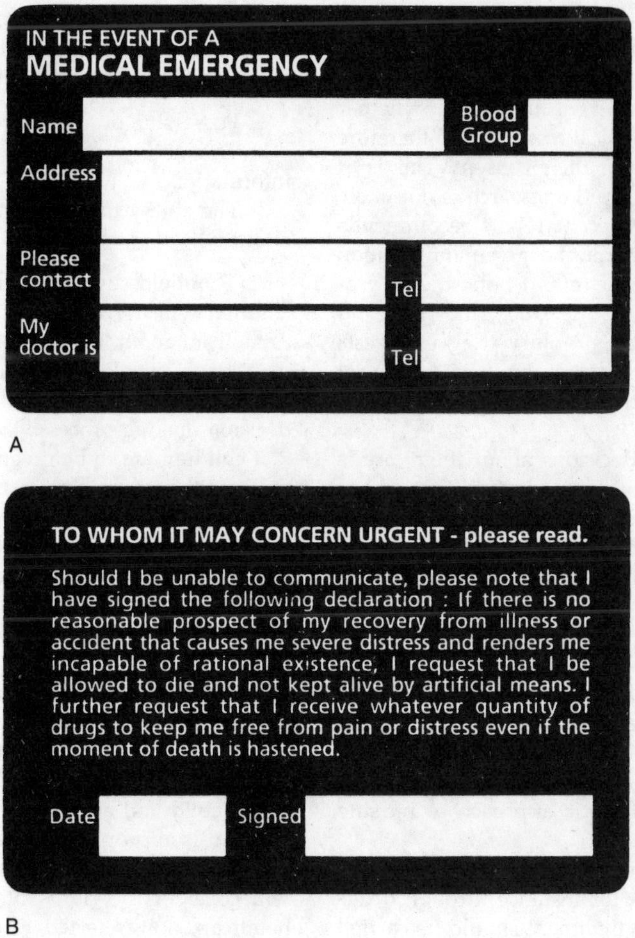

IN THE EVENT OF A
MEDICAL EMERGENCY

Name _____   Blood Group ___

Address _____

Please contact _____   Tel _____

My doctor is _____   Tel _____

A

TO WHOM IT MAY CONCERN URGENT - please read.

Should I be unable to communicate, please note that I have signed the following declaration : If there is no reasonable prospect of my recovery from illness or accident that causes me severe distress and renders me incapable of rational existence, I request that I be allowed to die and not kept alive by artificial means. I further request that I receive whatever quantity of drugs to keep me free from pain or distress even if the moment of death is hastened.

Date _____   Signed _____

B

Fig. 2.1 Living Will Alert Card

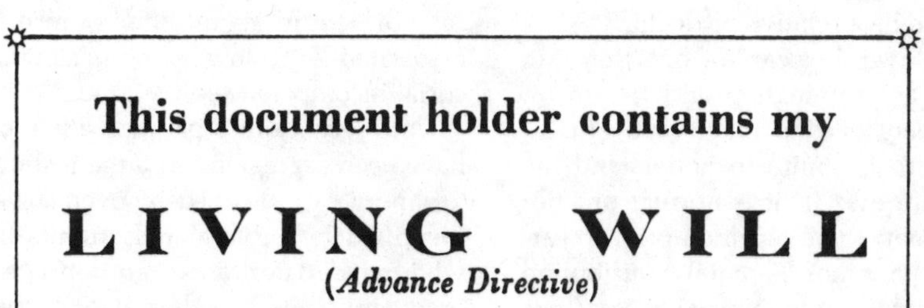

This document holder contains my

LIVING WILL
(Advance Directive)

In the event that I am incapacitated in any way please read the enclosed document concerning my health care

Fig. 2.2 Living Will medical records sticker

and this includes, as we have already discussed, the right to give or withold his consent to medical treatment.

Patients also have the right to decide whether or not to participate in medical research and therefore should always be asked for their consent. This is of particular importance where the research is not likely to benefit the patient. A recent report recommends that research subjects should be given information sheets which are clear, concise and honest, and provide information regarding the study, the risks and any insurance cover in case of injury. It also suggests the subject should be informed about any financial benefits to the researcher, subject or institution (Neuberger 1992).

Involving patients in decisions about their care is not only a requirement for the medical profession but for all health care providers within the NHS. Whereas previously nursing care reflected a medical approach based on a patient's clinical diagnosis and task allocation, such as bathing, dressings and medications, current nursing practice is person centred and based on individual patient's needs and wants. This approach to nursing care is known as the systematic approach and is concerned with helping patients and clients meet their needs through a process of assessment, planning, implementation and evaluation. (Ch. 3 discusses the systematic approach to nursing care in detail.)

Where patients are unable to give consent due to a temporary incapability, for instance through drugs or alcohol, only essential treatment should be carried out by the doctor. Where a person is permanently incapacitated then a legal guardian or someone appointed by a court of law is necessary to give consent. This person is likely to be a relative or doctor.

When children are over 16 years of age they can validly give consent to examination and treatment. Under the age of 16 years it is dependent on the maturity of the child and their ability to understand the issues involved. Within the UK it is normal practice for the consent of parents to be obtained prior to carrying out treatment to a minor. Parental contribution must be asked for before any medical research is carried out on a child under 16 years of age. However, where the life of a child may be endangered by parental refusal of consent to treatment, such procedures may be carried out in the face of parental objections.

By using a systematic approach to nursing care the child is identified as a person in his/her own right and therefore should be afforded the rights of any patient to participate in making decisions about their own care.

Rumbold (1993) cites three attributes as identified in The Presidents Commission (1982) as being necessary in order to make decisions:

1. Possession of a set of values and goals.
2. The ability to communicate and understand information.
3. The ability to reason and deliberate about one's choice.

As Rumbold suggests, although infants and young children will not possess such attributes, some children, from about 7 years of age, the age of reasoning, may have developed these attributes to a degree to which they could and should be involved in the decision-making process.

If children are to be given the same rights as other patients then they have a need to be informed in a manner which will enhance their understanding of their condition, its treatment and consequences.

Rumbold proposes that a 'partnership model' as described by Bandman & Bandman (1990), which involves the nurse, parents and child as equal partners in decision making, should be adopted. This model would appear to be appropriate as whilst it enables the parent to retain some control, it also permits the child to develop moral values and the ability to reason. It also allows the nurse to act in the best interests of the child and assume the role of patient advocate where it is appropriate to do so.

To conclude our discussion on patients' rights, we will consider the rights of individuals with mental handicap, now referred to as persons with learning disability. People with a learning disability share similar needs, wants and problems with other individuals within the society in which they live. The condition may present in many different forms but it is always associated with slow learning, slow development and social incompetence.

Until recent times people with a learning disability have been segregated in large institutions away from 'ordinary people'. Their overall needs have been identified by professionals from varying disciplines who have determined appropriate forms of care. Frequently this care has denied the individual the opportunity to make choices about even very basic needs and in so doing has inhibited personal decision making (Rumbold 1993).

However, the acknowledgement of patients' rights has resulted in a growing concern for the rights of people with learning disabilities and their entitlement to live their lives within mainstream society. This has led to a provision of a variety of statutory and voluntary services to enable these individuals to live within the community, avoid institutional care and transfer, where appropriate and in the person's best interests, to a community setting.

It is now recognized that many people with a learning disability can develop the ability and have the right, to make decisions about their own lives. The systematic approach to nursing care has enabled nurses to care for people as individuals. Consequently the risk of depersonalization has been reduced and people with a learning disability are empowered to exercise their rights. The role of the nurse must be to provide individuals with information in terminology which they can understand, help them develop skills to make choices about activities of living and act as an advocate on their behalf to ensure their choices are respected.

Rumbold (1993) argues that having created autonomy, it is then important that it is respected. This may mean that health professionals may not always agree with the decisions being made. However, even people who are considered to be capable of rational thought sometimes make irrational decisions and despite attempts that might be made to change their minds their decisions must be ultimately accepted.

That same degree of freedom must therefore be afforded to those who may be less capable, provided it is neither seriously harmful to themselves or others. As ordinary members of society, people with learning difficulties are entitled to the rights of ordinary people. (Ch. 7 discusses in detail care implications for disorders of learning.)

LIFE TRANSITIONS

Human development

Development has been described as a series of episodes or periods of equilibrium with periods of disequilibrium in between – a series of stages and transitions brought about by continuing change. These changes occur throughout life and may be internal and external, the individual acquires new cognitive skills, moves job, gets married, has children, becomes ill and retires.

Each change requires the individual to adopt new information and a new set of circumstances. At certain times there is a need for greater adaptation to accumulating change, these times seeming to occur when the individual moves from one role to another as from childhood to adolescence, from young adult to middle age and subsequently into old age.

These changes have been variously described as 'crisis points', 'opportunities for significant growth'

and 'a point of passage from one stage to the next' (Sheehy 1976).

Adolescence

Although adolescence and puberty are commonly seen as synonymous, they are in fact quite different things. Both mark the transition from childhood to adulthood but each is a different part of the process.

Adolescence is a term given to an indefinite period of development in which psychological and social changes occur. It has no observable beginning or end and some of the problems arising from adjustments which have to be made during adolescence may take years to resolve. However it is generally accepted that this phase commences around 12 years of age and ends around 22 years of age.

In the industrialized western world, adolescence is a stage which marks the maturing individual's search for identity. The individual being no longer a child but not yet a man/woman.

Puberty, on the other hand, is a biological event which marks the physiological onset of adulthood. It has distinct observable stages and is usually considered to date from the onset of menstruation in girls and the emergence of pubic hair in boys. However these are only two small observable changes in what is a complex process involving many bodily functions.

Physical development Quite dramatic physical changes occur during adolescence due to hormonal activity (refer to Ch. 6, Care Implications of Disorders of the Endocrine System, for a full discussion on hormonal functioning).

These changes not only affect the reproductive system and secondary sex characteristics but also the cardiovascular and respiratory system. They also promote growth of bone and muscle which leads to the 'growth spurt', a term usually taken to refer to the acceleration rate in height and weight which takes place in early adolescence. This radical change in body size and shape frequently results in a period of clumsiness as the individual attempts to adapt to these changes.

The body changes not only in shape and size but also in function – a girl's first period or a boy's first ejaculation have to be understood. Theoretically, the adolescent is capable of producing offspring.

However, a wide variation exists between individuals when these changes begin and end. For girls the menarche can start between the age of 9 and 17 years. For boys sexual maturation may vary between 13 and 17 years.

Therefore education within the home and school environment, relating to 'what is happening', is essential if young adolescents are to be helped to cope with the myriad of changes affecting them during this time.

The effect such physical changes have upon identity is important. The formation of identity is not only dependent on being different from others, but also a sense of self, consistency and a firm knowledge of how one appears to the rest of the world (Coleman 1980). It is therefore not surprising that as the adolescent's physical characteristics continue to change during this period, so does his/her self-image.

It is suggested that one of the ways adolescents cope with this constant change is through their attachment to particular sports stars or pop groups on which they model their behaviour and appearance (Groenman et al 1992). This practice enables the young adolescent to pronounce, at least outwardly, who they are and provides a constancy at a time when physical appearance is of critical importance for both the individual's self-esteem and popularity.

Social and emotional development As the adolescent (for simplicity, the male gender is used) moves from childhood into adulthood he establishes himself as an individual separate from the family.

During this transitionary phase he may be beset with doubts and uncertainties regarding his ability to cope with the demands of maturity. Because he is unable to organize his experiences, thoughts and feelings into any kind of consistent pattern, his behaviour alternates between that of childhood dependence and outright rebellion.

It is this unpredictability of his behaviour that many parents find so frustrating to cope with. However both parents and society in general frequently add to the adolescent's confused status by their ambiguous expectations of what is acceptable behaviour during this period. At times a child-like obedience is demanded, at others the self-confidence and independence of an adult.

Therefore in search of certainty and security and feeling no longer able to rely on the wisdom of adults in general, the adolescent turns to those in a similar situation to himself – his peer group.

However it is suggested that since other members of the group are in a similar confused state as to their identity the group itself becomes all powerful. An outcome of this is that the group exerts even more pressure upon the group members than does most family groups. Coleman (1980) argues that peer group influences are only harmful when family influences are absent, and that in general parents and friends act together as mutually reinforcing agents of socialization. Peer groups therefore have an important role to play in enabling adolescents to learn new social skills.

Sexual maturation forms the physiological background to many social and emotional changes which occur during the early adolescent years. Sexual behaviour is associated with a multitude of worries and anxieties. The adolescent has to decide what his sexual behaviour will be.

Many changes have taken place over the last 30 years in the western world regarding sexual activity. These changes and the lack of guidance as to what may be regarded as appropriate behaviour can cause great conflict to teenagers when faced with making such decisions. Because adolescents can be vulnerable to group pressures they may be pushed into a course of action without having the opportunity to work out the consequences.

Despite an increase in knowledge about contraception amongst teenagers, current statistics show a rise in unplanned pregnancies and abortions and may reflect this conflict.

However as discussed previously, knowledge and behaviour are not necessarily consistent with one another. This has been shown to be true regarding AIDS. Plant & Plant (1992) state that AIDS has had a limited impact on people's behaviour and that amongst heterosexual teenagers and adolescents unprotected sex remains the norm. They identify a strong resistance to safe sex and condom use, subsequently the potential for widespread HIV is high amongst this group within the population. These facts suggest that sex education programmes should be preparing young people for potentially troublesome areas of their future and should be built into the general education programme to avoid such crises and allow young people to take more control of their lives (Coleman 1980).

Cognitive development During adolescence because of a combination of both physiological and environmental factors important advances are made in cognitive functioning. According to the Swiss psychologist Jean Piaget, a qualitative change in the nature of mental ability should be expected around puberty. At this point the adolescent has the potential to achieve formal operational thought. In other words, the adolescent is less restricted by given data – the concrete reality. He has the ability to theorize and appreciate a range of possibilities and future events. He is capable of abstract thinking.

These new intellectual powers enable the adolescent to think critically about previously held beliefs and values. This may result in him challenging his parents' views on life in general, their status on morality, the country's policies and the current global situation. He may view the world as being very unfair, and full of injustices. He has a burning desire to put things right. During this adolescent phase adolescents may become strongly influenced by the ideals of particular political and religious groups. Values which are formed at this time will influence the adolescent's decision making, the results of which may affect his future adult life. Therefore it is important that during this period the adolescent is provided with support and guidance from parents, teachers and significant others regarding decisions affecting careers, vocations and political or religious commitments.

Young adulthood: 20–40 years

The entry into adulthood is dependent on varying cultural norms. For some assuming the responsibilities and privileges of the adult may be in their early teens, for others not until their thirties. In British society the age of 18 years confers certain legal adult status, permission to marry (16 in Scotland) and the right to vote. For many it is the end of secondary education and the start of careers, the power to earn their own money. The beginning of independence.

This stage has been described as a time for 'pulling up roots', a time of detachment from the family both mentally and physically, a time for beginning the search for personal identity.

It is through a consideration of the ramifications of full independence such as getting a job, forming a stable relationship, starting a family that force the adolescent into confronting the problem of identity. During this stage there is little change in cognitive and physical development but major changes in social interaction and roles. The period is characterized by the major tasks of loving and working.

Physical development Within the first phase of this period, 20–30 years, the young adult reaches the peak of physical development and is frequently regarded as being at the 'apex of physical attractiveness'. The skin is unwrinkled, muscles are supple, joints are strong and flexible and the mind is quick and alert. Energy appears inexhaustible. The young adult presents 'a picture of health'.

Because growth is complete nutritional intake should both maintain health and body weight. Good dietary management and other positive health behaviours practised during this time can prevent body changes to the cardiovascular system which may result in serious disease at a later stage in life. Therefore

health promotion for this particular group should be clearly identified as an integral part of nursing practice.

After 30 in the second phase of this period, a gradual decline begins. There is an increase in fatty tissue and maintaining a stable weight becomes more difficult. Both movements and reactions become slower and it takes longer to recover from physical exertions.

Sexual changes also occur during this period. Males reach their highest sexual capacity at about 20 years of age, whereas females reach it around 25 years. From 25 years onwards the potential for childbearing very slowly declines. After the age of 35 years the possibility of a woman having a handicapped child increases. These facts have an important influence on couples and their decisions about when and if to start a family.

Appearance is also affected by signs of ageing. Both men and women may find their first grey hairs and premature hair loss may affect men under the age of 40 years. Laughter lines (wrinkles) occur around the eyes and skin begins to lose its suppleness. After the age of 35 the memory becomes less reliable and in general there is an increase in health problems. Aches and pains become more evident and the risk of serious illness increases. These changes which indicate approaching middle age cause anxiety in some individuals.

Cognitive development As with physical development, cognitive development reaches its peak in the first phase of young adulthood. Most young adults are capable of abstract thought, memory functions at an optimal level, thinking is carried out quickly and information is stored in an efficient manner.

The young adult is primarily involved in developing and applying the required practical and professional skills to ensure a satisfying adult life. Everyday thinking becomes more systematic, decisive and task directed.

In general young adults are full of energy, ambitious and forward looking. However, for some, issues of adulthood, such as conflicts about identity, dependence and independence delay full adulthood being reached as they continue to experience periods of indecision, rebellion and relative passivity in their lives.

After 30 there is a slowing down of the thought processes, memory gradually dims and learning new things becomes more difficult. However, although the thought processes may no longer be at their peak, any deficit can be compensated for by experience. These experiences affect the conflict of thought. Thoughts become deeper and each new experience influences personality development and affects the individual's thought perceptions.

As discussed earlier in the chapter, experiences affect value systems and the young adult learns how to deal with society's apparent or actual conflicting attitudes. He/she also learns respect for others as well as him/herself. During this stage of development individuals frequently spend a great deal of time and thought coming to terms with personal and social ethical issues.

Social development Two major tasks confront the young adult during this stage – committing themselves to an occupation and forming an intimate relationship.

In today's society work is still seen as a necessary requirement for young adults. Employment provides not only financial benefits but a certain status within society. Work also provides the individual with a vehicle to develop his/her talents and skills. In turn this can boost self-confidence and self-esteem.

In the late twentieth century there is increasing evidence of role and career reversal between the sexes. A growing number of women are entering what was formerly seen as male occupations, for example engineering, and men entering customary female occupations like nursing.

Although the range of job opportunities is widening for young adults, the high unemployment situation which exists at present denies many young people the possibility of achieving their life ambitions. Research findings indicate that unemployment is one of several important contributory factors associated with young people and risk-taking behaviours like alcohol and drug abuse (Plant & Plant 1992). For some young people such behaviour may be used as an escape from the trauma of unemployment. The other major task facing young adults during this period is the development of a long-term relationship. Erikson describes the conflict of young adulthood as 'intimacy versus isolation'.

To develop and maintain a personal relationship during adult life an individual must be able to satisfy the needs of another and be satisfied by them. This involves mutual understanding, respecting the other as an individual and not just as an extension of one's own needs and desires.

Intimacy is therefore about deep personal caring and sharing. Studies show that an intimate relationship has a positive contribution to make to an individual's physical and emotional health status. People who are unable to establish satisfactory relationships because of an inability to share or who are afraid of being emotionally hurt, risk self-imposed isolation.

During this period many young adults marry or form other types of intimate relationships. The options now available are greater in this decade than ever before. Cohabitation has become quite commonplace. For some it acts as a trial marriage with the 'knot being tied' around the birth of the first child. For others it is of a much longer duration, in keeping with any legalized relationship. Increasingly couples are choosing to have smaller families or no family at all.

Although the intimacy desired by young adults is normally a love relationship encompassing a sexual element, it is not exclusively so.

According to Erikson, intimacy need not be of a physical or sexual nature but involves the union of two identities; for example an emotional commitment between two adults, as in the relationship between mentor and protegee or tutor and student. Friendships are of particular importance during this period. The basic need is for 'closeness and real relatedness with another person' and this can be found in both heterosexual and homosexual relationships.

The thirties brings further change to men and women. The middle of the thirties is literally the midpart of life – the deadline decade. It is a time for major investments in personal, occupational and social aspects of life. New choices may cause turmoil and crisis. Divorce is at its highest at this time.

Women are aware of this inner cross-roads sooner than men. Whatever life patterns women have followed they may see it as their 'last chance'. A chance to review all the options that have been set aside and those that ageing and biology will end in the foreseeable future. For many women it is an exhilarating time, a time for self-development and self-actualization.

Men too feel the 'push' in their mid thirties. It brings about a burst of speed in an attempt to achieve success in the career race. There is a need to be recognized; to be his own man.

Whatever man has achieved he is unhappy ... 'Is that all there is?' He is concerned at how little value may be placed on his achievements. He may depart from life-long practices, including marriage, take a second career or he may become self-destructive. He may also allow his suppressed nurturing feelings emerge and become more caring.

However the crisis is resolved it leads to middle age.

The older adult 40–60 years

From 40 to 60 years has become an accepted period associated with middle life. It is a time when significant changes occur within the three main component parts of human development. Despite these changes for many men and women, middle age is a particularly peaceful time. According to Erikson it is a time which involves generativity, creativity and productivity in family life and career.

Physical development The physical changes which began in the thirties now become more obvious. Mobility and strength decrease, body fat is redistributed and may increase (middle age spread). There is a decline in eyesight and hearing, hair continues to grey and baldness, particularly amongst men, increases. Women cease to menstruate and men's sexual potency diminishes. There is also a decline in tasks which require short-term memory and speed.

However, as with changes that occur during adolescence, these changes do not all occur at the same time nor do they affect everyone at the same age. They may vary considerably due to the overall health status of the individual and are associated with general life-style, diet, exercise, stress, genetic factors and freedom from disease or disabilities. A great deal of time, effort and money is spent in the UK in an attempt to stop the ageing process or hide the physical effects of the ageing.

The main changes occur for females with the onset of the menopause and the cessation of reproductive abilities. It is considered that the reduction in oestrogen levels contributes to women becoming more assertive and aggressive at this time. However, it also coincides with the completion of childbearing and as children leave home the caring and nurturing qualities developed for that role are less in demand.

Many myths are associated with the menopause and many can be dispelled. The majority of women are in good health during this period, are sexually active and because of the freedom from pregnancy find sex more enjoyable. Loss of childbearing capacity does not appear to be a major trauma for most women.

For men the climacteric is more likely to be psychologically induced, although there is a reduction in testosterone and in sperm count. This reduction in testosterone may contribute to the more nurturing and affiliative behaviour exhibited by men during this period. However, it is more likely that, as with women, the demands associated with earlier adult life to achieve, particularly in the world of work, have changed, enabling those other qualities to be expressed.

Cognitive development It has been accepted that the ability to learn is influenced by both inherited and accumulated experience and knowledge. Therefore it is important not to see the elderly as a homogeneous group but to be aware of the great variability that exists within the group. However, in general there is little decline in cognitive capacity during this period, any changes which do occur are very slow.

Despite the fact that learning new information and skills takes longer at this stage of development, the motivation to learn is high. Particularly in the early phase of this stage, in order to advance their careers, many individuals have to develop new skills, for example administrative or teaching skills, or they may have to adapt existing skills to new practices. This is also relevant for individuals who are starting a second career either from choice or necessity.

Increasing numbers of women and to a lesser extent men return to education at a further or higher educational level with a view to widening their options in the job market. Studies show they frequently achieve higher grades than younger students. During this period the older adult often identifies this time as an opportunity to develop their recreational activities to the full. This may involve them in pursuing a wide range of activities such as art, music or personal interest projects within higher education establishments, thereby demonstrating that people have the potential for continuing development across their life-span.

Social development For many people the middle years are the most productive years. In general men in their forties are often at the peak of their careers. Because the demands to achieve have lessened they may become a mentor to a junior colleague or become involved in civic and social activities assuming a position of responsibility.

During this period as children leave home the middle aged may become more involved in the care of their parents. As parents begin to decline there is a change in the relationship – a filial maturity – a psychologically healthy relationship most adult children develop with their ageing parents. The adult child becomes more dependable to the needs of the parent.

This situation may be complicated by the fact that many women return to work at this time due to a reduction in their domestic responsibilities as their children leave home. The change in the adult, child, parent relationship may place the woman back into the caring role she has recently abdicated. A refilling of the empty nest.

Common health problems affecting this age group include heart disease, cancer, diabetes and visual disorders. It is therefore important to promote health by attending to diet, exercise, safety measures, rest and relaxation and ensuring prompt treatment of disease symptoms.

However, as already indicated, this is a more tranquil period for many middle-aged adults, particularly couples who find high levels of satisfaction within their marriage and work in this postparental period.

Ageing

The ageing process may be said to begin from the moment of birth. However, the decline in physical and psychological functioning does not occur until the early twenties and more noticeable changes do not occur until middle and old age. Geographical and individual differences cause a wide variation in the rate of ageing. The process of ageing may be accelerated in countries where poverty, disease and hunger is rife, whereas at an individual level, general lifestyle, including smoking, drinking and exercise habits, are major contributory factors.

Changes in old age fall into three main categories: physical, social and cognitive.

Physical changes

Physical changes occur as the body becomes unable to successfully maintain homeostasis. In general changes occur within all the body systems. As ageing progresses, changes in appearance become more obvious. The skin becomes thinner and drier, eventually developing a parchment-like quality due to a decrease in subcutaneous fat. There is a continuance of hair loss amongst men and some women may also be affected after the menopause because of hormonal changes.

Hormonal changes also contribute towards changes in the skeletal system. Bones become more brittle (decalcification), there is a degeneration of cartilage around weight-bearing joints and atrophy of intervertebral discs. The pressing together of the vertebrae results in a loss of height and this is further exacerbated by a tendency of the elderly to stoop. Muscles gradually become weaker and flabby, thereby contributing towards a general appearance of weight loss and frailty. However good nutrition and exercise may delay these changes whilst the prophylactic use of hormone replacement therapy (HRT) can aid in the prevention of osteoporosis (brittle bones).

A lessened elasticity of lung tissue leads to decreased vital capacity, this makes expectoration more difficult and dyspnoea (difficulty in breathing) on exertion. These conditions are further exacerbated if the individual smokes. There are also changes in the special senses. Although most older people need reading glasses, the loss of hearing is more prevalent than the loss of sight. The nervous system may also undergo changes, brain weight decreases and neurones are lost and not replaced, co-ordination, balance and temperature control becomes less efficient. Subsequently there is a danger of accidents, a slower response to physical and mental stimuli, an increased risk of hypothermia. However the basic assumption that intelligence and intellect declines at this time is unfounded.

Changes to the cardiovascular system also take place; a narrowing or obstruction of the arteries (atherosclerosis) is caused by a degeneration of the lining of the arteries which affects the action of the heart. Cardiovascular disease is the most life-threatening condition affecting the elderly. However the degree of severity varies from person to person. Although genetic factors are a major contributory influence, factors which accelerate the condition include obesity, high blood pressure, smoking, excess saturated fats in the diet, lack of exercise and stress.

Changes in the digestive tract may ultimately affect absorption of nutrients and lead to subclinical malnutrition. Therefore attention needs to be paid to any alteration in both the appetite and elimination habits of the older person and prompt investigations carried out.

A decrease in hormonal levels does not necessarily bring about a lack of interest in sexual activity or intimacy. Men have the capacity to produce children well into their late years. Women, although unable to produce children, frequently retain a sexual interest. It is important for nurses to appreciate that older persons are still sexual beings.

The main gender differences at this time are that women live longer than men. This difference is considered to be due to differences in life-styles rather than any biological factors. Recent information related to heart disease and cancer rates in women support this theory, as the number of women who work and smoke increase so have their disease rates.

Social changes

Several social changes occur in old age. Many older people have been found to go through a process of disengagement. Some aspects may be seen as social in nature due to changes in employment, for example retirement reduces activity and social contact. Therefore friendships are particularly important at this time. Other changes may include physical disabilities, reduction in income, death of acquaintances and may be considered unavoidable.

Psychological disengagement however is concerned with the individual becoming less concerned and involved with others and more preoccupied with himself. This form of disengagement is considered to occur before social disengagement.

Disengagement may also be seen as a disattachment process, a series of disengagements occurring throughout life.

Whilst it is true that as a group older people may become introverted and disengaged, many maintain active involvement in many roles and find satisfaction in them. Others may gradually disengage from various active roles and show satisfaction in a more introspective and less involved life-style. Still others may show dissatisfaction with disengagement. They may involve people who are involuntarily disengaged through the death of a partner or who would have preferred to go on working rather than retire.

In old age sex roles continue to blend and frequently greater harmony and sharing of interests and pursuits are achieved. Grandparents show both nurturing and caring qualities towards the young.

Increasingly the older person becomes more dependent on family members and society for care in declining years. However, many elderly remain fiercely independent and continue to live in their own homes, many live alone, and exercise the right to do so.

The acceptance of death is the final phase of disengagement and of resolving the ego integrity versus despair crisis through an adaptation to the ageing process.

Cognitive changes

Cognitive decline is not a necessary consequence of ageing but is inextricably linked to the individual's interaction with their social and historical circumstances. Since such interaction can vary, so can the pattern of development. This model of development has been called the **plasticity model** and shows that people have the potential for continuing development across their life-span. Intellectual stimulation has been shown to promote and maintain alertness (Tight 1983).

It is therefore important to be aware of the variability that exists between individuals. In youth, people in general perform better on tasks which require insight, short-term memorization and complex interactions. As they grow older any slowing down of the thought process is compensated for by their problem-solving ability gained from life experiences.

Acute illness

It is likely there are as many ways to define illness as there are ways to define health. As discussed in Chapter 1, health is frequently defined as the opposite of illness. However, just because an individual is not in possession of full health does not necessarily mean that he is ill. Ill health or the negative dimension of health may refer to illness, disease, injury, disability or handicap either as single entities or as a combination of several (Downie et al 1990).

Illness may also be considered to be synonymous with disease. However, whereas disease generally is of medical origin and can be identified by a set of signs and symptoms, for example diabetes mellitus, illness tends to have a social basis and can be described by quite wide ranging symptoms, such as headache, dizziness, nausea. However, both illness and disease indicate an imbalance in homeostasis, a disturbance in the body's equilibrium.

Another view of illness proposes that there must be some evidence of an organic nature. Using this definition, anyone who feels ill but has no organic signs of disease may not be defined as being ill. Alternatively, an individual may be diagnosed as having a particular disease but feels quite healthy.

It has also been proposed that illness is only present if the individual perceives him/herself to be ill. However, this rather narrow view of illness by definition excludes those whose perception has been altered, such as those in a comatosed state.

Illness is common in most people. Research suggests that throughout life, individuals are rarely asymptomatic, having on average a new 'illness' episode every 6 days (Redman 1988). Much of this type of illness is never brought to the attention of the medical profession, being either 'ignored, tolerated or self medicated'.

Acute illness is normally characterized by a rapid onset, often the result of bacterial or viral invasion, and usually amenable to cure. Treatment is of short duration and the condition resolves without apparent side-effects. An example of acute illness is uncomplicated influenza.

Chronic illnesses are typically diseases that are incurable, such as cancers, heart disease, diabetes mellitus. They require to be managed by both patient and practitioner. Some chronic illness is characterized by intermittent episodes of acute symptoms called exacerbations. These are followed by periods of remission, where symptoms abate, for example multiple sclerosis, arthritis and emphysema.

Chronic illnesses are the main contributors to disability and death within the population (Ellis & Nowlis 1981, Taylor 1991). A person's perception of illness is influenced by a number of factors such as the subculture to which he/she belongs and whose values have been internalized, his/her health beliefs and health practices. Self-concept and body image also play an important role, as does an awareness of available support systems and care facilities during this 'illness crisis'.

Illness brings about a loss of the control and autonomy a person normally has over his/her life, and can elicit certain responses from the patient, family, friends, carers and society in general. As already indicated every individual reacts to the threat of illness in their own particular way. Illness may impose necessary changes in an individual's life-style, changes which may affect the person's homelife, job and family, and may occur in both acute and chronic illness. Some of these changes will be of a temporary nature, whilst others will be more permanent.

When assuming the role of a sick person, individuals tend to relinquish their other roles, such as husband, father, worker. This role change, in some instances, brings with it losses, in others, gains.

Losses

Losses experienced through illness frequently involve a loss of functional capabilities, the person may be confined to a bed, unable to care for him/herself, and therefore dependent on others.

This loss of normality may bring with it a loss of self-esteem, self-respect and a loss of recognition from others. This may prove to be a very threatening situation and evoke very negative feelings.

There may be guilt because the person is unable to carry out his or her normal role, for example wage earner, thereby depriving the family of income, which in the long term may reduce the family's basic standard of living. This in turn may further reduce the person's level of self-esteem.

Patients may also suffer from anxiety and apprehension. This may be primarily due to a lack of understanding and knowledge of their illness and treatment. They may be fearful of the outcome of their illness, of pain, of surgery and the threat of disability. They may also fear that the illness will affect their personal relationships.

Patients often react to these anxieties by reverting to immature behaviour. For example, children may start to bed wet having been toilet trained, whilst adults become more self-centred, irritable and discontented. There is often a preoccupation with the self and the condition. As an illness progresses and becomes more serious less attention is paid to the outside world, self-preoccupation increases, behaviour becomes more demanding and attention seeking.

As anxiety levels continue to increase and overwhelm the patient, they may exhibit hostile behaviour, such as being verbally abusive towards family, friends and carers including nursing staff.

Gains

Illness may, on the other hand, bring certain rewards or gains to the individual.

The dependence state engendered by the illness may be used in a manipulative way to affect relationships. The ill person may receive attention and consideration which would not be received if it were not for the illness. It is difficult to be angry with the sick even if it appears deserved.

Normally an attempt is made to protect the ill from the stresses of everyday life. Therefore there can be an escape from family conflicts, domestic issues and the stress of work. There is an opportunity to think only of the self.

These factors may reinforce the illness and interfere with recovery. The patient may feign pain or exaggerate symptoms to gain further attention. Paid leave from work and the relief from work stresses may discourage an early return to work.

A person's return to work after an illness is frequently identified as an indication of their recovery.

Within western societies a person is permitted to behave in a sick manner under certain circumstances, that is to adopt a 'sick role'. This provides a legitimate excuse for non-attendance at work. However, being sick should create an awareness of being a burden to others and a response by getting better as soon as possible. Also there is an obligation to seek competent help and prevent illness where possible.

The concept of the sick role was developed by Talcott Parsons (1981) and provides an insight into the ways an individual is expected to behave if suffering from an acute illness. However it is less useful when considering chronic illness or disability where recovery is not possible, and this will be discussed in more detail in the next section. Whatever the situation there is a need to find out why the patient is behaving in a particular manner. Therefore nurses need to be aware of the responses and their causes, to encourage patients to gain autonomy and control of their lives.

Coping with stress

Stress can be defined as any condition that causes the individual to react by producing a stress response to cope with the source of stress. This may be achieved by:

1. eliminating or reducing the source of discomfort
2. altering ones appraisal of the stressor
3. managing or reducing the feelings of discomfort.
   (Murphy 1985 cited by Sutherland & Cooper 1990)

The resources available to help the individual cope with stress may be internal or external, and include such factors as age, gender, education, lifestyle, life experiences and social support. Illness whether acute or chronic is considered to be a stressful event for most people and features in the top ten of Holmes & Rahe (1967) Social Readjustment Scale, which lists a variety of potential stressful life events.

Helping clients/patients to manage stress can be considered to be an important function of nursing. To manage stress a person must be able to identify the source of stress. This may be achieved with patients by using a stress rating scale, such as the Hospital Stress Rating Scale which identifies stress related to hospitalization (Kneisl & Ames 1986). Being aware of the sources of stress can aid in the prevention or reduction of stress. People in general cope more effectively with stressful events when they are prepared for them. Therefore the role of the nurse is to help the patient to be aware of what stress is, the sources of stress, and positive ways of coping with stress.

Coping has been described as the process of managing demands that tax or exceed a person's resources (Taylor 1991). It is influenced by:

1. Primary appraisals of the stressor (stressful event) – is it harmful, threatening or challenging?
2. Secondary appraisals – what coping resources does the individual have to manage the event and how adequate are they?

Two forms of coping have been identified. One form is directed at *solving problems* – the stressful situation is evaluated and an attempt is made to solve it or it is avoided. The other form focuses on *regulating emotions* – the individual tries to reduce the anxiety without dealing with the anxiety-provoking event.

Most stressful events involve both types of coping. Not all problems can be solved as for example with chronic illness, therefore individuals need to reduce their emotional distress to enable them to cope with the situation. Because most stressful events incorporate a variety of smaller problems, which may require a range of coping strategies, the greater the number of coping strategies an individual possesses the greater the likelihood he has of being able to cope with at least some stressful events.

Although stress has become the 'in' word with both the lay public and professionals, many people fail to recognize stress when it occurs. Since stress and body tensions occur simultaneously, recognizing body tensions aids in the recognition of stress and anxiety (Kneisl & Ames 1986).

The ability to relax in times of stress is helpful in coping and a range of stress reduction techniques such as deep breathing, progressive muscle relaxation and visual imagery can be helpful in reducing somatic arousal. This includes a reduction in heart rate, skin conductance, muscle tension, and self-reports of anxiety and tension.

An increasing number of nurses are now incorporating such stress reduction strategies into the everyday care of their clients and patients to promote recovery and a sense of well-being.

Health choices

Whether functioning in hospital or in the community the nurse has a duty to assist clients to assume a responsibility for their own health care.

However, whilst nurses are able to identify the importance of assisting patients to work towards independence, with for example a colostomy or diabetes, for some reason the importance of teaching health protection behaviours goes unrecognized. Nevertheless enabling clients to convert health-damaging habits into health-promoting ones through making positive health choices can bring benefits to both client and nurse.

Not only does the client achieve the benefits that accompany a health-promoting lifestyle, but also the increased self-esteem for taking active control over part of their life; for example, being in control of a drug habit rather than the drug habit being in control of them. Therefore making a positive decision about health can be a self-empowering process (Ewles & Simnett 1992).

Using the process of self-empowerment involves altering the way people feel about themselves through improving self-awareness and understanding. It involves the nurse in helping clients to think critically about their values and beliefs and constructing their own values and belief system.

A range of methods can be employed to help clients achieve self-empowerment and includes individual counselling, group work, experiental learning, therapy and advocacy (Ewles & Simnett 1992).

Setting short- and long-term goals with the client is important. The nurse needs to make sure the client fully understands the health risks associated with the behaviour that has to be changed and is aware of the options for making these changes. Also the client needs to understand personal benefits associated with these changes.

The provision of health education literature can provide the clients with valuable information on how to care for themselves and avoid illness. In addition to being better informed about personal health care, the client can become more aware of how to make the best use of the health care system to promote personal health and well-being. Participation in self-help groups may also be of value in helping them assume responsibility for their own health care through the provision of emotional and informational support.

It is not easy to modify one's life-style. Attitudes and behaviour change may take a long time. However clients who believe they have more control over what happens in their lives are more likely to become involved in activities that reduce their risk of illness.

Chronic illness and disability

The primary causes of morbidity and mortality within advanced societies have been attributed to chronic health problems associated with degenerative disease and chronic illness. This is because people who would normally have died of acute infections and trauma in the past now survive and live into old age.

Although disability affects all age groups, chronic health problems related to disability are more prevalent in people over 50 years of age. These conditions range from relatively mild ones, such as partial hearing loss, to more severe conditions, such as cancer, circulatory disease and diabetes.

Chronic health problems bring about major changes in the life-style of individuals, their families and friends, affecting them physically, psychologically and socially. Nevertheless it is important to remember that people with chronic health problems are individuals and subsequently their health needs will be influenced by several factors including age, socioeconomic circumstances and family support.

Chronic illness and associated health problems can be placed into three main categories: impairment, disability and handicap. Despite the fact that these terms are frequently interchanged, an important distinction between the three exists.

- **Impairment** means any abnormality of structure or function.
- **Disability** means a reduction in a person's ability to carry out particular tasks, functions or skills.
- **Handicap** is the effect of the impairment or dis-

ability in preventing the individual from pursuing desired aspirations or goals in society.

However each category is not mutually exclusive; for example, damage to the spinal cord leading to limb paralysis could result in a young ballerina being denied her goal of becoming a prima ballerina, thereby affecting her quality of life.

Until recently assessment of quality of life for the chronically ill was carried out by the medical profession based on a measurement of length of survival and signs of presence of illness (Taylor 1991). Little consideration was given to psychosocial consequences of the illness and its treatment, or to the views of the patient and relatives.

Recent studies have shown that a significant discrepancy exists between the views of professionals and patients as to what constitutes a quality of life. Therefore it is suggested that since quality of life is a subjective experience it should be assessed by the patient.

Several quality of life scales or measures are available. Some have been developed to assess activities of living whilst others deal with specific diseases such as cancer. Some are dependent on professional observations but the majority are assessed by subjective reporting of the patient.

By studying the quality of life among the chronically ill, areas that require particular attention and rehabilitation following the diagnosis of a chronic disease can be highlighted. These include problems associated with particular diseases and treatments, help in policy-making decisions and the effectiveness and cost effectiveness of interventions (Taylor 1991).

As discussed in Part III on acute illness, definitions of chronic illness do not fit into the 'sick role' as depicted by Parsons. The experiences of a person with a chronic condition will differ markedly from those of the acutely ill. Chronic illness is a long-term event and instead of relinquishing the patient role it must be integrated psychologically into the patient's life if successful adaptation to the disorder is to take place (Taylor 1991).

A complete cure is not the goal for the chronically ill, but is, as suggested by MacKenzie (Hinchliff et al 1993), 'the maintenance of health to an optimum achievable level dependent on the disability of the individual and the social and psychological consequences of the handicap'.

Therefore the role of the nurse in providing health care for patients with chronic illness and associated health problems will be different from the provision of care to the acutely ill. (See relevant chapters for the care implications for specific disorders.)

Emotional responses to chronic illness

Patients have been found to exhibit a wide range of emotional responses to chronic illness. Such responses are considered normal, whereas a lack of response has been associated with a poor recovery.

Common responses include:

- denial
- anxiety
- depression.

Denial Is a defence mechanism used to avoid the implications of an illness. Denial can have positive benefits in that it enables the patient to control their emotional reactions to illness, particularly in the immediate period following diagnosis when they are at their most vulnerable.

On the other hand, it may have negative implications and interfere with the monitoring of the patient's condition, delay treatment being sought and reduce the patient's involvement in the management of his/her condition.

Anxiety Is the primary response to a situation appraised as threatening. Many patients are overpowered by the thoughts of potential changes to their lives and by the probability of death.

Anxiety also occurs intermittently throughout the disease process causing distress and interference with good functioning.

Anxiety levels can be increased by a range of events; for example, awaiting test results, going for check ups, experiencing side-effects of treatments. All of these indicate a need for a full assessment and treatment of anxiety in the patient with chronic illness.

Depression A common and often debilitating reaction to chronic illness. It has been found to increase with the severity of the illness and the extent of pain and disability.

Depression is also associated with factors other than those specifically related to the condition, such as social stress and lack of social support.

Long-term depression has been linked with poor recovery.

Emotional reactions to chronic illness therefore require to be carefully monitored during the recovery and adjustment period, to enable appropriate care and treatment. (For a full discussion on the care implications of disorders of mood and emotions, see Ch. 8.)

Coping with chronic illness

Most patients with chronic illness will suffer some acute psychological reactions as a result of their condition. The coping strategies used to alleviate this distress have been found to be similar to those employed to deal with other stressful life events.

Patients use both active and avoidant strategies to cope with a range of stressors. The use of multiple coping strategies has been shown to be more effective in coping with the stress of chronic disease than using one predominant coping strategy.

In general, the use of actual coping strategies is more effective than avoidant strategies in reducing stress, where the condition is amenable to using active coping efforts.

As discussed earlier, individuals who feel they have some control over their lives may be better adjusted than those who feel they have no control. The same would appear to be true for patients with chronic illness. In those who perceive they have control over their illness, its causes and controllability, their level of adjustment to their condition is higher than those without this belief. Therefore nursing interventions that attempt to instil feelings of control are an important part of the care of the patient with chronic illness.

Rehabilitation and chronic illness

To enable rehabilitation to have any chance of success the patient must be involved in his/her care from the outset and agree to any plan that is formulated.

The goal is to enable the patient to alleviate, manage or solve his/her identified chronic health problems, to help him/her gain independence where possible and to cope with dependency where it is not possible.

The main problem-solving tasks frequently encountered during the rehabilitation process are physical problems associated with illness, employment/vocational problems and social relationships.

Physical problems associated with chronic illness can be divided into two general types:

1. Problems which occur as a result of illness.
2. Problems which emerge as the result of treatment.

Physical problems which arise from the disease itself can be wide ranging and include pain, discomfort, breathlessness, metabolic and locomotor problems. Cognitive impairment may also occur, for example, as the result of a stroke, and includes language, memory or learning deficits.

Therefore the physical consequences of disease can dramatically alter the quality of an individual's life.

Difficulties in physical functioning also occur due to treatment of the primary symptoms and underlying disease. In some instances the patient may feel the effects of the cure to be worse than the disease. For example patients receiving chemotherapy treatment may have to endure nausea, vomiting, hair loss and skin discoloration. Certain medications may have side-effects which cause drowsiness, weight gain or impotence. Other treatments may impose changes to the patient's diet, smoking and drinking habits. For some patients these restrictions may seem intolerable.

Therefore any rehabilitation plan must take into account these illness and treatment-related factors that may affect the patient's level of functioning. For example building a pain control programme into the nursing care plan for the patient who is experiencing pain associated with a cancerous condition.

Physical rehabilitation also needs to address the issue of patient adherence to long-term medical and treatment regimens. Research findings indicate that where patients are knowledgeable about their condition, feel in control of their situation and enjoy good social support, they are more likely to adhere to their treatment regimens. This reinforces the point that has been made previously that patients with chronic health problems need to be active participants in their own care.

For many patients their chronic condition affects their vocational activities and employment situation. For some this may mean restricting or changing their occupation. The cardiac patient may no longer be able to cope with the stresses of a high-powered job that may have contributed to his/her condition. The stroke patient will not be allowed to return to his/her job as a bus driver because of his incapacitated condition.

For some patients the illness may result in retraining or redeployment within their existing organization. This will allow them the opportunity to develop new skills which are important for their self-esteem. For others they may find that they are discriminated against because of their illness. They may be passed over for promotion or denied the opportunity for any further professional development, being considered a 'poor bet' for investment due to their prognosis. The effect of this may be quite demoralizing for patients who may feel they have made good progress in their rehabilitation programme up to this point. Still other patients may be stigmatized because of their illness. For instance, AIDS can evoke feelings of fear and anxiety amongst other people and so lead to employment restrictions. Epilepsy may also incite a similar response. This discrimination may result in people failing to disclose any impairment when making job applications.

Chronic illness may reduce a person's capacity to earn. Lack of finance not only affects the person but also the family. As discussed previously, losing ones identity as the family provider can seriously affect the self-esteem of the patient and can inhibit recovery.

It is therefore important that these potential problems are assessed as part of the rehabilitation programme and appropriate help in the form of counselling, job retraining and advice on how to cope with discriminating practices is initiated as early as possible.

Chronic illness can affect a patient's social relationships. After diagnosis difficulties may arise in re-establishing relationships, patients frequently complain of being rejected or pitied by family and friends. It is considered this situation may be the result of the patient's own behaviour which causes these responses, by either withdrawing from all social contacts or by forcing themselves into social activities before they have adjusted to their diagnosis. Or it may also arise due to the behaviour of significant others, who verbally indicate warmth and affection but non-verbally, by the use of body language, show rejection and revulsion. The patient therefore finds it difficult to interpret these confused messages.

As indicated earlier, chronic disease does not just affect the patient but invariably affects the lives of others. The main effect is the increased dependency of the chronically ill person on the family. In particular the spouse or partner assumes increased family responsibilities. Children may also have to take on more responsibilities than would be normal for a particular age.

For some families the burden may be too great, particularly for the children, and they may respond to these increased demands by exhibiting rebellious behaviour such as truanting from school, using drugs and antagonizing other family members.

Where the patient is a child, healthy children may experience changes to their daily life-styles due to the upheaval of normal daily life. This may evoke feelings of rejection, isolation and confusion in the child. They may also experience feelings of resentment, jealousy and guilt and demonstrate a wide variety of behaviours including headaches, stomach pains and vomiting to gain their parents' attention (Byrne 1994). It is therefore suggested that siblings as well as the primary care givers (parents) need to be involved in the sick child's care to alleviate the effects of the stress of chronic illness on the whole family.

The social issues produced by chronic illness need

to be addressed in the rehabilitation programme. Some may require immediate attention and intensive action over a short period, for example after diagnosis; this may involve counselling for both patient and family members. Over the longer time period individual family members may require personal counselling. Family therapy may be advantageous for the patient and family members to help them work through their problems and difficulties with the help of a therapist.

Dying and bereavement

Within primitive societies death is accepted as a natural conclusion to life. But within contemporary western society death and dying has become an abstract concept primarily observed through the media which concentrates on the more violent aspects of death – murders, accidents and other types of disasters. Death has become something that happens to others but rarely thought about at a personal level.

This belief is reinforced by the facts that people now live longer than they used to, often to an advanced age, there are fewer deaths in children, and most deaths occur in hospital.

However, the main causes of death in the UK are diseases of the circulatory system, respiratory system and cancers and not as the result of acts of violence.

Therefore, although most people will suffer bereavement in their lives, it is unlikely to occur before young adulthood or until middle age. Consequently people are rarely prepared for their own death or the death of a loved one.

Stages of dying

Throughout life a person experiences many different types of loss. Loss has been defined as 'being deprived of a valued object or person' (Rambo 1984). Suffering loss of any kind evokes feelings of sorrow, hurt, pain and discomfort. Rambo describes death as a person's ultimate loss – the loss of life. Grief is the subjective response to loss, mourning the process through which grief and loss are finally resolved.

Even before the loss occurs, anyone faced with a serious loss starts to grieve. Therefore the person with a diagnosis of terminal illness begins to grieve for the ultimate loss – the loss of self. However for most people death does not come suddenly and they live for days, weeks or months before life comes to an end. During this period they have to cope daily with their feelings as they go through the grieving process. Elizabeth Kubler-Ross (1969) identified five stages,

the psychological stages of dying, through which a person passes during the grieving process. They are:

1. denial
2. anger
3. bargaining
4. depression
5. acceptance.

However it is important to remember that each death is unique. Therefore the stages may not correspond with each individual's personal experience. Some individuals may move back and forth through the stages, whilst others may miss stages or pass through each stage rapidly to the final stage of acceptance. Still others may never move beyond the stage of denial. Nevertheless the concept of stages provides a useful tool to help nurses recognize and deal with such reactions in whichever sequence they may occur.

The dying patient is more likely to be accepting of death if those who care for him/her enable honest communication to take place and have come to terms with their own concerns regarding death.

Family members, however, may be experiencing similar stages of grief to the patient before they can accept the prognosis. They may also be at a different stage in the grieving process to the patient, and this lack of synchronization may block the communication pathway, denying the patient much needed family support and understanding. Some patients may feel that their loved ones have already let go and that they are being left alone to face death. Nurses therefore need to be aware that in providing care for the patient they also address the needs of the grieving family to help them cope with the impending loss of a loved one.

Three major requirements have been identified in order to meet the needs of dying patients (Freiberg 1992):

1. The control of pain – many patients greatest fear is the inability to control pain, so much so that they may welcome or even seek death to avoid it. (See Ch. 4 for a full discussion on managing pain.)
2. The need to retain dignity or feelings of self worth – by allowing the dying person as much control over decisions affecting his/her death as the rest of his/her life-span, dignity can be maintained.
3. The need for love and affection – many patients have stated that their fears were not of death itself, but of being abandoned (Rambo 1984). Love and affection can be shown through the use of good com-

munication skills, both verbal and non-verbal. Listening, talking, reassuring the patient that a loved one will be present until the end, touching, stroking and holding hands are all ways of showing the patient they are surrounded by love and affection. (See Ch. 4 for further discussion on support of the dying patient and his/her loved ones.)

Bereavement

Bereavement refers to a state of loss resulting from the death of a 'significant person'. The loss of a loved one through death is probably the most upsetting and dreaded event of a person's life. Whether death occurs suddenly or has been anticipated as the result of a long illness, surviving individuals find it difficult to cope successfully.

Bereavement has been identified as a state of acute stress. It can produce major changes in the immune, respiratory, cardiovascular, endocrine and autonomic nervous systems, with resultant changes in physical and mental health.

Death rates among bereaved people have also been shown to be significantly higher than similar non-bereaved individuals.

Grief is the psychological response to bereavement. Parkes (1972) has analysed four stages of the grief reaction:

1. *Numbness and denial.* There is a feeling of emptiness, as if the world has stood still. There is disbelief and denial of the event.

2. *Yearning or pining.* There is a preoccupation with the image of the deceased person. The person may be said to be seen, spoken to or heard.

3. *Despair and depression.* There is an acceptance the deceased has gone forever. It is a period when behaviour may become disorganized – some people may find it difficult to concentrate on daily tasks at home or at work. There are frequently feelings of intense despair and at times depression.

4. *Reality or reorganization.* A realization that life must and can go on without the deceased. The loss becomes less painful and successful resolution of the grieving process enables the survivor to begin to move into the future.

However, as with the stages of dying, grief reaction is very personal and the stages may not be experienced in any natural order. Indeed at times they may overlap so that yearning and pining is experienced along with despair and depression. Also adjustment to the loss may be set back on the occasion of the first anniversary of the death or by a birthday or wedding anniversary. Normal grieving may last

several months or even years. Men and those whose loss was sudden and unexpected appear to suffer extreme grief reactions (Taylor 1991).

For some people who have been bereaved, their family and friends are able to provide all the necessary support required. Others may find their family doctor or minister of religion particularly helpful during this period. District nursing sisters and health visitors are also available to follow up care of bereaved families whose relatives have died either at home or in an institutional setting. National voluntary organizations such as CRUSE (for widowed people and their children), Compassionate Friends (for bereaved parents) and the Gay Bereavement Project are also available for bereavement counselling and additional support.

INDIVIDUAL UNIQUENESS

In discussing people and health the need for nurses to appreciate the uniqueness of each individual has emerged as a prerequisite for the planning, provision and acceptance of health care.

As identified previously, people's ideas of health and being healthy are wide ranging. They are fashioned by age and sex, social background, culture and life experiences, religions or belief systems, attitudes and values.

Because of these differences, nurses' perceptions of health and illness may be markedly different from that of their clients. These perceptual differences may account for a patient's or client's apparent uncooperative behaviour regarding his/her health care activities. Should a client's belief system interfere with his/her health care, it is the nurse's responsibility, whether in an acute or primary care setting, to discuss these beliefs with the client in a non-judgemental manner.

To enable nurses to sensitively assess the health needs of clients they first need to explore their own beliefs and attitudes and assess their own health perceptions. By gaining a greater self-awareness, nurses should then be able to appreciate their client's perception of personal health needs. This knowledge will enable them to negotiate an approach to care which will be acceptable to both client and practitioner.

Gradually, the concept of health and health care is shifting away from the idea that health is the absence of disease, and health care really means illness care. A more holistic approach to health and health care is beginning to infiltrate the more traditional medical care systems. The Patient's Charter (DOH 1991) reflects this change of approach to some extent. The concept of holistic care is characterized by a belief that health is a positive state to be actively achieved and acknowledges psychological and social influences in the development of illness and the achievement of health. It provides the client/patient with responsibilities for both his/her health and illness through his/her attitudes, behaviour and spiritual beliefs. It emphasizes the importance of self-help, self-healing and health education.

Most important is the change in the relationship between patient and practitioner, from one of practitioner domination to one that involves an open reciprocal relationship between practitioner and patient. As well as using the more traditional medicines and treatments, holistic practitioners are more likely to incorporate complementary therapies such as herbal remedies, acupuncture, massage and hypnotherapy as part of their overall patient care. An increasing number of nurses are also developing these complementary skills for professional practice. However, American research findings indicate that people from the lower socioeconomic groups appear not to have benefited from this more participative approach to health care, remaining more or less passive recipients of medical services. This lack of involvement in their care may account for the lack of adherence to treatment, resulting in the subsequent medical/health problems frequently found in patients who are in receipt of this form of medical care (Taylor 1991).

To enable the client to participate fully as a partner within the framework of health care, certain communication points need to be addressed by the health practitioner.

First, the practitioner must listen to the patient. Interrupting or directing the patient away from the main point of the discussion not only denies the patient the opportunity to voice his/her concerns, but may also lead to the loss of vital information.

Secondly, the use of jargon and technical language is another important factor leading to poor communication. Use of such language distances the practitioner from the patient and prevents any fruitful discussion from taking place. If technical or professional language cannot be avoided then appropriate explanations should be provided. However, where professional jargon is used, practitioners often revert to using infantile and simplistic explanations, reducing the client to the status of a helpless child, consequently, reducing the client's self-esteem. Depersonalization of the patient is often employed by practitioners to keep the patient quiet during examinations or treatments. Although this may have advantages to both practitioner and patient as it allows the practitioner to concentrate, it can also cause stress and anxiety to the patient. An example of depersonalization is when the patient is talked about as his condition, for example, Mr Jones, the fractured femur, or the fractured femur in bed ten. Furthermore, any discussion that takes place does not include the patient. This denies the patient his rights to be involved and informed of any decisions regarding his care and is dismissive of any partnership between practitioner and patient.

As changes occur in health care the traditional roles of the nurse as client advocate and health teacher assume even greater importance. To support the concept of self-care, nurses need to emphasize their central role of client educator to increase client autonomy of their condition or treatment.

When clients cannot understand medical jargon, nurses can help to bring about a difference in the patient's understanding and so maintain control of their medical condition. Clients and patients need to have information to enable them to make informed choices about their treatment and care. Nurses can provide this information through teaching, by providing relevant literature, by acting as a referral agent informing patients of self-help and support groups.

At the end of the twentieth century, teaching about health and illness is one of the most important functions of the nurse. Clients need and want to know about health, how to maintain health and prevent ill health. Nurses need to use their professional powers of caring not only to protect the rights of clients and their families they nurse but to preserve and protect the nursing profession (Kneisl & Ames 1989).

Suggested assignments

ACTIVITY 1
a. Choose any ethnic group and find out the following information.
  i dietary needs and preferences
  ii special hygiene practices
  iii religious beliefs and customs
  iv traditional health care system – (beliefs and healing practices)
  v traditional family structure
  vi gender defined roles
  vii life style.
b. Consider the ethnic group to which you belong, and apply the same questions.
  What are the similarities and differences between the two groups?
  How could this information be utilised by the nurse in planning nursing care?

(cont'd)

ACTIVITY 2
What is your opinion of 'living wills'? Do you consider a person should have the right to choose freely and lawfully the time, method and place of his death? Or do you believe that it should be left to a person's loved ones to determine whether life-sustaining apparatus should be retained?
Explain your answer.

REFERENCES AND FURTHER READING

Atkinson R L, Atkinson R C, Smith E, Bem D J, Hildegard E R (eds) 1987 Introduction to psychology. Harcourt Brace Jovanich, San Diego

Bandaman E L, Bandaman B 1990 Nursing ethics through the life span. Prentice Hall, Englewood Cliffs

Breslow L, Enstrom J 1980 Persistence of health habits and their relationship to mortality. Preventative Medicine 9: 469–483

Brigham J C 1991 Social psychology. Harper Collins, New York

British Medical Association 1993 Medical ethics today. Handbook. London

Byrne D 1994 Out in the cold. Nursing Times (Scottish Edition) 90(11): 38–40

Carlson N R 1990 Psychology. Allyn and Bacon, London

Coleman J C 1980 The nature of adolescence. Methuen, London

Cormack D 1991 Research process in nursing. Blackwell Scientific Publications, Edinburgh

DOH 1991 The Patients Charter. London: HMSO

Downie R S, Fyfe C, Tannahill A (eds) 1990 Health promotion models and values. Oxford University Press, Oxford

Ellis J R, Nowlis E A 1981 Nursing: a human needs approach. Houghton Mifflin, Boston

Ewles L, Simnett I 1992 Promoting health a practical guide. Scutari Press, London

Freiberg K L 1992 Human development – a lifespan approach. Jones and Bartlett, Boston

Fristinger L 1957 A theory of cognitive dissonance. Row Peterson, Evanston

Fromer M J 1981 Ethical issues in health care. CV Mosby, St Louis

Groenman N H, Sieven O D'A, Buckenham M A (eds) 1992 Social and behavioural sciences for nurses. Campion, Edinburgh

Hall J 1982 Psychology for nurses and health visitors. The British Psychological Society. Macmillan, London

Henderson V 1966 The nature of nursing – a definition and it's implications for practice research and education. New York

Hetherington E, Parke E 1986 Child psychology, a contemporary viewpoint. McGraw Hill, Singapore

Hinchliff S M, Norman S E, Schober J E (eds) 1993 Nursing practice and health Care. Edward Arnold, London

Kennedy L 1990 Euthanasia: the good death. Chatto and Windus, London

Kenworthy M, Snowley G, Gilling C (eds) 1992 Common foundation studies in nursing. Churchill Livingstone, Edinburgh

Kneisl C, Ames S A 1986 Adult health nursing. A biopsychosocial approach. Addison-Wesley, Reading

Kubler-Ross E 1969 On death and dying. Tavistock Publications, London

Lothian Community Relations Council 1988 Religions and cultures: a Guide to patients beliefs and customs for health service staff

Mason J K, McCall Smith R A 1991 Law and medical ethics. Butterworths, London

Neuberger J 1992 Ethics and health care: the role of research ethics committees in the UK. Kings Fund, London

Niven N 1989 Health Psychology. An introduction for nurses and other health care professionals. Churchill Livingstone, Edinburgh

Oppenheim C 1993 Poverty: the facts. Child Poverty Action Group, London

Parkes C M 1972 Bereavement studies of grief in adult life. Penguin Books, Harmondsworth

Parson T 1981 Definitions of health and illness in the light of American values and social structure. In: Capla A L, Englehart H T, McCartney J J (eds) Concepts of health and disease. Addison-Wesley, New York

Plant M, Plant M 1992 Risk takers – alcohol, drugs, sex and youth. Routledge, London

Rambo B J 1984 Adaption nursing assessment and intervention, international edn. W B Saunders, London

Redman B 1988 The process of patient education. CV Mosby Company, St Louis

Rogers R W 1975 A protection (motivation) theory of fear and attitude change. Journal of Psychology 91. 93–114(7)

Rumbold G 1993 Ethics in nursing. Baillière Tindall, London

Sheehy G 1981 Passages: a predictable crises of adult life. Bantam Books

Smith A, Jacobson B (eds) 1988 The Nation's health: a strategy for the 1990s. Kings Fund, London

Sutherland I 1979 Health education. Perspectives and choices. Allan and Unwin, London

Sutherland V, Cooper C 1990 Understanding stress: a psychological perspective for health professionals. Chapman Hall, London

Taylor S E 1991 Health psychology. McGraw Hill, New York

Tight M (ed) 1983 Adult learning and education. Croom Helm, London

Tschudin V 1992 Ethics in nursing — the caring relationship. Butterworth-Heinemann, Oxford

UKCC 1992 Code of professional conduct. UKCC, London

VESS 1993 The living will (advance directive). VESS, Edinburgh

Whitehead M 1989 The way we live (lifestyle, behaviour, the individual and health). Health Studies in Nurse Education. Discussion Paper One. SHEG, Edinburgh

3

The role of the nurse

Helen A. S. Dougan

INTRODUCTION

The unifying force of the new diploma course, on which student nurses, and in some cases midwifery students, share common foundation studies, has encouraged the identification of the commonly required caring skills. This chapter is concerned with introducing some of these skills at foundation level. A bibliography is provided to enable readers to pursue the content in more depth.

The philosophy of nursing in the 1990s is firmly rooted in recognizing people as individuals with specific wants and needs. Caring is the activity of assisting patients or clients to meet their needs. These needs may or may not be recognized by the individual, or the nurse, but together they will embark on a journey of exploration. The aim is to cope with the situation that has brought the person to seek help.

Traditionally, nurses have been actively encouraged not to get emotionally involved with their patients and families. This is now changing, and what is considered important is coping by being involved, with the emphasis on holistic care. Coping by being involved requires developing interpersonal communication skills, and learning basic counselling skills. This means becoming a caring communicator, which requires the ability to demonstrate warmth, respect, genuineness and empathy. It also means learning to question, to listen, and when and how to be assertive.

Communicating clearly and accurately, verbally and in writing, is necessary for the implementation of a systematic approach to nursing care, and for a safe working environment. This approach to nursing care, often referred to as the nursing process, promotes clinical practice in a planned orderly and logical way. Skills required to implement the nursing process are observation, assessment, planning, goal setting, decision making and evaluation, as well as a sound theoretical knowledge of models of nursing which provide a framework within which these activities can take place.

The present emphasis on achieving value for money in health care has accelerated the need for nurses to demonstrate the benefits of their intervention. Nursing research – the means of understanding, assessing, and evaluating what nurses do – must be studied, as must quality assurance and standard setting.

The role of the nurse also includes caring for colleagues and for self. Attention to health and safety at work, especially protection from occupational injury, is important (see Ch. 11). Other aspects, such as the handling of potentially infectious material and nurturing a healthy immune system, are discussed in Chapter 4.

COMMUNICATION

Modern nursing theory emphasizes the importance of holistic care, that is recognizing that the person has psychological and social needs, as well as physical needs. To begin to understand how these needs might be met the student must first understand how people communicate.

Human society is a network of relationships between people, the substance of these relationships being based on communication. This communication is not always helpful: people can dominate, humiliate, threaten or reject others without necessarily being aware of their actions.

People are born with communication ability but not communication skills. Throughout the years of childhood and young adulthood, learning occurs which enables them to follow the complex rules of social interaction. This learning does not usually expose the individual to communication with the dying and the confused during periods of acute distress, anxiety, fear and profound grief. Communicating in these situations is the role of the nurse.

This role often generates anxiety. Lees & Ellis (1990) 'identified relationships with patients and other nurses, lack of confidence, worries about incompetence, and changing wards', as being major stress factors facing student nurses. Growing competence in communication skills can promote self-confidence, and therefore reduce the discomfort and anxiety experienced by students, when they confront new and stressful situations.

Good communication in a team provides a supportive working environment, which promotes professional growth. Good communication between health professionals and patients has been shown to improve recovery rates, reduce demand for analgesia, and improve patient compliance with treatment (Hayward 1975, Boore 1978).

Communication involves sending and receiving messages between two or more people. A message has two parts: verbal and non-verbal.

VERBAL COMMUNICATION

Verbal communication is a solely human activity between people who speak the same language. The meaning of the words can vary, depending on how they are spoken, and what understanding the receiver has of the words. Consider the effects of varying the following aspects of speech.

Volume

Loud speech sounds angry, aggressive and dominant. Soft speech sounds warm, shy and unassertive.

Exercise 1

Shout out the question: 'What do you think you are doing?'

Now speak the question out quietly.

Pitch or tone

Low pitch sounds dominant. It is often perceived as a sign of sophistication, sexiness, security and a positive manner.

High pitch or tone is perceived as being submissive and weak. A raised voice pitch may be interpreted as a sign of not telling the truth.

Variation in pitch gives colour and emphasis. Monotone speech shows disinterest and is usually boring. An enthusiastic speaker will have variation in tone.

Rate

Rapid speech gives the impression of a nervous anxious person, as also does a slow rate of speech, and speech hesitation.

Exercise 2

Try to identify and interpret differences in pitch, tone, and rate of speech when listening to the radio.

Meanings of words

Words may have different meanings for different people. 'Abortion' to the staff nurse in a gynaecological ward means the end of a pregnancy before it is viable, but she is careful to use the word 'miscarriage' when speaking with a woman whose medical diagnosis is that of 'incomplete abortion'. This nurse knows that the word abortion, to most people, means an induced termination of pregnancy, but especially that it is a very emotive word.

Some words may have no meaning to people. A patient may relate in some distress that the doctor has told her she has a 'B9 tumour'. To this woman a tumour means cancer, and she has no understanding of the word benign.

Abbreviations and jargon may have a similar confusing effect. These terms are often only understood by a specific group of people, and use must be avoided when speaking to patients and relatives, and used carefully with junior colleagues.

NON-VERBAL COMMUNICATION

Non-verbal communication is also known as body language. It comprises facial expression, eye contact, posture, gesture, spatial behaviour, touch and appearance.

A knowledge of the different components of verbal and non-verbal communication, and of their effect on social interaction, can assist the understanding of the signals which individuals broadcast. This knowledge may be used for self-appraisal, or self-analysis if there is a communication breakdown.

Day-to-day social interaction is a complex mix of the components of communication. In the helping, caring, relationship, the ability to display warmth, respect and empathy are mutually beneficial.

Facial expression

Faces convey the most expressive body language. The six basic emotions listed in Box 3.1 are almost universally recognized. The blending of these emotions creates other facial expressions.

Examples of these are:

- looking smug: the mixture of the happy and angry expressions
- the 'wry smile', one corner of the mouth up, one down.

Although facial expressions are almost universally recognized, there are cultural rules about displaying

---

Box 3.1   The six basic emotions

- Happiness, smiling mouth, and wrinkles around the eyes
- Sadness, raised brows, lowered upper eyelids and a down-turned mouth
- Anger, lowered brows are drawn together, the lips are drawn together, the eyes may stare
- Disgust, the nose is wrinkled, the upper lip raised, the brows are lowered
- Surprise, the mouth opens wide and the jaw drops, the brows are raised and the eyes open wide
- Fear, the brows are raised and drawn together, the eyes are wide open, as is the mouth and the lips drawn back tightly

---

emotions physically. Social teaching of self-control may be taken to the extreme in some oriental cultures. Emotions may also be shown in a physiological way by blushing or sweating.

Eye contact

Eyes are the receivers and transmitters of information. As indicators of mood they are the most reliable of all our facial features. Eye contact varies between cultures and sexes. Too much eye contact can be embarrassing, but too little conveys shyness, disinterest or boredom. There is a commonly held belief that 'the person who does not look you in the eye has something to hide'. Good eye contact is an essential aspect of listening skill, and it is also part of the complex structure used in conversation. Therefore the visually handicapped are particularly disadvantaged in this aspect.

Posture

Posture can reveal status, attitude, emotional level and discomfort.

Dominance may be expressed by being at a higher physical level. This is recognized by the good nurse communicator, who avoids it by automatically pulling in a chair to talk with a bed-bound patient. Perception of dominance can also be characterized by arm posture. Hands on hips, or generally waving arms about, make the body seem bigger, and therefore more important. In contrast, making the body seem smaller, for example putting the arms behind the back, is frequently interpreted as being submissive.

Orientation, that is the pointing with parts of the body, especially the head, shows whom an individual likes or respects, or who has their attention. Pointing with the head shows attention, and pointing with the body as well reinforces the signal. The leader in a crowd may be identified by being the person to which the others orientate their bodies. Turning the head and body away may be a signal of dislike, disregard, disinterest, or a wish to break off communication.

Parents and teachers tell children to stand up or sit up straight, as this gives the impression of being interested, respectful and having a positive attitude. An interested listener will lean forwards, but when interest begins to fade the body moves back, and a hand may be used to support the head. When completely bored, the body has a backward lean with legs stretched out, or shoes may be kicked off or played with.

People who are concerned about what their body is signalling, and want to create a good impression, sit facing their correspondent and lean forwards. When people know and like each other they often echo each other's posture. Mirroring another's position can help form rapport: this is a technique that is useful in counselling.

Posture may reflect a much more powerful message than words regarding emotional state. Consider the extremely anxious preoperative patient sitting bolt upright in bed; or the wide-armed joy of the child on seeing her mother; or the drooping, listless, position of the elderly man with no visitors.

When an individual has pain or discomfort the body may be held in an awkward position to give relief. The observant nurse, witnessing this, may recognize the ineffectiveness of recently administered analgesia.

Gesture

Gestures can replace speech, in which case they are known as emblems (Table 3.1). They are often used when communicating at a distance, or when there is no common language.

Each culture has its own emblematic gestures, and cross-cultural communication of this kind can be confusing and could cause serious offence.

The thumbs up sign, which as shown in the table means success in Britain, is considered very insulting in Greece and Turkey. So too is an open palm, held facing an individual, with fingers extended, a gesture that elsewhere might be used across a crowded room to indicate five. The V sign, a sign of abuse in Britain, is commonly used to symbolize victory in other countries.

Gestures are also used to complement or illustrate speech; a good public speaker will use these to keep the attention of the audience and to convey enthusiasm, for example, emphasizing points by counting out with the fingers. Gestures can be unintentional, and may reveal more about an individual's feelings than words (Box 3.2).

Box 3.2 Gestures may reveal emotion

- Embarrassment – the hand over the mouth
- Shame – hands over the eyes
- Anxiety, nervousness – nail biting and hand wringing
- Aggression – fist clenching

Spatial behaviour

Marking territory is human behaviour that is thought to lie deep in evolution. Our ancestors established territories to ensure physical survival; today it is part of our social survival.

Territorial behaviour is considered to relate to personal space, that is the immediate area around the body, and personal territory, that is the larger area around which the individual moves. The distance

---

Box 3.3 Four recognized zones. (Adapted from Hall 1966)

- The intimate zone, 45 cm (18 in). Normally reserved for lovers and close family; touch is important; whispering can be heard
- The personal zone, 0.5–1.2 m (1.5–4 ft). Touch is less important; visual cues can be seen
- The social zone, 1.2–3.7 m (4–12 ft). For more formal contact, such as conducting business; may have a barrier such as a desk. Speech and visual cues are important
- The public zone; 3.7 m (12 ft) or more. This is the distance a public speaker is placed from an audience; speech is more important than visual cues, which are difficult to see

---

Table 3.1 Significance of gestures in communication

Gesture	Meaning
Fast hand clapping	Approval, encouragement
Slow hand clapping	Disapproval
Shaking fist	Anger
Shrugging shoulders	No idea
Thumbs up	Success
Thumbs down	Failure
Nod of the head ↑↓ ↔	Agreement Disagreement

at which individuals stand or sit gives different information, according to the social setting and the relationship between them (Box 3.3).

If spatial behaviour is different from that expected by a person, they may be disturbed. A lover who keeps a distance may be signalling that there is a problem. Likewise a stranger who gets too close creates discomfort. Nurses and doctors must at times invade the intimate zone. Potential embarrassment is checked by reducing eye contact and displaying a detached facial expression.

Examples of individuals marking territory are seen every day. Members of a family have their own chairs around the meal table. Students leave their belongings on desks to reserve places while they go for coffee.

Personalizing the home or the office expresses an emotional attachment to a place, and informs others who is in control. The seating arrangement in an office conveys the occupant's expectations about how a visitor should behave. The position of the desk is the most important signal. The desk that is placed between the occupant and the visitor reinforces the occupant's sense of control; the desk that is placed against a wall to allow the occupant to sit sideways to the visitor signals that they should feel welcome and at ease. In health-care settings the desk should not be used as a barrier.

In 'home' territory the host is relaxed, which creates an advantage. A visitor, even of a higher status, is at a disadvantage. The host can lead and maintain conversation and will often win an argument. This knowledge is used in the workplace, for example by a subordinate who wishes to obtain agreement from a senior colleague on a controversial matter. By strategically holding the meeting in the junior's office, the advantage of home territory will make a favourable agreement more likely.

The community nurse with an uncooperative new diabetic patient may organize an education programme at the health centre, hoping that territorial advantage will break the deadlock. Conversely the community psychiatric nurse is aware that visiting an individual at home increases the patient's confidence to seek help. Encouraging a new patient to mark personal territory around their bed space, by displaying family photographs, a soft toy or their own clothes, can assist them to adopt the new environment.

Touch

The need to touch and be touched is deep seated, rooted in infancy. How, where and when people touch can have a significant effect on a relationship. If the message conveyed is appropriate, touch is a powerful form of communication.

Touch may not be a form of communication when it is simply functional and has no personal message: the hairdresser cuts hair; the doctor examines the woman in pain. Appropriate touching varies widely from culture to culture. People from Mediterranean countries are more generous with touch than the British, the Japanese less comfortable. Social touching such as the handshake can appear to be a meaningless ritual, but if done with conviction, it can equalize status and open communication channels.

When it is difficult to express feelings with words, the comforting touch on an arm can open a channel of communication that may strengthen a relationship, and convey a feeling of warmth, support and concern. Research has shown that touch can help people talk about themselves and their problems (Pattison 1973).

Touch can be threatening if a vulnerable part of the body is touched and the threat is backed up by sexual or aggressive verbal and non-verbal language. Sexual harassment in the workplace is an example of the former.

Appearance

Physical attractiveness is an important factor in a wide range of social situations. Success in school, in business, at the job interview, may depend on physical appearance. The obese, elderly and the disfigured are at a disadvantage.

First impressions can influence assessment of personality and character, and may even affect the interpretation of what a person says and does. These impressions may prove to be wrong once all the other information is collected. Therefore physical appearance can affect communication by conveying false information.

Warmth

Warmth in people makes others feel welcome, relaxed and comfortable. Displaying warmth makes the workplace a more pleasant environment and increases communication. Warmth is displayed verbally and non-verbally.

When in conversation with others the voice should be soft and rhythmical, keeping pace with the speaker's breathing. The words used should not convey disapproval or be judgemental. Facial and body language are used to convey attentiveness, as is giving the appearance of having time and ignoring distractions. Comfortable eye contact is maintained, the mouth has a loose natural smile, the forehead is smooth and unfurrowed. The body is held upright and leaning forward slightly, facing the individual. No hunching of shoulders, folding of arms or distracting mannerism is employed.

Touching conveys warmth, for example, the firm handshake on meeting, the holding of a hand in time of stress and the affectionate hug when a goal is achieved. These actions should be done spontaneously – being self-conscious and unsure about touching can be embarrassing to all and may dissolve warmth. The rule is to be natural and sincere.

Respect

Showing respect to others conveys that they are valued. It makes them feel important, well cared for and worthwhile. Acknowledging another's presence, remembering names, keeping appointments, listening to the other's point of view, are all forms of showing respect.

Sadly, many people can relate an incident in a health-care setting which made them feel angry and rejected, such as doctors discussing a patient's condition, in their presence, without explanation. Or the anxious visitor trying to find her sister, and being ignored by nurses chatting about a social event, eventually to be told that her relative had been taken back to theatre.

People respond positively when consulted and involved. This is one of the strengths of primary nursing, which will be discussed later. It is also a strength in the nursing team, which can make the most junior member feel valued.

Ways of showing respect to others are listed in Box 3.4.

Box 3.4 Ways of showing respect to others
• When you meet for the first time, introduce yourself and shake hands • Give your undivided attention • Determine how the other person likes to be addressed, and make a conscious effort to remember their name • Refrain from gossiping about other patients or colleagues, which would question your ability to keep a confidence • Allow time for others to talk, ask for their views, do not interrupt • If you have a limited time announce this in advance • If you are late or have to cancel an appointment, explain the reason and apologise

Empathy

An understanding of the difference between sympathy and empathy is essential to be aware of how to help another in their distress or anxiety. The need to express sympathy and empathy both come from the desire to demonstrate concern for another. A sympathetic display of concern usually means uttering some reassuring words and touching the arm or shoulder of the individual. The concerned feels better; the distressed may be grateful; but nothing has changed. Empathy is displayed when the distressed is encouraged to express her feelings and unburden herself. Relief may come from the opportunity of release, and the feeling of being understood.

Example 1

An anxious patient who may have a tumour is waiting to go to theatre to have abdominal surgery. The sympathetic nurse is warm towards him, gives him a hug and tells him kindly, 'You'll be all right'. She feels that she has reassured him. The patient in his misery thinks, 'It's okay for her'.

The empathetic nurse is warm towards him. She says, 'The thought of going down to theatre is a bit frightening. What's worrying you in particular?' The patient has an opening, and he may blurt out, 'My real fear is the anaesthetic. I feel stupid, but, you see my father died under anaesthetic 30 years ago'. This conversation may continue for some minutes, the patient being relieved by the nurse's understanding of his fear.

Self-disclosure (revealing one's own thoughts and feelings) may be used when striving to let another know they are being understood.

Example 2

A colleague who has returned to work after the death of her mother is near to tears at coffee break. As well as giving her an opening to talk about her feelings, the listener may disclose her feelings on her own mother's death. This will only help if it is a similar situation (for example, the death of a dog would be unsuitable) and the disclosure is brief, giving the bereaved a good hearing. Guidelines to form an empathetic response are given in Box 3.5.

As a footnote to these two examples, it has to be said that the learner who is trying to help should not be upset when she displays sympathy in place of empathy. This is certainly more acceptable to the patient

> **Box 3.5   Steps to guide an empathetic response**
>
> - Ignore distractions
> - Give full attention to the speaker
> - Be aware of your own non-verbal communication
> - Be receptive of the speaker's verbal and non-verbal communication
> - Ask yourself, 'what does this person want me to hear?'
> - Ask an open question

or colleague than the unsympathetic response, which might be:

- Example 1 (the patient apprehensive about going to theatre).
  The unsympathetic nurse says, 'Cheer up, it'll soon be over'.
- Example 2 (the colleague who has returned to work after the death of her mother). The unsympathetic nurse says, 'You'll have to pull yourself together, time will help'.

ASKING QUESTIONS

The helping nature of the nurse's role means continually asking questions, from the admission procedure, through everyday consultation, to discharge planning. The patients, and to some extent their relatives, are questioned. Within the nursing team, questions are asked up and down the hierarchy. Knowledge of effective questioning technique may provide more useful information and save time.

Being adept at asking questions and listening are basic requirements of being a competent and considerate nurse.

Open and closed questions

Closed questions are focused to elicit a brief reply, usually yes or no. A closed question is adequate for many everyday enquiries, such as, 'Would you like a cup of tea?' or 'Do you have false teeth?'

Open questions provide more information, and so they are phrased in such a way that the respondent cannot answer yes or no. 'Do you live alone?' is replaced by 'Who is there at home?' The respondent may now talk about her sick husband, her very dear cat, or if she does live alone, her sister who lives down the street.

Open questions may usefully be started with: Who, What, Why, How, When and Where.

Exercise 3

Rephrase the following as open questions:

- *Are you on any medicines?*
- *Are you deaf?*
- *Do you have any pain?*

A line of questioning may start with a closed question – 'Have you any children?' and continue to open questions – 'How many?' and 'Where do they live?' If a closed question is used unintentionally it can be rephrased and repeated – 'Do you live on a pension?', 'What kind of pension do you have?'

Gentle questioning

Assaulting respondents with a barrage of questions is to be avoided. 'Mrs Scott, there are some things we need to know to help your stay here. Did your doctor arrange your admission? Does your daughter know that you were being rushed in? Did you get time to pick up your things? What about your pills?' The individual will become confused, and not know which one to answer first.

Mr Robb has been advised by the doctor to stay in bed, but he continually gets out of bed and walks about the ward. His nurse, getting annoyed by his behaviour, demands to know, 'Why are you refusing to follow instructions?' Mr Robb responding to her annoyance shouts, 'Mind your own business'.

The gentle approach is to ask in a quiet voice, 'What is it that prevents you from following instructions?' The reply to this is more likely to get to the root of the problem, for example, 'I once had to lie in bed before and got so constipated, it was agony'.

LISTENING

In interpersonal communication, listening is a crucial skill. In order to respond to others it is necessary to pay attention to the messages they are sending out. Effective listening incorporates empathy, warmth and respect. The listener does not judge, pass opinion or give advice.

Passive listening

Sitting quietly with someone who is anxious or upset, using touch appropriately, may satisfy the need for comfort. Silences in social conversation can be uncomfortable, therefore learning to listen takes self-discipline. When trying to help, the listener must be receptive to all the communication the speaker is demonstrating. This is more easily achieved if the listener is not thinking what to say. Silences allow time for the speaker to decide how to continue, to judge how much the listener can be trusted, and how much to reveal.

Active listening

Active listening is when an environment is created to encourage an individual to talk and seek help. It is achieved when the speaker is made aware of having the listener's direct attention, encouraged by the listener's verbal and non-verbal communication. Feelings of warmth and empathy are transmitted by eye and facial cues, body posture, and the absence of distractions. Encouraging signals used are the nod of the head, and sounds such as Mm'nn, Uh uh, Yea, Really and Okay.

The listener may refer to statements that the speaker has made, and may match his verbal comments closely, so that they follow on in a coherent fashion, reflecting the feeling or content of what the speaker has said. The main points arising from the thoughts, ideas, facts and feelings may be summarized, to help the speaker focus on the main problems.

The receptive listener may become aware that the words being said do not match the non-verbal cues. This is called incongruent behaviour, and the non-verbal cues are usually to be believed.

ASSERTIVE COMMUNICATION

The constant state of change of the last decade has made it necessary for nurses to become more forceful, and on some occasions to function as the patient's advocate. These roles require the ability to tackle confidently issues which have the potential for disagreement. Some understanding of human behaviour, in this type of communication, is necessary before studying confrontation.

Communicating assertively means speaking out about one's thoughts and meanings in a clear direct manner which does not cause offence. This approach builds self-confidence and promotes respect. In contrast unassertiveness is a failure to stand up for one's rights, and possibly those of others. It means communicating in an unsure, uncomfortable, manner which encourages others to disregard the content of the communication, and lowers self-esteem.

Communicating aggressively means acting in a manner which is loud and forceful, by the individual determined to win, even at the expense of others. This form of communication is embarrassing, hurtful and usually unproductive.

These different forms of behaviour are illustrated in Box 3.6.

Box 3.6 Characteristics indicating assertive, non-assertive and aggressive behaviour

Verbal:
- The assertive voice is firm, warm and confident, with clear direct words
- The unassertive voice is weak, wavering, apologising, failing to say what is meant
- The aggressive voice is tense, shrill, loud and authoritarian, with superior haughty words and accusations

Non-verbal:
- Assertive messages are warm and honest, eye contact is good, posture is relaxed
- Non-assertive messages are incongruent, that is, not meaning what is signalled. The eyes are averted, downcast, and the stance is stooped, uncomfortable and fidgety
- Aggressive messages are flippant, superior, sarcastic. Eyes are cold, narrowed and staring. Stance is tense and rigid, and may have hands on hips

Behaviour:
- Assertive behaviour means making one's own decisions, being direct and fair in confrontation, and creating a good impression without putting others down
- Non-assertive behaviour means letting others make one's decisions, not facing up to confrontation, and putting oneself down
- Aggressive behaviour means making decisions for others as well as self, assaultive in confrontation, and putting others down

---

Example of saying no to an unreasonable request

In a very busy ward, Student Nurse Fox is determinedly struggling to meet her patients' needs. Staff Nurse asks her to run to pharmacy to collect non-urgent drugs. She wants to refuse without causing offence.

Non-assertive refusal:
'Um well okay if you say so'.
(Nurse Fox feels cross, frustrated, and put upon.)

Aggressive refusal:
In a loud cross voice, 'Why do you always pick on me, you allocate me the most difficult patients, and now you want me to go on an errand, to stop me getting on with my work.'
(Nurse Fox thinks 'Well that's done it, just when I need a good assessment')

Assertive refusal:
Using a firm pleasant voice and good eye contact, 'No, I can't go just now, my patients are needing a

lot of help, it must be important or you wouldn't have asked, I'll go later if that would help.'
(Nurse Fox is pleased as Staff Nurse understands.)

Guidelines to help when saying no to unreasonable requests are given in Box 3.7.

Exercises 4 and 5

4. *A friend asks you to lend her money. You have carefully budgeted your money and have none to spare. Phrase an assertive refusal.*
5. *A married senior colleague asks you to go out on a date. Your social life is going through a dull patch, and you know the marriage is troubled, but you do not want to go. Phrase an assertive refusal.*

CONFRONTATION

Aggressive confrontation may be hurtful, destructive and generally unhelpful. Avoiding confrontation may produce feelings of guilt, regret and frustration. Assertive confrontation is necessary when another's behaviour is potentially damaging or when they are invading the rights of others.

Example of assertive confrontation

You notice that on several occasions, your colleague, Joan, has breached Health Board Policy, by giving the controlled drug key to the house doctor without accompanying him to check the drug. You realize that any discrepancy would place her in line for disciplinary action. This is your assertive confrontation (good eye contact, a clear strong voice):

Joan, I've noticed that you've let the doctor have the controlled drug key, without going with him to the cupboard. You know that's against the rules. I'm concerned that you'll get into trouble if a mistake is made, or if a drug goes missing. I'd like you to stop trusting him with the

---

Box 3.7   Useful steps when saying no to unreasonable requests

In a steady clear warm voice, maintaining good eye contact:

- State your refusal very near the beginning of the reply
- Indicate briefly your reason
- Communicate your understanding of the requester's problem
- Suggest an alternative solution

Box 3.8   Useful steps in assertive confrontation

1. Be specific about the behaviour
2. State why the behaviour is a problem
3. Ask for a change of behaviour
4. Stress the benefits of change or the consequences of not changing

---

keys, as it would be a dreadful experience for you to be disciplined.

Box 3.8 lists useful steps in phrasing assertive confrontation.

Example showing the steps of assertive confrontation in use

Mr Scott is on a very low calorie diet which is essential for his health. His ward mate Mr Robb frequently tempts him with rich food brought in by his visitors. Requests to stop this behaviour have gone unheeded. Mr Scott has asked to have his bed moved, but this is difficult. Assertive confrontation is the alternative.

Mr Robb, I've noticed you tempting Mr Scott with sweet food (step 1), that's not very kind when his doctor wants him to lose weight (step 2). I would like you to stop teasing him (step 3), and help him instead (step 4).

SUMMARY

Nurses cannot *not* communicate, therefore they must, from the very beginning, understand the complexity of human communication. Caring communication comes from an awareness and sensitivity of the verbal and non-verbal messages being broadcast, knowing how to listen, and demonstrating warmth, empathy and respect. On occasion it calls for the ability to communicate assertively, and how to manage confrontation.

THE PRACTICE OF NURSING

In the 1990s nursing is changing fast while it develops as a profession and as an academic discipline. A universally accepted definition of nursing, one which would articulate clearly the roles and functions of the nurse, does not exist. A multitude of attempts at phrasing a definition have been made. One of the classical definitions has been formulated by Virginia Henderson (1966):

The unique function of the nurse is to assist the individual, sick or well, in the performance of those activities contributing to health or its recovery (or to a peaceful death) that he would perform unaided if he had the necessary strength, will or knowledge. And to do this in such a way as to help him gain independence as rapidly as possible.

A profession must have control over the performance of its members. In the UK the right to practice as a nurse depends on registration granted to an individual by the statutory body, that is the United Kingdom Central Council (UKCC). An Act of Parliament, The Nurses, Midwives and Health Visitors Act 1979, and orders under the Act, set out the legal position by which entry to the profession is controlled. To protect the public a register is maintained of those who have qualified and registered as nurses. Legally

therefore, the professional nurse is accountable for her actions to the statutory body as well as to the law of the land.

The professional responsibility of the nurse is however wider than working within the law. Ethical and moral responsibility are also demanded, and the professional nurse is expected to function within the code of conduct as published by the statutory body (Box 3.9).

A working group commissioned by the Scottish Office Home and Health Department to review and report on the role of the professional nurse was of the view that professional nursing practice must be grounded in *health* rather than in *illness*. Though it

---

Box 3.9   Code of Professional Conduct for the Nurse, Midwife and Health Visitor. (Reproduced with permission from UKCC 1992)

Each registered nurse, midwife and health visitor shall act, at all times, in such a manner as to:
- safeguard and promote the interests of individual patients and clients;
- serve the interests of society;
- justify public trust and confidence and
- uphold and enhance the good standing and reputation of the professions.

As a registered nurse, midwife or health visitor, you are personally accountable for your practice and, in the exercise of your professional accountability, must:

1   act always in such a manner as to promote and safeguard the interests and well-being of patients and clients;

2   ensure that no action or omission on your part, or within your sphere of responsibility, is detrimental to the interests, condition or safety of patients and clients;

3   maintain and improve your professional knowledge and competence;

4   acknowledge any limitations in your knowledge and competence and decline any duties or responsibilities unless able to perform them in a safe and skilled manner;

5   work in an open and co-operative manner with patients, clients and their families, foster their independence and recognise and respect their involvement in the planning and delivery of care;

6   work in a collaborative and co-operative manner with health care professionals and others involved in providing care, and recognise and respect their particular contributions within the care team;

7   recognise and respect the uniqueness and dignity of each patient and client, and respond to their need for care, irrespective of their ethnic origin, religious beliefs, personal attributes, the nature of their health problems or any other factor;

8   report to an appropriate person or authority, at the

earliest possible time, any conscientious objection which may be relevant to your professional practice;

9   avoid any abuse of your privileged relationship with patients and clients and of the privileged access allowed to their person, property, residence or workplace;

10   protect all confidential information concerning patients and clients obtained in the course of professional practice and make disclosures only with consent, where required by the order of a court or where you can justify disclosure in the wider public interest;

11   report to an appropriate person or authority, having regard to the physical, psychological and social effects on patients and clients, any circumstances in the environment of care which could jeopardise standards of practice;

12   report to an appropriate person or authority any circumstances in which safe and appropriate care for patients and clients cannot be provided;

13   report to an appropriate person or authority where it appears that the health or safety of colleagues is at risk, as such circumstances may compromise standards of practice and care;

14   assist professional colleagues, in the context of your own knowledge, experience and sphere of responsibility, to develop their professional competence, and assist others in the care team, including informal carers, to contribute safely and to a degree appropriate to their roles;

15   refuse any gift, favour or hospitality from patients or clients currently in your care which might be interpreted as seeking to exert influence to obtain preferential consideration and

16   ensure that your registration status is not used in the promotion of commercial products or services, declare any financial or other interests in relevant organisations providing such goods or services and ensure that your professional judgement is not influenced by any commercial considerations.

acknowledged that this could represent a major shift in conception among non-nurses, where the prevailing image of the professional nurse is often associated with nurse's work in acute sectors, this view does not lessen in any way the important contribution of the professional nurse to the diagnosis and treatment of disease. It is, however, the basis from which the wider role and function of the professional nurse in our society must be understood if professional nursing skills are to be most effectively and efficiently utilized and a quality nursing service offered to patients.

The working group in its report 'The Role and Function of the Professional Nurse' (Scottish Health Service Advisory Council 1992) identified the following key elements of the role and function of the professional nurse:

- The planning of nursing required for each individual patient.
- The delivery of direct care.
- Identifying when it is appropriate for the nursing care of patients to be undertaken by those without a professional nursing qualification.
- Preparing and supporting those who do not have a professional nursing qualification to undertake such activities that are delegated to them by the professional nurse.
- The effective and efficient management and organization of resources of personnel, equipment and services directly controlled or requested by the professional nurse.
- Standard setting, nursing audit and clinical audit.

Striving to grasp the unique function of the nurse in our society is difficult because of the changing expectations of that society. The nursing profession exists to meet the health-care needs of the people. Therefore as health-care needs change, so must health care. Changes have occurred in family structure and life-style. Great scientific and technological advances have been made. All of these have altered the pattern of disease and the traditional therapeutic approach, as well as the expectations society has of health professionals. Traditionally many health-care systems, including the British National Health Service, have been illness systems. However the current trend is towards prevention, and the promotion of a healthy life-style.

Changes have also come about because of the work of nurse theorists and researchers, who, over the past three decades, have built a body of knowledge unique to nursing. This has nurtured confidence within the profession, enabling the nurse to take a more appro-priate place in the health-care team than that of the physician's assistant. Models of care are examples of the work of nurse theorists, and are included in the next section.

THE SYSTEMATIC APPROACH TO NURSING CARE

The systematic approach to nursing care is often referred to as the nursing process. The nursing process is a framework of nursing philosophy, concerned with the health and well-being of the whole person. It considers the patient's physical, psychological and social needs. The systematic approach is problem oriented, and based on the four steps assessment, planning, implementation and evaluation; this is a structure which analyses the individual's situation, gives direction to nursing care and estimates the effectiveness of the care.

Understanding the nursing process starts by recognizing that all human beings are unique, and therefore it is unrealistic to give identical care to patients because they share a medical diagnosis.

A regimen that dictates a standard mobilization plan following a physical illness denies that the person's psychological state (e.g. anxiety), and their social experience (e.g. no previous hospital admissions), are relevant to the speed of their recovery. It may also create frustration and a feeling of failure. A patient needs a mobilization plan tailored to personal needs.

The second area of understanding is in relation to the four steps previously mentioned:

- *Assessment* means recording facts relevant to the individual's life before and after seeking health care. Physical, psychological and social aspects are all considered.
- *Planning* means identifying problems, setting priorities and/or goals, and writing a care plan.
- *Implementation*, or intervention, is working with the patient, giving or assisting with nursing care.
- *Evaluation* means to ascertain the worth of this care. Is it helping the patient? If the answer to this question is no, the four steps must be repeated.

This approach to nursing care is replacing a system based on instinct and tradition, which concentrated on diagnosis and standard practice, not on the individual. To better understand this, it is useful to look back at traditional nursing routines, that is task allocation. Then the modern methods of patient allocation and primary nursing are examined for comparison.

Task allocation

The example used is a medical ward, but the routines described were common to many clinical areas. Ward 1 is a busy female medical ward with 26 beds, in a large general hospital; the year is 1970. Twenty-two of the beds are in the main ward, set out Nightingale style – one row on each wall facing each other. The staff, who work a 44-hour week, consists of one ward sister, four staff nurses, eight student nurses and two part-time nursing auxiliaries. This is a very efficient well-organized ward; it is always clean and tidy; the patients get meals, medicines and treatments on time.

Nursing regimens pertaining to a medical diagnosis are neatly printed and pinned on the office wall, as in Box 3.10.

Throughout the day the staff do tasks relating to seniority. Sister takes the night report, liaises with the house doctor, answers the telephone, takes the consultants around the ward. Staff nurse gives out medicines, does any dressings or other technical treatments. The third year student nurse will bed bath the ill patients, take blood pressures, test the diabetic urines. Second year students will bed bath less ill patients, take temperatures, give oral hygiene, be re-

sponsible for intravenous drips. First year students will do bed-pan rounds, give out commodes, do pressure-area-care rounds, test urine, feed patients. Auxiliary nurses will clean lockers, supervise tub baths, make beds, put out soiled linen. A good shift is when everything is done quickly, everyone working efficiently, the ward is always tidy, and the patients cooperative. The patients have different needs met by different nurses, and at the end of the day the sister writes the nursing report.

Patients are treated very kindly in a motherly way, they are often called 'love' and 'dear'. Doctors are called 'Sir', and very few people ever disagree with them. Patients trust them implicitly. Patients or relatives who do not cooperate, who are so miserable that they cry, moan, ask questions or complain, are likely to become unpopular.

What is wrong with task allocation? It was a method of organization that placed the institution in the centre, that is the institution was considered more important than the patient. The patient had to fit in to what was expected of their diagnosis. Many nurses did not reach their full potential, and were frustrated with routines and petty restrictions.

Ward 1 may be left behind without regret. People have changed, patients demand involvement in their diagnosis, treatment and care. Nurses demand the responsibility of caring for all of their patient's needs, of being accountable and of being involved.

Patient allocation

One method of implementing the systematic approach to nursing care, is to organize patient care by allocating small groups of patients to individual nurses. This may be done on a shift by shift basis or for some days at a time.

Ward 2 is a mixed medical ward. The year is 1985.

The ward, which has 26 medical beds, is in a large teaching hospital. There are five four-bedded rooms and six single rooms. The day duty staff consists of one charge nurse, six staff nurses, two third year student nurses, two second year students, two first year students and four nursing auxiliaries.

The patients are allocated to their nurses for a few days at a time. To enable the trained staff to supervise the students, the allocation is arranged in pairs, a trained nurse with each student. The nursing auxiliaries circulate throughout the ward making empty beds, and assisting with patients as required.

On the early shift the nurse in charge of the ward has an allocation of four patients, those in the room adjacent to the nurses' station being the most suitable. Each staff nurse and student are allocated 11 patients,

---

Box 3.10   Nursing regimens

Coronary thrombosis

Day 1:   Bedrest, with two pillows. Patient dependent for all care, pressure areas rubbed 4 hourly, must be fed, bowels should not move, must not smoke, pain relief 6 hourly. Allowed one visitor for half an hour.

Days 2 and 3: Identical to Day 1

Day 4:   Sit upright with five pillows. May wash face, clean teeth and eat without help. Aperient to be given at 8 o'clock. Allowed two visitors.

And so on until discharge on day 14.
Ward routine (again neatly printed out for guidance):

5 a.m.   Bedfast patients turned and changed.

5.30 a.m. Bed pan round. Diabetic urines collected, tested and charted.

6 a.m.   Lights on, morning tea, and medicines.

6.30 a.m. Beds tidied, counterpanes on, blinds up, ward tidied.

7 a.m.   Temperatures done by junior student, senior student takes sister round.

And so on

NB. Patients should not be encouraged to have bedpans between official bedpan rounds.

NB. Students should not waste time speaking to patients, cleaning lists are on noticeboard in the sluice.

that is two four-bedded rooms and three single rooms. The staff nurses allocate patients to students, within their area, depending on the student's ability. For example, a junior student may be allocated five patients and would not be allocated a patient who required a dressing to be done.

The morning's work starts with the nurses talking with their patients and reading the care plans. This enables care to be prioritized, which means patients will feel cared for most of the time and not attended to in conveyor belt fashion. The whole shift will be utilized. No longer is quality care judged by the speed at which it is done.

All the nursing care a patient requires will be done by their own nurse. If that nurse is a student, medicine administration will be supervised by the staff nurse. At the end of the shift the nurses write the reports for their own patients.

One criticism of this method of organization is that registered nurses are assisting patients with personal hygiene and elimination, which are tasks that could be done by untrained nurses. However, this view misses the essence of modern nursing. To provide psychological and social support one has to know an individual, that is to spend time with them. The caring nurse assisting the patient to bathe is not just involved in social chit chat, but is also involved in listening, assessing and problem solving.

Primary nursing

To many, primary nursing seems a natural progression from patient allocation. This type of ward organization means that a patient has the same few nurses for the duration of their illness. One of these nurses is the primary nurse. Helped by associate nurses, this nurse is accountable for implementing the four steps of the nursing process with the patient, and is the patient's named nurse. The primary nurse liaises with the multidisciplinary team, and deals directly with the medical staff, not through the charge nurse.

A major difference of this method of organization is in the role of the charge nurse. This changes from total control of clinical practice, to that of consultant, adviser, teacher, counsellor and researcher. To fulfil this central supportive role, the charge nurse does not usually function as a primary nurse, but in the less demanding role of an associate nurse.

Ward 3 is the children's surgical ward in a district general hospital. The year is 1993. The ward has 24 beds, arranged in five rooms of four and four single rooms. Elective surgery is carried out four days a week; emergencies and transfers from the intensive care unit may be received daily.

The staff consists of one charge nurse, four primary nurses, five associate nurses, two student nurses (following the children's branch) and two care assistants. Students from the university, and on foundation studies, are attached to the ward in a supernumerary capacity. The four primary nurses and four of the associate nurses work together for some months at a time. The other associate nurses move around weekly, to accommodate fluctuations in staffing due to study leave, holidays and so on.

A balance of around six patients for each primary nurse is maintained, occasional imbalances being adjusted quickly due to the rapid turnover of patients. The primary nurse's name is placed with that of the patient's and consultant's names, above the child's bed.

The child and parents usually meet the primary nurse on the day of admission, an earlier meeting in the clinic or the ward being easily arranged if the child or parent wishes. The parents are given visiting information cards, which include the primary nurse's name and shift rota. Parents are encouraged to be involved in their child's care, being taught and supervised in the more technical aspects by the primary nurse.

Primary nursing is not just a new way of organizing the workload. It is also a method of stretching the professional nurse's knowledge, interpersonal, technical, management and teaching skills. It is challenging and demanding.

Summary

The nursing process is based on the belief that all human beings are unique. Nursing care is therefore not only dictated by the patient's diagnosis, but by many other factors such as previous experience of illness, cultural background, pain threshold and so on. A framework of the four steps, assessment, planning, implementation and evaluation, is used to integrate this uniqueness into an organized structure for nursing. To create a climate in which to respond to individualism, task allocation must be abandoned, and replaced by patient allocation or primary nursing.

SKILLS REQUIRED TO IMPLEMENT THE NURSING PROCESS

Assessment

Acute observation skills

Acute observation skills using all of the senses, sight,

hearing, smell and intuition, are needed. Physical, psychological and social signs are observed and recorded. Some examples of these would be:

- Physical signs: colour of skin, i.e. flushed, pale or cyanosed? Is patient clean or unkempt, any smell? Temperature, pulse, respirations and blood pressure.
- Psychological signs: is patient anxious or frightened, lucid and orientated?
- Social signs: what is the patient's level of understanding? How warm is the relationship with family and friends?

Interviewing skills

A knowledge of interpersonal communication, discussed earlier in this chapter, will be of use in this section.

Explain the purpose of the interview to the patient, which is to collect information to compile a patient profile. If this is a first meeting, introductions will be made. The time and environment should be chosen to avoid interruptions. Give good eye contact, display warmth, sit facing the individual in an open position.

A form may be used to ensure that essential information is collected. The questions should be asked in order of priority (determined by the patient's condition) and in the order that is likely to facilitate a response, i.e. factual, non-embarrassing issues first.

Use open-ended questions, that is, questions starting with when, how, why and what. When a question yields an incomplete answer, rephrase it to allow a fuller response. Whenever possible use a common word or expression instead of medical terms, and never use abbreviations. Reflecting the patient's previous statement, or repeating what has just been said, will encourage more information. Do not interrupt or criticize, but do employ active listening.

If the patient is tiring, stop. Information can be added when the patient has rested. At the end of the interview, be sure to give the patient the opportunity to bring up additional information or ask questions.

Planning

Identifying problems

The patient's profile is read carefully.

Problems may be found in relation to:

- a risk factor, e.g. obesity or smoking
- a sign or symptom, e.g. pain, breathlessness
- a social factor, e.g. worried about dog
- a psychological factor, e.g. fear of dying.

It is important that the problems are written as the patient's problems, not the nurse's. For example: Mr Smith is paralysed from the waist down, the problem statement should be, 'cannot bear his weight', not that, 'he needs two nurses to help him out of bed'.

Setting goals or aims

Goals are formulated in response to identified patient's problems. Therefore there is recognition that the current state is not satisfactory, either to the patient or the nurse, and there is need for change. Goals are devised before nursing intervention is carried out. Goals should be described in behavioural terms. A framework may be used to devise goals (Box 3.11).

Using this framework the need to 'push fluids' with a patient becomes the measurable goal: 'The patient (1) will drink (2) at least six cups (3) of fluid, of his/her choice (4) between 8 a.m. and 6 p.m. each day' (5).

Implementation

Nursing intervention is planned and carried out in response to the patient's problems, needs and goals. Many practical and technical nursing skills are required to implement care, as can be seen in the care plans later in this book.

Prioritizing is a work practice skill that needs to be learned in the ward. An example of prioritizing care would be:

1. A very ill patient who has had a poor night, may be given oral hygiene, have her intravenous infusion and catheter checked, and have her position changed. Then she can be left to sleep, to be bed bathed later when there is more time and she is rested.
2. Then the lady due in physiotherapy at 9.00 a.m. can be helped to shower and get into her track suit on time.
3. The man who has a great deal of pain when his varicose ulcer is dressed will be consulted regarding

---

Box 3.11 The five elements that make up a goal. (Adapted from Binnie et al 1984)

1. WHO is to demonstrate the desired behaviour
2. The ACTUAL BEHAVIOUR
3. The RELEVANT CONDITIONS under which the behaviour will be performed
4. The STANDARD that will be used to evaluate behaviour
5. By what TIME the expected behaviour will be achieved

a suitable time to do the dressing; analgesia will be offered half an hour before.

Evaluation

This is done in an informal way throughout the time a nurse works with the patient. They may sit down together to discuss the progress being made in meeting the set goals. Formal evaluation requires the skill of writing a concise, legible, accurate report.

A written report should be specific and descriptive. Before committing anything to writing, the nurse should think:

- What have I heard?
- What have I seen?
- What do I think?
- How did the patient respond? There may be a change or a lack of change in the patient's condition when expected, or a new problem.

MODELS OF NURSING

A model of nursing is a detailed description that reflects the common understanding of what a group of nurses are trying to achieve. It is a conceptual model, that is built of ideas, beliefs and knowledge. These need to be discussed, analysed and written down in such a way that everyone shares the same perception of the model.

Understanding of the term model, in this context, may be helped by the reader thinking of being given instructions by a friend on how to find him in a large building which the reader has only seen from outside. As instructions are given, each person has an idea in their mind, a model, of how the building is laid out, where the main corridors run, and so on. If the two friends have different mental models, then the instructions given will be hopelessly confusing. But if they have the same mental model, the communication will be efficient and accurate, and the friend will be found with ease.

All nurses have an image of what nursing is, that is their own model:

- Nurse 1 may see it as a series of tasks to be got through in the quickest possible time; she may consider her colleague who explains and listens to her patients as inefficient.
- Nurse 2 may see her role as that of a surrogate mother, washing, dressing and speaking to her patients like children.
- Nurse 3 may believe that patients should be involved in their care, and that health education promotes a change in life-style.

If models were no more than images in nurses' heads, then it might well be asked if it is necessary to consider them any further. The problem is that images do not simply remain in the head – they are acted out.   (Wright 1990)

A patient being cared for by the three nurses above may have a confusing time, as may students, having to learn each supervisor's internal model. To prevent this confusion, the nursing team must discuss together what they think nursing is in the context of the work they are presently engaged in. When they decide as a group what they think nursing is and write it down, then that is the basis of a nursing model. The group may then go on to develop this model, but it is more likely that they will adapt an existing model which closely reflects their own feelings and the patient's needs. Box 3.12 lists some benefits of implementing an agreed model.

The nursing process provides the four-step framework for a systematic approach to care; a model decides the approach and content of the nursing. Together they provide the basis for quality nursing practice.

To aid comprehension it is useful to look back at what is being replaced, that is the medical model.

The medical model

The medical model has for many years been the basis of nursing and medical education and practice. The medical model concentrates on the anatomy and physiology of the human body, and how the body systems work together to create the balance that is seen as good health, that is biological homeostasis. Psychological and social aspects of the person are not emphasized, in fact any disturbance in these may be considered to be caused by a physical problem.

The medical model is concerned with diagnosis and treatment, and therefore places great emphasis on the ability to recognize signs and symptoms, to make a

---

Box 3.12 Reasons for implementing an agreed model. (After Pearson & Vaughan 1986)

- Lead to consistency of care, preventing confusion
- Give rise to less conflict within the team
- Give direction to nursing care within the area, since the goals will be understood by the whole team
- Improve understanding of the nursing care, within the multidisciplinary team
- Act as a major guide in decision and policy making because the components of the model chosen can act as a guide against which to check decisions

diagnosis and cure, or alleviate the disease. This approach has some merit when cure is possible, but if cure is not possible there may be a feeling of failure.

The medical model requires the patient to fit in to what is expected of their diagnosis, and denies their individuality. It gives status to high technology, and encourages a hierarchy of tasks in the ward. It denies the patient involvement with decision making and planning of their care. Therefore it can no longer be considered as a possible choice when nurses are selecting a model.

Three models in current use

There are many models and categories of model described in nursing literature. In this book it has been decided to concentrate on three in current use: Roper, Logan and Tierney's activities of living model; Orem's self-care model, and Peplau's model.

To enhance the understanding of each model, the text is presented under the headings:

- theories
- the goals of nursing
- the model integrated with the steps of the nursing process.

The activities of living model (Roper, Logan and Tierney)

Theories

Nursing is concerned with helping people at all stages of their life-span to achieve their optimal level of health. It is also concerned with helping people to overcome, or adjust to and cope with problems in their activities of living caused by trauma, disease and so on.   (Roper et al 1983)

The essence of this model is in understanding that all individuals are involved in Activities of Living (ALs), as in Box 3.13, which help them live and grow.

Box 3.13   Activities of living

- Maintaining a safe environment
- Communicating
- Breathing
- Eating and drinking
- Eliminating
- Personal cleansing and dressing
- Controlling body temperature
- Mobilizing
- Working and playing
- Expressing sexuality
- Sleeping
- Dying

Some of the activities of living are essential to survival, others increase the quality of life. The independent performance of these activities is affected first by the position of the person in their life-span, the very young and the elderly being more likely to be dependent. Secondly the dependence/independence continuum for each activity may be influenced by age, inborn disabilities, ill health or environment (Fig. 3.1).

Three further broad activities are identified as being used by individuals in living; these are preventing, comforting and seeking. For example, a preventing activity would be giving up smoking to improve health. A comforting activity would be to relieve a worry by sharing it with a friend. A seeking activity would be to go to the library to search for information.

This model of nursing is based on a model of living:

Nursing is viewed as helping patients to prevent, alleviate or solve, or cope with problems (actual or potential) related to the Activities of Living (ALs). Recognition of the fact that the patient's problems may be actual or potential means that nursing not only responds to existing problems but is also concerned with preventing problems, whenever necessary.   (Roper et al 1980)

The goals of nursing Nursing concentrates on enabling the individual to alleviate, manage or solve problems associated with their ALs, to help them regain independence, or to cope with being dependent. Identifying potential problems enables the individual to carry out preventing activities, and the nurse to be involved in the promotion of health. Helping the individual to regain independence also means working in close cooperation with other members of the health-care team.

The model integrated with the steps of the nursing process *Assessment* aims to ascertain what the patient can or cannot do in each of the 12 ALs, which will enable the usual routines to be discussed and problem areas to be identified. Physical, sociological and psychological aspects will be considered, for example if the patient confides that constipation is a constant problem, the nurse may gently enquire about the amount of roughage consumed in the diet, the privacy of the toilet, and what the patient usually does to overcome this problem.

At the initial assessment it may be inappropriate to discuss expression of sexuality, or dying, unless the patient volunteers the information. The authors of the model consider assessment to be a continuous process, therefore relevant information on all the activities may be added to or altered as the nurse – patient relationship grows.

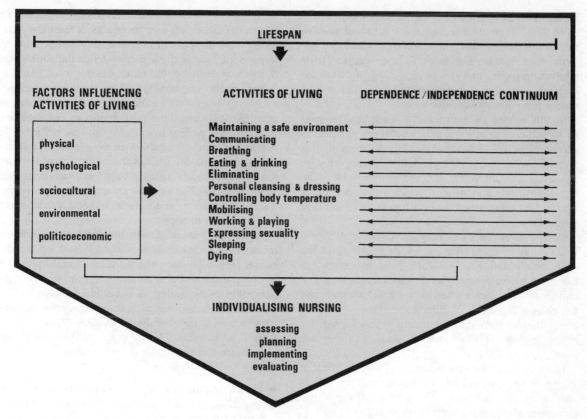

Fig. 3.1 Diagram of the model for nursing. (Reproduced with permission from Roper et al 1990, figure 5.1)

In summary, collect information on each AL by establishing:

- What does the patient normally do?
- What does the patient do or not do now?
- What actual and potential problems exist?

Planning care is done after the initial assessment. Actual and potential problems relating to the ALs are identified and written on the care plan. Potential problems often relate to the medical diagnosis and therefore may be anticipated, e.g. the postoperative bedfast patient at risk from a deep venous thrombosis. For each problem a related goal is devised, towards which the patient and nurse can work. These may be short-term, or long-term goals. The goal must be phrased in terms of patient behaviour, and not in the nursing actions needed to achieve the goal.

The nursing action may now be written. This is planning the intervention which will achieve the goal, and eliminate or reduce the problem.

In summary, when planning care:

- identify and write down patient's actual and potential problems
- set goals, describing patient's expected behaviour
- write the nursing actions to be taken.

Implementation of the care plan will comfort the patient, and enable him to receive help with dependent living activities, and prevent potential problems.

Evaluation focuses on establishing if the set goals have been achieved, in whole or in part. As stated, assessment in this model is considered to be a continuous process, therefore evaluation may include a re-examination of the patient's dependence/independence in performing ALs.

Orem's self-care model of nursing

Theories This model is based on the belief that individuals have an innate ability for self care, that is to initiate and perform activities on their own behalf in maintaining life, health and well-being. In the

1990s, many people are demanding more control over their lives. They are rejecting the traditional passive role of the patient, wishing to retain personal and parental responsibility for health, to have access to their medical records, and to be involved in decision making, planning and evaluating care. This radical model promotes this involvement.

In this model the individual's needs are referred to as self-care requisites. When self-care demand is greater than the individual's ability to meet it, this is referred to as a self-care deficit. Some self-care requisites are universal, as listed in Box 3.14; some developmental, and others, which arise out of ill health, are categorized as health-deviation self-care requisites.

Developmental self-care requisites Orem identifies a wide range of circumstances, which might affect the individual's ability to self-care. First the stages of life must be considered: the developmental stages of childhood and adolescence, the pregnant woman and the elderly. Secondly conditions which may adversely affect human development must be considered, for example, loss of employment, loss of a partner, poverty or disability.

Health-deviation self-care requisites These arise out of injury, disease or disability. Additional self-care needs may relate to changes in the individual's physical structure, physical function or to changes in behaviour. For example, the person with a swollen inflamed limb due to a deep vein thrombosis has a change in physical structure, finds weight bearing on the limb unbearably painful, and so has loss of function. The pain, discomfort and apprehension about the condition make sleeping difficult, that is a change in behaviour.

In summary, self-care deficits arise when an individual is unable to meet universal, developmental or health-deviation self-care requisites. It they are cared for by a parent, partner or friend, this is referred to as dependent care. If the self-care deficit cannot be met in this way, nursing will be required.

The goals of nursing This model encourages nurses to work with patients and their families to promote self care. This partnership works together, to enable the patient to increase self-care ability or to reduce self-care demands, with the objective of eliminating self-care deficits. That is, when a patient and his family/friends cannot cope without help, the nurse steps in. The aim of nursing is to improve the patient's situation, or to guide and teach the patient and his carers to cope.

The model integrated with the steps of the nursing process *Assessment* in this model is done by the nurse, helped by the patient, relatives and friends. It is considered to be a continuous process, with information being added as it becomes available. The universal, developmental and health-deviation self-care requisites are considered, to identify areas where there is an imbalance between the individual's ability to self care and the demand being made.

This may be done by:

- Identifying the individual's usual self-care abilities.
- Identifying the limitations on these due to present circumstances.
- Determining if problems or potential problems exist due to self-care deficits.
- Establishing if a deficit is due to a lack of skill, knowledge or motivation.
- Identifying what the patient should or should not do in meeting self-care demands in the present circumstances.

Planning Once self-care deficits, and perhaps the reasons for these, have been identified, care planning in the form of patient-centred goals and intervention may be set down.

As the long-term goal of this model is the restoration of the balance between self-care abilities and self-care needs, the extent of nursing intervention which an individual requires will only be partly dictated by their present condition. The willingness and ability of the individual, their family, and friends, to be involved will be a significant factor when writing the care plan. For example, the mother of a mentally handicapped teenager, admitted for major surgery, may indicate that she would like to bathe and care for him during this acute illness.

The nurse will help individuals meet self-care demands, by using one of these three nursing systems:

Box 3.14 Orem's universal self-care requisites

- The maintenance of sufficient intake of air
- The maintenance of sufficient intake of water
- The maintenance of sufficient intake of food
- The provision of care associated with elimination processes and excrements
- The maintenance of balance between activity and rest
- The maintenance of balance between solitude and social interaction
- The prevention of hazards to human life, human functioning and human well-being
- The promotion of human functioning and development within social groups in accordance with human potential, known human limitations, and human desire to be normal

- Wholly compensatory, e.g. the dependent acutely ill patient following major bowel surgery.
- Partly compensatory, e.g. the patient who requires assistance in managing a new colostomy, and wound dressing.
- Supportive educative, e.g. the patient coping with a colostomy, needing questions answered, and problems solved.

Intervention This is the action carried out by the nurse to enable the patient to eliminate self-care deficits.

Orem (1985) has identified six nursing actions which may assist individuals to meet their needs. These are:

- doing or acting for another
- guiding or directing another
- providing physical support
- providing psychological support
- providing an environment which supports development
- teaching another.

Evaluation is done by the nurse and the patient, who assess the extent to which the balance between the ability and the demand for self care has been achieved. The patient's perception of how care is progressing is of paramount importance in this model.

The patient-centred goals are examined to evaluate what has been achieved. It may be possible to observe the patient progress from wholly compensatory care, through partly compensatory, to supportive educative care. Alternatively new actions may have to be planned if progress is not being made.

Peplau's model

Theories The essence of this model is the need to establish and nurture the nurse – patient relationship, without which nursing would not be helpful or therapeutic. The nurse needs a clear understanding of how, and what, she communicates with the patient. She must be schooled in the arts of warmth, empathy and self-awareness, to enable her to form a close relationship with her patient.

Illness is viewed as a potential learning and growing experience for the patient and the nurse. Health allows the individual to have a feeling of well-being that enables him to live productively within society.

Failure to meet life's problems may cause frustration, stress, illness and a lack of growth. Nursing may foster growth by guiding the individual to positive behaviour.

The goals of nursing This model perceives the nurse as providing the patient with the ability to seek the best possible quality of life, or to cope with chronic illness, or dying. The nurse will also help the individual to understand his health problems and to learn from the experience of illness.

In the role of counsellor, the nurse gives the patient the opportunity to gain a greater understanding of self, to recognize their reaction to stress and to identify their coping mechanisms. This growth may enable the individual to avoid future illness. The nurse may grow through an increased understanding of the effects of stress on different individuals.

The model integrated with the steps of the nursing process This model has four phases through which the nurse – patient relationship progresses. These phases may be likened to the steps of the nursing process:

- Phase of orientation – assessment.
- Phase of identification – planning.
- Phase of exploitation – implementation.
- Phase of resolution – evaluation.

Phase of orientation – assessment Because of the nature of the model, that is, being based on the unique relationship between the individual and the nurse, there is no formal pattern to follow in this assessment. The inexperienced nurse may find it useful to refer to a mental checklist of human needs during the initial discussion.

Information is collected so that problems may be identified. Subjective and objective observations are made and documented. Subjective data is the description of the situation as perceived by the patient, objective observations are those made by the nurse.

In this phase the patient may be very anxious in his new environment and with the new experience of being ill. The nurse must employ skilful interaction, to foster trust and nurture the relationship.

The identification phase – planning This phase begins for the patient when a trust builds up with the nurse, and he begins to understand his problems more clearly. The nurse will be observing the patient for signs of behavioural change, which may give an understanding of what the patient is thinking and feeling.

At this phase of the model, the nurse will plan the care and set the goals without involving the patient, the reason being that at this stage of the illness, what the patient wants may be different from what he needs. As the relationship develops the patient's wants should get closer to his needs.

The exploitation phase – implementation In this phase

the patient is making full use of the resources around him, seeking information about his problems, and working closely with the nurse to achieve the set goals. He has a clearer understanding of his needs.

The nurse–patient relationship changes as the patient moves from dependence to independence. Care planning and goal setting are now cooperative processes.

The resolution phase – evaluation   The patient becoming independent is meeting goals, preparing to leave hospital and to lead a healthy life at home, or live independently without the community nurse's intervention. The nurse will now evaluate the situation, having learned from the experience.

The termination of the nurse–patient relationship must be planned. The sense of loss will, for the patient, be counteracted by the joy of regaining health and independence, and for the nurse, by the pleasure of helping this process.

While each phase can be discretely described, in practice the four phases also tend to overlap, and earlier phases may be repeated as dictated by changes in the patient's needs. Nurses who are observant and aware of the current phase in the nurse patient relationship tend to be more effective than nurses who are unaware of this.

Simpson (1991)

Models have been developed to give nurses a framework in which to practice. Many models have been developed by nurse theorists, then taken and adapted to suit the needs of a particular group of patients. Examples of the three models described here are illustrated in later chapters of this book.

The many facets of the nurse's role

It is difficult for many people to understand the true worth of the professional nurse of the 1990s. The gradual rejection of task allocation, in favour of patient allocation, has enabled her to remain at the bedside. As she attends to the patient's needs (often needs that a healthy person carries out in private), she is using her scientific knowledge, for example by observing the side-effect of a medicine; her technical skill, in positioning the patient; and, as the relationship develops, counselling and teaching skills.

The expert nurse at work is not difficult to recognize as she manages complex clinical situations in a caring efficient manner. Her experience and wide knowledge base enable her to make clinical judgements quickly, without having to waste time on the alternatives. The right words, those which inform, inspire and comfort, are readily available. This clinical expertise has not been adequately documented by

Box 3.15   Domains of nursing practice (Benner 1984)
1. The helping role 2 The teaching – coaching function 3. The diagnostic and patient-monitoring function 4. Effective management of rapidly changing situations 5. Administering and monitoring therapeutic interventions and regimens 6. Monitoring and ensuring the quality of health-care practices 7. Organizational and work-role competences

nurses and therefore is not widely appreciated outwith the clinical environment. Dr Patricia Benner's research in 1984 and 1989 moves some way to correct this deficit. Benner interviewed experienced clinical nurses, identified the many roles of the nurse, and these roles were then documented as the domains of nursing practice (Box 3.15).

To increase the reader's understanding of the role of the nurse, an example of the care given to one patient and his family over a few days is described in Case History 3.1. Benner's domains of nursing are identified by printing the appropriate number alongside the text. This example illustrates some of the practitioner role skills of the professional nurse, the dominant role when assuming responsibility for the nursing needs of the patient and their family. The modern nurse must integrate into this role the information from research findings as a component in achieving high quality nursing care.

RESEARCH

The research role of the nurse is not reserved for academics and teachers, it is a role that must be accepted by all practising nurses. Although not all nurses are required to initiate and implement research studies, they are however required to identify researchable problems, to assist with the collection of data and to implement research findings.

The primary task of nursing research is to develop nursing theories that serve as the scientific basis for the practice of nursing. Without research the science of nursing would not grow. Folklore and tradition would prevail, to the detriment of the quality of nursing as well as to the best use of skilled manpower.

Nurses, as professionals, accept legal responsibility for their actions and defend them on the most recently available knowledge. To be credible, this knowledge must be generated by research. Nurses must therefore

Case History 3.1

Fiona Scott is the grade F staff nurse in a 22-bedded oncology ward in a large Scottish teaching hospital. Fiona is mentor to Gillian, the third year student nurse presently shadowing her 'on duty' pattern.

This week Fiona has eight patients, one of these patients, Mr Walter Dumfries, is a 59-year-old married schoolteacher from a small town 80 miles away. Mr and Mrs Dumfries are coming to terms with his diagnosis of cancer of the larynx. He has been admitted for radical radiotherapy, which will consist of 20 treatments over a period of 4 weeks.

3   On meeting Mr and Mrs Dumfries, Fiona observes by their body language that the couple have a close loving relationship, and they are both very apprehensive. She also notes that Mr Dumfries has had a massive weight loss (his clothes are too big). In discussion she realizes that they have a sound knowledge of the diagnosis, but little understanding of radiotherapy. Over a period of 10 minutes Fiona kindly and skilfully obtains the information she requires to write her patient's care plan.

3   In writing the plan, Fiona identifies two problems
&   that will require assistance from other members of
7   the multidisciplinary team. These are nutritional requirements from the dietician, and breathing exercises from the physiotherapist. As she identifies the latter of these problems she is aware that her patient may require an emergency tracheostomy, and in the event of this unusual complication happening, knowing the physiotherapist previously will benefit Mr Dumfries.

1   Another problem identified is the distance
&   between the hospital and home. Many patients go
3   home at the weekend during radiotherapy treatment, and this is what the Dumfrieses were anticipating. Fiona is cautious – her assessment of this patient, in these circumstances, alert her to encourage the couple to consider alternative plans, which would include Mrs Dumfries being around much of the time.

2   Later, Fiona and Gillian sit down with Mr Dumfries to listen to his fears and answer his questions. The next day he will go to have his treatment planned. The medical staff have explained this, and Fiona must ascertain if this has been understood. Using pictures, diagrams and a booklet, she works with Mr Dumfries, and Gillian, to increase their knowledge.

4   On the Wednesday of the second week of
&   treatment Mr Dumfries is becoming increasingly
7   breathless, and finding swallowing more and more difficult. Fiona alerts the medical staff, and asks her colleague to take over the administration of the ward and reallocate her patients temporarily.

2   Helping her patient into a comfortable position
3   well propped up with pillows, she records his vital
&   signs every 15 minutes. Gradually he becomes
4   cyanosed. Sitting on the bed holding his hand, she reminds him of the possibility of a tracheostomy being necessary because of the swelling of the tissue in response to treatment. The medical staff efficiently assess the situation and prepare for surgery.

1   Fiona leaves her patient with a colleague for a few minutes to speak to Mrs Dumfries personally, and explain what is happening. Knowing the lady has spent time in the chaplaincy centre she suggests, gently, that she might spend the next hour in there. Going back to her patient she prepares him for the anaesthetic and, recognizing the fear in his eyes, explains confidently how previous patients she has nursed with this complication have been up moving around the room the following day.

6   Her patient having gone to theatre, Fiona
&   resumes her role as nurse in charge. She liaises
7   with the nursing officer regarding the increased workload Mr Dumfries will give the night staff and suggests that an overnight stay in the intensive care unit might be arranged. Unfortunately a bed is not available in the intensive care unit, therefore the patient must return to the ward.

5   On return from theatre with a tracheostomy tube in position, Mr Dumfries is in pain. Intramuscular diamorphine has been prescribed, and Fiona and Gillian administer this controlled drug.

3   Over the next few days the tracheostomy tube
&   requires clearing with suction, and the dressing
5   requires changing. Fiona teaches Gillian to do this. Parentral nutrition is started due to the patient's continued weight loss. Fiona ensures that his vital signs are recorded 4 hourly, in anticipation of infection due to these invasive procedures.

---

be continually aware of studies that are directly related to their own area of clinical practice. The findings of these studies must then be employed in an attempt to improve patient care. The future of nursing science depends upon the active involvement of all nurses in the implementation and utilization of nursing research.

The ability to read and comprehend research, and to understand the research process, begins by learning some research terminology. For this purpose a terminology relating to research is provided in the glossary at the end of the book.

RESEARCH DESIGN OR METHOD

Research design or method are the terms used to describe the approach adopted to undertake a research project. Three methods are commonly used:

- experimental or quantitative
- descriptive or survey
- interpretative or qualitative.

Nursing as a discipline draws knowledge from a wide range of sources each with its own style of research. The potential choice of research styles or methods for nursing research is therefore very wide and ranges from the highly quantitative methods of the biological and medical sciences, through the social sciences and humanities to more qualitative methods.   (Couchman & Dawson 1990)

Experimental research is concerned with the collection of facts and the study of the relationship of one set of facts to another. Scientific techniques are used, and the data is produced in the form of statistical analysis. This research, which produces hard facts, is familiar to nurses in the role of assisting with medical research. Most experimental · research designs are based on an experimental and a control group, as in drug trials.

This scientific approach is a problem-solving model:

- a problem is stated
- a possible explanation, that is a hypothesis, is written
- data is collected
- the data is interpreted to see if the hypothesis was right
- conclusions are drawn.

An example of nursing research might be in relation to patient education. The nurse researcher, Staff Nurse Quest of the cardiac unit, identifies that many postmyocardial infarction patients are unreceptive to health education. The hypothesis is that anxiety, regarding the possibility of sudden death in the short term, makes the patient deny the need for life-style changes. A research programme is designed, a sample of patients is chosen, and the measurement of some variables is made. Half of the patients are taught relaxation techniques, the other half (the control) are not, then the measurements are repeated. The aim of the experiment would be to see if helping the patients relax would make them more receptive to the need for life-style changes.

An advantage of this type of research is that strong conclusions may be demonstrated regarding the effects of intervention. One disadvantage is the ethical issue of withholding from a group of patients help which would generally be thought to be beneficial.

Descriptive research is the term used to describe what is going on, a survey being done to obtain information which can be analysed. Large groups of people are often used, the main purpose being fact finding. In surveys, the aim is to obtain answers to the same questions from a large number of individuals, to enable the researcher not only to describe but also to compare, and to demonstrate patterns in certain categories. The census is an example of descriptive research. In a health-care setting, a survey may be undertaken to obtain information on the effectiveness of nurse–patient communication in a ward, or department.

Information is collected by means of questionnaires, or checklists administered by the interviewer. Great care has to be taken to ensure that the respondents are truly representative of the population being surveyed. For example if 75% of the patients attending a clinic were over 70 but most of the completed questionnaires were done by those under 50, this would clearly be unsatisfactory. Wording of the questionnaire is crucial: it must be tested by doing a pilot study to ensure that all questions mean the same to all respondents.

On this occasion Staff Nurse Quest would devise a questionnaire to seek information from the patients, based on their needs for health information and relaxation classes. The questionnaire would be piloted and changed as necessary. This done, all the post-myocardial infarction patients passing through the unit would be encouraged to complete a questionnaire. At the end of a pre-arranged time-span, the researcher would have facts and statistics to assist with the setting up of a teaching programme tailored to the patients' needs.

Descriptive research is a relatively cheap way of fact finding. If the survey is well structured and piloted, it can provide answers to the questions what? when? how? and where?, but not why? Causal relationships cannot be proved by a survey – to find an answer to why? requires interpretative research.

Interpretative research is concerned with seeking insight rather than statistical analysis. It originates from the social sciences and humanities. It is based on the rationale that understanding the individual's perception and interpretation of events is the way to understand human behaviour. The two main methods of collecting qualitative data are observation and interview, the results produced therefore being words and descriptions rather than numerical data.

The case study approach is an example of this type of research. It is a detailed account of a specific instance or experience, and gives an opportunity for one aspect of a problem to be studied in depth within a limited time-scale. It allows the researcher to reveal new information, which may prove crucial in understanding the success or failure of a situation. An example of this in a health-care setting might be the introduction of a new appointment system in the diabetic clinic. The case study researcher would identify the common and unique features of that particular organization, to show how they affect the implementation of the new system.

Staff Nurse Quest, using this method of research, might arrange to carry out in-depth interviews with a few former patients of the cardiac unit. This may assist in gaining some insight into what enables some postmyocardial infarction patients to make life-style changes, while others do not. The difference between this and a survey is that the patients may reveal innovative information, which the staff may then use to help others. One of the great disadvantages of this research method is that it is very time consuming.

It is possible for these results to be analysed to produce some quantitative data which can be subjected to probability analysis, enabling proactive as well as retrospective action to be taken.

EVALUATING PUBLISHED RESEARCH

The aim of reading research critically is not to be destructive, but to make a reasoned judgement about it. The checklist given in Box 3.16 provides a method of ensuring that published research is of a high quality. However before considering implementing the findings, the nurse would first search for other research reports which replicate the results. Secondly she would assess the clinical significance of the results for her patients – for example, an improvement in the patients' comfort of 5% may not be worth the upheaval of changing practice, whereas an improvement of 60% would. Lastly she would need to discuss the cost implications and the effect on manpower within the multidisciplinary team.

QUALITY ASSURANCE

Historically there has always been a commitment to provide quality of nursing care. Measuring quality of care informally has been a traditional exercise for experienced nurses, each having internalized standards which allow the recognition of good and bad nursing care.

The present political emphasis on achieving value for money in the Health Service, the increased expectation of the consumer and the desire of the nursing profession for individual accountability, have accelerated the need for nurses to measure the standard of their care in a formal manner.

Box 3.16   Checklist for reading research

What was the study about?
- Is the research problem and/or the hypothesis stated clearly?
- Is the title descriptive?
- Is there an abstract?
- Was the research worthwhile?

Why was the study done?
- Does the paper show why the writer chose to study that particular question?
- Who funded it? Could that have caused a bias?
- Is the author an experienced researcher?

How was it done?
- What design of research was used? Some examples are:
  descriptive – use questionnaires and interviews to survey a topic
  experimental – measure variables in a controlled setting
  interpretative – use observations and interviews in natural settings
- Why was the design and method chosen?
- How were the research tools developed and are there examples of them?
- What was the response rate?
- Were changes made on the basis of a pilot study?
- If relevant, how were ethical issues taken into account?
- Are the references up to date?

Are the findings explained, justified and relevant?
- What statistical tests have been conducted? Can they be easily understood?
- How do the conclusions and recommendations relate to the research aims?
- If all the research aims have not been met, has this been discussed?
- Has the hypothesis been proven?

Setting explicit standards, writing them down, and reviewing and updating them regularly, may ensure that everyone is working together to provide the best possible care for the patient.

A quality assurance programme, or nursing audit, is a systematic approach that enables nurses to measure the quality of their care, identify good and bad practice, and where necessary plan and implement improvements.

In order to measure and evaluate, or make a judgement, about such a complex activity as nursing, it is important to see the task in some organised way. In simple terms, quality assurance involves deciding what should be, comparing what should be with reality, and identifying the gaps and taking action.   (Pearson 1987)

Quality assurance as a discipline has generated its own terminology; to enhance understanding of this section a brief glossary is provided.

QUALITY ASSURANCE PROGRAMMES

There is a choice of how a quality assurance programme may be set up, that is, whether to use a commercially developed package or to write in-house standards. The former include Qualpacs, (Wandelt et al 1974) and Monitor (Goldstone et al 1983). These are methods of measuring current nursing practice against predetermined standards.

Qualpacs

The Quality Patient Care Scale was developed by Wandelt & Agar at the College of Nursing, Wayne State University, USA (Wandelt & Agar 1974). It is a method of concurrent audit, a tool based on how nursing care is being delivered to patients at the time of delivery. It includes a review of patient records, interviews with patients and staff, and direct observation of patient and staff behaviour. The information is gathered by specially trained observers (who work in pairs to reduce observer risk), who relate the information to predetermined criteria. The interaction records contain 68 items that are arranged in six subsections:

- psychosocial: individual – 15 items
- psychosocial: group – 8 items
- physical – 15 items
- general – 15 items
- communication – 8 items
- professional implications – 7 items.

Each item is scored on a scale of 1 (poorest care) to 5 (best care), and a list of cues is provided to clarify how each item should be interpreted. Patients are randomly selected – usually 15% of the unit population. The observers spend 2 hours directly observing care and 1 hour inspecting the nursing records. It is therefore a time-consuming method, with a rather complicated scoring system.

It is generally considered that the greatest strength of this system is that the use of direct observation provides valuable data that cannot be collected by any other method.

Monitor

Monitor was developed by Goldstone, Ball and Collier 1983 (Newcastle upon Tyne Polytechnic) as an adaptation of the Rush-Medicus System. It is a method of concurrent audit, utilizing patient and nurse interviews, direct observation and the examination of patient records. Two approaches are taken to examine quality of care, that is 'Patient Monitor' in direct pa-

tient care and 'Ward Monitor' in ward procedure and management.

The audit is carried out by specially trained observers who are familiar with the tool. A random sample of patients with different levels of dependency would be invited to take part. Patient Monitor, which is described briefly in this text, uses a framework similar to that of the nursing process. Information is documented of each patient's experience in these four areas:

- assessment and planning
- meeting physical needs
- meeting psychological, emotional and social needs
- evaluation of the care.

Patients are classified into dependency categories according to their independence/dependence in the following:

— personal care
— feeding
— mobility
— nursing attention
— other circumstances (which takes into account preparation for surgery/procedures, or episodes of incontinence, etc.).

The categories are:

- category I – minimal care
- category II – average care
- category III – above average care
- category IV – maximum or intensive care.

Different questionnaires are used for each dependency category in each of the four areas. They direct the observer to ask the patient or the nurse for information, or to seek the information from the patient records. The scoring system is 1 for yes and 0 for no, not applicable is removed from the list. Therefore the nearer the score is to 100% the higher the standard of care being carried out.

Monitor has been used successfully in the UK for some years. It is labour intensive, which makes it expensive, but it is a system which has demonstrated that there are aspects of nursing care which are valid and reliable indicators of quality, and can be objectively measured.

A quality assurance programme using in-house standards

To enhance understanding of this section, the example of a quality assurance project undertaken in a palliative care ward (hospice ward) by Charge Nurse Best will be used. Jim Best and his colleagues adopted the ethos of the Dynamic Standard Setting System (DySSSy) as developed at the Royal College of Nursing by Alison Kitson (1989).

DySSSy is a problem-solving approach to audit which may be described as 'bottom-up', that is, the nurses who will use the standards set, monitor and evaluate them. Standards written this way should be practical and achievable, and are owned by the nurses who write them. They are patient centred, and have the potential for multidisciplinary use.

Using this approach requires the practising nurses in a clinical area to write their philosophy of care. In doing so they need to explore their approach to nursing in relation to holistic care and individualism, the code of professional conduct, and the spirit of the health unit in which they work. Box 3.17 shows the philosophy devised by Jim Best and his colleagues.

Objectives

The nurses identify key objectives, that is, what they hope to achieve through the programme. These will be in relation to improving quality of nursing care, making efficient use of resources, creating a climate of enquiry and promoting professional development.

We believe that a quality assurance programme:

- will demonstrate to patients, team members, and managers, that we deliver an excellent standard of care.
- will identify any problems in achieving excellence and in so doing, help us overcome the said problem.
- will encourage us to utilize research to overcome our problems.
- will lead to a sense of achievement that will maintain staff morale.

Box 3.17 Philosophy of hospice ward

We aim to keep the atmosphere on the ward as comfortable as possible, one in which everyone, be they patient or staff, is valued

Physical care and symptom control, although being of paramount importance, will not overshadow the importance of giving psychological, social and spiritual support to our patients and their loved ones

We are flexible in the care delivered to each individual, taking account of the patient's priorities and fitting in with whatever the patient feels like doing

Communication and accountability within the team are each individual's responsibility, but we recognize the need to support each other at all times

---

The quality assurance cycle

This is a series of steps that is used as a guide when setting, monitoring and evaluating standards. The cycle is circular to signify that the process may need to continue until a good standard is written.

Setting standards The first step is to identify the *topics* and *sub-topics* of the standards. The topic, that is the broad category of the standard to be set, is identified. This is a useful way of grouping standards together in an organized fashion. In this example pain control is the topic.

Sub-topics may then be identified. These are more specific areas in which it should be possible to promote and demonstrate an improvement with an identified care group. In this example the sub-topic is the use of opiates.

The next step is to identify *standards* and *criteria*, that is to describe nursing in measurable terms (the following is adapted from Kemp & Richardson 1990).

Standards, which are often written down as standard statements, should be:

- realistic, that is, achievable
- understandable – clear, simple language must be used
- measurable – suitable to be used with an audit tool
- appropriate and acceptable for a particular group of patients.

Criteria should be:

- related to the response one would expect for the standard being measured
- descriptive of nursing responsibility, patient involvement and/or relevant resources
- reliable, so that the data is consistent, accurate and suitable for statistical analysis
- valid and free from bias.

There are usually three types of criteria described – structure, process and outcome (the following is adapted from Sale 1990).

Structure refers to factors in the organization that enable the work to be carried out, such as:

- the physical environment
- equipment
- staffing, including skill mix and numbers
- educational facilities
- ancillary services
- management and personnel.

Process refers to the performance, that is the care the nurse gives to the patient. Process criteria describe what action must take place in order to achieve the standard:

- the assessment techniques and procedures
- methods of delivery of nursing care
- methods of patient education
- methods of communication
- methods of documenting
- how resources are used
- evaluation of competence of the staff carrying out nursing care.

Outcome is the end result of care and performance – what is expected and desirable, in a specific and measurable form, in relation to:

- patient behaviour
- patient response
- level of knowledge
- health status.

Standard statement and criteria from the hospice ward

Topic: pain control.

Sub-topic: use of opiates.

Care group: terminally ill patients.

Standard statement: each patient's pain will be kept at what he/she considers an acceptable level without causing stupor or confusion.

Structure criteria:

- the nurse has a knowledge of pain assessment and control in patients with terminal cancer, the drugs and the methods of administration
- the patient's prescription is clearly written and the indication stated
- the ward will have a stock of the full range of opiate drugs and the appropriate equipment for administration, including syringe drivers
- the skill mix will reflect the number of registered nurses required to administer controlled drugs promptly
- the nurse has access to current literature on pain control.

Process criteria:
The nurse will:

- observe the patient's body language when still and on being moved
- discuss pain control with the patient using a pain assessment tool
- liaise promptly with the medical staff regarding uncontrolled pain

- alleviate the patient's fears and concerns regarding opiate analgesia
- monitor bowel movements and administer regular aperients
- acknowledge and investigate observations made by relatives, domestics, etc.

Outcome criteria:
The patient will:

- discuss any fears regarding uncontrolled pain
- understand the need to take regular aperients when taking opiates
- recognize circumstances and activities which increase pain, and discuss avoidance of these
- recognize and ask for help immediately before pain reaches an unacceptable level.

The standard will now be discussed within the ward team. Changes may be made and once agreement is reached the standard will be implemented, care being taken that the structure criteria have been met.

Monitoring To monitor the standard an audit tool is used. Audit tools are data collection systems which use either concurrent information, that is, whilst the nursing is still in progress, or retrospective information, after the nursing is completed.

Methods of *concurrent* information collecting include:

- Open chart auditing, comparing the patient's charts and nursing notes against pre-set criteria.
- Patient interview, or completion of a questionnaire.
- Direct observation of nursing care, either of the care given by one nurse or a group of nurses.

Methods of *retrospective* information collecting include:

- Audit of the patients' charts and nursing notes – an agreed percentage of the records of patients who have been discharged are examined by an outside agent.
- Post-care conference – audit of patients' charts, nursing notes, progress and outcome of care, carried out by an in-house team.
- Post-care patient interview or questionnaire.

In this example Nurse Best and his colleagues opted for a retrospective, monthly post-care conference. Each of the ten registered nurses in the ward examined the charts and notes of one patient (approximately 20% of all patients). The process of data collection required the nurse to note any incidence of uncontrolled pain or constipation from each patient's notes and records.

Evaluation   If the data demonstrates that the standard is being met, then the exercise has been successful. If it has not been met, the review of the data should indicate where the problem is, and that area of care can be improved. It is essential to ensure that the care is given according to the agreed standard: 'If this vital last step is not taken, then there has been little point in the exercise, and there will be no improvement of patient care. Where standards are found to be low, or there is poor quality of care, action must be planned and taken to change practice.' (Sale 1990.)

Charge Nurse Best opted for an in-house method of quality assurance which he found brought a high level of commitment and cooperation within the team. As the work progressed confidence and morale grew, as well as a realization that this was a continuous process that would have no end.

There is a tendency to consider monitoring of quality in nursing practice to be management responsibility. In the present climate, if clinical nurses do not take the initiative to monitor their own standards of care, it will be done for them. This would then be a missed opportunity, as a quality assurance programme can be an effective means of generating change to improve patient care, as well as producing an audit.

The trained nurse has been well prepared by her education to give quality care at the bedside, in the clinic and in the home. Those who would confine her to the role of manager, or supervisor of care assistants, fail to understand that to ensure the standard of care the consumer expects it is necessary to ensure the skill mix is heavily weighted in favour of trained nurses. Higgins & Dixon (1992) confirmed that 'investment in employing qualified staff, providing post qualification training and developing effective staff methods of organising care pays dividends in providing quality care'.

Suggested assignments

1. Students are often encouraged to keep a clinical diary for the purpose of reflection. Material from this diary can be used with the guidelines in this chapter as an exercise on how an empathetical response might be phrased. Take an entry from your diary in which a sympathetic or an unsympathetic response has been made. Using the guidelines in Box 3.5, phrase an empathic response.
2. Read the Code of Professional Conduct for the Nurse, Midwife and Health Visitor in Box 3.9. You may want to make some notes. Discuss the implications of the Code for students of nursing and midwifery.
3. Having read the section on Models of Nursing, identify the nursing model being used in your clinical area. Compare and contrast the theory with the reality.
4. With at least one other colleague, select a piece of research from a nursing journal. Working independently, read the piece of research critically using the checklist in Box 3.16. Meet up with your colleague and spend some time contrasting and comparing your impression of the published paper.

REFERENCES AND FURTHER READING

Benner P 1984 From novice to expert: excellence and power in clinical practice. Addison-Wesley, California

Benner P 1989 The primacy of caring: stress and coping in health and illness. Addison-Wesley, California

Binnie A, Bond S, Law G, Lowe K, Pearson A, Roberts R, Tierney A, Vaughan B 1984 Systematic approach to nursing care. Open learning package. Open University Press, Milton Keynes

Boore J 1978 A prescription for recovery. Royal College of Nursing, London

Couchman W, Dawson J 1990 Nursing and health care research. Scutari, Harrow, ch 5, p 43

Falconer A 1992 Effective interaction with patients. Churchill Livingstone, Edinburgh

Goldstone L, Ball J, Collier M 1983 Monitor: an index of the quality of nursing care for acute medical and surgical wards. Polytechnic Products Ltd, Newcastle upon Tyne

Hall E J 1966 The Hidden Dimension. Doubleday, New York

Hayward J 1975 Information – a prescription against pain. Royal College of Nursing, London

Henderson V 1966 The nature of nursing. Macmillan, New York

Higgins M, Dixon P 1992 Skill mix and the effectiveness of nursing care. Nursing Standard 7 (4): pp 18–21

Kemp N, Richardson E 1990 Quality assurance in nursing practice. Butterworth-Heinemann, Oxford, pp 32, 33

Kitson A 1989 Dynamic standard setting system (DySSSy). Royal College of Nursing, London

Lees S, Ellis N 1990 The design of a stress management programme for nursing personnel. Journal of Advanced Nursing 15: 948–950

Nelson-Jones R 1990 Human relationship skills, 2nd edn. Cassell, London

Orem D 1985 Nursing: concepts of Practice, 3rd edn. McGraw Hill, New York

Pattison J 1973 Effects of touch on self exploration and the therapeutic relationship. Journal of Consulting and Clinical Psychology 40: 170–175

Pearson A 1987 Nursing quality measurement. Quality assurance methods for peer review. John Wiley, Chichester, ch 1, p 2

Pearson A, Vaughan B 1986 Nursing models for practice. Butterworth-Heinemann, Oxford, ch 1, p 5

Porritt L 1990 Interaction strategies, 2nd edn. Churchill Livingstone, Edinburgh

Roper N, Logan W, Tierney A 1980 The elements of nursing. Churchill Livingstone, Edinburgh

Roper N, Logan W, Tierney A 1983 Using a model for nursing. Churchill Livingstone, Edinburgh

Sale D 1990 Quality assurance. Essentials of nursing management series. Macmillan, London, ch 2

Scottish Health Service Advisory Council 1992 The role and function of the professional nurse. Scottish Office Home and Health Department, Edinburgh

Simpson H 1991 Peplau's model in action. Macmillan, London, ch 2, p 10

UKCC 1992 Code of Professional Conduct for the Nurse, Midwife and Health Visitor, 3rd edn. UKCC, London

Wandelt M, Ager J 1974 Quality patient care scale. Appleton Century Crofts, New York

Wright S 1990 Building and using a model of nursing, 2nd edn. Edward Arnold, London, ch 1, p 2

Wright S 1990 My patient – my nurse. The practice of primary nursing. Scutari, Harrow

4

Science and the art of nursing

Anne Waugh

INTRODUCTION

The aim of nursing is to provide holistic patient care and, in order to achieve this, the nurse must understand the patient or client and his perception of health and ill health (see Ch. 2). This must be considered in relation to the point on the health–illness continuum at which the health problem has arisen (see Ch. 1). Nursing assessment (see Ch. 3) is carried out at the beginning of the nurse–patient relationship and thereafter at appropriate intervals. This should identify actual and potential problems related to the circumstances that brought the patient or client into the health-care system. Care planning should then take into account management of these problems in an appropriate order of priority. Life-threatening situations must be resolved first and then other concerns according to their short- or long-term significance.

In order to achieve this, the nurse must understand the principles of nursing practice and adapt them to meet individual patient requirements. She must also be familiar with the pathology of common disorders and her caring role before and after investigations and various forms of treatment. This chapter provides an introduction to these aspects of nursing under the headings:

- optimizing nutritional status
- maintaining fluid balance
- balancing needs of rest vs mobility
- managing pain
- preventing spread of infection
- knowing the nature of common disorders
- knowing the nature of investigations
- understanding the nurse's role regarding prescribed treatments

The common patient problems and general principles of practice introduced here are then developed and applied appropriately to specific care situations throughout this book.

OPTIMIZING NUTRITIONAL STATUS

Nutrition is concerned with the processes by which we take in material from the environment and use it to maintain and promote body function. Eating, digestion (mechanical and chemical), absorption and utilization of nutrients are all involved in nutrition. A **nutrient** is any substance which is digested, absorbed and utilized to promote body function. The main groups are:

- carbohydrates
- fats
- proteins
- minerals
- vitamins.

It is important to bear in mind that when **eating**, the focus is often on the food which makes up the **diet** rather than its underlying purpose of providing **nutrients**. A **balanced diet** provides appropriate amounts of all nutrients to meet body requirements and contributes to well-being in specific ways described in this section. The main functions of nutrients are production of heat and chemical energy, and promotion of tissue growth and repair.

Eating is considered a pleasurable activity by most people. It is not only a vital activity for health but is also an important aspect of social behaviour which is influenced by many factors which will be considered. The role the nurse plays in helping people meet their nutritional requirements in health, and also when they are ill, or unable to eat is discussed at the end of this section.

ENERGY

Metabolism describes all chemical activity which takes place within the body. Chemical breakdown of large compounds into smaller ones is called **catabolism**. Conversely, **anabolism** describes metabolic processes in which simple substances are combined into more complex compounds.

Units of energy

Energy is produced as a result of catabolism of carbohydrates, fats and proteins. In 1960, the International System of Units (SI units) was introduced and the **joule** replaced the calorie as the unit of energy:

1 kilojoule (1 kJ) = 1000 joules (used for food portions)
1 megajoule (1 MJ) = 1000 000 joules = 1000 kJ (used for daily energy requirements)

Energy requirement

This is determined mainly by basal metabolic rate (BMR). BMR is the amount of energy required to maintain involuntary functions (e.g. cellular respiration, heartbeat, breathing) at rest. BMR is measured at rest in a warm environment, several hours after a meal. Factors which affect BMR are shown in Table 4.1. Daily energy requirement is determined by the same factors that effect BMR. Values for daily energy requirement are shown in Table 4.2.

NUTRITIONAL STATUS

This term denotes the state of health produced by a person's dietary intake.

Table 4.1 Factors which affect basal metabolic rate (BMR)

Factor	Effect on BMR
Primary factors	
Sex	Greater in men than women
Age	Greater in children, decreased in elderly people
Muscular activity	Increase in relation to both intensity and duration of exercise
Secondary factors	
Digestion	Greater after meals (specific dyanamic action of food), decreased in starvation
Thyroxine	Thyroid hormone which increases BMR
Fever	Increases BMR
Pregnancy and lactation	Increase BMR
Mental state	Acute anxiety and other emotional states increase BMR, severe depression reduces BMR

Table 4.2 Daily energy requirements		
Activity level	Men (MJ)	Women (MJ)
Sedentary	10.50	8.80
Moderately active	12.50	10.50
Active	14.75	12.50
Very active	17.85	15.75
Pregnancy (last 3 months)		11.50
Lactation		12.50

Nutritional assessment

This process is used to measure nutritional status. Accurate assessment is based on several types of data:

- physical measurement
- biochemical data
- nutritional history.

The nurse often makes a judgement of a patient's nutritional status using her observation and interview skills. Signs of poor nutritional status are shown in Box 4.1.

NUTRIENT GROUPS

Carbohydrates

This group of nutrients includes all dietary sources of sugar and starch. Such foodstuffs include bread, potatoes, cereals, biscuits, confectionery, milk, preserves, fruit and sugar itself. Carbohydrates are the major dietary source of energy, providing 16 kJ per gram.

Box 4.1 Features which may indicate poor nutritional status

Dietary history
  Nutrient groups not all taken in diet
  Inappropriate energy intake
Physical assessment
  Overt obesity or emaciation, muscle wasting
  Body weight 20% greater or less than suggested weight for height
  Skin: dry or scaly
  Gums: swollen or bleeding
  Teeth: discoloured, decayed broken or missing
  Lips: cracked, swollen or inflamed
  Eyes: sunken; pale conjunctiva
  Hair: dull, brittle, sparse, dry hair
  Nails: ridged, easily broken, irregularly shaped
  Behaviour: listless, lethargic, confused, depressed
Symptoms
  Anorexia, indigestion
  Constipation, diarrhoea
  Short-term weight loss or gain

Carbon, hydrogen and oxygen are the elements from which carbohydrates are formed. Carbohydrates are classified according to the size of the molecule:

Monosaccharides are simple sugars: glucose, fructose and galactose. Simple sugars are absorbed into the circulation from villi in the small intestine.

Disaccharides consist of two chemically bound monosaccharides. Disaccharides are maltose, lactose and sucrose. Enzymes must divide disaccharides into monosaccharides before they can be absorbed.

Polysaccharides are composed of many thousand monosaccharide units and include starches, glycogen and cellulose. Dietary sources include cereals, pulses and vegetables. Not all polysaccharides are digestible, although some are rendered so by cooking. If undigestible, they remain in the gastrointestinal tract as fibre. Digestible polysaccharides are broken down to monosaccharides which can then be absorbed into the circulation.

Fibre

It is now recognized that fibre plays an important function in many parts of the gastrointestinal tract. Fibrous food requires more chewing and promotes salivation. Both of these activities in turn promote healthy teeth and gums. Gastric emptying is delayed and the appetite is satisfied for longer. The hygroscopic nature of fibre increases the bulk of the residue within the gastrointestinal tract, which in turn promotes peristalsis and reduces the occurrence of constipation.

The highly refined diet characteristic of the Western world has been implicated as a predisposing factor in the high incidence of diverticular disease and possibly large bowel cancer. Contemporary health education therefore aims to increase dietary fibre in Western countries.

Fate of absorbed monosaccharides

Blood containing nutrients absorbed from the gastrointestinal tract travels to the liver via the hepatic portal vein. In the liver, fructose and galactose are converted into glucose.

Fate of glucose

Blood glucose levels are maintained within a narrow range irrespective of energy requirements and meal times. This is achieved by endocrine hormones, predominantly insulin and glucagon, which are secreted from the Islets of Langerhans in the pancreas. Following a meal, the blood glucose level rises and insulin is secreted in response to this rise and reduces blood glucose levels (see Ch. 16).

When blood glucose levels fall, glycogen stores in the liver and skeletal muscles are mobilized mainly under the influence of glucagon. This restores blood glucose levels to normal limits and meets increased demand.

Blood glucose levels can also be maintained when short-term glycogen stores are exhausted by either catabolism of fat (stored in adipose tissue) or tissue protein.

Glucose is continually required by all cells as a substrate for energy production. Entry into most cells requires insulin and energy production is most efficient in the presence of oxygen. Complete metabolism of glucose results in production of chemical energy (stored in chemical bonds as adenosine triphosphate, ATP), heat, carbon dioxide and water. Water formed in this way is known as 'metabolic water'.

In the absence of insulin, plasma glucose levels rise and symptoms of diabetes mellitus arise (see p. 568). Excessive carbohydrate intake predisposes to obesity in the long term.

Proteins

These large molecules contain the elements carbon, hydrogen, oxygen and nitrogen. Dietary protein is the only source of body nitrogen. Proteins may also incorporate elements such as sulphur and phosphorus. During digestion proteins are broken down into their constituent units: amino acids. These are absorbed into the circulation from the villi in the small intestine.

Twenty different amino acids exist and the body is able to synthesize many of them by converting one into another, a process known as **transamination**. Those amino acids which cannot be synthesized in the body must be eaten in the diet, and are called **essential amino acids**. After absorption, amino acids are reassembled within body cells into the proteins needed for cellular growth and repair. Proteins play a vital role in metabolism, as all enzymes and some hormones are proteins. Blood clotting and muscle contraction also depend on the presence of specialized proteins.

In the absence of other substrates, proteins are used as a source of energy yielding 17 kJ per gram. Amino acids can be converted into glucose by the liver, a process known as **deamination**. The amino group is converted into ammonia and then urea which is excreted in the urine. Disruption of liver function can result in accumulation of ammonia which has serious

consequences (see p. 535). If urea cannot be excreted due to renal failure, its accumulation causes uraemia (see p. 595).

Nitrogen balance

As protein is the only source of dietary nitrogen and excess amino acids cannot be stored, a regular protein intake is necessary to prevent breakdown of existing protein to meet metabolic requirements.

Negative nitrogen balance is present when dietary protein intake does not meet body needs and may be a result of either increased requirement (e.g. lactation, growth spurts and illness) or decreased intake (e.g. starvation, fasting, dietary imbalance or major loss). Sources of dietary protein are more expensive than other nutrient groups and therefore poverty frequently predisposes to a low protein intake and negative nitrogen balance. Consequences of inadequate protein intake and negative nitrogen balance include poor wound healing, muscle wasting and loss of strength. **Positive nitrogen balance** is achieved by providing protein in excess of minimum requirements to prevent or manage these situations.

Fats

Ingested fat is broken down by digestion to fatty acids and glycerol which are absorbed into the lymphatic system by lacteals in the villi. After entering the circulatory system via the thoracic duct, utilization begins. Fatty acids and glycerol provide heat and energy. Complete metabolism yields 37 kJ per gram, which is twice the energy yield of carbohydrates and protein. Excess is converted to triglycerides and stored in adipose tissue. Retroperitoneal deposits of fat protect the abdominal organs and subcutaneous deposits provide insulation. These deposits are also long-term energy stores. Fats play an important role in the transport of fat-soluble vitamins and form the major part of cell membranes.

Additionally, fat makes the diet more palatable and prevents the rapid return of hunger after a meal as it reduces the rate of gastric emptying.

Two types of fat are recognized: saturated and unsaturated. Saturated fats are typically hard and sources include fatty meat, butter, cream and cheese. Unsaturated fats are softer and sources include vegetable oils and nuts.

Minerals

A summary of minerals and trace elements and their

functions is found in Table 4.3. These essential constituents of the skeleton, body fluids and soft tissue must be included in the diet as they cannot be synthesized within the body. The trace elements chloride, magnesium, phosphorus and sulphur are all present in living matter and therefore very seldom pose a dietary problem.

Water

All metabolism activity requires a fluid medium, and water constitutes 65–70% of adult body weight.

Sources include fluids taken, and many foodstuffs have a high water content. Small amounts of 'metabolic water' are formed as a waste product of energy production.

Vitamins

Vitamins are essential for health and must be taken in the diet as they cannot be synthesized in the body. They are classified according to their solubility: water-soluble vitamins, B group and C (Table 4.4); and fat-soluble vitamins A D E and K (Table 4.5). These

Table 4.3 Major minerals

	Functions	Daily requirements	Sources	Excess	Deficiency
Sodium	Principal extracellular cation, maintains osmotic pressure of extracellular fluid Along with calcium, gives bone its rigidity Salts assist in maintaining homeostatis of acid–base balance, e.g. sodium bicarbonate Makes the diet palatable	Not established	Table salt, meat, fish, most processed foods, used as a preservative	Rare in health as excess excreted in urine If present causes oedema	Rare in health as depletion is prevented by action of aldosterone on the renal tubules Occurs in Addison's disease, severe diarrhoea and vomiting
Potassium	Principal intracellular cation maintains osmotic pressure of intracellular fluid Required for muscle contraction and conduction of impulses along nerves	Normal diet provides 2.5 g RDA not established	Fish, meat, vegetables, fruit (especially citrus fruits and grapes)	Occurs in renal disease Results in cardiac arrhythmias	Occurs following severe diarrhoea, diabetic (hyperglycaemic) coma and diuretic therapy Results in muscle weakness and cardiac arrhythmias
Calcium	Major constituent providing strength to bones, teeth Required for muscle contraction, conduction of nervous impulses, normal heart rhythm, blood clotting	500 mg 1200 mg in pregnancy and lactation	Milk, cheese, eggs, cereals, green leafy vegetables	Arises from tumour of parathyroid gland Results in kidney stones (calculi)	Results in tetany, ulcers, osteomalacia, (adults) rickets (children) bruising
Iron	Required for formation of haemoglobin	Male 10 mg Female 12 mg Pregnancy 13 mg Lactation 15 mg	Red meat, liver, egg yolks, oatmeal, pulses, green vegetables, chocolate		Iron deficiency anaemia (see p. 487)
Iodine	Required for synthesis of thyroid hormones	0.15 mg	Shellfish, vegetables grown near the sea, iodized salt	Decreased synthesis of thyroid hormones	Cretinism (children) Myxoedema (adults) (see p. 560)
Fluorine	Constituent of teeth and bones	1.5–4.0 mg	Fluoridated water	Mottling of teeth	Dental caries (tooth decay)

Table 4.4 Fat-soluble vitamins – A, D, E, K

Vitamin	Daily requirement	Functions	Dietary or other sources	Deficiency symptoms
A (*retinol*) Precursor- carotene 1) Converted to Vitamin A in walls of small intestine	750 µg	1. Assists in the synthesis of mucous secretions which prevent epithelial tissues from hardening 2. Maintains normal vision in dim light. Visual purple (rhodopsin), present in the rods of the retina is decomposed in bright light and restored by Vitamin A 3. Promotes good tooth structure by producing ameloblasts (enamel-producing epithelial cells) 4. Promotes normal growth in children	Animal sources – liver, chicken, kidneys, eggs, whole milk, butter, fish liver oils, fortified margarine Plant sources – (precursor) carrots, leafy green and yellow vegetables, fruit	Follicular hyperkeratosis Xerophthalmia. Nyctalopia (night blindness, poor adaptation to dim light) Prone to infection of mucous membranes. Poor tooth formation.
D (*calciferol*)	2.5–10 µg	1. Aids normal skeletal development 2. Facilitates absorption of calcium and phosphorus	Action of ultra-violet rays of sunlight on skin Dietary sources – eggs, butter, oily fish, cod-liver oil Artificial sources – produced by irradiation of plant sterols – medications, fortified margarine	Rickets in children Osteomalacia in adults Poor teeth Lowered blood calcium and phosphorus levels Poor posture
E (*tocopherols*)	20 mg	1. Helps in formation and function of red blood cells 2. May protect red blood cells from haemolysis 3. Protection of essential fatty acids 4. Anti-oxidant	Vegetable oils, green leafy vegetables, wholegrain cereals, wheatgerm, egg yolk, nuts	Not recognized
K (*phytomenadione*)	Very small amount met by dietary intake and bacterial synthesis.	Assists in the formation of prothrombin in the liver Necessary for the coagulation of blood	Green leafy vegetables, wheatgerm	Prolonged clotting time of blood Haemorrhagic disease of the newborn

tables also show the functions of vitamins and their deficiency states.

Water-soluble vitamins, as their name suggests, readily dissolve in water and are easily excreted. They are not therefore stored in the body and accumulation is not a problem. In contrast, fat-soluble vitamins cannot leave the body dissolved in water and if intake is excessive, they may accumulate.

Processes used in the preservation and storage of foodstuffs can inactivate their vitamin content.

EATING AND DRINKING

When a person is unable to carry out these physical requirements there is clearly a role for a carer to assist. This may arise as a result of ill-fitting dentures, absence of teeth, or a disorder of the mouth or gums. Difficulty with chewing or swallowing also poses problems. However in addition to practical help with these activities the nurse must also be aware that there are psychological and social factors which influ-

Table 4.5   Water-soluble vitamins – B complex, C

Vitamin	Daily requirement	Functions	Dietary sources	Deficiency symptoms
B₁ (*thiamine*)	0.4 mg for every 4200 kJ of intake	Necessary for complete metabolism of carbohydrates	Meat (especially pork) Liver Nuts Wholegrain and enriched cereals and bread Brown rice and wheatgerm Milk, dairy foods, eggs Brewer's yeast	*Beriberi* with symptoms: polyneuritis anorexia, fatigue, depression, irritability, pain, weakness and incoordination of leg movements abnormal carbohydrate metabolism
B₂ (*riboflavin*)	1–2 mg	Necessary for cell oxidation and reduction processes and efficient use of carbohydrates, proteins and fats	Wholegrain and enriched cereals Milk, dairy foods Liver Eggs Leafy vegetables Liver concentrates	Greasy, scaly skin Stomatitis Cheilosis Bloodshot eyes, blurred vision Glossitis
B₃ (*niacin, nicotinic acid nicotinamide*)	10 mg	Essential for tissue oxidation and needed by central nervous system to maintain mental health	Meat, especially liver and kidneys Fish and poultry Wholegrain and enriched cereals Pulses Nuts Milk and eggs	*Pellagra* with symptoms: depression or dementia dermatitis diarrhoea
B₆ (*pyridoxine*)	Trace	Important in metabolism of amino acids Regulation of nervous system	Lean meats Wholegrain cereals, Dried yeast Walnuts Leafy green vegetables	In infants, convulsions
B (*folic acid*)	Trace Increased need in pregnancy	Essential for development of red blood cells	Green leafy vegetables Yellow fruits and vegetables Yeasts, meats Nuts, milk	Megaloblastic anaemia
B₁₂ (*cyanocobalamin*)	Trace	1. Necessary for formation and maturation of red blood cells (see Ch. 14) 2. Needed for functioning of all cells particularly of bone marrow, nervous system and gastrointestinal system	Animal sources – liver, kidneys, fish, beef, milk and dairy products	Megaloblastic anaemia due to: 1. inadequate intake of Vitamin B₁₂ (e.g. vegetarians) 2. deficiency of intrinsic factor (e.g. Addisonian pernicious anaemia, total gastrectomy) 3. bacterial or parasitic interruption of normal absorption in alimentary canal 4. malabsorption syndromes
C (*ascorbic acid*)	30–70 mg	1. Production of collagen 2. Necessary for growth and tissue repair 3. Aids absorption of iron in gastrointestinal tract 4. Formation of red blood cells in bone marrow	Citrus fruits, tomatoes, leafy green vegetables, potatoes, small berry fruits	1. Weakness, proneness to infection, pains in limbs and joints 2. *Scurvy* – prolonged deficiency

ence them. When buying and preparing food, it is important to remember that for most people, food and not nutrients is the focus of activity.

Psychological factors

Knowledge about different foodstuffs and their place in a balanced diet is needed to enable appropriate selection of food. This may be influenced by emotion resulting in treats or indulgence for comfort. Eating disorders such as obesity or anorexia nervosa (see Ch. 9) may also affect selection of food. Fatigue, lethargy and depression may lead to neglect of shopping, preparing and eating. These activities may also be affected by locomotor functioning and facilities at home for storing and cooking food. The influence of the media is important in reinforcing knowledge about what good food is. However, food advertising is frequently targeted at fast foods and convenience foods which often are not as healthy as they are claimed to be. Such foods frequently have a high content of sugar, salt or saturated fat.

Social factors

Eating is a social activity, initially governed by culture, family background and sometimes religious requirements. Mothers have significant influence on dietary intake in the early years of life. They not only select food for their children but also determine how it is prepared, presented and eaten. This will frequently depend on availability and budget. When a child goes to school, other factors begin to influence his choice. These include catering arrangements for school meals and preferences or habits of his peers.

During adolescence, independence from home requires independent decisions about buying and preparing food. A working knowledge of basic nutrition is then necessary to maintain health. Throughout life, changing circumstances may require changes in eating habits. In the later years, reduced mobility, low pension and loss of one's spouse (especially in men) can predispose to poor nutrition in elderly people.

HEALTH EDUCATION

Education about good nutrition is important in order to enable people to make healthy choices in selecting the food they eat. This targets many places:

- school
- media
- hospital.

In a wide variety of settings the nurse is in a position to influence and also educate her clients about many aspects of health including eating.

Recommendations on dietary intake have been made in order to improve health and reduce the incidence of illness caused by poor eating habits in the UK. The report of The National Advisory Committee on Nutrition Education, (NACNE) (1983) and of the DHSS Committee on Medical Aspects of Food Policy (the COMA report) (Department of Health and Social Security 1984) contain recommendations on which health education regarding dietary intake should be based. These include reducing dietary fat and sugar, increasing fibre, and preventing obesity.

MODIFIED NUTRITIONAL REQUIREMENTS

For some patients, freedom to determine their own dietary intake is restricted according to their specific nutritional requirements. This is frequently a modification to an oral diet. In these situations, the nurse plays an important role in reinforcing dietary advice. Other means of maintaining nutritional status include nasogastric feeding and parenteral nutrition and it is a nursing role to manage such regimens.

Modified diets

Some diseases result in specific dietary requirements and the nurse must be aware of these in order to provide an appropriate dietary intake:

- diabetes mellitus (see Ch. 16)
- diseases of the liver and biliary tract (see Ch. 15)
- diseases of the kidney (see Ch. 17)
- diseases of the cardiovascular system (see Ch. 12)
- anaemia (see Ch. 14).

Obesity

This condition is present when a person weighs 120% of his ideal weight. Obesity develops as energy intake continually exceeds requirements, the excess being converted to fat and stored in adipose tissue. Once gained, extra weight often proves hard to shed. Success requires increased energy expenditure and reduced energy intake. Unless there is substantial motivation to lose weight, a patient will require a great deal of reinforcement and encouragement to adhere to a reducing diet.

Predisposing factors include excessive intake of carbohydrate and fats which may arise for a variety of reasons, such as economy, habit or comfort derived from eating. Adoption of a less energetic lifestyle, either in employment or leisure activities, will also lead to weight gain unless energy intake is reduced.

Obesity is a predisposing or precipitating factor in many illnesses including diabetes mellitus, cardiovascular diseases and joint disorders. In addition risks associated with surgery increase. It is therefore important to maintain body weight within limits determined by one's height.

The value of drugs and surgery in treating obesity is questionable.

Nasogastric feeding

A nasogastric tube may be passed in order to meet fluid and nutritional requirements when a patient cannot swallow safely but has a functioning gastrointestinal tract. Such situations include blockage of the oesophagus, unconsciousness or impairment of the swallowing reflex.

Appropriate feeds are usually commercially prepared and provided by the dietitian according to individual requirement. Continuous feeding given via a fine bore tube at a constant rate over several hours each day may be used. Alternatively, intermittent bolus feeds are warmed to 37°C and administered every 2–4 hours via a wider bore tube. In either situation it is considered physiologically beneficial to rest the gastrointestinal tract overnight and feeds are therefore given during the day. Principles of practice are listed in Box 4.2.

Total parenteral nutrition

Also known as hyperalimentation, total parenteral nutrition (TPN) involves infusion of a solution of sterile nutrients into a central vein in order to meet individual nutritional requirements. The solutions used are chemical irritants, especially to small peripheral veins, and are therefore infused into a large central vein to minimize this problem. TPN contains all the necessary nutrients in a readily utilizable form: energy as glucose and/or a lipid emulsion, nitrogen source as amino acids, trace elements and vitamins.

Indications include negative nitrogen balance, for example after extensive burns and major trauma or surgery. Long-term parenteral nutrition is sometimes necessary in some cases and patients are carefully taught how to manage their own treatment at home.

Principles of nursing practice are listed in Box 4.3.

Box 4.3   Principles of nursing practice – TPN

- Maintain constant infusion rate by using a volumetric pump to prevent fluid overload or hyperglycaemia
- Maintain a fluid balance chart
- Record blood glucose levels frequently to detect hyperglycaemia until insulin requirement is accurately identified
- Prevent infection:
  Never use the line for administering drugs or other fluids
  Use aseptic technique when dressing the entry site
- Detect infection promptly by recording temperature, pulse and respirations 4 hourly
- Offer frequent mouthwashes or oral hygiene to counter reduced salivation
- Collect 24-hour urine specimens as requested to monitor electrolyte and nitrogen balance
- Provide psychological support to enable the patient to adapt to loss of psychological, social and physical pleasures associated with eating
- Provide care of a central venous line

Box 4.2   Principles of nursing practice – nasogastric feeding

- Before administering feed, check correct position of the tube by either:
  Aspirating gastric contents and testing its acidity by observing blue litmus paper turn red, or
  Injecting air down the tube and listening for bubbling through gastric juice using a stethoscope over the stomach
- Follow principles of good hygiene to prevent contamination of the feed
- Record volumes given on the fluid balance chart
- Record when the patient's bowels have opened as there is increased risk of constipation as the feed does not contain fibre
- Provide frequent oral hygiene (see gastric aspiration above)

MAINTAINING FLUID BALANCE

In health homeostasis, or balance of body fluid and electrolytes, is maintained. Excess fluid intake is excreted in urine which is formed by the kidneys. Although its main constituent is water, urine also contains electrolytes and metabolic waste products including urea and creatinine. The minimum daily volume of urine required to excrete waste products is 500 ml, and a healthy person passes 1000–1500 ml of urine per day, depending on fluid intake.

Should the control mechanisms be unable to maintain homeostasis, signs of imbalance appear and serious consequences may arise. These include oedema and dehydration and the nurse is frequently in a position to observe the onset of the signs and symptoms. A fluid balance chart may be required to monitor fluid intake and output. Sometimes fluid intake is maintained by giving fluid through a nasogastric tube or an intravenous infusion. A urinary catheter may be required to monitor urine output. The nurse's role in these situations is explored at the end of the section.

DEHYDRATION

Dehydration occurs when fluid intake does not meet body water requirement. In an attempt to conserve fluid and maintain the blood volume and its composition, depletion of extracellular fluid occurs. Fluid losses are then minimized and signs of dehydration (Box 4.4) may arise.

In severe cases, circulating blood volume may also decrease causing signs of shock, tachycardia, hypotension, pale, clammy skin, which may be accompanied by anxiety and restlessness. Coma and death can follow.

Dehydration has more serious consequences in children and elderly people who have less body water and can therefore withstand water losses less easily. Pyrexia, or fever, increases water loss through sweat and signs of dehydration may arise if fluid intake is not increased to compensate for increased loss.

OEDEMA

This term describes accumulation of interstitial fluid and is accompanied by swelling of the affected tissues. Commonly oedema is a result of systemic disease (often a cardiac or renal disorder) or local trauma.

Box 4.4 Signs of dehydration

Thirst – experienced and relieved by increasing fluid intake

Dry mouth – the tongue and oral mucosa dry out as salivation decreases. Furring of the tongue and discomfort follow

Skin – appears flaccid as extracellular fluid becomes depleted and dry as sweating is reduced

Low urinary output – occurs as water reabsorption in the distal renal tubules is maximized. Urine becomes more concentrated, appearing darker than its normal pale amber colour

Constipation – occurs as water absorption from the large intestine increases

Sunken eyes – may be observed as extracellular fluid around the orbit is depleted

---

Formation of tissue fluid

Normally the volume of plasma and interstitial fluid remains constant as a consequence of continuous movement of fluid out of and into capillaries. Blood entering the capillaries from the arterial circulation is propelled both along and through the capillary walls. Blood pressure, or hydrostatic pressure at the arterial end, is greater than at the venous end of the capillary. Osmotic pressure is exerted by the plasma proteins and acts as an inward force, drawing fluid into the capillary.

At the arterial end of the capillary, the outward hydrostatic pressure exceeds the inward osmotic pressure and the net effect is movement of water from the capillary to the interstitial space.

At the venous end of the capillary, the inward osmotic pressure exceeds the outward hydrostatic pressure and the net effect is movement of water from the interstitial space into the capillary. Small lymphatic vessels also play an important role in returning interstitial fluid back into the circulation.

When this mechanism of continual fluid exchange is disrupted, fluid may accumulate in the interstitial space causing oedema. Causes of oedema are shown in Table 4.6.

Sites of oedema

When **dependent oedema** occurs, the location is determined by gravity and the person's position. In an ambulant or sitting position, it occurs initially in the feet and ankles. With increasing severity, it may also affect the legs. In some cases **pitting** is observed on affected areas. This means that when firm finger pressure is applied, an indentation in the skin remains when the finger is removed.

In pulmonary oedema (see Ch. 12) congestion of the venous capillaries in the lungs causes accumulation of fluid in alveoli. The patient experiences acute breathlessness. This is accompanied by a productive cough and frothy sputum is expectorated.

Localized oedema may occur at many other sites and examples are given in Table 4.6.

Irrespective of the cause, it is important to recognize that oedematous or swollen tissue is susceptible to damage. Accumulation of interstitial fluid impairs capillary blood flow into oedematous tissue and the cells receive less oxygen and nutrients. Metabolic waste products accumulate in affected tissue. Should this tissue then be compressed between a bony prominence and a firm surface such as a bed or chair, capillary blood flow is further impaired. The potential

Table 4.6 Causes of oedema

Mechanism	Effect and examples
Increased arterial hydrostatic pressure	More fluid is forced out of the circulation than is able to return, e.g. overtransfusion of IV fluids, caused by salt and water retention, circulatory overload, particularly susceptible are those with cardiac or renal failure
Decreased plasma osmotic pressure	General depletion of plasma proteins, e.g. nephrotic syndrome
Increased capillary permeability to plasma proteins	Localized effect, e.g. inflammation
Increased venous hydrostatic pressure	Localized venous obstruction impedes return of fluid to venous capillary, e.g. tight stockings, bandages, plastercasts, sitting with legs crossed at the knee, sitting with bend of the knee at the edge of a chair Impaired skeletal muscle pump of lower limbs causes pooling of blood in veins, e.g. bedrest
Impaired lymphatic drainage	Local obstruction of lymphatic drainage prevents return of interstitial fluid e.g. diseased lymph nodes or following surgical removal of lymph nodes (see Mastectomy p. 632).

for development of pressure sores (see p. 235) is increased in such situations. Oedematous areas, particularly those over bony prominences, must therefore be carefully assessed for early signs of pressure sores.

USE OF A FLUID BALANCE CHART

When it is likely that physiological fluid balance cannot be achieved, a record is kept of all fluid intakes and outputs over each 24-hour period in order to monitor fluid status. In hospital, some patients may have additional sources of fluid intake and loss (Table 4.7).

This data is of great diagnostic significance and its accuracy is a major nursing responsibility.

Fluid intake

It is sometimes necessary to encourage extra fluids

Table 4.7 Intakes and outputs recorded on a fluid balance chart

Intakes	Outputs
Oral fluids Intravenous infusion (blood transfusion, parenteral nutrition)	Urine Gastric aspirate or vomit Diarrhoea Wound or other drainage (e.g. chest aspiration, ascitic fluid)
Nasogastric feeding (jejunostomy tube)	Insensible loss (sweat, water vapour from lungs)

and the nurse will have to provide drinks very frequently. This may be facilitated by offering a varied selection of fluids rather than many glasses of room temperature water from the patient's water jug.

In other cases restriction of oral fluid is necessary. The challenge to the nurse is to provide small amounts spaced over the 24 hours, remembering that some fluid is also required to swallow drugs. Providing ice cubes to suck and frequent oral hygiene can alleviate the sensation of thirst.

When a patient is unable to drink, dehydration is prevented by administering fluid via a nasogastric tube or an intravenous infusion.

24-hour balance

This is calculated at the same time each day and is the difference between total intake and total output. The balance may be positive or negative. Negative balance arises when more fluid has been lost than taken in, and is often the aim when treating oedema. Positive balance means that more fluid has been taken in than lost. This is the aim of treatment in dehydration.

Daily weight

When recorded before breakfast this provides an accurate indicator of fluid lost or gained in the previous 24 hours.

URINARY CATHETERIZATION

A catheter may be passed into the urinary bladder for many reasons including:

- accurate monitoring of urinary output in seriously ill patients
- investigation or treatment of the urogenital tract
- control of haemorrhage following prostatic surgery
- maintenance of a dry environment in urinary incontinence where other measures have proved ineffective.

A variety of catheters is manufactured and appropriate selection depends on the sex of the patient, its purpose and expected length of use. Longer catheters are needed for males (40–45 cm) as the urethra is longer than the female urethra for which a 20–25 cm catheter is used. Catheters designed for long-term use are more expensive but have a silicone coating to reduce urethral irritation. Diameter, balloon size and tip shapes also vary.

Indwelling catheters have at least two lumens, one

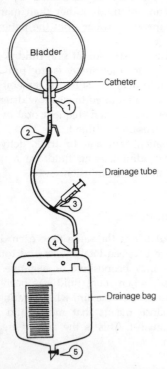

Fig. 4.1 Points at which bacteria can enter a urinary drainage system. 1, the urethral orifice; 2, connection of catheter and drainage tube; 3, where sample of urine taken; 4, connection of drainage tube and collecting bag; 5, drainage bag outlet. (Reproduced with permission from Roper et al 1990, figure 10.4)

to inflate a balloon keeping the catheter tip within the bladder and another for drainage of urine. This lumen is connected to a drainage bag forming a sterile closed circuit (Fig. 4.1). A third lumen if present is used to introduce irrigation fluid. Principles of nursing practice are listed in Box 4.5.

INTRAVENOUS INFUSION

An intravenous infusion is used to maintain adequate fluid intake in the following situations:

- when oral and nasogastric routes are unavailable
- when it is unsafe for a patient to swallow, e.g. unconsciousness
- when absorption from the gastrointestinal tract is impaired
- for administration of drugs.

A cannula is inserted into a peripheral vein, usually in the hand or forearm. In children the scalp vein is commonly used. There are situations where access to the superior vena cava or right side of the heart is required. A central vein is cannulated to:

- measure central venous pressure
- administer total parenteral nutrition
- administer some drugs
- insert a temporary pacemaker.

Fluid infused fall into two main categories, clear fluids and blood products. Blood and its products include plasma and synthetic substitutes, platelets and clotting factors. Blood transfusions require additional specific care and are explained on page 493. Clear fluids including 5% dextrose, Normal saline (0.9% saline) and Hartmann's solution are given to meet requirements for fluid and electrolytes, in contrast to parenteral nutrition which also meets nutritional requirements.

The following formula is used to calculate the rate of flow for prescribed intravenous fluid:

$$\text{Drops per min (Flow rate)} = \frac{\text{Volume to be infused (ml)} \times \text{drops per ml}}{\text{Time of infusion (min)}}$$

The number of drops per ml delivered by a particular administration set is indicated on its wrapper.

Principles of care are shown in Box 4.6.

Box 4.6   Principles of care for an intravenous infusion

- check infusion fluid according to local policy
- check prescribed flow rate is correct at least hourly
- exclude air from the circuit to prevent entry to the bloodstream and air embolism
- maintain system intact to prevent haemorrhage and introduction of infection
- provide frequent oral hygiene to ensure oral mucosa remains moist as salivary flow, normally increased by eating, will be reduced
- ensure the comfort and security of line by applying splint and bandage as necessary
- anticipate increased dependence due to restricted function of limb used for access
- anticipate finite lifespan of the infusion and observe for pain and inflammation at the site.

NASOGASTRIC TUBES

A nasogastric tube is passed via the nose and oesophagus into the stomach for one of the following reasons:

- to aspirate gastric contents, or
- to feed a patient.

Gastric aspiration

This is carried out to prevent nausea and vomiting due to accumulation of gastric secretions which occurs when peristalsis is impaired. This is often called paralytic ileus. Gastric aspirate decreases as peristalsis and bowel sounds return. Accurate recording is the nurse's role, and is an important diagnostic aid.

The nasogastric tube may be attached to a drainage bag to allow continuous drainage or it may be closed off with a spigot as aspirated using a syringe at regular intervals. Principles of care are as follows:

- provide frequent oral hygiene to compensate for mouth breathing and reduced salivation
- record volumes of aspirate on the fluid balance chart

- record characteristics of the aspirate in the nursing notes
- always ensure the tip of the tube is in the stomach before putting fluid into the tube (Box 4.2).

Nasogastric feeding

Indications for nasogastric feeding and related principles of care are explained on page 99.

BALANCING NEEDS OF REST VS MOBILITY

The ability to move about enables us not only to meet our basic needs such as eating and drinking, but also to work and carry out leisure activities which maintain our social contact and self-esteem. Additionally, exercise promotes well-being, fitness and optimizes functioning of the locomotor system. Rest and sleep are also required to maintain health. Sleep is discussed in Chapter 8.

Complete rest in bed may be dictated by unconsciousness, critical illness or physical confinement due to traction. While such patients may not be in a condition to fully appreciate loss of the benefits of mobility, they become dependent on nursing staff both to meet their needs and to prevent them developing the following hazards of immobility:

- stiffness of joints leading to restricted movement and eventually contractures
- pressure sores
- deep venous thrombosis and pulmonary embolism
- chest infection
- constipation
- boredom and loss of self-esteem due to increased dependence.

Mobilizing increases oxygen requirement which is met by increased cardiac output and respiratory effort. In health there is capacity for increases in both of these parameters to meet increased demand. However, for those patients who already have impaired reserves due to cardiac or respiratory problems, exercise may lead to further compromise in function and exacerbation of the original problem. In such cases, a doctor may recommend less exertion and more rest.

Other patients may benefit from increased rest. During fever, there is already an increased demand for oxygen, and patients are encouraged to rest in order to prevent further increases in demand for oxygen. Patients with painful conditions exacerbated by movement may be encouraged to rest, for example to promote healing of a damaged limb. Other patients who are in pain, for example postoperatively, may voluntarily reduce their attempts at mobility to minimize pain which will predispose them to other potential problems. A similar situation may occur in people who are suffering from fatigue, lethargy or depression who may be inclined to spend much time sitting around.

Patients may therefore either benefit from reduced mobility or voluntarily reduce exertion and in both cases are at increased risk of developing hazards of immobility.

It is important to identify any restrictions imposed on mobility and to plan nursing care appropriately. Following a period of bedrest a programme of gradual mobilization (Box 4.7) is implemented with the aim of promoting mobility without over-tiring the patient. Criteria indicative of tiring are identified for each patient depending on their underlying problem. These criteria may include breathlessness, palpitations, perspiration, sweating and pain on exercise. It is important to tailor the amount of planned exercise to the patient's condition and to increase this as his condition permits. If an exercise-related symptom returns, more rest will be necessary and the gradual mobilization plan adapted appropriately.

Box 4.7   Example of a programme of gradual mobilization

Days 1 and 2	Bedrest
Day 3	Up to sit in a chair for half an hour (twice)
Day 4	Up to sit in a chair for an hour (twice)
Day 5	As day 4, plus walk to toilet or bathroom, wheeled back on a chair
Day 6	As day 5, plus walk back from toilet
Day 7	Mobilize freely in the ward
	As able before discharge: take an immersion bath, climb stairs

---

MANAGING PAIN

Pain is a distressing experience arising from actual or potential tissue damage. The physical sensation may be accounted for by physiological theories which will be considered later. However, perception of pain also has subjective components: psychological and social. For the nurse an appropriate definition is:

pain is what the patient says it is, existing when he says it does   (McCaffery 1983)

It is important for the nurse to learn to assess pain effectively and to provide pain relief whenever possible. These issues are examined in this section.

TYPES OF PAIN
Acute pain

This is characterized by sudden onset and frequently accompanies organic disease. When the underlying cause is dealt with, the pain ceases. Acute pain is highly localized, that is, its site can be located precisely. When severe, acute pain is accompanied by increased pulse and blood pressure. The patient may also appear pale, anxious and restless. These signs are a result of increased activity of the sympathetic nervous system. Other symptoms may be associated with the experience of pain or its disappearance, for example, exercise or nausea and vomiting. These relationships may be of diagnostic significance.

Chronic pain

In contrast to acute pain, chronic pain is a long-term sensation, and is often defined as having lasted more than 6 months. The feeling may be constant, spasmodic or recurrent and its site diffuse, having unclear boundaries. The onset of chronic pain is insidious and there is often no organic cause apparent. The patient may adapt to chronic pain by appearing withdrawn, depressed or listless. Signs of increased sympathetic nervous system activity which accompany acute pain are usually absent. Causes of chronic pain include cancer, arthritis and slow-healing injuries such as burns, although for many sufferers, no cause is identified.

Referred pain

This is present when pain arising from an internal organ is perceived as coming from another area of the body. Pain in the left arm is often a sign of cardiac disease.

FUNCTIONS OF PAIN

Pain has a **protective** function. Children learn by experiencing pain not to repeat certain behaviours which will cause them harm; for example, touching hot or sharp objects. Its presence following physical injury will result in resting a sprained ankle thereby promoting healing. Rest also relieves the pain of angina (see Ch. 12). Severe pain in any part of the body is likely to result in the sufferer seeking medical advice for treatment of the underlying cause.

Health-care professionals use the presence of acute pain as a **diagnostic tool**, its nature and location being in some cases characteristic of a particular condition. Changes in severity of the pain may be indicative of improvement or deterioration of the underlying cause. The nurse's skill in observation may assist accurate diagnosis and facilitate effective management.

THEORIES AND PATHWAY OF PAIN

A painful stimulus results in activation of receptors for noxious stimuli known as nociceptors. Not only do physical stimuli such as heat, pressure and sharp objects but also chemical substances released during the inflammatory process (see p. 118) activate nociceptors usually found in the skin.

Activation of nociceptors results in the generation of nervous impulses in a sensory nerve which are conducted to the spinal cord and then upwards to the brain (Fig. 4.2). Transmission of impulses across synapses between neurones is mediated by chemicals called neurotransmitters. Within the brain, the thalamus is the seat of pain sensation and it has neural connections with other areas including the limbic system (concerned with memory and emotion), the basal ganglia (concerned with movement) and the cerebral cortex which localizes and integrates incoming signals. Complex mechanisms mediate perception of and reaction to pain, and involve many sites within the brain.

The specificity theory

This theory postulates that different types of nociceptor exist for the sensations of touch, heat and pain. The nociceptor then relays impulses to discrete centres within the brain which distinguish between touch, temperature and pain.

The intensity theory

In this theory it is proposed that only one type of nociceptor exists and that the intensity of its stimulation and subsequent input to only one centre in the brain allows distinction between degrees of pressure and extreme pressure which causes pain.

The gate theory

This theory, devised by Melzack and Wall in 1965, proposes the existence of gates in the pain pathway.

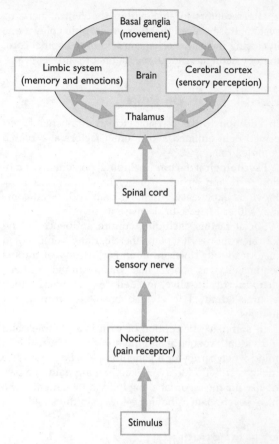

Fig. 4.2 Diagrammatic representation of the pain pathway

These gates, within the spinal cord, can either be open or closed. When the gate is open, pain impulses pass through and are transmitted to the brain. The gate can also be closed. In the same way that a swing door may be opened from either side, both downward influences from the brain and upward impulses to the brain may close the gate. Stimulation of sensory nerves by gentle rubbing near the site of pain is thought to close the gate preventing transmission of upward impulses in the pain pathway. Downward impulses from higher centres can also close the gate, for example feelings of relief may reduce the impact or severity of perceived pain.

This more elaborate theory can explain the influence of emotions on perception of pain, and also the observation that rubbing a painful area can bring pain relief.

Many neurotransmitters have been identified within the pain pathway. These include endogenous opiate-like substances including endorphins which act on opiate receptors located within the central nervous system. It is believed that these endorphins play a role in closing the gate mechanism within the spinal cord, thereby acting as central mediators of pain.

PERCEPTION OF PAIN

In addition to the physiological component of perceived pain outlined above, other factors also play a complex role.

Psychological factors including personality, emotion, fear and anxiety can heighten perceived pain. Previous experience of similar pain and its outcome may either increase or decrease its severity.

Social factors, including culture, influence behavioural responses to pain, the Spartans being noted historically for stoicism. In an early study of trauma victims, it was shown that war-wounded soldiers, thankful to be alive, needed less analgesia than victims admitted to civilian hospitals with similar injuries.

In summary, perception of pain is a complex and individual experience and the nurse must bear this in mind when caring for a patient in pain. She must also make every effort to avoid stereotyping pain to a particular diagnosis, or labelling individual patients who have severe pain as having a low pain threshold.

PAIN ASSESSMENT

Because perception of pain is an individual experience, and pain assessment is a skilled nursing role which must be based on good communication, in order to assess pain, the nurse must find out its characteristics in relation to the factors listed in Box 4.8.

Tachycardia, hypertension and pale, sweaty skin are signs of increased activity of the sympathetic nervous system which may also be apparent.

In addition to the information gained from verbal interaction, the nurse must also observe for apparent non-verbal cues. A patient in pain may grimace or frown, clutch or rub the affected area or adopt an unusual posture such as the fetal position to protect the affected site.

The nurse then compares verbal and non-verbal clues to make her interpretation of the situation. This observation skill is particularly significant when the patient is unable to communicate verbally; for example, young children, people with learning difficulties, or those with impaired speech following cerebral damage.

It important to remember that when a patient describes characteristics of pain that this is then subject to interpretation by the nurse before action is taken. Use of a pain assessment tool enhances objectivity by allowing the patient to make his own judgements about his pain.

PAIN ASSESSMENT TOOLS

For the reasons above, the use of pain assessment tools is highly desirable. Many such tools are available and include linear rating scales with either numbers or adjectives which act as prompts, or for children, frowning or smiling faces (Fig. 4.3). In each case, the patient indicates the point on the scale which represents his pain.

More complex assessment can be carried out using The London Hospital Pain Observation Chart (Fig. 4.4). In addition to assessment of severity, many sites and means of pain relief can be included enabling a pain profile to be identified and then evaluation of nursing interventions.

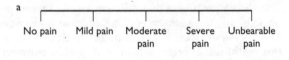

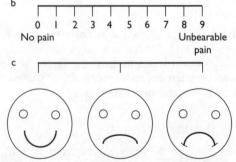

Fig. 4.3 Pain assessment tools (see also Fig. 4.4)

Box 4.8 Factors considered in pain assessment

- Location(s)
- Severity
- Nature, e.g. sharp, throbbing
- Duration – continuous or intermittent
- Precipitating factors, e.g. eating, exercise
- Associated symptoms, e.g. nausea, vomiting, fainting
- Effective methods of pain relief

The London Hospital
PAIN OBSERVATION CHART

This chart records where a patient's pain is and how bad it is, by the nurse asking the patient at regular intervals. If analgesics are being given regularly, make an observation with *each* dose and another *half-way between* each dose. If analgesics are given only 'as required', observe two-hourly. When the observations are stable and the patient is comfortable, any regular time interval between observations may be chosen.

To use this chart, ask the patient to mark all his or her pains on the body diagram. Label each site of pain with a letter (i.e. A, B, C, etc).

Then at each observation time ask the patient to assess:

1. The *pain in each separate site* since the last observation. Use the scale above the body diagram, and enter the number or letter in the appropriate column.
2. The *pain overall* since the last observation. Use the same scale and enter in column marked *overall*.

Next, record what has been done to relieve pain. In particular.

3. Note any *analgesic* given since the last observation, stating name, dose, route and time given.
4. Tick any other *nursing care* or *action taken* to ease pain.

Finally note any *comment on pain* from patient or nurse (use the back of the chart as well, if necessary) and initial the record.

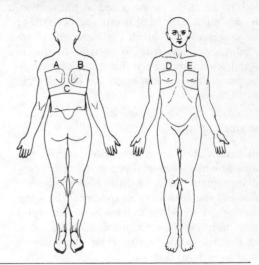

Date _____ Sheet number _____   Patient identification label

Time	Pain rating										Measures to relieve pain (specify where started)										Initials
	By sites								Overall	Analgesic given	(Name, dose, route, time)	Lifting	Turning	Massage	Distracting activities	Position change*	Additional aids*	Other*	Comments from patients and/or staff		
	A	B	C	D	E	F	G	H													

Adapted from the London Hospital Pain Observation Chart

Fig. 4.4 Pain observation chart. (Adapted from the London Hospital Pain Observation Chart)

NURSING MANAGEMENT OF PAIN

The aim of nursing intervention is to provide effective pain relief. Various strategies which may be employed by the nurse are described in this section. In acute pain rapid pain relief is often achieved, and analgesic drugs can be given 'as required'. With chronic pain, however, relief is usually harder to achieve and often requires continued use of medication. The principles of management for chronic pain are outlined below.

Relief of fear and anxiety

Fear and anxiety often accompany pain. Sources may be identified by using active listening, direct eye contact and appropriate touch which all help the patient to feel safe and able to express his concerns. The nurse may either be able to help with these herself or report them to a more experienced member of the team. Ensuring that the call button is within the patient's reach reassures him that he can seek assistance quickly when necessary.

Relaxation techniques

Teaching a patient to use relaxation techniques including yoga and meditation is sometimes useful in alleviating pain. Rhythmic breathing exercises are taught to expectant mothers at prenatal classes to alleviate pain during childbirth.

Comfort measures

These include positioning and repositioning the patient by turning or lifting him up in bed. Supporting or applying a splint to a painful limb may alleviate pain. Elevation of an oedematous limb encourages drainage of excess fluid by gravity, relieving swelling. Massage may bring relief by increasing circulation to the affected area. Hot applications, for example a kaolin poultice, also increase circulation to an area where they are applied. Cold applications such as ice packs can bring relief by reducing the temperature of a painful area.

Patient environment

The environment should minimize noxious stimuli, such as bright lights, loud noises, odours. The environment should feel fresh, not stuffy. Providing appropriate pleasant environmental stimuli such as radio, television and visitors can enhance well-being.

Other techniques

Doctors may also recommend the use of transcutaneous electrical nerve stimulation (TENS), nerve blocks and occasionally neurosurgery to alleviate pain. As mentioned in Chapter 1, many people find complementary therapies helpful in relieving pain. While there may be no recognized scientific explanation for their effect, health-care professionals must accept their perceived benefits non-judgementally.

Analgesia

It is an important nursing role to consider the value of the strategies outlined above prior to administering analgesic medication to relieve pain.

Before administering analgesia pain assessment is carried out. However, it is also important to listen to what the patient is saying about his pain before suggesting the need for analgesia. The patient should be reassured that analgesic drugs can be given when they are needed within the prescribed limits, at any time – not only during medicine rounds. If prescribed medication is not effective in controlling pain, this must be reported to the medical staff.

Other drugs which relieve pain

Drugs used to relieve pain are usually referred to as analgesics, however it is important to recognize that in certain situations other drugs are also used:

- non-steroidal anti-inflammatory drugs (NSAIDS) for painful inflammatory conditions, e.g. arthritis
- glyceryl trinitrate (GTN) for angina
- local anaesthetics for minor surgical procedures.

Management of pain in terminal care

When pain is a consequence of a condition which cannot be cured, all these measures are taken and analgesia is administered with the aim of complete pain relief. It is important to assess the effect of analgesia given and to recognize recurrence of chronic pain. Analgesic drugs are administered as regular doses usually every 4 hours, not 'as necessary'. The strength and dose of analgesia are increased when required. When possible, the oral route is used as this reduces effects associated with parenteral administration of strong opiates including respiratory depression and sedation. Other routes used in terminal care are sublingual, rectal and, increasingly, subcutaneous infusions.

ANALGESIC DRUGS

These drugs can be considered according to their principal site of analgesic action, either within the central nervous system (the opiates) or peripherally (aspirin, paracetamol and the non-steroidal anti-inflammatory drugs).

Opiates

These are naturally occurring substances derived from opium and also synthetic compounds which produce their analgesic effect by acting on opiate receptors in the brain and spinal cord.

The desired therapeutic effect is usually analgesia, but may also be sedation and euphoria. As with many drugs, other effects and/or side-effects may also occur and the nurse must make further observations on a patient receiving continuing doses of these drugs, especially when they are given by injection (Table 4.8).

Opiates are often categorized according to their potency – strong, intermediate and mild. Strong opiates include the controlled drugs morphine, diamorphine, papaveretum and pethidine. Dihydrocodeine has intermediate analgesic properties. Mild opiate analgesic drugs include dextropropoxyphene and codeine. Codeine is also used for 'side-effects' of opiate action, namely to treat diarrhoea and as a cough suppressant.

Two close relatives of the drugs above are pentazocine and buprenorphine. They also have analgesic properties but unlike the above drugs, their effects cannot necessarily be reversed by the opiate antagonist naloxone.

Aspirin, paracetamol and non-steroidal anti-inflammatory drugs

These drugs act by inhibiting synthesis of prostaglandins, chemicals which, among their many actions, mediate the inflammatory response (of which pain is a cardinal sign) and the temperature thermostat in the hypothalamus. When drugs from this category are given, inhibition of prostaglandin synthesis accounts for their actions (Table 4.9).

PREVENTING SPREAD OF INFECTION

Since the legendary days of Florence Nightingale, emphasis on the tenets of cleanliness and hygiene have been central to the nurse's role in preventing spread of infection. During the following century revolutionary advances in knowledge and social conditions, particularly sanitation and housing, have changed not only the impact of infection but also its control and treatment. Infectious illnesses which were a major cause of death and long-term ill health at the beginning of this century are now largely eradicated (e.g. smallpox) or prevented by immunization (Table 4.10) or can be effectively treated when they do occur. However, more recently recognized infectious diseases, in particular AIDS, now pose an ever-increasing challenge to mankind.

Babies are normally born free of microbes, however they rapidly acquire a resident microbial population which is retained and added to throughout life. For the most part, these acquired microbes do not cause harm or disease and are referred to as **commensals**. Sometimes however microbes do cause disease, and in these situations, they are referred to as **pathogens**. The reason that we do not all suffer and die from repeated infections is the existence of defence mechanisms which confer resistance to many infections (see p. 484).

Microbes come from a source or reservoir, and once an infection is acquired it can be transmitted to other people. The newly infected person is known as the **host**, who may then act as a potential source.

In everyday life, our health depends not only on our body defences but also on general hygiene measures. Hygiene measures require modification in an institutional setting. Within a hospital, further precautions must be taken to minimize the occurrence of infectious outbreaks or epidemics.

Table 4.8 Side-effects and other effects of opiates, and related nursing implications

Other effects	Related nursing implications
Central nervous system	
Respiratory depression	Observe respiratory function
Hypotension	Observe blood pressure
Cough suppression	Encourage deep breathing to reduce stasis of secretions
Nausea and vomiting	Consider concurrent use of an antiemetic
Peripheral nervous system	
Decreased peristalsis	Observe for paralytic ileus or constipation
Contraction of smooth muscle	May exacerbate conditions e.g. renal or biliary colic

Table 4.9   Actions, side-effects and contraindications of aspirin, paracetamol and non-steroidal anti-inflammatory drugs (NSAIDS)

Drug	Effect	Side-effects	Related contraindications
Aspirin	Analgesic Anti-inflammatory Antipyretic Reduces platelet aggregation	Gastric irritation Acute or chronic intestinal bleeding Allergy (bronchospasm) Reduces platelet aggregation Reye's syndrome Salicylism (in overdose)	Peptic ulcers (CI) Inflammatory bowel diseases (CI) Asthma (SP) Warfarin therapy (INT) Haemophilia and other blood clotting disorders (CI) Children under 12 years (CI)
Paracetamol	Analgesic Antipyretic	Liver toxicity (may be irreversible and fatal in overdose)	Liver dysfunction (SP)
NSAIDS e.g. *ibuprofen,* *indomethacin,* *naproxen,* *mefenamic acid*	Anti-inflammatory Analgesic Effective in dysmenorrhoea	As for aspirin, and water retention Skin rashes	Peptic ulcers (CI) Inflammatory bowel diseases (CI) Asthma (SP) Warfarin therapy (INT) Haemophilia and other blood clotting disorders (CI) Children under 12 years (CI) Many other drugs (INT)

CI = contraindication; SP = special precautions taken; INT = interacts with

In this section, the nature of micro-organisms and the chain of infection are examined and then the nursing measures used to minimize spread of infection are explained. Later in the section, control of body temperature is outlined and the mechanism of fever described. Finally, principles of care for patients with a disorder of body temperature are discussed.

The nature of micro-organisms

Pathogenic human micro-organisms are most commonly bacteria, viruses and fungi.

Bacteria

These unicellular micro-organisms can be visualized as colourless organisms under a light microscope. They vary in length between 0.3 and 14 µm. Bacteria replicate by binary fission in a favourable environment producing two identical daughter cells. They can exist in a wide variety of environments although most human pathogens find the following body characteristics conducive to replication:

• temperature around 37°C
• moisture

Table 4.10   Routine UK Immunization Schedule (Department of Health 1992)

Vaccine	Immunization against	Age
D/T/P *Polio* Hib	Diphtheria, tetanus, pertussis (whooping cough) Poliomyelitis *Haemophilis influenzae* b (meningitis)	3 doses of each between 2 and 6 months
MMR	Measles, mumps, rubella (German measles)	12–18 months
Booster D/T and Polio	Diphtheria, tetanus } 4th dose Poliomyelitis	4–5 years
Rubella	Rubella (German measles)	Girls only: 10–14 years
BCG	Tuberculosis	10–14 years
Booster tetanus and polio	5th dose	15–18 years

Table 4.11   Characteristics used for classification of bacteria

Characteristics	Features
Gram staining	Gram-positive or gram-negative (dependent on composition of the cell wall) Hospital-acquired gram-negative bacteria can be very difficult to treat
Morphology (shape)	Bacilli – rod shaped, some can adapt and survive adverse conditions in resistant forms called endospores Cocci – spherical Coccobacilli – very short rods Spirochaetes – spirals
Arrangement	Diplo – pairs, e.g. diplococcus Staphylo – clusters, e.g. staphylococcus Strepto – chains, e.g. streptococcus
Oxygen requirement	Obligatory aerobes – oxygen is essential for multiplication Obligatory anaerobes – complete absence of oxygen necessary for multiplication Facultative anaerobes – can replicate with or without oxygen

- availability of nutrients
- slight alkalinity
- appropriate gaseous requirements.

Classification of bacteria is based on three main characteristics shown in Table 4.11, which enables identification of a pathogen and then appropriate treatment.

Treatment of bacterial infections

Antibiotics are used when clinically indicated, however there is no one antibiotic capable of killing all types of bacteria. Appropriate selection is determined by a microbiologist who cultures the organism and tests it for antibiotic sensitivity. Broad spectrum antibiotics are effective against a variety of groups whereas a narrow spectrum antibiotic is effective against a limited group only. Sometimes a combination of antibiotics which act in different ways is prescribed.

For some patients at risk of infection, a course of prophylactic antibiotic therapy may be prescribed. This may be appropriate following major surgery or to prevent chest infections in patients with chronic bronchitis during the winter months.

It is important to ensure that narrow spectrum antibiotics are used when possible and all the prescribed treatment is taken. This minimizes the risk of bacterial resistance to antibiotics developing and in such cases another antibiotic must be used. Resistance to antibiotics can be transferred between bacterial species and it is an increasing problem which poses a serious threat to effective treatment of bacterial infections.

Viruses

These micro-organisms are much smaller than bacteria, being 10–30 nm in size, and they cannot be seen under a light microscope. Viruses are responsible for many infections including the common cold and influenza. There is also evidence that viruses play a role in the occurrence of some types of cancer.

A virus consists of a strand of deoxyribonucleic acid (DNA) or ribonucleic acid (RNA) surrounded by a protein coat called a capsid. It may also have a further protective protein layer referred to as an envelope.

Viruses, unlike bacteria, can only reproduce within a living cell although they can exist independently. Once inside a living cell, viral nucleic acid diverts the metabolism of the host cell into producing viral components: nucleic acid and protein coats. These are assembled into many new viruses which can cause death of the host cell after their release. Each new virus may then invade and destroy more host cells.

Classification of viruses is based on the type of nucleic acid they contain and their shape as seen by electron microscopy.

Treatment of viral infections

Only a few antiviral drugs are available. None are effective against colds, influenza or AIDS.

Vaccines are available to confer resistance against some viral illnesses.

Fungi

These micro-organisms include yeasts and moulds and may be visible to the naked eye. They rarely cause serious illness except in a host with compromised immunity, for example patients with AIDS (see p. 499), leukaemia (see p. 494) or receiving systemic steroid therapy (see p. 567).

In most cases fungal infections affect superficial tissues, often the skin, hair, nails or mucous membranes, e.g. athletes foot, ringworm.

Candida albicans is a commensal micro-organism which causes thrush in the mouth and vagina. This condition is usually associated with compromised immunity but is also common following antibiotic treatment which destroys commensal bacterial flora.

Treatment of fungal infections (mycoses)

Antifungal drugs are available to treat minor infections by local application and also for systemic use in serious cases.

THE CHAIN OF INFECTION

The chain of infection is the process by which infection can be acquired and transmitted. The following factors predispose to spread of infection in hospital:

- large number of people in close confinement
- many reservoirs of pathogens
- more virulent pathogens
- iatrogenic portals of entry and exit
- population comprises many susceptible hosts.

The links which form the chain of infection are considered in turn and then nursing measures involved in breaking each are discussed (Fig. 4.5).

Reservoirs

Pathogenic micro-organisms originate from many sources or reservoirs in hospitals. They may be animate or inanimate (Box 4.9). It is essential for the nurse to be aware of both actual and potential reservoirs to ensure appropriate measures are used to prevent transmission of pathogens from such sources.

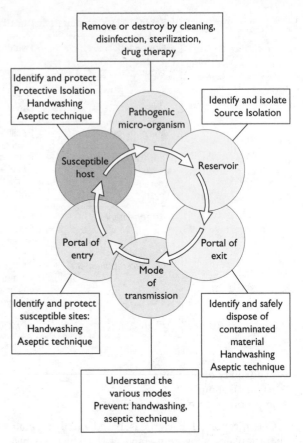

Fig. 4.5 The chain of infection (nursing measures used to break it are shown in the boxes)

Box 4.9   Reservoirs of micro-organisms

Animate
  Hosts
  Carriers
  Insects including cockroaches, fleas and mosquitoes
  Animals including rats
Inanimate
  Contaminated airborne droplets
  Contaminated food and fluids
  Dust which may be contaminated by airborne droplets, or shed from clothing, bedlinen, skin and hair
  Fomites – are all articles which have been in contact with an infected person and must therefore be disinfected or sterilized to prevent transfer of micro-organisms to others

A potential reservoir must always be handled as though it is an actual reservoir. Source isolation, and safe disposal, sterilization or disinfection (considered later) of all material in contact with reservoirs is necessary to break this link in the chain.

Mode of spread

Several routes of spread are recognized:

Direct personal contact either from one person to another or from one site to another on the same person. The latter is referred to as endogenous infection.

Indirect contact by contaminated fomites.

Vectors may be vermin or insects which harbour micro-organisms which are pathogenic if they spread to humans.

Airborne by contaminated moisture droplets or dust.

Vertical by spread in the placental circulation from mother to foetus.

Portals of entry and exit

Spread of pathogens also requires an exit site from the host or other reservoir, and a site of entry into the next victim. Table 4.12 shows common portals of entry and exit.

Susceptible host

Patients at increased risk of infection can be identified amongst the hospital population. Such patients include those having limited immunity and include babies, young children and elderly people. Patients receiving chemotherapy or immunosuppressant drugs may fall into this category along with those having radiotherapy. Additionally, invasive treatments may compromise or bypass defence mechanisms and are also listed in Table 4.12.

Following infection, signs of inflammation (see p. 118) may be apparent. If invasion is followed by systemic signs of infection the patient may experience further problems discussed later in this section.

CONTROL OF INFECTION IN HOSPITALS

Many hospitals have a Control of Infection Committee Team which includes microbiologists and nurses who determine local policies governing practice when there is an infection risk to staff or patients. The aim is to minimize hospital acquired or **nosocomial** infection. Effective implementation involves educating staff about any activities they undertake which may pose an infection hazard to patients, themselves or other staff. Strategies adopted for such policies are based on breaking the chain of infection. Areas of infection control policy are:

- cleaning methods which minimize raising dust.
- disinfection of fomites, in particular, reusable items including bedlinen, cutlery, crockery and sanitary utensils, or use of disposable items.
- waste disposal, including contaminated materials and sharp objects.
- immunization programmes are implemented to reduce 'at risk' staff contracting serious infectious illnesses, e.g. hepatitis B.
- other measures which primarily involve nurses and are outlined in the text.

Table 4.12 Portals of entry and exit		
System	Portal of entry	Portal of exit
Respiratory tract	Inhalation of contaminated air or droplets Tracheostomy or endotracheal tube	Expiration of droplets especially when coughing or sneezing
Alimentary tract	Ingestion of contaminated fluid or food	Excretion in faeces
Urinary tract	Urinary catheter, instrumentation Poor genital hygiene	Excretion in urine
Integument	Inoculation of broken skin, e.g. abrasions, lacerations, wound, drain, IV infusion, open sores	Leakage from broken skin, e.g. serous fluid, blood
Mucous membranes	Inoculation	Discharge from mucous membranes
Reproductive tract	Penis or vagina during sexual intercourse	Penis or vagina during sexual intercourse

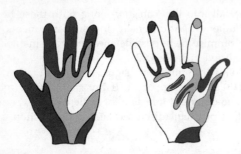

Fig. 4.6 Areas most neglected when handwashing: palm (right) and back of hand (left). Key: black = most frequently missed areas; grey = less frequently missed areas. (Reproduced with permission from Chandler 1991, figure 38.3)

Handwashing is the single most important measure which all staff must carry out after patient contact. This is because the hands not only carry resident flora but may also have acquired other micro-organisms, referred to as transient flora. Transient flora are frequently pathogenic but are more easily removed by handwashing than resident organisms.

Research by Taylor (1978) showed that some areas are commonly missed during handwashing. These include the thumbs, nails, fingertips and areas between the fingers (Fig. 4.6). Particular attention should be given to these areas when handwashing. It is also important to dry the hands thoroughly to prevent chapping and breaks in the skin.

Good personal hygiene dictates that handwashing is carried out before meals and after using the lavatory. Nurses play an important role in facilitating this practice for bedfast patients and those who are unlikely to carry this out voluntarily (those who have learning difficulties, children and some people with mental health problems), although Pritchard & Hathaway (1988) suggest this is not routine practice for all patients in hospital.

Use of gloves when handling body fluids prevents accidental inoculation of broken skin with infected fluids which may contain the viruses which cause hepatitis B and AIDS.

Cleaning, disinfection and sterilization are used in situations where there is potential for contamination. A spectrum (Fig. 4.7) can be devised with good housekeeping principles at one end and a sterile environment at the other.

It is impossible to maintain a sterile environment around living beings, as sterilization kills all living matter including micro-organisms and bacterial spores. Autoclaving is a widely used technique for sterilizing heat-resistant material that can be subjected to pressurized steam. Irradiation is used commercially for disposable plastic items that cannot withstand high temperatures.

Disinfection removes and destroys many micro-organisms but is ineffective against bacterial spores; some disinfectants are toxic to tissue. The process involves use of soap, chemicals and sometimes heat, used according to local policy.

Cleaning removes surface contamination and should be carried out before either disinfection or sterilization.

Aseptic technique is a non-touch technique used to prevent direct and indirect transfer of micro-organisms between the hands and a wound or other susceptible site. The actual technique may vary but it is based on the following principles:

- maximize cleanliness by using a clean treatment room or by avoiding dust-raising activities in the area for at least an hour beforehand.
- handwashing before and after procedure.
- use of sterile equipment and lotions on the treatment area to prevent direct contact between the nurse's hands and susceptible sites.

Source isolation involves nursing a patient who has a virulent infectious condition in a cubicle with the aim of containing the pathogen and therefore minimizing its spread. After considering the route of

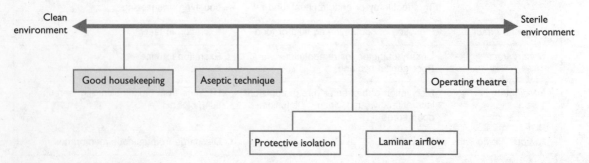

Fig. 4.7 The cleanliness spectrum

transmission, specific precautions will be taken for individual patients with particular emphasis on disposal and disinfection of all material from the cubicle. These precautions vary according to the route of spread, e.g. airborne (tuberculosis, see p. 457), excreta (food poisoning, see p. 545) or body fluids (hepatitis, see p. 546).

Protective isolation also involves nursing the patient in a single room, but with the aim of preventing the introduction of infection. It is required by patients who would be at significant risk from contracting an infection. Nursing principles dictate that the precautions taken ensure that everything entering the room is as clean as possible.

A summary of nursing measures which may be taken to break the chain of infection is shown in Figure 4.5.

TEMPERATURE CONTROL

Precise control of body temperature is a prerequisite for homeostasis. Outwith narrow limits, metabolic dysfunction occurs, in particular enzyme and biochemical function is disrupted. Continuous heat production and loss are finely balanced, maintaining temperature within normal limits despite a wide range of external temperatures and activity levels. The mechanisms of heat production and heat loss are summarized in Figure 4.8.

The control centre for body temperature acts as a thermostatic mechanism and is situated in the anterior hypothalamus of the brain. It regulates heat loss or production according to body temperature, thus maintaining homeostasis.

During any 24-hour period, a diurnal variation in temperature is observed with highest recordings during the evening and lowest during the night.

Pathophysiology of fever

Pyrexia or fever is a sign of an underlying disorder, commonly infection, but is also caused by trauma, neoplasms and metabolic disorders.

During fever, the temperature thermostat is reset to a higher level by chemical mediators. These include pyrogens and prostaglandins released from damaged cells. Heat production is then increased to exceed heat loss and body temperature rises. The response to conservation of heat may be accompanied by physical appearance of pallor and feeling cold. When body temperature reaches the new higher level, the patient may feel hot and sweaty, and appear flushed. Basal metabolic rate rises increasing the demand for oxygen and is accompanied by increased pulse and respiratory rate.

Nursing measures used to assess presence and course of infection

Terminology associated with temperature recordings is shown in Box 4.10. Temperature is recorded on admission and if outwith the normal range, recordings of temperature, pulse and respiratory rate are carried out at least 4 hourly. If the patient is seriously ill, blood pressure recordings may also be carried out.

In addition to the features described above, the pyrexial patient often feels lethargic and generally unwell. Other symptoms such as nausea and headache may also be present.

The nurse should also observe the patient for other common signs of infection:

- onset or presence of cough and the nature of any sputum expectorated
- excretion of cloudy or offensive smelling urine, dysuria
- redness around wound, drain or any other site, e.g. intravenous infusion
- presence of a rash.

Patients who would be at significant risk should they contract an infection require very close obser-

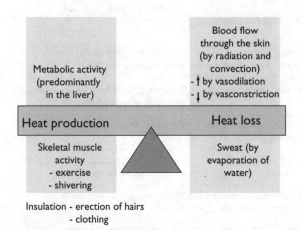

Fig. 4.8 Factors involved in homeostasis of body temperature

Box 4.10 Interpretation of body temperature measurements	
Normal range	36–37°c
Pyrexia	above 37.5°C
Hypothermia	core temperature below 35°C
Core temperature	usually measured in rectum
Peripheral temperature	usually measured orally, or per axilla

vation for any sign of infection throughout their admission, even if they remain apyrexial.

Principles of nursing care for a pyrexial patient

Problems which are commonly experienced by a pyrexial patient and their related nursing care are identified in Nursing Care Plan 4.1. Some of these principles are expanded further below.

Progress is monitored by recordings and observations described above, their frequency being determined by the patient's condition. It is important to recognize that dehydration is a consequence of fever

Nursing Care Plan 4.1 A pyrexial patient			
Actual or potential problem	**Aim**	**Nursing care**	**Rationale**
Fever	To monitor course Minimize heat generation Lower body temperature	❐ Record temperature, pulse and respiratory rate ❐ Nurse in bed ❐ Ensure area is well ventilated, but draught free, bed-clothes are loose fitting ❐ Indirect fanning ❐ Administer antipyretic drugs as prescribed	Evaluate treatment and nursing measures Minimizes skeletal muscle activity Encourages heat loss by radiation Increases heat loss by connection and conduction Lower level of temperature thermostat (see Box 4.10)
Sweating	Prevent damage to skin	❐ Wash gently dry affected areas ❐ Cotton or natural fibres for linen ❐ Change linen as necessary	Maintains skin clean, dry and intact
Dehydration	To maintain fluid balance To prevent or correct dehydration	❐ Observe for signs of dehydration especially young children and elderly people ❐ Encourage 2.5–3 litres of oral fluid ❐ Maintain fluid balance chart ❐ Administer IV fluids if prescribed ❐ Carry out frequent oral hygiene	Early detection if dehydration developing – are more susceptible to effects of dehydration Compensates for increased losses Monitor progress with increased intake, adequate output Patient may be unable to take adequate intake orally Maintains moist oral mucosa
Anorexia	To optimize nutritional status	❐ Provide an appetizing easily digested diet high in protein and energy ❐ Supplement with nourishing fluids	More appealing to patient Meets increased energy requirement and promotes tissue healing
Malaise	Provide a restful environment	❐ Allow planned periods of rest, interspersed with periods of gentle stimulation, e.g. TV, radio, visitors ❐ Leave call bell within easy reach	Permits rest and sleep, reducing fatigue and irritability Enables patient to seek assistance promptly when required
Dependent for elimination needs	Maintain dignity Prevent constipation	❐ Offer toilet facilities every few hours and provide privacy at this time ❐ Record when bowels open in the nursing notes	Reduces embarrassment and anxiety Bedrest, dehydration and light diet all predispose to constipation
Confusion	Maintain patient safety	❐ Nurse in a bed positioned where close observation is possible	Minimizes risk of accidents or injury
Infectious condition	Prevent spread	❐ Identify potential route of spread and appropriate nursing care required	Confines pathogenic micro-organisms to host

and that children and elderly people have less body water and are therefore more susceptible to the effects of dehydration. In children, high temperature may also predispose to fits and active intervention is therefore desirable to reduce this risk.

When a pyrexial patient feels cold, he should be given another blanket and observed closely until he feels warm again. An excessive peaking of temperature is apparent when a patient experiences a **rigor**. This is characterized by exaggerated shivering, chattering of the teeth and the patient feeling very cold despite being pyrexial. These symptoms are the result of increased heat production and then heat conservation in response to a sudden rise in the level of the temperature thermostat. When signs of a rigor are apparent, the patient's temperature is recorded, the doctor is informed and the patient observed closely. When shivering stops, the patient's temperature is recorded again. A peak in temperature will have occurred and this is followed by a period of heat loss characterized by profuse sweating as the patient's temperature falls. Blankets are then removed and other methods of cooling employed as necessary.

If a microbial cause of pyrexia is suspected, specimens are collected as requested. Appropriate drug treatment may be prescribed after sensitivity is established.

Hypothermia

Awareness of the predisposing factors and giving appropriate advice or practical help can often prevent hypothermia.

Predisposing factors include inadequate protection against heat loss or inefficient heat-generating mechanisms. Young children and elderly people are susceptible to both of these situations. Exacerbation of the situations above may occur as a result of low environmental temperature which is further compounded by dampness and wind. This predisposes to hypothermia in poorly clothed hill walkers and climbers. Low income also renders many people, especially the elderly who live in cold climates, susceptible as their homes may be inadequately heated and insulated. Principles of care are shown in Box 4.11.

KNOWING THE NATURE OF COMMON DISORDERS

ALLERGIC DISORDERS

Internal recognition of a foreign protein, known as an allergen, results in production of antibodies to neutralize its effect. Subsequent exposure to the allergen results in allergic symptoms. These may be minor but troublesome, such as a skin rash or running eyes or nose, but can also be sudden and catastrophic resulting in laryngeal oedema (causing respiratory obstruction) or severe shock (causing death from anaphylactic shock).

AUTOIMMUNE DISORDERS

The body fails to recognize an endogenous substance as its own and forms antibodies against it. This response results in the body then destroying its own affected tissues resulting in loss of their functions.

DEGENERATIVE DISORDERS

These disorders include those of diseased tissue with little regenerative capacity in young and middle-aged people. In older people, there is an increased incidence of such conditions due to the physiological processes of ageing which result in slower regeneration of tissue. Degeneration is associated with loss of structure and/or function of affected tissue. This category includes disorders of the nervous system, locomotor system and the circulatory system.

CONGENITAL ABNORMALITIES

A congenital abnormality refers to any defect with which an infant is born. The causes are:

- chromosomal abnormality
- genetic inheritance
- environmental factors
- multifactorial.

Most human cells have 46 chromosomes – 44 autosomes, or body chromosomes, and two sex chromosomes which determine the sex of an individual.

Box 4.11 Principles of care for a hypothermic patient

- prevent further cooling
- promote gradual rewarming } to prevent sudden vasodilatation which may
- avoid direct heat } lead to shock
- monitor progress by hourly measurement of core temperature and vital signs
    rising pulse and falling blood pressure are indicative of shock
- maintain or restore fluid balance
- maintain pressure areas intact
- provide education to prevent another episode.

Unlike other body cells, gametes (ova and spermatozoa) have 23 chromosomes. Following fertilization of an ovum 46 chromosomes are present which can be identified as 23 pairs. Autosomes are identical pairs, while the sex chromosomes may be different. A female has 2X chromosomes (denoted XX) while a male has one X chromosome and a smaller Y chromosome (denoted XY).

Chromosomes contain the chemical template for expression of genes which determine many physical characteristics including skin, hair and eye colour. Genes act as the template for all proteins essential for metabolic and biochemical processes. (See Ch. 7).

Chromosomal abnormalities

In these conditions autosomes or sex chromosomes can be affected. The fertilized ovum has an abnormal number or structure of chromosomes.

Autosomes Abnormalities have serious implications when they affect the body chromosomes. The presence of too few chromosomes usually results in spontaneous abortion of a fetus. Down's syndrome is associated with the presence of an extra or abnormally formed autosome.

Sex chromosomes may also be affected with either an extra or missing sex chromosome. Abnormalities of sex chromosomes are not usually life threatening but result in recognized syndromes: Turner's syndrome, Klinefelter's syndrome.

Genetically inherited disorders

These conditions arise when one or both parents have an abnormal gene which is passed on via the gametes. Autosomes or sex chromosomes may be affected and these defects may or may not be expressed. An abnormal gene which is not expressed can nevertheless be transmitted and affect other offspring. The parent may then be identified as a carrier of a particular genetic abnormality. Inheritance of these disorders is determined by characteristics of the gene itself and whether it is carried on an autosome or sex chromosome. The probability of inheritance can then be predicted and this forms the rationale for genetic counselling.

Environmental factors

A range of these are implicated in causing abnormal fetal development.

Infection during pregnancy, especially by viruses, predisposes to a high incidence of serious fetal abnormalities. In the UK an immunization programme against the rubella virus (German measles) is used to minimize its risk. Other harmful viruses are usually ingested in susceptible foods which should therefore be avoided during pregnancy. Expectant mothers are given dietary advice to minimize this risk.

Ionizing radiation was recognized to be a cause of physical deformity after the atomic bomb at Hiroshima.

Chemicals including drugs (e.g. thalidomide) may cross into the fetal circulation causing physical malformation. Such chemicals are known as **teratogens** and it is now standard practice to avoid prescribing drugs during pregnancy unless serious medical circumstances dictate otherwise.

Multifactorial causes

In these situations an interplay of environmental and complex genetic components is implicated but their roles cannot be precisely distinguished.

Congenital malformations of multifactorial origin include cleft lip and palate, spina bifida, congenital dislocation of the hip and congenital heart defects.

OTHER DISORDERS

Iatrogenic conditions arise as a result of medical treatments for other conditions.

Idiopathic disorders are of unknown cause.

INFLAMMATION

Inflammation is the physiological response to tissue damage. An inflammatory condition can be recognized from the Latin suffix *-itis* and some examples are shown in Table 4.13.

Causes include trauma, exposure to extremes of temperature, ultraviolet and ionizing radiation, and presence of foreign bodies including micro-organisms.

The acute inflammatory response

There are five cardinal signs of inflammation:

- redness
- heat
- swelling
- pain
- loss of function.

These are easily recognized when superficial areas are affected.

The immediate response to tissue damage is short-lived constriction of capillary vessels. Damaged cells

Table 4.13 Inflammatory conditions	
Inflammatory condition	Affected organ
Appendicitis	Appendix
Laryngitis	Larynx
Dermatitis	Skin
Hepatitis	Liver

then rapidly release chemical mediators including histamine, serotonin, bradykinin and prostaglandins. In particular, histamine causes prolonged dilatation of the surrounding capillaries, resulting in increased blood flow through them causing redness and heat in the area of injury.

The capillary walls which are normally only freely permeable to water and other small molecules then become permeable to larger molecules, including the plasma proteins albumen, globulin and fibrinogen. As these proteins accumulate in the extracellular fluid their osmotic effect retains more fluid in the area causing local oedema and swelling. The effect of swelling in the area compresses sensory nerve endings leading to perception of tenderness and pain. Chemicals, including prostaglandins, potentiate the sensitivity of the nerve endings to painful stimuli. Swelling also leads to restriction or loss of function of the damaged tissue.

A fibrin wall formed from plasma fibrinogen may be laid down around the inflamed area to protect adjacent tissue from damage.

Leucocytes migrate from capillaries by chemotaxis (chemical attraction) to the extracellular fluid. Neutrophils and tissue macrophages ingest foreign material and cell debris into intracellular vacuoles. Digestion of these vacuoles occurs by the action of enzymes released from intracellular inclusions known as lysosomes. This process is called phagocytosis and results in removal of damaged tissue and foreign material from an inflamed area.

Outcomes

Resolution

Regeneration of tissue occurs as new cells are laid down and fibrin strands are degraded by enzyme action. Other waste products are removed by the lymphatic and circulatory systems. An areas of fibrous tissue, recognized externally as a **scar**, remains.

Suppuration (pus formation)

Suppuration may delay healing. Pus is a collection of dead phagocytes, cell debris, fibrin, inflammatory exudate and live or dead micro-organisms liquefied by the action of lysosomal enzymes. Abscess formation then occurs. A superficial abscess or boil can rupture externally discharging pus before resolution occurs. A deep abscess usually requires surgical drainage to reduce the risk of secondary complications.

Wound healing (regeneration)

Wound healing occurs following loss of tissue associated with inflammation. A wound may arise following inflammation, from a surgical procedure or as a result of trauma. Lacerations, burns and pressure sores are also wounds. Principles of wound healing are outlined here and explained fully on page 232. During the process of wound healing, several overlapping stages are identified. The initial phase of wound healing closely resembles the inflammatory response and rids the affected area of cellular debris and foreign matter. Thereafter, new tissue is laid down in the area of tissue loss. This is then re-modelled and strengthened with collagen fibres. The size of the permanent scar is related to the extent of tissue loss.

Systemic response

A systemic response may accompany a local inflammatory reaction, especially following invasion by pathogenic micro-organisms. Toxins may be released during the local response producing general systemic effects including fever, general malaise, anorexia, headache and lethargy.

Additional symptoms due to inflammation of a specific organ arise as its functional ability is decreased or lost during the inflammatory process. For example in hepatitis, failure to conjugate bile in the liver causes increased levels in the circulation which is observed as jaundice.

Chronic inflammation

This process is physiologically similar to the acute process but characteristically lasts longer and is less severe. The area of tissue destruction is larger, and therefore during resolution more fibrous tissue is laid down. Subsequent loss of function is usually more extensive following a chronic inflammatory process.

Anti-inflammatory drugs

These fall into two categories: corticosteroids and

non-steroidal anti-inflammatory drugs (NSAIDs). All of these drugs reduce the rate of wound healing due to their anti-inflammatory effects.

Corticosteroids When used systemically, these drugs may have serious side-effects which are discussed on page 567.

Non-steroidal anti-inflammatory drugs These drugs are more commonly used for inflammatory conditions as their side-effects are less serious than corticosteroids. Their mode of action is outlined in Table 4.9.

METABOLIC DISORDERS

These conditions result in signs and symptoms caused by disordered metabolic function producing a wide range of recognized conditions. The causes are:

- excess or deficiency of an endocrine hormone
- an enzyme deficiency
- failure to eat or overeating, either total intake or of a specific nutrient
- ingestion of chemicals including alcohol.

TRAUMA

Accidental injuries are a significant cause of morbidity and mortality. In addition to complete recovery or death, long-term disability can also occur. Injuries sustained can be minor and dealt with using principles of first aid, or catastrophic in nature. Trauma results in tissue damage and is followed by inflammation and then healing depending on the regenerative capacity of the affected tissue. While most accidents are associated with physical events, other causes include radiation, chemicals and exposure to extremes of temperature. Commonly, accidents occur at home, at work or on the street.

Major incidents

Each Purchasing Authority coordinates a plan to maximize efficient use of resources following a large untoward event which results in many casualties, e.g. plane crash, explosion, etc.

TUMOURS

A tumour or neoplasm is an abnormal tissue mass which evades the processes which normally regulate cell division. A tumour may be either benign or malignant. Table 4.14 highlights distinguishing characteristics of these two tumour types.

While the differing characteristics of benign and malignant tumours dictates their treatment and outcomes, the type of tumour is also important. Tumours are further classified according to the tissue from which they arise: epithelium, connective, muscle or nerve.

It is important to recognize that the term 'carcinoma' correctly refers only to malignant tumours arising from epithelial tissue and is therefore not synonymous with the term 'cancer'. Any malignant tumour may be referred to as 'cancer'. The term 'new growth' also correctly describes any growth, benign or malignant. It is essential for the nurse to be aware that the diagnosis of cancer frequently arouses very negative attitudes and feelings.

Table 4.14 Characteristics of benign and malignant tumours

Characteristic	Benign	Malignant
Growth rate	Slow	May be fast growing
Invasion of surrounding tissue	Does not occur	Common
Spread	Does not occur	Occurs by local invasion, via lymphatic system, via bloodstream
Resemblance to parent tissue in structure and function	Common, i.e. differentiated cells	Often poor, i.e. undifferentiated cells
Recurrence	Rare	Common
Adherence to superficial tissue	Mobile on palpation	Fixed on palpation
Associated pain of a superficial lump	Often tender	Usually painless in early stages
Threat to host	Usually favourable	Depends on extent at time of diagnosis
Long-term effects if untreated	Compression of adjacent structures causing symptoms due to their dysfunction (some symptoms are life threatening depending on their location)	As for benign tumours Effects of spread to other organs Carcinomatosis in terminal stage

Growth, spread and effects of malignant tumours

A tumour starts from one abnormal cell which divides at a rate greater than that which is necessary for tissue regeneration. It enlarges by continuation of this accelerated mitotic process. The lowest limit of clinical detection is around 0.5 cm^3, the tumour weighing around 1 g and comprising 10^9 cells. A superficial lump is detected more easily than an internal one which may not be found until it causes symptoms.

A malignant tumour may then spread:

- directly into adjacent tissue
- via the bloodstream
- via the lymphatic system.

The structure and function of nearby tissue is impaired by direct invasion. Detached cells may carried in the bloodstream to distant locations and become lodged in these organs. A secondary tumour known as a metastasis then grows causing further problems. Other detached cells, cleared by the lymphatic system, may become lodged in lymph nodes which enlarge impairing drainage of fluid from distal areas.

In some cases, presenting symptoms at the time of diagnosis are caused by secondary growths, or metastases, the primary site remaining asymptomatic. For many tumours the sites of metastases are predictable, for example, spread from intestine to the liver via the hepatic portal vein is common in tumours of the bowel. Like their primary tumour, the growth of metastases also impairs the structure and therefore function of affected tissue, commonly causing the problems shown in Table 4.15.

Some benign endocrine tumours produce hormones in the absence of the normal stimulus and homeostatic controls. High levels of hormones will then circulate in the bloodstream with consequent ill effects (see Ch. 16).

Further progression of a tumour without treatment eventually impairs systemic body metabolism resulting in a state known as carcinomatosis. This terminal state is characterized by anorexia, malaise, cachexia (disproportionate weight loss), anaemia and fever. It is accompanied by disruption of physiological and biochemical function. These late systemic effects are unrelated to the site and type of primary tumour or its metastases.

Early signs of cancer

Early diagnosis of a malignant tumour facilitates treatment as spread may not have occurred. Health education has been directed at self-recognition of early signs and seeking prompt medical advice if any of the changes in Box 4.12 occur.

For some cancers, early detection may be improved by screening people most at risk. Such programmes are intended to provide curative treatment to any diagnosed cases. Investigations used must be reliable, relatively inexpensive and neither time-consuming nor distressing to the client to maximize voluntary uptake. A rigorous follow-up system for non-attenders must be in place to ensure that all the target population is tested, and recalled at stated intervals. An effective system is required for communicating results to GPs and patients, ensuring that all those requiring treatment or follow-up are notified.

Staging

It is recognized that as the disease spreads, treatment is less effective and the prognosis worsens. Staging is used to determine the extent of a tumour and its spread, enabling appropriate treatment to be identi-

Table 4.15 Common symptoms caused by tumour or metastases	
Affected organ	Symptoms
Partial or complete obstruction of the alimentary tract	Nausea, vomiting, constitipation, intermittent diarrhoea
Compression of bronchi or bronchioles	Recurrent respiratory tract infections Breathlessness
Bone	Pain Pathological fracture
Skin	Ulceration
Brain	Nausea, vomiting Headaches, visual disturbances Personality change
Liver	Jaundice

Box 4.12 Early warning signs of cancer
Change in bladder or bowel habit A sore which does not heal Unusual bleeding or discharge Thickening or lump in breast or elsewhere Indigestion or difficulty in swallowing Obvious change in a wart or mole Nagging cough or persistent hoarseness

fied. Investigations are usually needed to complete accurate staging. Staging is carried out not only to identify the most effective treatment, but also to determine effectiveness of treatment given.

KNOWING THE NATURE OF INVESTIGATIONS

There are many types of investigations available and while they may be useful in reaching a diagnosis, many are invasive and expensive.

Investigations may be carried out for a variety of reasons:

- results may confirm a provisional diagnosis
- results may exclude the presence of a particular disorder
- results may suggest that further investigations are necessary
- results may reveal the presence of an undiagnosed disorder
- monitoring of therapeutic effects of treatment
- screening for early signs of treatable conditions in groups of 'at-risk' individuals.

A nurse must be familiar with common investigations used to enable her to explain to the patient why the investigation is required and how this is related to his present situation. She must be competent in preparing the patient so he knows what to expect before, during and afterwards. Appropriate psychological and physical care may also be required before, during and after the investigation. It is often the nurse's responsibility to ensure that any specimens collected do not pose a hazard to others who may transport, handle or test them.

This section contains an outline of some common investigations which are expanded upon where relevant in Chapters 5–17.

BIOCHEMISTRY

Chemistry is a precise science and in relation to living matter it is known as biochemistry. Accurate measurement of constituents of body fluids are made in the laboratory to ensure that there is a vary narrow range of error, thereby optimizing the validity and reliability of the scientific method. Results obtained are then interpreted by comparison against a range for normal people in relation to sex and age.

Biochemical specimens are commonly blood and urine, but any other body fluids can also be analysed.

Types of analyses vary but are usually related to homeostatic parameters, including levels of electrolytes and enzymes or blood gases and acid base balance.

Common biochemical investigations which are carried out by nurses are described in Box 4.13.

HAEMATOLOGY

Blood samples are sent for microscopic analysis of characteristics and number of its cellular constituents.

MEDICAL MICROBIOLOGY

Investigations of this nature attempt to identify pathogenic micro-organisms, usually bacteria, fungi and viruses. Bacteriology specimens are also tested for sensitivity to antibiotics. Specimens which a nurse should be able to collect include midstream and catheter specimens of urine, sputum, faeces, swabs and exudates from a wound, drain or other sites.

In addition to general principles of specimen collection, it is vital not only to prevent inadvertent contamination of samples but also to minimize risk of infection to self and other staff.

ENDOSCOPY

By inserting an instrument into a hollow organ or body cavity, the area is lit and inspected for patency and other abnormalities including inflammation and

---

Box 4.13 Biochemical investigations carried out by nurses

Urinalysis – simply carried out using reagent strips and is commonly undertaken by nurses. The results however are only as accurate as the observations made on the reagent strip. Therefore, despite being a routine task, it is essential to follow the manufacturer's instructions precisely

Plasma glucose testing – reagent strips are available and may be used by nurses and diabetic patients. Before carrying out this procedure, the user must be taught about sampling technique and implication of measurements made as they determine subsequent treatment

24-hour urine collection – an investigation in which the nurse is often responsible for ensuring the patient complies with instructions to ensure accuracy of the specimen. Use of a container incorporating specific preservatives may be necessary

ulceration. A rigid tube was used before development of the flexible, fibreoptic instruments. The latter are less distressing for the patient and can be inserted further into the body. Such instruments allow visualization of the duodenum and colon. A small fragment of tissue, known as a biopsy, may be taken and sent for histological examination if abnormalities are observed.

The organ should be empty to maximize visual inspection and specific preparation is therefore required. Most of these procedures are carried out under sedation (e.g. gastroscopy, colonosopy) or general anaesthesia (e.g. bronchoscopy, cystoscopy and laparoscopy).

X-RAYS

These invisible rays penetrate tissue, the extent being determined by the relative densities of tissue within the irradiated area. A photographic plate is developed and dense tissue such as bone is readily identified. Observing loss of continuity of bone enables diagnosis of fractures. Soft tissue is not usually seen on a plain X-ray but by introducing a dye into the lumen of a hollow structure outlines of the gastrointestinal tract, blood vessels and chambers of the heart can be observed. The dyes used are referred to as radio-opaque or contrast media and by reducing X-ray penetration they show up as pale areas on the X-ray film.

Preparation requires removal of all metal objects to prevent deflection of X-rays and masking of abnormalities. Further nursing care is also required before and after procedures using contrast media.

Unless medical circumstances dictate otherwise, women who are, or may be pregnant should not receive X-ray as the fetus is at risk of developing deformities. The radioprotection precautions required by staff to minimize their exposure to X-rays are outlined on page 128.

CT SCAN

Computerized axial tomography, referred to as a CT scan, is an expensive but very useful investigation which is available in large hospitals. A computer records information taken from serial X-rays and displays precise images which reveal the anatomical size and relationship of internal structures in transverse section or 'slices'. This non-invasive X-ray technique is used to visualize internal structures of the brain and abdomen.

ULTRASOUND

This non-invasive investigation utilizes high frequency sound waves which penetrate and are reflected by tissues. A probe placed on the skin acts as both a source and receiver of reflected sound waves. A computerized image is then sent to a visual display unit. This scanning technique is used to enable visualization of internal tissue, often a fetus, kidney or the heart.

PATHOLOGY

In the pathology department, the anatomical structure of cells, tissues and organs is studied. Investigations range from microscopic examination of a small tissue fragment, or biopsy, to autopsy.

Visual and microscopic observation of tissue often leads towards diagnosis. Microscopic examination allows distinction of cellular features characteristic of inflammation, degeneration and tumours (benign and malignant).

UNDERSTANDING THE NURSE'S ROLE REGARDING PRESCRIBED TREATMENTS

It is often considered that treatment of a disorder will lead to a permanent cure. However this may neither be the intended aim nor outcome of some forms of management. Box 4.14 illustrates the range of purposes.

Box 4.14 Forms of medical management not associated with cure

Preventive or prophylactic treatment – the aim is prevention of a disease, e.g. immunization
Palliative treatment – symptoms secondary to a disease can be alleviated, increasing quality of life when no cure is possible
Conservative treatment – an ethical decision may be undertaken to withhold active medical treatment allowing nature to take its course. All nursing measures to promote comfort and well-being continue
Control – signs and symptoms can be reversed by changes in lifestyle and, or lifelong drug treatment, e.g. diabetes mellitus.

There is a wide range of treatments available but choices are determined by considering the nature of the disease and its effect on individual characteristics of a particular patient, e.g. age, general fitness, pre-existing disease, quality of life. Treatments and related nursing issues included in this section are:

- patient education
- diet
- drug therapy
- radiotherapy
- surgery (including principles of anaesthesia and preoperative and postoperative care).

PATIENT EDUCATION

An informed person who understands his illness and how it will or may affect him is more likely to act rationally on advice he is given. The importance of good communication and relationship building with patients has already been emphasized but will enable a patient to follow advice or instructions particularly where a major change in life-style is sought.

The behaviour of nurses and other health-care professionals is also important as it may be used by a patient either consciously or subconsciously as a good example. The influence that a nurse has on patients by acting as a role model cannot be underestimated.

Providing a patient with written information is very useful. It is a permanent record and reinforces verbal advice which, even if it is understood at the time, is easily forgotten. Specific education and its importance in particular disorders is discussed in the following chapters.

DIET

The importance of maintaining body weight appropriate to height was highlighted on page 99. A patient may need advice on how to achieve this if he is either overweight or underweight. Many health-care professionals including nurses are in a position to provide this information and to reinforce progress made.

Patients may require a modified diet as part of managing a particular medical problem (see p. 98). A dietitian or skilled nurse may initially advise patients about appropriate foods and all other nurses then play an important role in reinforcement and as role models.

DRUG THERAPY

Administering drugs and or facilitating compliance with prescribed medication are integral to the nurse's role in any setting. Medications are numerous and the actions of some common drug groups are listed in Table 4.16. Many different routes and preparations can be used, and therefore safety is of utmost impor-

Table 4.16 Common drug groups and their actions

Drug group	Action
Anaesthetic	Produces loss of all sensation
Analgesic	Relieves pain
Antacid	Counteracts gastric acidity
Anti-anxiety	Relieves anxiety
Antibiotic	Combats bacterial infection
Anticoagulant	Reduces rate of blood clotting
Anticonvulsant	Prevents or relieves fits
Antiemetic	Relieves nausea and vomiting
Antipyretic	Lowers elevated body temperature
Antipsychotic	Modifies symptoms of severe mental illness
Aperient or laxative	Stimulates peristalsis and evacuation of the bowel
Cytotoxic	Kills rapidly dividing malignant cells
Diuretic	Stimulates urine production
Hypnotic	Promotes sleep

tance. To use drugs safely requires familiarity with legislation and understanding of the pharmacological and professional concepts outlined in this section. The nurse is responsible for expanding her knowledge of specific drugs, their actions and side-effects in each new clinical area.

Nursing implications of legal, professional and health board documents

In order to maximize patient safety and to prevent errors due to overdose or omission there are legal, and professional frameworks laid down regarding the supply, storage and use of medications.

The Medicines Act (1968) identifies three categories of drugs shown in Box 4.15. Non-prescription medicines and the general sales list include many remedies

Box 4.15 Categories of drugs laid down by the Medicines Act (1968)

Prescription Only Medicines	– are dispensed by a pharmacist on receipt of a prescription
Non-prescription Medicines	– may be sold directly by a pharmacist after patient consultation
General Sales List	– can be bought over the counter at many outlets including newsagents

used for everyday ailments, such as indigestion, constipation, colds and minor aches and pains.

Drugs in all the categories have potential side-effects and may interact with each other even though they are perceived as safe by many people. It is therefore vital to ask patients about all medications they regularly take whether they are prescribed or not.

The Misuse of Drugs Act (1971) dictates more stringent precautions to be taken when dealing with drugs known to have addictive properties. These drugs are referred to as controlled drugs, and in a hospital the charge nurse or her deputy is legally responsible for their safe storage and administration.

Controlled drugs include strong analgesic drugs, some opiates, some barbiturates and amphetamines. Their potential for addiction is seldom realized in clinical practice but they create significant problems when they are abused. Drug addiction is not only associated with physical problems due to tolerance, dependence and withdrawal but also has a complex psychological component which compounds the difficulties associated with treating the problem (see p. 339).

In addition to these legal requirements, the UKCC (1984) issued professional guidelines (see Ch. 3). From these sources managers devise and update their own policy for safe handling, storage and administration of medicines. Each nurse must then ensure she conforms to employers' requirements when dealing with any aspect of drug treatment.

Nursing implications of pharmacological concepts

An understanding of some basic concepts as they apply to nursing will enable the nurse to explain her actions in relation to administering drugs and patient teaching.

Absorption The rate at which drug levels in the bloodstream rise determines the rate of onset of action. Levels rise immediately after intravenous administration and more slowly after injections into muscle or subcutaneous tissue. Following oral administration, absorption is slower than by injection. The rate is determined by the chemical characteristics of the drug, the functioning of the gastrointestinal tract and the extent of first pass metabolism.

First pass metabolism Drugs which are absorbed into the bloodstream from the gastrointestinal tract travel to the liver via the portal vein before reaching the heart and the systemic circulation. Some drugs are extensively metabolized by the liver and therefore never reach the systemic circulation if they are given orally. This is known as first pass metabolism, and when it occurs at a significant rate, another route must be used.

Therapeutic range This term describes the lower and upper plasma levels of a drug for safe therapeutic effect. Under the lower limit therapeutic action may not occur and above the upper limit side-effects or toxicity may occur. For some drugs the therapeutic range is narrow, the upper limit being only just under the level where toxicity occurs. In such cases, plasma levels may be measured to ensure they are within the limits of the therapeutic range. This not only ensures effectiveness, but also minimizes the risk of side-effects or toxicity which may be serious or permanent.

Distribution After absorption has occurred, the drug is taken in the bloodstream to its site of action. For some drugs, certain barriers to tissue distribution exist, for example many drugs do not cross the blood–brain barrier. Another barrier may be the placenta; however many drugs cross this barrier and cause harm to the developing fetus. Drugs which have this effect are referred to as **teratogenic**. It is for this reason that drugs are not prescribed during pregnancy except after careful consideration.

The length of drug action and therefore dose intervals also depend upon the drug's chemical characteristics which determine the rate of clearance from the body. **Metabolism**, or breakdown of drugs, renders them water soluble and occurs in the liver.

Elimination into the urine, or excretion, of most drugs takes place in the kidneys. Drugs which are metabolized and/or excreted rapidly are given more frequently. Immaturity or impairment of renal or hepatic function predisposes to accumulation of drugs within the body. Impaired function can be due to disorder of these organs but is also a feature of the ageing process. Children and elderly people are therefore prone to effects of drug accumulation, and are usually prescribed lower doses than adults.

Tolerance is associated with repeated use of some drugs, a larger dose being required to produce the same therapeutic effect after several doses. In this situation, the synthesis of liver enzymes which metabolize these drugs may be increased, thereby reducing their therapeutic effect and duration of action.

Dependence is present when a person must continue taking regular doses of a drug to prevent the occurrence of withdrawal symptoms.

Withdrawal symptoms are psychological and physical problems experienced by a person who stops taking a drug on which he is dependent. Physical symptoms can be explained physiologically but are unrelated to psychological effects or perceived benefits of such drugs. Management of drug dependency is discussed in Chapter 10.

Routes of administration, preparations used and related nursing implications

Many routes are available for administering drugs, and these fall into two categories: systemic and local. Systemic routes result in the drug circulating in the bloodstream around the whole body including the site of action. However, it is sometimes possible to deliver a smaller dose of a drug directly to the site of action, and in such cases the route used is referred to as local. For example, an inhaler may be used to

Table 4.17 Routes of drug administration, preparations used and related nursing implications

Routes	Preparations used	Nursing implications
SYSTEMIC Oral	Tablets, capsules linctus, suspensions	Requires absorption from and therefore functioning of small intestine Follow instructions on label to ensure optimal action, e.g. before meals when stomach is empty, swallow whole to enable slow release of contents Pour liquids away from the label to prevent staining which may render label unreadable Shake liquids before use to ensure thorough mixing of ingredients Unsuitable route if there is no swallow reflex (e.g. unconsciousness), vomiting, drugs which are protein or acid sensitive (inactivated in stomach)
Sublingual	Tablets	Absorption only occurs when oral mucosa is moist
Parenteral	Injection equipment and ampoules Subcutaneous injection Intramuscular injection Intravenous injection	Aseptic technique used to minimize risk of infection when penetrating skin Suitable for self-administration of small volumes at suitable sites Rate of absorption (usually 10–30 min) is related to blood flow through suitable muscle (greatly reduced in shock) Depot preparations of oily substances available for long-term release over several weeks Rapid onset of action and therefore side-effects, intravenous injections are only given by doctors and suitably qualified registered nurses Parenteral route of choice for patients who are shocked or have a bleeding tendency
Rectal	Suppositories Enema	Absorption slower than oral route but overcomes a difficulty if oral route cannot be used Cultural acceptancy of this route varies Also used as a local route, e.g. haemorrhoids
LOCAL **Rectal**	Suppositories Enema	Absorption slower than oral route but overcomes a difficulty if oral route cannot be used Cultural acceptancy of this route varies Treatment of local conditions
Vaginal	Pessary, cream	Require applicator to administer
Inhalation	Steam alone, or with aromatic oils Metered dose inhaler Nebulizer	Patient requires supervision to prevent injury from scalds Patient must be able to coordinate activating inhaler and perform deep inspiration to receive a preset dose of the drug Requires supply of pressurized air or oxygen to deliver the drug in droplet form from container via a face-mask Effective in patients with acute respiratory distress as it is inhaled over several minutes
Topical skin	Cream, ointment, liquid	Use of gloves is recommended as long-term exposure to staff may result in side-effects caused by absorption through the skin of the hands
Ears	Drops	Use a separate labelled bottle for each ear
Eyes	Drops, ointment	Use a separate labelled container for each eye

relieve breathlessness caused by constriction of bronchiolar smooth muscle. When absorption of an inhaled drug occurs, plasma levels will be much lower than they would have been if a systemic route was used to achieve the same therapeutic effect. Local routes are used when appropriate as the incidence of dose related side-effects is significantly reduced. Routes of administration, the preparations used and related nursing implications are shown in Table 4.17.

Maximizing compliance

Compliance

This term means that a patient takes his medication as it has been prescribed. It is increasingly recognized that this is often not the case and patient consequences of non-compliance are ineffective treatment, which may arise either from omission or overdose. Non-compliance is also wasteful of already stretched financial Health Service resources. Factors which predispose to poor compliance are shown in Box 4.16.

Polypharmacy

Polypharmacy is present when a drug regimen consists of many drugs. It is often the result of multiple prescribing for coexisting and unrelated problems and is prevalent in elderly people. Several factors may be involved:

• prescribing by several different doctors
• presence of multiple pathologies
• repeat prescriptions being given on demand without regular assessment of all drug therapy.

The consequences of polypharmacy are serious. The risk of side-effects and drug interactions increases with the number of individual drugs taken. The likelihood of treatment being taken correctly

---

Box 4.16   Factors which predispose to poor compliance

• Polypharmacy
• Lack of knowledge about prescribed treatment
• Presence of side-effects
• Improvement or relief of symptoms, especially if the time-scale of treatment is not understood
• Complex regimens, e.g. before AND after meals
• Physical difficulties – getting to a chemist, opening containers, poor vision so unable to read instructions or count drugs
• Psychological – lack of understanding or memory; idiosyncrasies, e.g. sharing drugs or hoarding until the problem is really severe

---

decreases. Polypharmacy may account for about 10% of admissions to care of the elderly wards.

Nursing role in facilitating compliance

When admitting a patient, an accurate record of all medications taken is established. It is also important to ask the patient about any remedies bought 'over the counter' that they may take, as these and the contraceptive pill are not considered as 'medicines' by many people. This action enables identification of the potential problems of polypharmacy and poor compliance. Evaluation of overall drug treatment is then carried out by a doctor. While listing the drugs, the nurse can assess what that patient already understands about his medication and determine a baseline for any further education needed. This should start after admission, and not just prior to discharge.

The nurse then has an informed point from which to plan necessary interventions when administering medication. The patient is shown the number of drugs and their appearance at each treatment time. Later this is reinforced by asking which drugs he should be having at that time. Effects and side-effects are also discussed. The teaching process continues with reinforcement until the patient is familiar with the prescribed regimen. A card detailing drug treatment is a useful *aide-memoire* and can be given to the patient for reference after discharge.

Compliance aids   Blister-wrapped calendar packs can be used, although many older people cannot get the contents out easily.

Memory boxes with separate compartments designed to accommodate a week's supply of treatment can be used. These too remind the patient if he/she has taken drugs due at a particular time, but they need to be refilled at least weekly.

Self-medication programmes are used in some clinical areas, notably those with elderly patients on several drugs. The patient assumes responsibility for compliance with prescribed medication, initially under close nursing supervision. Such programmes have proved effective in achieving high rates of compliance, which are maintained after discharge.

Before introducing a self-medication programme, it is necessary to determine how the practical differences in storing many drug supplies on one ward can be adapted within Management Policy for storage of medicines.

Drug treatment is often an expected consequence of seeking medical advice. Compliance with this treatment is of paramount importance and the nursing role in optimizing this has been discussed.

The nurse should be able to answer patients' queries regarding their drugs and reinforce explanations given by others, and therefore be knowledgeable about drugs commonly used in the area in which she is working. Sometimes extra information is needed by patients receiving drug treatment in order to minimize interactions with certain foodstuffs or commonly used remedies bought from a pharmacy. In other cases it may be necessary for the patient to carry a card or wear an identity bracelet outlining treatment. Specific examples are included under the management of particular situations in the following chapters.

RADIOTHERAPY

Radiotherapy is used in the management of malignant tumours and is carried out in specialized regional centres. It utilizes invisible high energy radiation known as ionizing radiation which penetrates and destroys living tissue.

The ionizing radiation used in radiotherapy comes from two main sources:

1. Beams of high energy X-rays which are produced by a large machine called a linear accelerator.
2. Gamma rays emitted from radioactive sources, called radioisotopes.

Ionizing radiation, irrespective of its source, causes tissue damage by the same process and although the characteristics of tissue penetration vary, the principles of nursing management and care are the same.

Tumours vary in their sensitivity to radiotherapy. Rapidly dividing cells are most sensitive to ionizing radiation, or radiotherapy. This is because cells are most sensitive to damage by ionizing radiation immediately before cell division. The rationale of treatment is to administer a lethal dose to malignant cells with minimal exposure of surrounding healthy tissue. Side-effects, discussed later, are also most apparent when nearby healthy tissue with a rapid rate of cell division falls within the field of treatment. Factors associated with radiosensitivity are:

- rapid growth rate
- poorly differentiated cells
- vascular tumours with good oxygen supply
- small size
- early stage
- ability of surrounding tissue to withstand ionizing radiation.

Diagnosis and accurate staging is carried out prior to commencing radiotherapy. The aims of treatment may be any one of the following:

Curative or radical: radiotherapy is the only treatment planned to maximize destruction of the tumour.

Adjuvant: radiotherapy is combined with surgery or chemotherapy with the aim of destroying the tumour.

Palliative: radiotherapy is used to relieve distressing symptoms with the aim of increasing quality of life when no cure is available. Lower doses are used and side-effects should not occur. Common symptoms which may be relieved by this means include bone pain, haemoptysis and others caused by compression of the respiratory or alimentary tracts.

Radioprotection

The International Radiation Symbol is displayed prominently to alert staff in areas where ionizing radiation, including X-rays, is used. As the characteristics of ionizing radiation are such that tissue penetration and damage result, staff working in the proximity of ionizing radiation must protect themselves from its potential risks. Radioprotection precautions must be taken in such areas, as indicated by local guidelines which are based on the following principles:

- maximize distance from the source
- use of protective shielding materials such as lead or concrete
- restrict time of exposure to irradiation.

These principles are applied to any particular situation which involves ionizing radiation (and includes plain X-rays) to ensure the safety of staff involved. During X-ray procedures, it is necessary for staff in the vicinity to wear lead aprons if they must remain with the patient. Women of child-bearing age must not be exposed to ionizing radiation after day 10 of the menstrual cycle if there is a possibility of pregnancy, in order to prevent congenital abnormalities caused by exposure of a fetus. Exposure of personnel is monitored to ensure the amount of radiation received over periods of time remains less than agreed international safety levels.

Types of radiotherapy treatment

External beam therapy

External beam therapy is also known as teletherapy or deep X-ray therapy (often abbreviated to DXT). The patient is exposed to a carefully controlled beam or beams of ionizing radiation. This is carried out in a room with thick concrete walls to contain ionizing radiation generated. The patient remains alone during treatments surrounded by large pieces of machinery. There is a two-way communication system between the patient and staff, and although the treatment itself is painless, it is a lonely and potentially frightening experience for the patient.

Treatment is prescribed after taking the following factors into account:

* patient – age, general fitness
* tumour – type, size, stage, location
* field(s) of treatment – see below.

Use of more than one field, or beam (Fig. 4.9), directed towards the tumour will cause less destruction of surrounding healthy tissue than constant exposure of the same skin and underlying tissues. With two beams directed towards the tumour site, this area receives a larger dose of radiation than the tissue between the tumour and the two skin sites. This technique also allows protection of sensitive tissue, for example, the spinal cord. Accurate positioning of the beams may be achieved either by marking treatment fields on the skin or by using a custom-made latex shell as a guide.

The total dose is then prescribed detailing the number of treatments, or fractions, their length and sites to be used. A record of treatments is kept as the effects of radiotherapy are cumulative. Tissue becomes less sensitive to repeated irradiation and overdose can cause tissue necrosis.

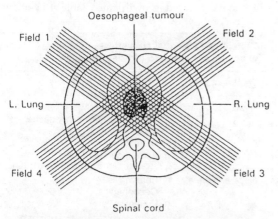

Fig. 4.9 Multi-field irradiation technique used to treat oesophageal carcinoma. The spinal cord is avoided, and although a portion of the lungs is unavoidably involved in the irradiation zone, the dose received is lower than the dose delivered to the tumour. (Reproduced with permission from Boore et al 1987, figure 16.1)

Internal radiotherapy

A radioisotope which emits ionizing radiation may be inserted internally, in close proximity to tumours in some locations.

Patients receiving internal radiotherapy are a potential source of irradiation to all others and are nursed in areas where radioprotection is available, often in a protected cubicle whose walls do not allow penetration of ionizing radiation. Nursing care is carried out expediently and as far from the radioactive source as is practicable. The impact of physical and social isolation can be dramatic and this may be alleviated by communicating via an intercom and providing appropriate diversional therapy. A radioactive hazard sign and specific radioprotection precautions to be taken by staff are clearly displayed on the cubicle door.

Interstitial therapy Small implants of a radioisotope are inserted into tissues delivering a localized dose of ionising radiation. Needles, wires or small seeds are used as sources to treat certain tumours of the tongue or breast.

Intracavitary therapy Radioactive implants are inserted into hollow organs such as the uterine cervix using special applicators.

Management of a patient receiving radiotherapy

A multidisciplinary approach is essential when caring for a patient receiving radiotherapy. Good teamwork between all health-care professionals will enhance relationship building with the patient, who in the recent past is likely to have had to deal with the diagnosis of cancer followed by meeting a new team of doctors and nurses. It is vital to be aware that lay people equate radiotherapy treatment with cancer irrespective of other information, including euphemisms, which may have already been given. A nurse caring for these patients must develop sensitive communication skills and the ability to face a diagnosis of cancer with an honest and optimistic attitude.

Common fears of a patient with cancer

The nurse plays an important role in alleviating many of the anxieties her patients will have. Diagnosis of cancer is often associated with fear, fright, pain, suffering and expectation of death. These fears arise for a variety of reasons:

* lack of knowledge and presence of false beliefs
* challenge to one's beliefs and values about the meaning of life and death
* change in family role and responsibilities
* unfulfilled business
* unachieved goals
* feelings of shame, guilt or anger
* insomnia.

Preparation for treatment

A patient is prepared for the radiotherapy treatment by providing information about its nature and possible side-effects. Optimism and reassurance that the impact of any side-effects can be minimized, and that their occurrence is now less common with advances in technology, is helpful. The nurse can enable her patient to overcome many of his anxieties by allowing their expression and reinforcing explanations given by other members of the multidisciplinary team.

Anticipation and early recognition of side-effects enables appropriate moral support and early nursing intervention if necessary. Side-effects or reactions are related to the site and dose of radiotherapy.

Potential side-effects

Skin reactions These affect skin of treatment fields and may be compared to sunburn of varying severity:

1. Inflammatory – manifest by erythema and slight oedema.
2. Dry desquamation – temporary reduction in activity of sweat and sebaceous glands causes drying, flaking and itching. The patient may also complain of a burning sensation.
3. Moist desquamation – blistering and oozing from the skin occurs and may be accompanied by peeling. Further treatment may be postponed until epithelial repair is evident.
4. Late effects – occur a few years after high doses of irradiation and include depilation (hair loss), telangiectasis (damaged epithelial capillaries are seen as tiny red outlines on the skin), atrophy and fibrosis.

Skin care for treatment fields Advice must be sought before applying anything to treated skin as many soaps, creams and lotions contain zinc and other metals which may sensitize the treated areas.

Areas of treatment are gently washed with plain warm water and patted dry using a soft towel to prevent trauma. Markings around treatment areas should be avoided. Adhesive tape must not be used as it causes peeling of treated skin. Loose-fitting clothing will reduce the risk of chaffing.

Fatigue and anorexia These side-effects appear during the first week of treatment and disappear a few weeks after treatment is finished. The patient often feels depressed and may associate these problems with worsening of the cancer rather than the radiotherapy. They arise as the removal of dead cells and debris takes place. This process increases the body's energy requirements. Repair of healthy tissue makes further demands on energy supplies and, consequently, fatigue and lethargy often result.

Nutritional intake frequently does not meet increased energy requirements even if anorexia is not a problem. Side-effects of radiotherapy may include stomatitis, nausea, vomiting, dysphagia or indigestion which if present will exacerbate poor nutritional intake caused by anorexia.

The nursing challenge is to provide appetizing meals which provide sufficient protein and energy to meet increased demand for tissue repair. Nourishing fluids and dietary supplements can add to solid intake. Total fluid intake should be at least 2000–3000 ml per day to facilitate excretion of nitrogenous waste products.

Altered body image This problem may arise in a patient with cancer for a variety of reasons, including alopecia, surgical amputation, sudden weight loss and skin reactions.

The skills used by the nurse to enable a patient to come to terms with a problem of this nature are discussed on page 531. Practical interventions include anticipation of this potential problem and ensuring the availability of appropriate appliances.

Local reactions These side-effects arise due to tissue damage within healthy organs inside the treatment field and are most marked in those tumours which have a rapid growth rate. Table 4.18 shows

Table 4.18 Potential side-effects following exposure of organs to ionizing radiation	
Treatment field	Potential side-effect
Head	Alopecia Cerebral oedema (headache, nausea, irritability) Stomatitis Altered sense of taste
Neck and chest	Pharyngitis Oesophagitis Pnuemonitis
Abdomen	Gastritis (nausea, vomiting, indigestion)
Pelvis	Colitis (diarrhoea) Cystitis Vaginitis (bleeding, discharge)
Flat bones, e.g. skull, pelvis, sternum	Bone marrow suppression (decreased formation of erythrocytes, leucocytes, thrombocytes (platelets)

potential side-effects arising from exposure of specific areas to radiotherapy.

Discharge planning

A course of radiotherapy can be carried out either as outpatient, inpatient or both. In each case, the patient should be given written information about commonly experienced problems and how help can be sought.

SURGERY

This specialized branch of practice involves procedures carried out in conjunction with anaesthesia. The procedures, often referred to as operations, are usually classified according to their anatomical location with an appropriate suffix (Box 4.17).

Principles of anaesthesia

An anaesthetic is given to cause reversible loss of all sensation from an area involved in surgery and is categorized as general or regional. During a general anaesthetic, a patient is unconscious and during regional anaesthesia consciousness is maintained unless sedative drugs are also given.

General anaesthesia

To enable surgery to be carried out, a general anaesthetic must induce the following effects:

- sleep or unconsciousness
- analgesia
- skeletal muscle relaxation.

The depth of anaesthesia required depends on factors related to the specific nature of the surgery being performed, including the location and length of the procedure. In the past, one anaesthetic agent was administered until the patient was sufficiently anaes-

---

Box 4.17	Classification of surgical procedures by suffix
-ectomy	removal of
-ostomy	creation of an opening to or from
-oscopy	visualization of
-pexy	fixation of
-rraphy	suturing of
-plasty	refashioning of
-desis	binding or fusion of

Box 4.18	Categories of anaesthetic drugs
Short-acting anaesthetic agents*:	
thiopentone	(Intraval)
methohexitone	(Brietal Sodium)
propofol	(Diprivan)
etomidate	(Hypnomidate)
ketamine	(Ketalar)
Volatile agents:	
halothane	
enflurane	
isoflurane	
Gas:	
nitrous oxide	

*Proprietary names are given in parentheses.

---

thetized to enable specific surgery to be carried out but this was accompanied by significant mortality. Current practice involves the use of combinations of drugs to induce and then maintain the levels of unconsciousness, analgesia and muscle relaxation required.

Induction of anaesthesia is usually achieved by administering an intravenous injection of a fast-acting anaesthetic agent (Box 4.18) which puts the patient to sleep, and produces unconsciousness.

To maintain sleep, further intravenous injections of fast-acting drugs may be used for short procedures. For longer procedures, gas or vaporized volatile agents (Box 4.16) are mixed with oxygen and inhaled through the rebreathing circuit of an anaesthetic machine.

To induce and maintain analgesia intravenous injections of strong opiate drugs are frequently given, although spinal or epidural routes may also be employed.

To produce and maintain skeletal muscle relaxation intravenous injections of muscle-relaxant drugs are given. These drugs affect all skeletal muscles including the respiratory muscles and the patient will require assisted ventilation. An endotracheal tube is used to intubate the patient and respiratory function is then supported by mechanical ventilation.

When surgery is complete, the anaesthetic is reversed and the patient then requires appropriate postoperative care to facilitate a safe recovery.

Regional anaesthesia

This category includes several techniques or routes by

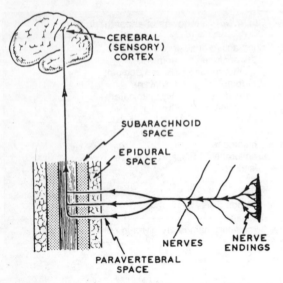

Fig. 4.10 The pathway of pain: the course of painful impulses from a wound to the brain is illustrated. The passage of impulses can be interrupted at any of the sites indicated by the arrows. (Reproduced with permission from Campbell & Spence 1985, figure 1.1)

which local anaesthetics may be administered. Local anaesthetic drugs include lignocaine, bupivicaine and cocaine. Irrespective of where they are applied in the pain pathway they act in the same way. This is by producing reversible blockage of nervous impulses at the point of application, thereby preventing transmission of nervous impulses in pain fibres from distal locations to the cerebral cortex. Figure 4.10 illustrates the various sites within the pain pathway at which regional anaesthesia is used. The extent of anaesthesia is determined by the area from which anaesthetized neurones receive their sensory input.

Nursing care for patients receiving spinal and epidural anaesthesia is explained in Ch. 5, for the other techniques it is discussed on page 133.

Nursing care of the surgical patient

Surgery may be carried out either electively, following planned admission from a waiting list, or as an emergency at short notice. Sometimes surgery is further distinguished as 'major' or 'minor'. While there is no clear-cut distinction between the two, in general, minor surgery is associated with a straightforward procedure and a short period of hospitalization. Increasingly, minor surgery is carried out on a day basis.

Aims of nursing care

- To promote optimal psychological well-being before, during and after surgery.
- To promote optimal physical well-being before, during and after surgery.
- To minimize the risks of complications associated with surgery.

In order to achieve these aims, detailed assessment of the patient must be carried out in relation to the specific surgery planned and the type of anaesthesia to be used. This enables identification of actual and potential problems with which the nurse working in a surgical ward must be familiar. She must also know the specific nursing care which will minimize the occurrence of these problems and their early signs. This enables early detection of problems or complications should they arise.

Preoperative nursing care

Preoperative care starts when it is decided that surgery is necessary. This may be at an outpatient consultation with advice being given about life-style changes which will enhance both the surgery itself and the subsequent period of convalescence. Advice may include reducing weight and stopping smoking, in addition to controlling pre-existing illness.

Preoperative nursing care is carried out to meet the broad aims above. Nursing Care Plan 4.2 explains the nursing care required by a patient going for surgery under general anaesthesia. Several key areas of preoperative and postoperative care are explained in more detail below. In the following chapters these principles are applied and explained in more detail in relation to specific types of surgery.

Psychological preparation A patient admitted for elective surgery can largely plan his domestic and employment situations around his incapacity. However a patient admitted as an emergency is likely to experience anxiety related to both situations above and also the sudden onset of a condition requiring imminent surgery. This patient is also likely to require medical and nursing intervention to stabilize his physical condition before surgery.

By using effective communication skills (Ch. 3), the nurse can identify specific fears for individual patients and then build up their trust. She can then assist her patients to overcome many of their worries. Fatigue and insomnia compound anxiety and it is important that the nurse enables the patient to have periods of rest. A sedative may be prescribed to promote sleep on the night before surgery.

Nursing Care Plan 4.2   Principles of preoperative care

Problem	Aim	Nursing action	Rationale
1. Anxiety regarding forthcoming operation	To optimize psychological preparation of the patient and family for surgery	**COMMUNICATING** ❏ Display kind, caring approach to patient and family ❏ Identify causes of anxiety (see text) ❏ Encourage patient to express his feelings and concerns and deal with them appropriately ❏ Explain operation and its implications to patient and family using appropriate language, involve relevant sources of support, e.g. medical social worker, chaplain, specialist nurses ❏ Explain the need for postoperative equipment such as oxygen, suction, intravenous infusion	Helps to establish a good rapport with patient and family Sharing these should help the patient to feel more relaxed and increase his trust in the team Helps to remove fear of the unknown, and ensures patient is knowledgeable about the surgery and its likely outcome By being forewarned, all equipment is seen as a predictable necessity rather than meaning that something has gone wrong in theatre
2. Patient may not be physically fit for surgery	To optimize physical preparation of the patient prior to surgery	**MAINTAINING A SAFE ENVIRONMENT** ❏ Prepare patient for preoperative investigations: i. chest X-ray ii. electrocardiograph (ECG) iii. blood sampling ❏ Measure and record patient's temperature, pulse respirations and blood pressure, weight and height ❏ Perform and record urinalysis results Physiotherapist to teach patient: i. deep breathing exercises ii. how to cough postoperatively iii. leg exercises	Preparation for and explanation of these investigations will allow patient to understand and gain confidence that surgery is being planned and carried out meticulously Enables detection of abnormalities which could complicate surgery Gives a baseline measurement for postoperative period Allows for identification of abnormalities prior to surgery Postoperatively reduces complication of chest infection by preventing sputum retention and encouraging full chest expansion Reduces the risk of deep vein thrombosis
3. Patient to have a general anaesthetic	To prepare patient to ensure his safety prior to, during and after anaesthesia	❏ Prepare patient's skin according to local policy ❏ Fast patient for 4–6 hours prior to operation ❏ Inform patient when fasting starts and remove all food and fluids from locker. Place fasting card above patient's bed ❏ Take time to sit and talk to patient about fears or concerns ❏ Carry out appropriate bowel preparation	Purpose of skin preparation is to remove micro-organisms from the surface of the skin to prevent wound infection Failure to do so would put the patient at risk of vomiting or regurgitating gastric contents when anaesthetized predisposing to aspiration pneumonia. Informs all staff that patient is fasting By allowing patient to express him/herself any unrelieved anxieties may be discussed Prevents constipation in the days after major surgery

Nursing Care Plan 4.2 (*cont'd*)			
Problem	**Aim**	**Nursing action**	**Rationale**
3. (cont'd)			For some surgery on the alimentary tract bowel preparation over several days is required to minimize the risk of intraoperative contamination
		❏ Administer night sedation if prescribed	Helps the patient to relax and hopefully obtain a good night's sleep prior to theatre
		MORNING OF OPERATION ❏ Patient to have shower prior to theatre, ensure skin, hair, nails and umbilicus are clean	These areas can harbour micro-organisms
		❏ Remove nail varnish and make-up	These conceal early signs of cyanosis or shock during and after surgery
		❏ Help dress patient in theatre gown and modesty pants	These are made of cotton. Nylon is not permitted in theatre as it can cause static electricity which would be a hazard since there are anaesthetic gases and oxygen present
		❏ Patient encouraged to rest in clean bed	Reduces further potential skin contamination
		❏ Complete the nursing checklist prior to theatre	Ensures safety of patient
		i. Remove any dentures, note crowns or loose teeth	Dentures could slip backwards and occlude the airway during anaesthesia. Crowns and loose teeth must be reported to anaesthetist so that extra care may be taken to prevent them being dislodged and entering the airway
		ii. Remove contact lenses or glasses	Contact lenses dry out on the cornea causing damage. Glasses are kept safely in the ward
		iii. Remove all jewellery except wedding ring which is taped to finger using non-allergic tape	Jewellery is removed because: (a) it harbours micro-organisms; (b) if diathermy machine is used in theatre and patient's jewellery comes in contact with metal of the operating table, electricity may go through the jewellery to earth, causing a diathermy burn
		iv. With patient's permission, deal with their valuables according to hospital policy	Keep patient's property safe and reduces another potential source of anxiety
		v. Record presence of prostheses not removed ie. artificial eye, wig, hearing aid	Theatre staff should be aware when prostheses are still in situ so that they can be removed when the patient is anaesthetized. A hearing aid is particularly important to aid pre- and postoperative communication

Nursing Care Plan 4.2 (*cont'd*)

Problem	Aim	Nursing action	Rationale
3. (cont'd)		vi. Check that the consent form is fully completed	Ensures that the patient is knowledgeable about the surgery and likely outcome and is agreeable to this. Report any indecision or omission to the medical staff before premedication is given as the patient's right to refuse must be accepted
		vii. Check the patient's identity by asking him/her for full name and date of birth. This information should be checked with identity band on patient's wrist	Asking the patient to identify himself ensures correct identification. Identity band allows correct identification when the patient is unable to respond
		viii. Ask patient to empty his/her bladder approximately 1 hour prior to surgery	Patient's bladder should be empty prior to receiving anaesthesia, as muscle-relaxing drugs would cause incontinence
		❐ Explain purpose of and administer premedication as prescribed	Premedication helps to relax patient and reduce anxiety. It also facilitates induction of the anaesthetic
		i. Warn patient that the drugs may cause drowsiness, light headedness and produce a dry mouth. Patient also warned that he/she should not attempt to get out of bed alone as he/she may fall	Preparing patient to expect these effects, reduces anxiety and maintains patient's safety
		❐ Accompany patient to theatre with his/her notes and X-rays, according to hospital policy	Maintains the comfort and safety of patient

Many known stressors create anxiety prior to surgery:

● fear of the unknown
● fear of death, hospitals, anaesthetics
● fear of scars or mutilation
● lack of knowledge or understanding about the nature of the operation and its outcome
● loss of control over one's life
● loss of normal support mechanisms.

Hayward (1975) found that patients who had been given relevant information preoperatively experienced less pain and anxiety postoperatively than the control group of patients who were encouraged to talk but were not given details of realistic postoperative recovery. In another study, Boore (1978) found that effective psychological and physical preparation reduced both postoperative stress and recovery time. It is therefore apparent that effective preoperative nursing care has psychological and physical benefits.

Physical preparation

Fasting   It is important to check with the anaesthetist which regular drugs should be given to a patient who is fasting.

Fasting is required for 4–6 hours preoperatively to minimize aspiration or regurgitation of gastric contents into the lungs during anaesthesia when the cough reflex is absent. A nasogastric tube may be used to empty the stomach prior to emergency surgery. Hamilton Smith (1972) found that this fasting period was often greatly exceeded by nurses in order to fit in with ward routines rather than the comfort and well-being of individual patients.

During periods of fasting plasma glucose levels remain constant as glycogen stores are broken down. When these reserves are exhausted, protein and fat are then broken down to provide energy. Fat breakdown leads to accumulation of ketones which are excreted in the urine (ketonuria) and may also cause nausea.

Skin preparation Traditionally, hair has been removed by shaving the area around the incision preoperatively. However, it is now thought that this process may result in tiny lacerations which then act as a source of infection if they become contaminated. Some hospitals reduce this risk by using depilatory cream rather than shaving.

Running water from a shower removes microorganisms more effectively than soaking in a bath, however some patients may not be fit enough to stand under a shower. Sometimes antiseptic agents are used for cleaning the skin at this time.

Postoperative nursing care

Principles of managing any seriously ill or unconscious patient dictate the priorities of:

- maintaining a clear *airway*
- assessment of effective *breathing*
- assessment of adequate *circulation*.

These priorities are applied in the immediate postoperative period. Care initially takes place in the recovery room and if there is a recovery suite available patients do not return to the ward until they are easily roused by speech.

The principles of postoperative care following surgery under general anaesthesia are explained in Nursing Care Plan 4.3.

Observation of respiration and circulatory function A baseline set of recordings is important to detect subsequent changes or trends. The frequency of these is reduced or increased again as the patient's condition dictates.

Haemorrhage Primary haemorrhage occurs when there is substantial blood loss during surgery. Haemorrhage may also occur when the blood pressure returns to its preoperative level a few hours after surgery and may be due to incomplete haemostasis or a slipped ligature. The patient may have to go back to theatre to deal with this type of bleeding. Risk of haemorrhage is not completely over until some days postoperatively, especially after certain types of surgery, and in these circumstances it is usually associated with a wound infection.

Vigilance is therefore necessary for some time after surgery. This enables detection of both overt haemorrhage and its consequence, hypovolaemic shock.

Eating and drinking Nausea and vomiting may occur as a side-effect of anaesthetic drugs and fluids cannot be given until the patient is fully conscious again. Oral fluids are therefore withheld for a few hours postoperatively in most cases. Instead, mouthwashes can be given to moisten the oral mucosa and relieve the dry mouth commonly experienced after fasting and drugs given for premedication.

Paralytic ileus occurs when the bowel has been handled during surgery causing the peristaltic activity of the smooth muscle to be lost. Stasis of the bowel contents within the handled area occurs and leads to accumulation of intestinal secretions. A nasogastric tube is inserted to drain or aspirate gastric contents, thus preventing vomiting in such circumstances. Fluid intake is maintained by intravenous infusion until peristalsis returns. At this time bowel sounds have returned and flatus is passed. Oral fluids are recommended and when well tolerated, a diet which is easily digested can be introduced.

Pain Frequent assessment using a pain chart is carried out, and prescribed analgesia is given as required. Opiate drugs are used by injection until nausea and paralytic ileus subsides. Situations which increase pain include bed-bathing, physiotherapy and mobilizing. Timing these activities appropriately with the administration of analgesia to minimize discomfort is an important part of care planning.

Intramuscular injections may be given and increasingly patient controlled analgesia (PCA) is being used. PCA is administered intravenously via a small pump and the patient can self-administer his analgesia as required. This method has proven effective despite concerns of addiction or overdose. Respiratory rate is monitored hourly to detect signs of respiratory depression.

Mobilizing Early mobilization is beneficial for many reasons. The risk of chest infection and deep venous thrombosis is reduced and it provides a psychological boost to the patient. Exercise and mobility are usually increased gradually. Following major surgery increasing exercise levels must continue for some time after discharge until previous fitness levels are regained.

Discharge planning and convalescence This process facilitates a comfortable and complete recovery after a period of convalescence. Effective planning is increasingly important as the trend for early discharge continues.

Nursing Care Plan 4.3   Principles of postoperative care

Actual/potential problem	Aim	Nursing action	Rationale
1. **Airway obstruction**	To prevent or detect, and report promptly	**BREATHING** ❑ Nurse patient in the recovery position until conscious ❑ Observe for stridor	Maintains airway patency and prevents the tongue occluding it Indicates partial airway obstruction
2. **Inadequate breathing**	To detect and report promptly	❑ Observe rate, depth and effort of breathing ❑ Observe skin for pallor or cyanosis	Changes may indicate inadequate respiratory function Indicates hypoxia
3. **Potential hypoxia**	To maintain normal oxygenation	❑ Administer oxygen therapy as prescribed ❑ Ensure mask is comfortable and reasons for its use are reinforced to patient ❑ Explain the safety precautions required when oxygen is in use to both patient and family i. No smoking while oxygen is in use ii. Oil or grease should not be used around any oxygen connections iii. Fire extinguisher should be readily available iv. Unnecessary electrical devices should not be used whilst oxygen is in use ❑ Give regular oral hygiene to prevent oral mucosa becoming dry	Additional oxygen will increase level of oxygen available to tissues, thus preventing hypoxia If the mask is uncomfortable it may cause sores and will not be tolerated by patient Oxygen supports combustion and all staff, patients and visitors should be aware of the dangers Appliances like electric razors and hairdryers should not be used The oral mucosa dries quickly when oxygen is used and can soon become sore and infected unless kept moist
4. **Development of haemorrhage or hypovolaemic shock**	To detect early signs and report promptly	❑ Record blood pressure, pulse, respiration as instructed ❑ Observe the patient's skin and report pale, cold, clammy skin ❑ Observe wound site for signs of oozing or leakage ❑ Observe drain(s) for nature and amount of drainage	These would be detected by falling blood pressure readings and a rising pulse rate Indicates the presence of shock Increasing leakage can indicate haemorrhage. May require the application of pressure dressing or further attention from the surgeon Increasing drainage can indicate haemorrhage
5. **Anxiety and fear following surgery**	To reassure patient by explaining all procedures at a level of the patient's understanding	**COMMUNICATING** ❑ Explain all procedures prior to them being performed using terms the patient understands	Continues philosophy of having a well-informed patient. Research has shown that patients who are well informed are more likely to have an uncomplicated and speedy postoperative recovery

Nursing Care Plan 4.3 (*cont'd*)			
Actual/potential problem	**Aim**	**Nursing action**	**Rationale**
5. (cont'd)		❑ Repeat explanations as necessary	Disorientation is common in the immediate postoperative period after general anaesthesia
6. Postoperative pain	To control pain by effective use of analgesia	❑ Give analgesia as prescribed, particularly prior to known painful events, i.e. visit by physiotherapist ❑ Monitor effect of analgesia with the aid of a pain chart	Patient who is pain free will be able to cooperate with physiotherapy and move around in bed more. Pain-free patient will also benefit psychologically If analgesia is not controlling pain the medical staff should be asked to review prescription
7. Dehydration or fluid overload	To maintain fluid balance	**EATING AND DRINKING** ❑ Maintain accurate record of fluid intakes and outputs ❑ Monitor rate and flow of intravenous infusion if present ❑ Monitor intravenous cannula site for signs of infiltration ❑ Observe for presence of, and report increasing dyspnoea, cyanosis, tachycardia and expectorating frothy sputum ❑ Offer patient sips of water when permitted	Enables evaluation of fluid balance Important to ensure that the patient receives correct amount of fluid to maintain normal hydration If infiltration of the tissue occurs, the medical staff are informed so that they may resite intravenous infusion These indicate pulmonary oedema which can arise from fluid overload Increases patient's oral comfort and promotes gradual return of absorptive function of alimentary tract. When fluids are well tolerated intravenous infusion can be discontinued
8. Postoperative nausea	To minimize or alleviate	❑ Administer antiemetics as prescribed ❑ Aspirate nasogastric tube if present	Recognize that opiate analgesia and anaesthetic drugs cause nausea Minimizes gastric contents
9. Impaired nutritional status caused by prolonged fasting	To regain nutritional status	❑ Introduce easily digested diet when fluids are tolerated	Re-establishes oral intake, providing energy and protein required for wound healing
10. Wound or other infection	To prevent infection occurring	**MAINTAINING BODY TEMPERATURE** ❑ Administer prophylactic antibiotics as prescribed ❑ Monitor patient's temperature 4 hourly. Note and report pyrexia, confusion and restlessness	Greatly reduces the possibility of infection occurring after major surgery These are signs of infection. Early identification and reporting allows prompt treatment

Nursing Care Plan 4.3 (*cont'd*)

Actual/potential problem	Aim	Nursing action	Rationale
10. (cont'd)		❑ Observe wound and other susceptible sites for signs of infection; local pain, redness, increased warmth, presence of purulent exudate. Send specimen for culture and sensitivity if infection is suspected	Any developing infection must be identified and treated promptly
		❑ When fully conscious and vital signs are stabilized, patient should be assisted into an upright position well supported by pillows	The upright position aids fuller chest expansion and minimizes stasis of secretions which predisposes to chest infection or atelectasis.
		❑ Encourage patient to perform deep breathing hourly as taught preoperatively by physiotherapist	
		❑ Encourage patient to support abdominal or thoracic wound when coughing	Any increase in stress on the wound could lead to wound breakdown and delayed healing
11. Patient unable to maintain his own hygiene in the short term	To maintain a good standard of hygiene	**PERSONAL CLEANSING AND DRESSING** ❑ On return from theatre once vital signs are stable, patient is assisted to wash his face and hands, and helped into own nightclothes	Helps the patient to feel fresher and more comfortable
		❑ Patient may require a bed bath on the first day. Attention paid to all his hygiene needs	Patient too ill to have anything other than a bed bath. Maintains the patient's usual standard of personal hygiene
		❑ Patient can begin to take a more active part in his personal hygiene as his condition improves	Restores a feeling of being more in control of events, and therefore has a positive effect on morale
		❑ As the patient's condition improves, patient can progress to an immersion bath or preferably a shower	A shower is preferable as there is less risk of infection occurring as the patient is not sitting in potentially contaminated water
12. Patient immobile and prone to complications until he is able to resume full mobility	To prevent the complications of immobility	**MOBILIZING** ❑ Prevent the formation of a deep vein thrombosis:	
		i. on return from theatre, implement passive leg exercises until such time as the patient is able to exercise his legs independently	Encourages venous return to right side of heart by use of calf muscle pump. Prevents stasis of blood in deep veins thereby preventing clot formation
		ii. Encourage deep breathing	Facilitates the removal of anaesthetic gases from lungs and aids venous return to the heart
		iii. Administer heparin if prescribed	Heparin is an anticoagulant and thus prevents the formation of clots in the blood vessels
		iv. Apply antiembolism stockings if prescribed	Aids the venous return from the legs
		v. Observe calves and report swelling, complaints of calf tenderness or pain, redness or increased heat	These are indicative of deep vein thrombosis

Nursing Care Plan 4.3 (*cont'd*)

Actual/potential problem	Aim	Nursing action	Rationale
12. (cont'd)		☐ Prevent the formation of pressure sores: i. perform 2-hourly pressure area care to coincide with turning ii. use pressure-relieving aids as appropriate ☐ The patient is helped to sit out of bed when his condition permits, and encouraged to mobilize gradually thereafter (Box 4.6)	Allows regular (2 hourly) evaluation of effectiveness of nursing action and reassessment and planning as required Prevents formation of pressure sores Improves morale and improves expansion of lungs reducing the risk of chest infection. Promotes increased independence
13. Urinary retention	To prevent or detect	**ELIMINATING** ☐ Monitor and record urine output ☐ Report to medical staff if patient has not passed urine 6–8 hours postoperatively ☐ Encourage patient to pass urine regularly	Allows monitoring of fluid balance Patient may be underhydrated or have retention of urine. Recognition of either allows prompt treatment This reduces stasis time in bladder. Stasis predisposes to urinary tract infection

Patient education is based on the areas identified in Nursing Care Plan 4.3 and will promote uncomplicated convalescence and recovery. When possible information booklets should be given to reinforce verbal information. Such booklets are also a very useful reference source after discharge when there is no one readily available to answer queries. Factors which are taken into account when planning discharge of a surgical patient are:

- where and when sutures will be removed
- date and time of follow-up appointment
- availability of drugs or other supplies needed
- need for other treatments, e.g. physiotherapy
- nutritional requirements to promote wound healing
- specific advice on lifting, sexual intercourse, mobility, exercise, returning to work
- need for aids, prosthesis or appliances

- contact with specific counselling or support groups
- need for community services, e.g. district nurse, home help, meals on wheels
- availability of information booklets to reinforce information given verbally.

Suggested assignments

1. Relate the nursing measures used to prevent or minimise spread of infection to the chain of infection.
2. Consider the effectiveness of methods you have seen used to assess and manage patients' pain.
3. Compare and contrast the needs for rest and mobility in a small group of patients. Consider how each patient's care is implemented to maximise the benefits of both.

REFERENCES AND FURTHER READING

Barker H M 1991 Beck's nutrition and dietetics for nurses, 8th edn. Churchill Livingstone, Edinburgh

Bond M R 1984 Pain – its nature, analysis and treatment, 2nd edn. Churchill Livingstone, Edinburgh

Boore J 1978 Prescription for recovery. RCN, London

Boore J et al 1987 Nursing the physically ill adult. Churchill Livingstone, Edinburgh

Brunner L S, Suddarth D S 1989 The Lippencott Manual of Medical Surgical Nursing (2nd edn). Harper Row, London

Caddow P (ed) 1989 Applied microbiology. Scutari Press, Middlesex

Campbell D, Spence A A 1985 Norris and Campbell's anaesthetics, resuscitation and intensive care, 6th edn. Churchill Livingstone, Edinburgh

Chandler J 1991 Tabbner's nursing care: theory and practice, 2nd edn. Churchill Livingstone, Edinburgh

Clark J, Sage C, Attree M 1988 Essential Nursing Care (Letts Study Aids). Letts, London

Department of Health 1992 Immunisation against infectious disease. HMSO, London

Department of Health and Social Security (DHSS) 1984 Committee on Medical Aspects of Food Policy. Diet and disease (The COMA Report). HMSO, London

Evans D M D 1989 Special tests – the procedure and meaning of the commoner tests in hospital, 13th edn. London: Faber and Faber, London

Hamilton Smith S 1972 Nil by mouth? RCN, London

Hancock B, Bradshaw J D (1986) Lecture notes on clinical oncology, 2nd edn. Blackwell Scientific Publications, Oxford

Hayward J 1975 Information – a prescription against pain. RCN, London

Hinchliff S M, Montague S E 1988 Physiology for nursing practice. Baillière Tindall, London

Jamieson E M et al 1992 Guidelines for clinical nursing practice, 2nd edn. Churchill Livingstone, Edinburgh

Kinsey Smith M D 1980 Fluids and electrolytes: a conceptual approach. Churchill Livingstone, Edinburgh

Marieb E M 1992 Human anatomy and physiology, 2nd edn. Benjamin Cummings, California

McCaffery M 1983 Nursing the patient in pain. Harper and Row, London (adapted for UK by B. Sofaer)

National Advisory Committee on Nutrition Education (NACNE) 1983 Guidelines for health education in Britain. London: Health Education Council, London

Pritchard V, Hathaway C 1988 Patient handwashing practice. Nursing Times Vol 74(2) p 84(36): 68–72

Roper N, Logan W W, Tierney A J 1990 The elements of nursing. Churchill Livingstone, Edinburgh

Spector W G 1989 An introduction to general pathology, (3rd edn.) Edinburgh: Churchill Livingstone

Stockwell F 1972 The unpopular patient. RCN, London

Taylor L J 1978 An evaluation of handwashing techniques. Nursing Times Vol 74(2) p 54–55

Trounce J R 1990 Clinical pharmacology for nurses, 13th edn. Churchill Livingstone, Edinburgh

Royle J A, Walsh M 1992 Watson's medical-surgical nursing and related physiology, 4th edn. Baillière Tindall, London

Wilson K W 1990 Ross and Wilson's anatomy and physiology in health and illness, 7th edn. Churchill Livingstone, Edinburgh

Nursing care principles for specific disorders of health

Nursing care principles for specific disorders of health

SECTION CONTENTS

The chapters in this section cover the specialised areas of nursing care and reflect the changing pattern of disease, with an increased emphasis on common care strategies.

5

Care implications of disorders of the nervous system

Isobel M. Gibson

In order to give nursing care to patients suffering from the effects of injury to or disease of the nervous system and, equally important, to appreciate the significance of observations which the nurse will be asked to make, an understanding of the structures involved and how they function is essential. A brief description is given below, and readers are referred to Tortora and Grabowski *Principles of Anatomy & Physiology*.

ANATOMY AND PHYSIOLOGY

The functional units of the nervous system are neurones supported by glia, the connective tissue. The neurone (Fig. 5.1) consists of a cell body and its processes – dendrites through which impulses are received and an axon which transmits the impulse via other dendrites to another neurone. The axon is usually covered by myelin which acts as a conductor. Along with its conduction property, nerve tissue also has the property of irritability, responding to partly electrical/chemical stimulation.

The propagation of a nerve impulse, i.e. the action potential, is an electrochemical process. This however is too weak to cross the synaptic gap (between axon and dendrites) therefore a chemical neurotransmitter is released, e.g. acetylcholine, dopamine, noradrenaline which excites the next neurone initiating another impulse. The chemical is then neutralized thus inactivating the synapse.

For descriptive purpose the nervous system can be divided into:

- the central nervous system (CNS)
- the peripheral nervous system.

The brain enclosed within the cranium, or skull, can be anatomically divided into the cerebrum,

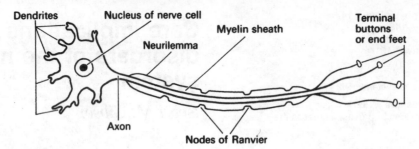

Fig. 5.1 A neurone

cerebellum and brain stem (Fig. 5.2). It is covered and protected by three membranes, the dura mater, the arachnoid mater and the pia mater, known collectively as the meninges (Fig. 5.3).

The dura mater has two layers, the outer attached to the under surface of the skull, the inner forming notably the tentorium cerebelli which separates the anterior and middle fossae of the skull from the posterior fossa, and the falx cerebri which incompletely separates the anterior and the middle fossae. The extradural space is found between the skull and the dura. Between these two layers are the venous sinuses (Fig. 5.3).

Following head injury blood may collect in the extradural and subdural spaces forming haematomas (see Fig. 5.12A,B).

The arachnoid mater is a serous membrane lying beneath the dura between which is a potential space, the subdural space. Web-like processes extend from this to the pia mater which is firmly attached to the surface of the brain. The subarachnoid space containing cerebrospinal fluid (CSF) is found between these two layers.

The brain stem

This is an elongated structure, which passes from the cerebrum through the tentorial hiatus to the posterior fossa where it connects with the cerebellum. There are three anatomical divisions, midbrain, pons varolii and medulla oblongata (Fig. 5.2). Deep within the medulla groups of cells the vital centres – respiratory, cardiac and vasomotor – associated with reflex activity are found. There are also reflex centres for coughing, swallowing and vomiting.

From the medulla via the brain stem to the cerebral cortex is a network of nerve cells and their fibres, the reticular formation. This functions as a filter, determining which sensory information will be allowed to reach the cerebral cortex. A state of arousal within the cerebral cortex is activated by the reticular formation

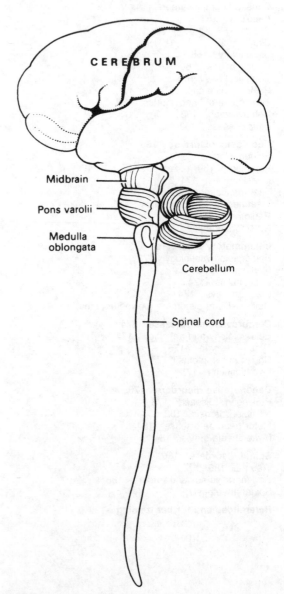

Fig. 5.2 Cerebrum, cerebellum and brain stem relationships. (Reproduced with kind permission from Wilson 1990.)

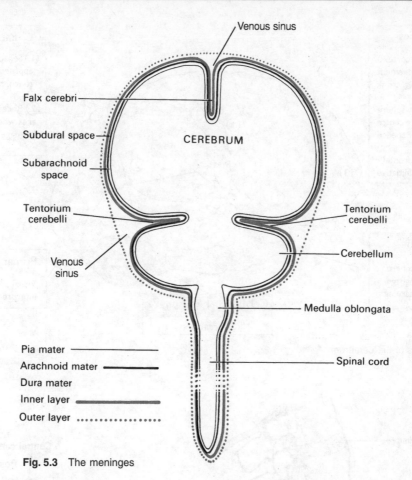

Fig. 5.3 The meninges

and any factor, for example head injury, which impairs this function will result in altered consciousness. Figure 5.4 details the functions of the various areas of the brain.

Spinal cord

The spinal cord surrounded by the meninges is a direct continuation of the medulla oblongata lying within the vertebral canal of the vertebral column, extending from the 1st cervical to the 1st/2nd lumbar vertebra. It is divided into segments: eight cervical, twelve thoracic, five lumbar, five sacral and one coccygeal.

In cross-section the spinal cord resembles an H-shaped mass of grey tissue surrounded by white matter arranged in tracts. The posterior horn of the H receives sensory impulses from the peripheral nerves whereas the anterior horns receive voluntary motor impulses from the motor cortex within the cerebrum (Fig. 5.5B).

Thirty-one pairs of spinal nerves arise from either side of the cord, emerging from the vertebral canal through the intervertebral foramina (Fig. 5.5A). A typical nerve has a mixture of sensory and motor fibres derived from the anterior and posterior nerve roots. Although the spinal cord ends at the 1st lumbar vertebra, the meninges extend as low as the 2nd sacral vertebra, and the spinal nerves arising from the lower end of the cord hang within the theca until they leave at their appropriate levels.

Motor pathways

The motor pathways should be considered as an integrated system. However, they can be understood more easily if considered as the pyramidal tract and the extrapyramidal tract, the two parts working in co-ordination.

The pyramidal tract

This pathway arises in many parts of the cerebral cortex but predominantly within the motor area of

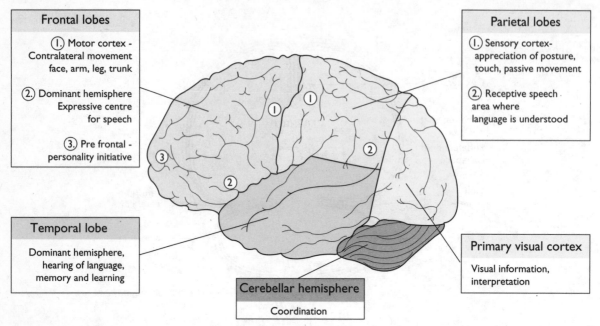

Frontal lobes

(1.) Motor cortex -
Contralateral movement
face, arm, leg, trunk

(2.) Dominant hemisphere
Expressive centre
for speech

(3.) Pre frontal -
personality initiative

Temporal lobe

Dominant hemisphere,
hearing of language,
memory and learning

Parietal lobes

(1.) Sensory cortex-
appreciation of posture,
touch, passive movement

(2.) Receptive speech
area where
language is understood

Primary visual cortex

Visual information,
interpretation

Cerebellar hemisphere

Coordination

Fig. 5.4 Functions of the cerebrum

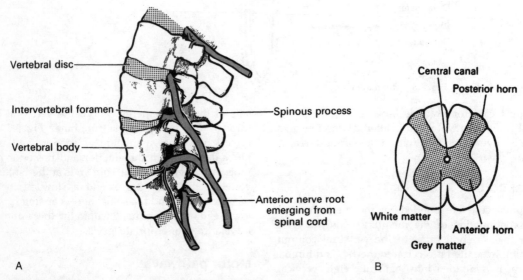

Vertebral disc

Intervertebral foramen

Vertebral body

Spinous process

Anterior nerve root
emerging from
spinal cord

Central canal

Posterior horn

White matter

Anterior horn

Grey matter

A

B

Fig. 5.5 (A) Spinal nerves emerging through intervertebral formamina. (B) Section through spinal cord

the precentral gyrus of the cerebral cortex. The fibres pass through the internal capsule to the midbrain, some also travelling to the medulla and motor nuclei of cranial nerves. The majority of fibres cross in the medulla innervating the motor nuclei on the opposite side; some fibres innervate the motor nuclei on the same side, for example the motor nucleus of the facial

nerve branch controlling the upper face. Thus damage within the left hemisphere will cause a right lower facial weakness, the upper branch from the uncrossed fibre being uninvolved.

The crossed medullary fibres then descend in the white matter (corticospinal tracts) of the spinal cord between the anterior and posterior columns of grey matter. The remaining uncrossed fibres descend in the white matter between the anterior columns of grey matter crossing to the opposite side at the level of termination.

The extrapyramidal tract

This is composed of fibres arising from:

1. widespread areas of cortex, especially frontal and parietal lobes
2. the cerebellum
3. the basal ganglia.

These are masses of grey matter embedded in the white matter of the cerebral hemisphere, the main centre being the corpus striatum. The particular contributions of the corpus striatum are:

- Provision for automatic-type motor activity including emotional responses.
- Relaying the influence of the cerebral cortex onto voluntary muscles.
- Exercising an influence on fibres of the pyramidal and extrapyramidal tracts.

Extrapyramidal fibres arising from the cortex, cerebellum and basal ganglia, descend in the white matter of the spinal cord and terminate within the anterior horn cells. These fibres exert their influence by modifying the muscle fibres in the muscle spindle thereby altering responses to change in tension. Without this, smooth normal movement would be impossible and balance and posture maintenance would be affected.

Final common pathway

The pyramidal pathways convey impulses to alpha cells whose axons are distributed to muscle fibres of motor units, whereas the extrapyramidal impulses are conveyed to gamma cells whose axons are distributed to the muscle spindle in muscle fibres, both pathways constituting the upper motor neurone. The alpha neurone constitutes the final common pathway forming the lower motor neurone.

Sensory pathways

An awareness of our internal/external environment reaches the sensory cortex of the brain via sensory pathways, the nature of the sensation transmitted determining the pathway taken. Within the skin are types of receptors, sensitive to touch, pain, temperature, and from the joint capsule, position sense and

the degree of muscle contraction are conveyed. These stimuli travel via sensory cranial nerves or peripheral spinal nerves.

Nerves conveying sensation of touch or proprioception enter the posterior column of white matter to the medulla where they synapse, crossing to the opposite side and then travelling to the thalamus. A further synapse occurs, the impulse travelling to the sensory cortex.

Nerves conveying pressure, temperature and touch also enter the posterior horn of grey matter but synapse here crossing at this level, then ascend to the thalamus and then onto the sensory cortex. The thalamus, a mass of nerve cells which is also part of the basal ganglia, is thought to perceive sensation but is unable to discriminate between or interpret these stimuli.

The meninges

These consist of three membranes, the dura mater, the arachnoid mater and the pia mater, covering and protecting the brain and spinal cord.

The dura has two layers. The outer layer is attached to the under surface of the skull. The inner layer forms folds, notably the tentorium cerebelli which separates the anterior and middle fossae of the skull from the posterior fossa, and the falx cerebri which incompletely separates the anterior and middle fossae (Fig. 5.6). Between these two layers are the venous sinuses.

The arachnoid is a serous membrane lying under the dura between which is a potential space, the subdural space. Web-like processes extend from this to the pia mater which is firmly attached to the brain. The subarachnoid space containing cerebrospinal fluid (CSF) is found between these two layers.

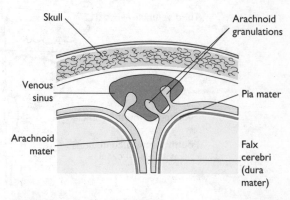

Fig. 5.6 Arachnoid granulations

The ventricles

Within each cerebral hemisphere can be found the right and left ventricles. These communicate with the third ventricle via the intraventricular foramen. The third ventricle communicates with the fourth ventricle via the aqueduct of midbrain.

Within the ventricle can be found vascular fluid processes called choroid plexuses which are involved in the formation of CSF. This circulates through the ventricular pathway leaving via the roof of the fourth ventricle to enter the subarachnoid space.

Since the fourth ventricle is continuous with the central canal of the spinal cord, a small amount of CSF flows into the canal (Fig. 5.7). Absorption back into the venous circulation occurs through arachnoid granulations found around the venous sinuses. Obstruction within the ventricular system results in accumulation of CSF, dilatation of the ventricles and an increase in intracranial pressure (ICP).

Peripheral nervous system

This has two components, the cerebrospinal and the autonomic system.

The cerebrospinal system

The cerebrospinal system is composed of the cranial and spinal nerves. There are 12 pairs of cranial nerves that are either sensory or motor fibres or both. Some also carry fibres from the autonomic system.

The autonomic system

This comprises sympathetic and parasympathetic components. The sympathetic system is particularly active in states of stress and fear, the fibres emerging with motor fibres between the 1st thoracic and 2nd lumbar segment, which they leave to join the sympathetic chain.

The chemical transmitter noradrenaline when released at sympathetic nerve endings causes dilatation of pupils, acceleration of the heart, constriction of skin and blood vessels thus increasing blood pressure.

The parasympathetic system is sometimes referred to as the 'emptying system' as it speeds up digestion and elimination. Parasympathetic fibres emerge with some cranial and sacral nerves and are activated by acetylcholine.

In most circumstances sympathetic and parasympathetic actions are mutually antagonistic, circumstances determining which action will predominate.

INTRACRANIAL PRESSURE

ICP is maintained automatically within a set of normal limits (0–10 mmHg; 80–180 cm H_2O) for most individuals, fluctuating continually to accommodate certain activities.

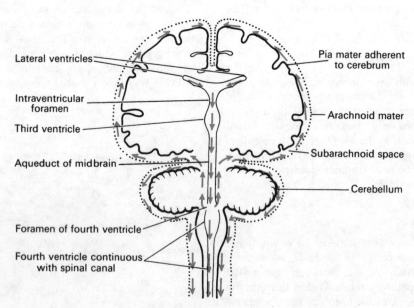

Fig. 5.7 Flow of cerebrospinal fluid

Lateral ventricles

Intraventricular foramen

Third ventricle

Aqueduct of midbrain

Foramen of fourth ventricle

Fourth ventricle continuous with spinal canal

Pia mater adherent to cerebrum

Arachnoid mater

Subarachnoid space

Cerebellum

Sharp rises occur during coughing, sneezing and straining at stool (the Valsalva manoeuvres (p. 157), afterwards falling again rapidly to normal, whereas standing upright lowers ICP. The three intracranial components are held therefore in a state of equilibrium and fundamental to understanding ICP is the modified 'Munro Kellie hypothesis' which states;

the skull a rigid compartment is filled to capacity with essentially noncompressible contents, brain matter, intravascular blood, and cerebrospinal fluid. If any of these three increase in volume, another must decrease or else intracranial pressure will rise.

Changes therefore in intracranial pressure may be as a result of:

1. Increases in brain tissue volume: tumour growth, abscess formation, intracellular bleed, increases in tissue fluid (oedema as a result of anoxia, trauma, inflammation).
2. Expansion of cerebral blood volume, as a result of carbon dioxide retention or obstruction to venous overflow.
3. Increase of circulatory CSF, caused by ventricular obstruction or CSF reabsorption impairment.

Normally therefore when an increase occurs within one of the components, reciprocal changes take place in the other two, thus allowing initially a degree of compensation without a change in ICP.

CSF volume can be reduced by increased absorption or reduced production. Compression of intracranial vessels will reduce the amount of the circulating cerebral blood volume and cerebral tissue can also become compressed, this however is limited. With unequal pressure differences within the brain compartments increasing, increased ICP exerts its effect by distorting and shifting cerebral tissue from the area of high pressure to an area of low pressure – brain herniation – and by reducing the effective perfusion of the brain (Fig. 5.8).

There are different types of herniation syndromes dependent on whether the area of high pressure is above the tentorium (supratentorium) or below (infratentorium). Increased pressure above the tentorium causes part of the temporal lobe to herniate through the tentorial hiatus, thus compressing the brain stem, further depressing consciousness and changing pupillary reaction.

Infratentorial herniation, although less frequent, is due to a pressure gradient in the posterior fossa which forces part of the posterior cerebellar hemisphere, the cerebellar tonsils, through the foramen magnum, compressing the medulla oblongata, leading to respiratory and cardiac arrest. Children's skulls can expand, so they have this additional compensatory mechanism to accommodate increasing intracranial volume and are thus partially protected from extremes of ICP.

Raised ICP can be accompanied by a variety of clinical features, early-morning headache, vomiting and papilloedema, the 'Cushing Triad'. Since their presentation may be of late onset or in some patients may not be present, one of the most reliable indicators in the detection of a rise in ICP is an alteration in the level of consciousness.

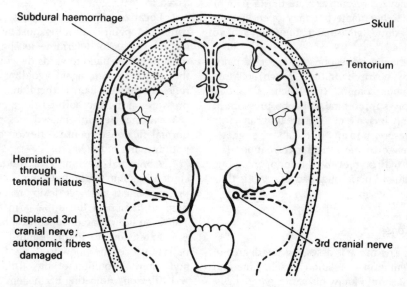

Fig. 5.8 Displacement of brain

Consciousness means the awareness of, and the attention to, surroundings and depends on the interaction between the cells of the upper brain stem, the reticular activating system, (arousal mechanism) and the cerebral hemispheres. Any interruption to this will lead to depressed consciousness and impairment in the arousal mechanism.

If neurological observations are to reflect such deterioration or improvement in a patient's condition every nurse must perform them similarly. Different assessment charts have been used, often proving unreliable, as terms such as drowsy, semicomatose, stuperous can be ambiguous.

Jennett & Teasdale (1974) introduced a coma scale now internationally known and accepted as the Glasgow Coma Scale (GCS) (Fig. 5.9). This provides an objective method of assessing consciousness using three modes of behaviour, eye opening, verbal response and motor response. Each mode is independently assessed, and the patient's best response to specific stimuli recorded in graphic format. Stimuli used include supraorbital pressure, ear lobe pressure and pressing a pen on the nailbed.

Eye open

1. Spontaneously. Note if eyes open when patient is approached without stimulation from the nurse. This suggests that the reticular formation of the cells in the medulla is functioning.

2. To speech. If the eyes are closed the nurse addresses the patient by name, increasing sound as necessary to achieve a response. Note that a patient may not recognize her name but may open eyes in response to the sound, also that patients may have hearing difficulties.

3. To pain. If there is no response to speech a painful stimulus may be used, initially touch/shaking, increasing to a more painful type such as nailbed pressure. To apply supraorbital/ear lobe pressure at this stage may only increase eye closure by grimacing.

4. None. No response to any of the above suggests a degree of damage to the reticular formation. The patient however, may be prevented from opening one or both eyelids due to periorbital oedema and is thus recorded as C, i.e. Closed.

Best verbal response

1. Orientated. The nurse is assessing the degree of the patient's orientation in relation to self, time and place. The patient should know his name, where he is,

i.e. hospital, town, month and year. The questions should allow for minor mistakes and should be varied in their presentation to avoid rote repetition.

2. Confused. If the patient answers one or more of the above questions wrongly the patient is recorded as confused. It is important that incorrect answers should be corrected.

3. Inappropriate words. The patient cannot hold a conversation. Minimal verbal responses are used, 'yes and no' or obscenities, often in response to painful stimulus.

4. Incomprehensible sounds. In response to verbal or painful stimulus, usually moans and groans.

5. None. No sounds are made in response to pain. Note should be made however of reasons why patients may be unable to respond verbally, for example deafness, inability to understand the language, speech difficulties or the presence of endotracheal/tracheostomy tubes. This is recorded as T on the chart.

Best motor response

Motor activity is the third mode of behaviour assessed. If response in the arms is different then the best response is recorded. The leg response is not noted here since this may be purely a reflex action.

1. Obeys commands. The patient is assessed by being able to obey simple commands – 'lift up your arms,' 'put out your tongue'. Squeezing the assessor's fingers is not reliable since it may represent a grasp reflex, however if it is used the patient should be asked to 'leave go'.

2. Localize pain. If no response is forthcoming to command, painful stimulus must be instituted to note the response. To determine localization the patient must move his hand towards the chin area, to remove the source of pain, again avoiding the possibility of reflex responses. Pain is therefore inflicted either by pressure on the supraorbital ridge or ear lobe.

3. Normal flexion. Nailbed pressure should elicit a normal flexion response – flexion at the elbow and withdrawing of the hand.

4. Abnormal flexion. This subdivision is not included in some Glasgow Coma Scale charts. Nailbed pressure elicits a slower flexion response but, in addition, adduction of the upper arm and wrist occurs. This is an indication of subcortical brain involvement.

5. Extension to pain. Painful stimulus to the nailbed causes the elbow to straighten with adduction and internal rotation of the arm, accompanied by wrist flexion, indicating brain stem involvement.

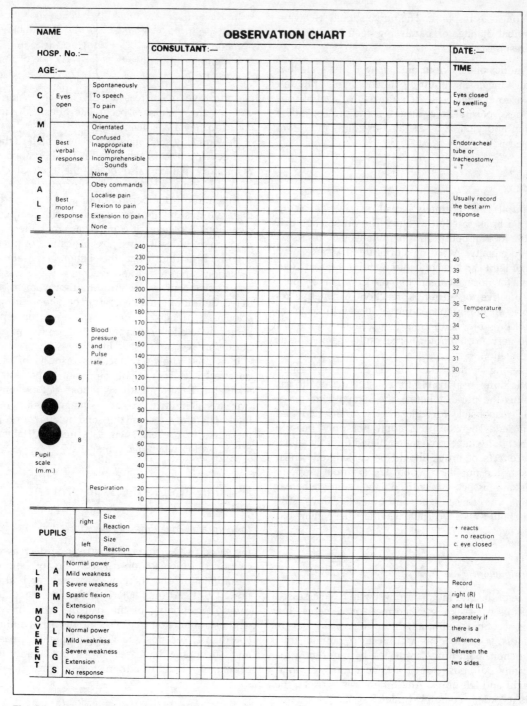

Fig. 5.9   Neurological observation chart

6. None. No response. The nurse should be aware that spinal damage or paralysing agents may result in no response.

All modes of behaviour are arranged in a scale that indicates increasing brain dysfunction, and although the Glasgow Coma Scale determines the level of consciousness, observations made on the pupils, motor function and vital signs are also useful as indicators of raised ICP.

Pupils

The pupils are normally equal in size (2.5 mm), having a brisk reaction to light. The nurse should if possible look at both pupils simultaneously to assess size and equality. Avoiding a brightly lit area, a small beam of light can be shone into each eye separately to observe the normal constriction reaction. This is noted as + (positive) or – (minus) reaction. A negative reaction is an important feature as it may indicate increased pressure/herniation displacement on the 3rd cranial nerve, oculomotor nerve, on the same side as the herniation.

Travelling within the 3rd nerve are parasympathetic fibres responsible for constriction of the iris and thus the pupil, whereas the sympathetic nerve supply responsible for dilatation is unaffected and unapposed. Therefore the pupil not only fails to constrict but will become more dilated than the other.

The effects of drugs should be considered whilst assessing the pupillary action. For example pinpoint pupils are associated with opiate usage, whereas atropine can cause fixed and dilated pupils. The nurse should also ascertain whether the patient has a glass eye!

Motor function

The use of the best motor response will have assessed upper limb weakness/abnormal movements but in this section actual strength, normal, weak, severe weakness, is assessed as a guide to pyramidal tract dysfunction. Both limbs are tested by requesting the patient to 'pull, push', against the examiner, comparing right and left limbs. Any differences between the two is recorded separately under R or L.

Vital signs

Although the triad of:

- bradycardia
- increase in the systolic blood pressure
- widening of the pulse pressure

} Cushing response

is indicative of increased ICP, in the majority of patients these changes occur late after the patient's conscious level has deteriorated.

How quickly such signs occur are related to the rate and development of the raised ICP. Alterations in the respiratory pattern also occur, the type of change related to the level of brain dysfunction.

Alteration in temperature can also occur as hypothalamic dysfunction is associated with temperature elevations. However, it is important that attempts are made to exclude all other possible causes of infection.

It is important that the patient's baseline observations are known and that repeated assessments are carried out to determine improvement or to detect deterioration. Recognition of deteriorating consciousness, unequal pupils, etc., should be reported promptly to allow intervention and to prevent further brain damage and to save life.

It is now known that certain aspects of nursing do affect ICP. This is not important in patients with normal ICP but for those whose ICP is unstable even transient increases can be dangerous and may be fatal. Therefore recognizing and taking appropriate measures to prevent such rises must be taken into consideration when planning care.

Nursing interventions to prevent increases in ICP

Inadequate airway maintenance

Increased CO_2 (hypercapnia) and decreased O_2 (hypoxia) due to obstructed airway stimulates vasodilatation and therefore increases cerebral blood flow (CBF) and thus ICP. This should be avoided by careful positioning of the patient. When necessary gentle oral suction may be employed but limited to less than 15 seconds, since coughing will increase ICP and suctioning increases any hypoxia and hypercapnia. O_2 should be administered as prescribed.

Obstruction to venous return

Raising the head of the bed 15–30 degrees unless otherwise instructed will help lower ICP due to improved venous drainage. Again body position is important, the head kept in a neutral position avoiding rotation and flexion of the neck.

Valsalva manoeuvre

This should be recognized (exhaling against a closed epiglottis) and prevented since this involves increasing intrathoracic/intra-abdominal pressures which in turn increases central venous pressure leading to increased ICP. It is important that the patient does not become constipated, so if possible a high fluid and high fibre intake should be encouraged and if necessary a prescribed stool softener administered to prevent straining at stool.

Prevention of pain/loud noises

Both may increase restlessness in the patient and may initiate an increase in systemic blood pressure, in turn increasing CBF and hence ICP and so should be avoided. Procedures should be well planned to allow undisturbed periods of rest. If possible prevent overstimulation and minimize painful procedures by giving adequate analgesia. Never allow the patient to be startled and ensure that the environment is as quiet as possible keeping conversation regarding the patient out of their earshot.

Management of ICP

There are various ways in which raised ICP can be managed, obviously related to the underlying cause:

1. Surgical intervention may be performed, for example to evacuate a haematoma, to relieve hydrocephalus or to decompress a tumour (see p. 172).

2. Medical management

Use of steroid therapy (dexamethasone) is particularly effective in relieving inflammation and oedema around tumours, although not so effective in head injury. (For uses and side effects see Ch. 4.)

Osmotic diuretic A hypertonic solution, for example Mannitol 20% given intravenously, will attract fluid from oedematous brain tissue into the vascular compartment resulting in a diuresis thus removing excess fluid.

Patients should therefore be catheterized to monitor closely output and fluid balance since such diuresis may cause fluid and electrolyte imbalance and a further deterioration in consciousness.

Controlled ventilation Hyperventilation may be used to maintain adequate oxygenation and to control the patient's ICP. This reduces the Pa_{CO_2}, inducing cerebral/vasoconstriction which lowers the cerebral blood volume and thus the ICP.

It is important to remember that it is often the nurse who detects alteration to consciousness through frequent observations and who should report such so that intervention may take place.

HEAD TRAUMA

The majority of head injuries are mild, only one in five attending an accident and emergency department require admission, the majority being discharged within 2 days. Less than 5% of the 100 000 admitted to general hospitals require transfer to a neurosurgical unit; morbidity and mortality however remain problematical in this group. Since the majority of survivors are under 30 years of age permanent damage causes social, financial and economic restraint.

Causes of craniocerebral trauma

The majority of craniocerebral injuries result from a number of traumatic causes, as shown in Box 5.1.

Aetiology

Head injuries are usually caused by either the head coming to a sharp stop such as hitting a windscreen

---

Box 5.1   Causes of craniocerebral trauma

Road traffic accidents (RTAs)	Almost three-quarters of all severe head injuries including pedestrians are a result of RTAs
Accidental Industrial Sport injuries	Injury occurs often as a result of falling from a height or caused by swinging objects
Assaults Peacetime	Assault on the head with a hammer results in a blunt non-penetrating type head injury whereas a knife, axe or low-velocity bullet lodged within the skull or brain results in a penetrating injury
Wartime	High-velocity missile wounds with a small entry wound and large exit give rise to extensive and devastating brain damage with high mortality

after travelling at considerable speed, deceleration force, or by an object such as a golf ball travelling at speed and striking the head at acceleration force.

Craniocerebral trauma may involve in any combination:

- scalp
- skull
- brain.

Scalp

Scalp lacerations, contusions and haematomas are not in themselves significant, apart from being a source of haemorrhage or infection. However they may be important as a guide to underlying possible brain damage.

Skull

A fractured skull can occur at the point of impact or at a distance from it (Fig. 5.10).

Simple skull fractures

These are linear and non-displaced – they travel in straight lines crossing a point of weakness. No specific treatment is required, however if an underlying blood vessel is torn, for example the middle meningeal artery, blood will escape resulting in the formation of an intracranial haematoma between the skull and dura mater. This is called an extradural haematoma. Some linear fractures may also extend into the irregular sharp base of the skull as a result of which the dura mater is torn causing cerebrospinal fluid (CSF) leakage from the nose, (rhinorrhoea) or ear (otorrhoea), with an increased risk of meningitis.

Compound fractures

The overlying scalp is lacerated. Adequate wound debridement and closure is necessary.

Depressed skull fracture

This often occurs due to localized trauma, such as a blow to the head from a hammer. As a result a fragment of bone is depressed below the normal skull table and the inner table could penetrate the dura and brain tissue.

The scalp may or may not be lacerated, but if it is there is an increased risk of introducing infection. Surgical elevation is required early to elevate the

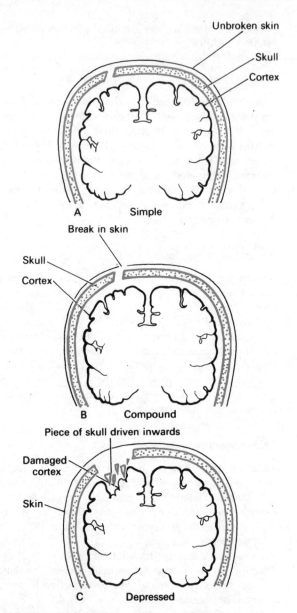

Fig. 5.10 Fractures of the skull

indriven bone and to repair any dural defect. It is important to realize that brain damage can occur without a defect on the scalp or a skull fracture.

Brain injury

Primary brain damage occurs at the time of injury as a result of the acceleration/deceleration forces on the brain substance causing neuronal damage. Rotational forces also cause shearing and tearing of the brain tissue, especially between grey and white matter.

Concussion is manifested by temporary dysfunction often clearing within 24 hours. Loss of consciousness as a result of transient distortion of the brain stem often but not invariably accompanies concussion, with amnesia for the event being common. Such patients need not be admitted provided they or significant others are available at home to observe and follow hospital instructions (Fig. 5.11). Irritability, temporary lethargy, poor memory and concentration may continue for some time afterwards, although the reason is not fully understood.

Contusion

Contusions are often found on the brain surface as a result of the brain tissue hitting the inside of the skull. The brain may be damaged directly under the point of impact, coup injury, on the same and/or opposite the point of injury, contre-coup injury. Although the skull comes to an abrupt halt the brain continues to travel within it, striking one side of the skull, and moving in the opposite direction to strike the other side, and as a result both sides suffer. The frontal and temporal lobes are more susceptible, due to the rough edges around the sphenoid and orbital bones of the skull.

Laceration

In combination with concussion, laceration may occur. The brain may be lacerated as a result of rapid movement and shearing of the brain tissue.

Little can be done to prevent brain damage at the time of injury. Some measures – seat belt legislation,

---

IMPORTANT ADVICE AND INSTRUCTIONS ABOUT HEAD INJURIES IN CHILDREN

PATIENT'S NAME: ....DATE OF BIRTH...

THIS FORM SHOULD BE GIVEN TO A RELATIVE OR FRIEND

Any child who has suffered even a minor head injury, including a simple fall, blow to the head, or being knocked down, may take several hours to recover. For the 24 hours after the accident the patient should be watched carefully, roused and spoken to frequently, and must be brought back to hospital immediately if:

THE PATIENT BECOMES UNCONSCIOUS OR DIFFICULT TO ROUSE

THE CHILD BECOMES CONFUSED, IRRATIONAL OR DELIRIOUS

CONVULSIONS OR JERKING OF THE FACE OR LIMBS OCCUR

THE CHILD COMPLAINS OF PERSISTENT HEADACHE OR DEVELOPS A STIFF NECK

VOMITING OCCURS FREQUENTLY

BLEEDING FROM THE EARS OCCURS OR IF THERE IS A WATERY DISCHARGE FROM THE EARS OR NOSE.

HOSPITAL: ....

DEPARTMENT: ....

DOCTOR'S SIGNATURE: .... Date: ....

Fig. 5.11   Instructions about head injuries in children.

use of protective headgear – have helped to prevent or alleviate primary brain damage occurring at impact, however, little can be done to prevent brain damage at the time of injury. Basic first aid in maintaining a clear airway may however, prevent the secondary complications of hypoxia and hypercapnia (see p. 156) which increase ICP. Any external haemorrhage should also be stopped since hypovolaemia will also lead to subsequent brain damage.

The main aim of care is therefore directed at the recognition and prevention of secondary complications which arise as a consequence of changes to ICP, due to haematoma, oedema formation, hypoxia and hypotension.

Investigations

The following may be used as an aid to assessing the degree of damage sustained following a head injury:

Plain skull X-ray: These should be of good quality and will demonstrate any fracture.

CT scan: This is a non-invasive X-ray procedure which allows the densities of a transverse slice of the brain to be seen by producing an image at any given level. The scanner employs conventional X-rays but instead of using a film, produces a computer picture (see Ch. 4).

Complications

Haematoma

Bleeding may occur outside the dura (extradural), under the dura (subdural) or into the brain cortex (intracerebral/subarachnoid haemorrhage). Although haemorrhage can occur within minutes of the injury, it may be hours/days before clinical features are evident and it is for this reason that nursing observations of ICP are so relevant (see pp. 154–156).

Extradural haematoma This is as a result of a skull fracture to the temperoparietal region of the skull with associated laceration of the meningeal vessel (Fig. 5.12A). If the haemorrhage is mild to moderate the patient may not be unconscious at the time of injury, but as the clot expands impairment of consciousness, with the development of progressive focal deficits occur, for example contralateral paralysis/speech dysfunction. Should the middle meningeal artery be ruptured the progress is inevitably rapid with eventual tentorial herniation.

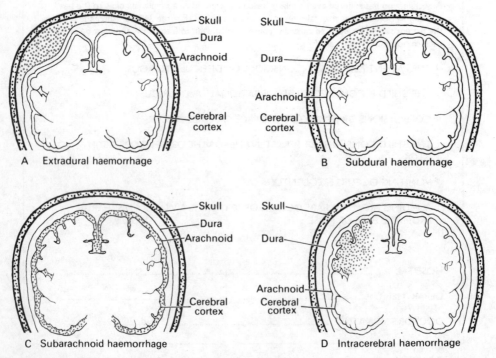

Fig. 5.12 A–D. Types of intracranial haemorrhages

Subdural haematoma (Fig. 5.12B) This occurs as a result of torn bridging veins and can be classified according to the length of time between injury and onset of symptoms: acute within 24 hours; subacute 1–14 days, and chronic after 2 weeks.

Acute subdural haematoma This is usually follows a blow of considerable violence which also causes significant damage to the brain tissue. Again the brain can become compressed quickly and failure to recognize changes in ICP will result in tentorial herniation.

Subacute haematoma This is associated with a less severe head injury but the patient fails to improve.

Chronic subdural haematoma This may result from a very minor head injury, often not remembered, with a lapse of weeks sometimes months between the injury and the presentation of clinical features. This often occurs in the elderly and alcoholic patient where due to cerebral atrophy more space is present to allow expansion of the clot before the brain becomes compressed.

Intracerebral haematoma (Fig. 5.12D) Since most haemorrhages occurring within the cortex result in extravasation of blood into the subarachnoid space producing a traumatic subarachnoid haemorrhage, (Fig. 5.12C) the two conditions can be discussed together.

The clinical features will depend on the severity of damage and resulting haemorrhage. These range from headache, neck stiffness, irritability, photophobia, to progressive impairment of consciousness. As can be seen regardless of the type of haematoma, the effects of it are similar in that compression of brain tissue, with a rise in ICP, tentorial herniation and mid-brain distortion ensue.

The urgency for immediate surgical treatment is dependent on the clinical findings on admission or subsequent observations. A small intracerebral haematoma may be left to reabsorb. If however, the patient should deteriorate quickly as a result of an expanding extradural haematoma, burr holes may be made directly over the haematoma to evacuate it and to ligate the bleeding vessel. This may need to be followed up by a craniotomy – the skull is opened and the bone reflected to enable an intracerebral haematoma, tumour or abscess to be evacuated.

Postoperative care

The patient recovering from cranial surgery spends his first 24 hours under the constant care of one nurse, so it is important that the nurse is skilled at assessing and interpreting the patient's neurological status and vital signs (see pp. 154–156).

The patients face many complications, epilepsy, infection and increases in ICP, the most important initially being the detection of ICP alterations. Postoperatively raised ICP is often the result of three main structural complications, cerebral oedema, haemorrhage and hydrocephalus.

Cerebral oedema, develops in response to traumatic or ischaemic brain damage either pre-, intra- and/or postoperatively.

Cerebral haemorrhage can occur within the first 48 hours after cranial surgery, the causes vary, but it may be due to coagulation dysfunction or as a result of surgical trauma.

Hydrocephalus, a gradual accumulation of CSF, with a progressive dilatation of the ventricles, may occur as a result of obstruction to CSF flow or malabsorption of CSF by the arachnoid granulations (Fig. 5.6). CSF can become obstructed in and around the fourth ventricle due to haematoma/oedema following posterior fossa surgery and blood in the subarachnoid space may block the arachnoid villi preventing the absorption of CSF.

Thus all three structural complications above have the potential to raise ICP in the postoperative period.

Maintenance of the airway

Respiratory status is always important post anaesthesia but in the neurological patient this is even more crucial, particularly in relation to surgical cerebral trauma and its effects on the vital respiratory centre. Depression of the respiratory centre will result in respiratory acidosis recognized by increasing dyspnoea, restlessness, agitation and tachycardia. Prolonged anaesthesia and the inability to maintain a clear airway may have a similar effect.

Such symptoms are likely to increase blood pressure, contributing in turn to cerebral oedema. The patient should be nursed in the recovery position, oxygen being given to promote respiratory exchange and to 'wash out' anaesthetic nitrous oxide.

The oral cavity should be kept clear of secretions by gentle suction given as required. Following posterior fossa operations the reflexes of the cranial nerves involved with swallowing and gagging may be impaired. These reflexes should be assessed prior to giving oral fluids, to reduce the risk of aspiration of fluids/food.

Fluid balance

Close monitoring of fluid intake and output is also vital in the postoperative phase. The aim is to avoid fluid retention, which could contribute to cerebral oedema, and to prevent dehydration and thus impaired cerebral blood flow as a result of excessive fluid loss.

Following frontal craniotomy, damage around the hypothalamus and pituitary gland may occur, interrupting the normal production or secretion of the antidiuretic hormone, resulting in the development of diabetes insipidus. Polyuria, with low urinary specific gravity and polydipsia, are the presenting features and require early prompt recognition. Thus patients at risk have specific gravity measurements made on every specimen of urine and accurate intake and output maintained. Replacement antidiuretic hormone can be administered when required.

Epilepsy

Epileptic seizures increase cerebral metabolic demands which may further compromise cerebral integrity. This is more common after supratentorial surgery but should be recognized early, and prompt action taken during any seizure to maintain the airway (see p. 164). Anticonvulsants are not usually used prophylactically but will be given following an initial seizure.

Temperature control

Hyperthermia also increases the metabolic requirements and may be in response to hypothalamic damage or postoperative infections, the commonest being chest, wound and meningitis. Whatever the cause, the aim is to detect any pyrexia early, to treat the cause and lower the temperature. Specimens from obvious potential sources of infection, for example sputum, urine, should be obtained and sent to bacteriology for culture and sensitivity.

Measures should be taken by the nurse to reduce the temperature (see Ch. 4).

Periorbital oedema

As a result of prolonged retraction on the frontal lobes, swelling around the eyes is fairly common. This puts pressure on the eyes and prevents normal eyelid function, often making the patient feel isolated and disorientated. Furthermore, damage to the 5th cranial nerve or altered consciousness may cause incomplete eyelid closure with increased risk of corneal abrasion.

Eye care in the first 24 hours is thus essential, the eyes being bathed with sterile normal saline as often as necessary. Artificial tears/eye drops may be prescribed and ointments that reduce bruising may be applied. The patient should be encouraged as soon as possible to open and exercise the eyelids which will help reduce some swelling.

Pain relief

Codeine phosphate is the preferred analgesic since this does not affect the level of consciousness. Constipation may become a problem, therefore fibre/mild aperients may need to be prescribed.

Wound care

The wound is closed by sutures or staples and covered by a dressing which may be removed after 24 hours and replaced by a plastic protective dressing. Any drain is removed as soon as drainage is minimal. Sutures/staples are removed around the 7th day.

Following cranial surgery the patient is at risk from many potential complications, therefore the earlier such complications are identified the sooner treatment can be given with less risk to the patient of disability or loss of life.

The course of head injuries

Fortunately most patients make a spontaneous recovery and can return to their homes and occupations with little if any change in their previous pattern of living. There are others however, who will suffer from some disturbance which may affect their daily living. The following are some of the problems.

Post-traumatic epilepsy

Two stages are described.

1. Early epilepsy Occurs 1–7 days following initial head injury, usually taking the form of focal epilepsy (see Ch. 7), and is commonly associated with a depressed fracture or intracranial haematoma. Some patients will also develop status epilepticus. Anticonvulsants need to be taken for 12–18 months.

2. Late epilepsy This usually occurs about 12 months following the initial injury, but in a small number of cases the first seizure may only occur 3–4 years post injury. Anticonvulsants should be given for 18 months to 2 years. Patients at risk of developing epilepsy should be advised not to drive, the onus being on the patient to inform the Driving Vehicle Licensing Centre (see Ch. 7).

Post-traumatic syndrome (postconcussional syndrome)

Until recently this was thought to be psychological in origin but it is now known that even the mildest head injury can cause diffuse neuronal damage. The symptoms may be behavioural; irritability and agitation, loss of self-confidence and loss of concentration; and organic, headache and vertigo. Vertigo is probably due to damage to the cochleovestibular apparatus. The patient should be reassured that symptoms will subside in time.

Rehabilitation

Not all patients make an uneventful recovery following head injury, for many, disability is a combination of behavioural and physical handicaps. The physical problems are mainly spasticity, gait disturbances and speech disorders. The behavioural problems however are not so noticeable; memory, cognition and especially personality changes are sometimes not recognized.

Apart from immediate postoperative rehabilitation, it is often difficult in general hospitals to give the time needed to such patients, since rehabilitation of the head-injured patient may be very slow.

Nervous tissue damaged at the time of injury is unable to regenerate, therefore both physical and behavioural rehabilitation is a relearning process. In co-operation with nursing staff, the following members of the health team have specific responsibilities for ensuring an adequate rehabilitation regime.

- **Physiotherapists** concern themselves with body movements; strength and mobility exercises, co-ordination and balance.
- **Speech therapists** help the patient to communicate, which in itself will help lessen frustration.
- **Occupational therapists** work closely with physiotherapists, co-ordinating restored movements into purposeful actions to achieve as far as possible independence in activities of living.
- **Clinical psychologists** are involved in helping to restore intellectual and memory processes.
- **A social worker** will collect information regarding the patient's home circumstances and any financial problems that may arise as a result of injury. Education of the patient's family members is also vital, since they must have a clear understanding of any deficits from which the patient is suffering or may suffer. Family members can also learn the exercises most advantageous to the patient so that they can

be continued at home, and guidance should be readily available from hospital and/or GP as to how they can best offer support during difficult times.

Some disorders, for example epilepsy, physical and mental handicap, following head injury (Nursing Care Plan 5.2) can cause mixed emotional reactions in others such as pity, fear and hostility. Defining certain kinds of illnesses as different/abnormal can separate patients and their relatives from the rest of society.

Such stigmatization may further disadvantage the patients. They may react by perceiving themselves as different, exacerbating their feelings of devaluation and increasing their lack of self-esteem. Many patients and their families have to accept not just a physical handicap but also a social handicap – that of social prejudice.

The patient and their relatives can also be introduced to HEADWAY, The National Head Injuries Association, a support group for the head injured and their families. Headway groups can be found all over the country, the main centre (HEADWAY, National Head Injuries Association, 7 King Edward Court, King Edward Street, Nottingham NG1 1EW; tel: 0602 240800) can give information regarding a local group.

Finally, time heals, the period of rehabilitation cannot be hurried. However, following severe head injury, not all patients will recover consciousness, as although the brain stem functions, the cerebral cortex remains inactive and is described as in the persistent vegetative state. In such circumstances care can be discussed as for the unconscious patient. Although there are many reasons for unconsciousness, the basic nursing principles underlying the care remains the same. In unconsciousness the normal protective reflexes are impaired or lost, and therefore the patient is dependent on others for his/her safety until normal function is resumed. Caring for the unconscious patient has two main broad aims:

1. To maintain the patient's life and well-being.
2. To make intelligent observations and assessments.

The priorities of care required by the unconscious patients are presented based on a problem-solving approach in Nursing Care Plan 5.1 using the framework of the activities of daily living (ADLs).

Ethical issues

Better emergency care at the site of the accident

Nursing Care Plan 5.1   Care of the unconscious patient using Roper, Logan and Tierney model

Problem	Goal	Nursing action	Rationale
1. Possible respiratory complications due to altered consciousness	Prevent respiratory obstruction	❏ Place in lateral/semiprone position, supported by pillows between legs and behind back	Position will prevent the lax tongue from causing airway obstruction
		❏ Maintain head in neutral position (especially brain diseases)	Head-down position and twisting of neck will increase ICP
		❏ Do not nurse head down (unless instructed) to achieve postural drainage	Respiratory depression is a common cause of deterioration in the unconscious patient
	Maintain adequate Po_2	❏ Administer O_2 at prescribed rate/%	Promotion of adequate gaseous exchange
		Ensure mask is placed and maintained correctly	
		Increase oral hygiene	O_2 will dry oral mucosa
	Respiratory rate remains within normal limits	❏ Observe respiratory pattern; rate, rhythm, depth	Respiratory pattern may alter indicating increased respiratory difficulty and may be associated with increased ICP
	Remains apyrexial	❏ Send sputum specimen to microbiology for culture and sensitivity	
	Maintains a clear airway	❏ Use oral airway if necessary changing 2 hourly	
		Give gentle suction as required to remove pharyngeal secretions	
		Do not tape airway in position	
		Record and report alterations in temperature and pulse	
2. Poor nutrition and fluid intake due to unconscious state	Maintain fluid intake of 1.5–2 litres daily or according to medical instructions	❏ Pass nasogastric tube (orogastric in head-injured patient) and commence feeding either continuously or by bolus method, according to patient's absorption	Gastric feeding using the more natural route is more advantageous over parenteral feeding with its inherent infection risk
		❏ Liaise with dietician/doctors to discuss type of feeding	In fractured base of skull nasogastric tube can inadvertently be placed into cranial cavity
	Achieve daily nutritional req. of 2000 Kcal + 50 g protein or according to medical instructions	Weigh patient if possible twice weekly and record	
		❏ Turn patient prior to feeding	Patient may regurgitate feed if turned following, increasing risk of aspiration
		❏ Prior to bolus feeding aspirate stomach contents, measure, record and check if contents are to be replaced	Aspiration indicates how effectively feed is being absorbed
			As aspirate contains important electrolytes most should be returned
		❏ Give oral hygiene following feed	Psychologically promotes comfort; preventing increased drying of oral mucosa
		❏ Nostril should be kept clean and free from crust formation	
		❏ Ensure feeding tube is anchored securely, tape and change as required	
	Urine output should be maintained at around 1–2 litres daily	❏ Observe urinary output	Lack of fluid/fibre will increase risk of constipation
		Initially hourly measurements may be requested	

Nursing Care Plan 5.1 (*cont'd*)

Problem	Goal	Nursing action	Rationale
3. Unable to control elimination due to unconscious state	Maintain skin integrity	❏ Keep skin clean and dry at all times	Incontinence increases skin contamination, therefore possible skin breakdown
		❏ If necessary condom drainage may be used on male patients: system changed daily	
	Satisfactory bladder/ bowel function	❏ Urinary catheterization may be required: a. to relieve urinary retention b. to assess accurately urine output Maintain closed urinary drainage system ❏ Give prescribed catheter care (see Royal Marsden Manual of Clinical Practice)	Change as soon as possible to incontinence appliance since increased risk of infection associated with indwelling catheters
		❏ A bedpan/urinal may be given at regular intervals	It is possible to establish a bladder training programme by observing the voiding pattern
		❏ Observe and report alterations to output and chart accurately	
	Avoid constipation	❏ Record bowel movements Bowel check every third day and if required give prescribed stool softener/suppositories	Lack of mobility, lack of fluid may cause constipation. This may in turn be a cause of urine by-passing the catheter
	Avoid diarrhoea	❏ Observe and report episodes of diarrhoea. Discuss possible alterations in nutritional regimen	Occasionally when nasogastric feeds are introduced, especially if highly concentrated, diarrhoea may result, thus further skin contamination
	Insensible loss kept to a minimum	❏ Maintain body temperature within normal limits	
4. Difficulty in maintaining a safe environment	Maintain a safe environment: a. Physiologically b. Psychologically	❏ Ensure adequate airway and emergency equipment at bedside and in working order	
		❏ Cotsides in all beds with padded protection if necessary, especially if patient is very restless or at risk of epileptic fits	Prevention of injury
		❏ Frequent eye care 2 hourly or more frequently. Treat each separately with cotton wool ball soaked in sterile normal saline. Clean from inner canthus outwards use fresh cotton ball for every application to eye. Instil prescribed drops/ointment	Diminished/absent corneal reflex may result in corneal abrasion. Lack of blinking present
	By determining at-risk patients, pressure sores are prevented	❏ Inspect skin at each turn especially over bony prominences. Determine 'at-risk' patients using accepted scale, i.e. Norton/Waterlow	Sense of pressure may be diminished/absent Norton/Waterlow scales assess various aspects related to patient, mobility, consciousness, incontinence
		❏ Patient position changed 2 hourly use of sheepskin, Spence mattress does not obviate the need for turning and repositioning	

Nursing Care Plan 5.1 (*cont'd*)

Problem	Goal	Nursing action	Rationale
5. **Communicating with other is difficult**	Continue communicating with the patient treating them no differently from any other patient	❏ Explain to patient prior to intervention, even when it may be difficult to realize if patient can acknowledge the information ❏ Speak normally, encourage others to do so ❏ Communicate by touch, holding hands ❏ Aromatherapy may be used ❏ Play personal stereo/radio turned to music liked by patient or use taped messages from friends ❏ Note any non-verbal cues from patient, e.g. restlessness, increase in pulse, respiratory rate, which might indicate an uncomfortable position or pain	Hearing may be last sense to be lost in unconsciousness Provides stimulation but is only valuable for short periods of time
6. **May not be cared for as an individual with their own personality/ sexuality**	Promote individuality	❏ Privacy of patient and significant others should be respected ❏ Explain to significant others the rationale of nursing both sexes together within the same ward area ❏ Dress patients as far as possible in their own clothes. Apply make-up if desired by significant others ❏ Respect varying relationships that may exist	This may be necessary in the acute areas when patient is critically ill to ensure best use of nursing expertise and equipment Accord the same understanding to heterosexual/homosexual relationships
7. **Inability to perform personal cleansing**	Maintain a high standard of personal hygiene	❏ Daily bed bath (as patient's condition improves immersion bath may be given) or more frequently as required ❏ Encourage significant others to participate ❏ Ensure nails are kept short ❏ Teeth/dentures kept clean ❏ Eye care (see 4 above) ❏ Shave patient if necessary ❏ Apply make-up if desired ❏ During menstruation increase vulval toilet and change sanitary towels as necessary ❏ Dress according to custom and significant others' preferences	Frequent washing may be required to eliminate sweat and freshen patient Skin damage can occur during periods of restlessness Dentures may be worn in long-term unconscious patient if well fitting
8. **Difficulty in controlling body temperature**	Maintain body temperature	❏ Record temperature as often as required ❏ Eliminate cause of any temperature rise, specimens to microbiology: a. sputum b. cerebrospinal fluid	Slight temperature elevations are not unusual, especially following brain damage. If, however, it is above 38°C this suggests infection or hypothalamic temperature regulating centre damage

Nursing Care Plan 5.1 (*cont'd*)

Problem	Goal	Nursing action	Rationale
8. (cont'd)		c. blood cultures d. urine specimens ❏ Reduce body temperature: a. fan patient b. tepid sponging c. use of antipyretic suppositories ❏ Do not allow patient to sweat	A temperature elevation increases the amount of O_2 required by the brain but if there is no corresponding increase in the inspired air volume, the volume of O_2 will not meet brain needs and as a result consciousness deteriorates Tepid sponging is helpful if sweating mechanism is lost as it allows by evaporation the loss of heat Sweat allowed to remain on the skin cools quickly and if the patient starts to shiver a further elevation in temperature results
9. Patient is immobile (prolonged immobilization results in joint stiffening)	Prevention of the development of contractions, foot drop, etc. which may mitigate against full rehabilitation	❏ Place patient in neutral position, supporting weak limbs by correct pillow positioning ❏ Turn patient 2 hourly ❏ Participate in passive limb exercises	Joints should be put through their full range of movements several times daily Nurses can complement work of physiotherapist by performing passive limb exercises at each turn
10. Deterioration in consciousness	Recognize any alteration, especially that of deteriorating consciousness	❏ Perform Glasgow Coma Scale assessment to assess degree of arousal and response according to need (see pp. 154–156) ❏ Allow patient to sleep	Assessment of consciousness may indicate deterioration and thus detection of ICP elevations Sleep is necessary for repair of body function (see Ch. 9)
11. Dying **Brain stem death**	Peaceful death with dignity	❏ Support patient and relatives ❏ Allow relatives to participate in care ❏ Accept that patients may become brain stem dead when ventilated	Death and dying can be traumatic for patient, significant others and nursing staff

has enabled casualties to reach an accident and emergency department in a better condition where the main priority is to maintain an adequate airway. Intubation and ventilation, whist intended to facilitate full recovery, may not be achieved and continued life support may result in a patient becoming brain stem dead.

For many years until the 1950s only conventional death was recognized; arrest of circulation and cessation of other vital functions. With advances in modern technology and the introduction of intensive care units it has been possible to save the lives of patients who would have otherwise died. However, such were these improvement in technology that machines could continue to inflate lungs and keep the heart beating and maintain ongoing biological functions even if brain stem death had occurred.

It was recognized that if the brain had died and in particular the brain stem, continued ventilation achieved nothing. In that time a 'conventional death' – 'ventilating until asystole' – would ensue usually around 14 days, often sooner. This was seen as

CHECKLIST OF CRITERIA FOR DIAGNOSIS OF BRAIN DEATH

Diagnosis to be made by two independent doctors one a consultant and the other a consultant or senior registrar. Diagnosis should not normally be considered until at least 6 hours after the onset of coma or, if cardiac arrest was the cause of the coma, until 24 hours after the circulation has been restored.

Name .... Unit No ....

PRE-CONDITIONS

Are you satisfied that the patient suffers from a condition that has led to irremediable brain damage? Specify the condition:

Time of onset of unresponsive coma:

Dr A ....

Dr B ....

Are you satisfied that potentially reversible causes for the patient's condition have been adequately excluded, in particular:

	Dr A	Dr B
Depressant drugs		
Neuromuscular blocking (relaxant) drugs		
Hypothermia		
Metabolic or endocrine disturbances		

TESTS FOR ABSENCE OF BRAIN-STEM FUNCTION

	Dr A		Dr B	
	1st testing	2nd testing	1st testing	2nd testing
Do the pupils react to light?				
Are there corneal reflexes?				
Is there eye movement on caloric testing?				
Are there motor responses in the cranial nerve distribution, in response to stimulation of face, limbs or trunk?				
Is there a gag reflex? (If the test is practicable)				
Is there a cough reflex?				
Have the recommendations concerning testing for apnoea been followed?*				
Were any respiratory movements seen?				

	Dr A	Dr B

Date and time of first testing ....

Date and time of second testing ....

(As stated in paragraph 30 of the Code of Practice the two doctors may carry out the tests separately or together.)

Dr A Signature .... Dr B Signature ....

Status .... Status ....

*Diagnosis of brain death. Br Med J 1976; ii: 1187–1188
See note (b) on page 35 of the Code of Practice

Fig. 5.13 Checklist of criteria for diagnosis of brain death.

causing continued distress to loved ones, was bad for staff morale and with limited facilities available, was judged not cost effective, inappropriate, denying such facilities to those who might otherwise benefit.

In essence if the brain is dead the patient is dead, the process being irreversible. Therefore the need arose to judge death by other criteria so that brain stem death could be recognized in the presence of continued circulation and artificial ventilation. In making such a decision certain *preconditions* must be met (Fig. 5.13). Here the patients must first be being artificially ventilated, the cause of the unconsciousness is known, it is irremediable and that potentially reversible causes have been excluded, such as hypothermia, overdose of drugs including neuromuscular drugs used to support ventilation, metabolic and endocrine disorders.

Having established the preconditions above, the second part of the criteria assesses brain stem reflexes. The patient is also disconnected from the ventilator long enough to allow the $Pa\text{CO}_2$ to rise above the respiratory stimulus threshold (6.7 KPa). Hypoxia during this procedure can be prevented by giving oxygen at 6 litres per minute via a suction catheter into the endotracheal tube. It is required that two doctors perform this and that the criteria are repeated after an interval. The time of death is at the conclusion of the second set of criteria.

Throughout this time significant others must be kept fully aware about what is involved, the possible outcome and options. It is often the nurses who will have to provide the emotional support during such a stressful time. Brain death may be a difficult concept to grasp, especially when the patient can be seen to be breathing, albeit assisted, with a heart beat displaying on a cardiac monitor. Human touch and kind explanations can provide much needed comfort but it should be appreciated that the nurse also will need support from colleagues and senior staff.

Although brain death and renal transplantation developed independently, they are closely associated and can at times be assumed, wrongly, to lead to a conflict of interest. It is only after the diagnosis of brain death has been made that it is appropriate to consider the suitability of the patient as an organ donor.

The diagnosis of brain death is made by those responsible for the patient's care. The request for organs can be obtained by the same staff or by a transplant co-ordinator, neither of whom are involved directly with the care of the recipient of the organ. Sometimes this is made easy by the relatives recognizing and accepting the results of brain stem function tests, and they may make the initial approach to staff, especially if the patient carried an Organ Donor Card, but prior to discontinuation of the support system. There is probably no best time to broach the subject. Each situation must be assessed individually, but it would appear that an approach made to significant others prior to the second set of brain stem tests allows the family time to consider their decision.

If the patient carries a signed donor card there is no legal requirement to request permission from the family although their views should be obtained. The decision to proceed with organ removal must be carefully assessed by medical staff.

If the answer to organ donation is no, this is accepted and a relative can stay with the patient following disconnection if they wish. If on the other hand permission is given following brain death certification, significant others will be encouraged to say farewells with the understanding that it is impossible to disconnect the patient from ventilation as it is better to remove organs from a heart-beating cadaver.

Following organ removal and transplantation, the transplant co-ordinator can inform the family of the outcome, if they have expressed that wish. No confidentiality is breeched, and many families gain comfort in knowing that some good has come from their loss.

NEOPLASTIC DISORDERS

Epidemiology

Brain tumours tend to occur before 10 years of age or within the 50–60 age group. Some six new neoplasms per 100 000 present yearly in the UK, accounting for just over 2000 deaths. The aetiology of brain tumours remains unknown. No hereditary causes or links with occupation, infection or head injury have been proven. There is a possibility of increased risk following scalp or cranial radiation used previously to alleviate tinea capitus, and an increased incidence of brain lymphomas following immunosuppressive therapy.

Pathology (Table 5.1)

Intracranial tumours can be described as benign or malignant, primary or secondary and can also be classified according to cellular origin and location. A tumour may be said to be benign histologically, encapsulated, confined to a specific area but it may be lethally positioned so that its removal is impossible. A malignant tumour, however, may grow quickly with poor differentiation and may infiltrate other tissue

Table 5.1 Pathological classification

Tissue	Characteristics	Prognosis
BRAIN TISSUE Astrocytoma	Commonest type of intrinsic brain tumour occurring in any age group, arising from astrocytes of the cerebral hemispheres A cerebellar astrocytoma is more common in childhood	Depends on site and grading. Cerebral tumours may be graded I–IV: grade IV being the most malignant. Prognosis dependent on the grading, grades I–II may live 6–7 years, whereas grade II–IV may only survive 12–23 months Relatively benign and complete removal may be achieved Note: Grading is only a reflection of the biopsy specimen and may not be a true indication of the whole tumour
Oligodendroglioma	These occur usually in the younger adult, arising mainly in the cerebral hemispheres, are slow growing, may infiltrate and adhere to the dura mater	If diagnosed early, prognosis is slightly better than that of astrocytomas
Ependymoma	Ependymal cells line the ventricles therefore these tumours can arise anywhere within the ventricular system, particularly around the floor of the fourth ventricle and cauda equina. Most occur in children and young adults	Again dependent on site and grading
Medulloblastoma	These arise in the cerebellar vermis and are highly malignant, invading the fourth ventricle, spreading to the third ventricle obstructing CSF flow. Seeding may occur into the subarachnoid space. More common in children	
MENINGEAL TISSUE Meningioma	Meningiomas arise from the arachnoid granulations and are therefore more common around the venous sinuses. They are extrinsic, growing outside the brain, but compress underlying brain tissue. Occasionally, spinal meningiomas may occur	Histologically meningiomas are principally benign tumours. Removal may depend however on site and location to the venous sinuses (Fig. 5.6)

SKULL TISSUE
  Primary
  ↓   ↓
Benign Malignant
  Secondary
	Primary tumours are quite rare and may be benign (**osteoma**) or malignant (**sarcoma**)
	
	Metastatic deposits form a primary breast or lung tumour or from direct invasion from nasopharynx are more common	

NERVE SHEATH TISSUE	A common example of an intracranial nerve sheath tumour is the **acoustic neurinoma** involving the 8th cranial nerve. Benign, slow growing	Total resection may be impossible due to close proximity to brain stem and other cranial nerves. 5th and 7th cranial nerve damage may occur during surgery

so total removal is also impossible. The majority of intracranial tumours are primary, that is they arise from the central nervous system (CNS) tissue or its supporting cells and very rarely metastasize outside the CNS. Less commonly secondary tumours arising from lungs or breast metastazise via blood, lymphatics or CSF to the brain.

In adults 70% of tumours occur supratentorially, and 30% within the posterior fossa, the incidence being reversed in children.

Tumours can arise in the following areas:

1. brain tissue
2. the meninges
3. the skull
4. peripheral and cranial nerves
5. pituitary gland and pineal gland (see Ch. 16).

Clinical presentation

Common features produced by intracerebral tumours (benign or malignant) are usually progressive over time. Occasionally the patient may present as an emergency due to haemorrhage within the tumour or as a result of hydrocephalus developing.

Generally the effect of tumour growth is as a result of:

1. **Raised ICP**. The patient complains of headache on wakening or with activities associated with increasing ICP (see p. 153). Projectile vomiting often unrelated to intake of food may occur, possibly due to pressure on the reflex vomiting centre in the medulla. Some patients may also demonstrate papilloedema as a result of obstruction to venous return causing swelling of the optic discs and retinal venous engorgement.

2. **Disturbed function due to tumour location**. The presentation and recognition of focal features may help in identifying its location (Table 5.2).

Table 5.2 Disturbed function due to tumour location	
Area of brain	**Disturbed function**
Frontal lobe	Personality changes Contralateral motor weakness Speech deficit (dominant hemisphere)
Parietal lobe	Perceptual problems Disturbed sensation
Occipital lobe	Visual field defect
Temporal lobe	Psycomotor seizure Auditory hallucinations
Cerebellum	Impaired balance and gait
Symptoms may be so slight as to be ignored or unnoticeable until activities of daily living are affected or a seizure occurs. Eventually the tumour may obstruct and compress the ventricular system/CSF circulation which allows CSF to accumulate, increasing further ICP.	

Investigations

Plain skull X-ray

This may be helpful because a tumour may cause bone erosion and calcification may be viewed.

Spine and chest X-ray

Metastatic brain deposits, such as a bronchogenic carcinoma, commonly arise from a primary lesion (see Ch. 13).

Computerized axial tomography (CT scanning) or magnetic resonance imaging (MRI)

Both are non-invasive procedures. CT scanning allows the densities of a transverse slice of brain to be viewed by producing an image at any given level. Any abnormality, for example tumour size, density and surrounding oedema, as well as ventricular size can be obtained.

MRI is more sensitive and uses radiofrequency transmission to magnetically align certain cell nuclei which then fall out of alignment. The signals transmitted from the realigned nuclei are formed into detailed brain pictures.

Angiography

This may occasionally be undertaken to demonstrate the abnormal blood supply in tumours, and/or to locate displacement of vessels associated with space-occupying lesions (see Ch. 4).

Radioisotope scanning

The procedure may be used in centres where CT/ MRI is not available. A radioisotope, usually technetium (^{99m}Tc) pertechnetate, is given intravenously. Any disturbances within the blood-brain barrier allow this radionucleide to pass through and accumulate in oedema around the space-occupying lesion. The gamma rays emitted by the isotope can be detected by a rectilinear scan, and recorded as dots on paper or on a polaroid film.

Therapeutic management

Surgical excision of the tumour is the aim although this is not always possible without causing disastrous neurological deficits. There is no justification for complete removal at the expense of disabling the patient totally.

Biopsy of the lesion may be undertaken for histological report only. If the lesion is contained within a lobe of the brain, it may be possible to perform a lobectomy without further damage to functional areas. A subtotal removal of the tumour will reduce the size of the lesion and thus relieve the ICP for a time. Cystic tumours if accessible can be drained and completely removed. A deep-seated lesion may be biopsied by stereotactically guiding a cannula aided by CT scanning to a predetermined site. If craniotomy has been performed routine postoperative care is given (see Ch. 4). The patient will be nursed as any unconscious patient until fully recovered from the anaesthesia. Many tumours are highly vascular and therefore some bleeding may occur postoperatively causing an extradural or subdural haematoma. Serial observations lead to the detection of this complication and allow measures to be taken to obviate their dangerous effects (see pp. 154–156).

As far as his condition allows the patient may be mobilized from the second postoperative day and encouraged to carry out everyday tasks. Posterior fossa operations may be performed to excise cerebellar tumours or acoustic neuromata. In general, the postoperative care is the same as that following craniotomy. In addition, because of the possibility of swelling around the brain stem, closer observations should be made of respiratory patterns.

Treatment of hydrocephalus

Hydrocephalus may occur at any time due to blockage of pathways by tumour invasion/oedema and increased pressure can be relieved by the insertion of a ventriculoperitoneal shunt (Fig. 5.14). Routine postoperative care should be instituted. Transient adynamic ileus may occasionally be a complication of peritoneal placement of the tubing and the nurse should be aware of the clinical features of this (see Ch. 15).

Radiotherapy

This is often combined with surgical treatment. This regimen will commence after suture removal and wound healing and may continue over a period of 4–6 weeks. Life expectancy following radiotherapy may be increased from months to years depending on the tumour grading. Since a medulloblastoma metastasizes into the CSF the spinal cord may also be irradiated, as well as the cerebellum and fourth ventricle.

The management of a patient undergoing radiotherapy is given in Chapter 4.

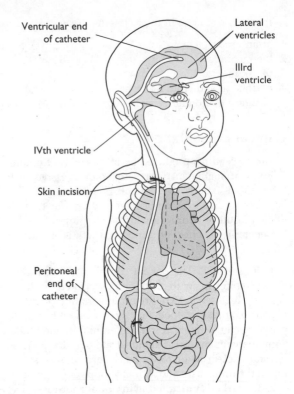

Fig. 5.14 Uniflow shunt system

Nursing strategies

Patients who have a poor prognosis require continuous support, as do significant others, from the time of the diagnosis and especially in the terminal stages of the patient's illness. The patient should be encouraged to go home for short periods of time and good liaison with the community services is essential for this to work well. Specialist nurses, stoma therapists, breast care nurses, and McMillan nurses can all be called upon for support.

Significant others should be made aware that they can communicate with the hospital staff for advice or a 'chat' when the patient is at home. Readmission can easily be arranged, and hospice facilities made use of. Self-help groups such as Cancerlink, Backup and Taktent (Scotland) are available nationally.

The patient should be kept comfortable and pain free as the condition deteriorates. Significant others should be encouraged to visit whenever they wish and help nurse their relative if they desire to do so. This may help relieve some feelings of guilt which may be present at not looking after the patient at home. The hospital chaplain may be involved with significant others throughout the care of the patient.

Table 5.3 Organisms invading the CNS	
Causative organisms	Route of entry
Bacterial Streptococcus pneumoniae	Blood Borne
Haemophilus influenzae	All blood borne, mainly from sinusitis, otitis media
Neisseria meningitidis	May be the result of a dural tear or contamination during or following an invasive procedure
Viral Coxsackie virus Mumps virus Herpes simplex	Associated with post viral infection, innoculation
Enterovirus	Spread from gastrointestiinal excreta

INFLAMMATORY DISORDERS

Epidemiology/aetiology

Various micro-organisms can invade the CNS and peripheral nervous systems (Table 5.3) leading to the development of meningitis, encephalitis, brain abscess and Guillain–Barré syndrome. Infants/children (3 months to 8 years) and the elderly, whose resistance is lowered, are most prone. Other associated factors are malnutrition, alcoholism and immunosuppression.

Meningitis

Common symptoms

Meningitis occurs when bacteria/viruses invade the meninges and/or the brain. The onset of meningitis may be insidious or abrupt. A primary infection, for example otitis media, may have already been identified and the symptoms of infection, fever, chills, headache, vomiting, may already be present. As the meninges swell and become irritated, signs of meningeal irritation develop, for example stiff neck, photophobia; seizures may also be present in the very young.

In meningococcal meningitis, associated with overcrowded living conditions and upper respiratory tract infection (URTI), a petechial rash may also be noticeable. Infection of the CNS can be life-threatening and early diagnosis and treatment to reduce swelling from inflamed tissue and therefore reduce ICP, will lessen the risk of hydrocephalus and tentorial herniation and will prevent death and disability.

Investigations

Diagnosis can be aided by history, including recent vaccinations and travel, and from physical examination and CSF estimated (Table 5.4). Other tests may aid detection of a primary source, for example chest X-ray, sinus X-rays.

Therapeutic management

Aggressive management with the appropriate antimicrobial drug commences, sometimes even before the causative organism has been identified. All strains tend to be resistant to penicillin G and chloramphenicol for those with penicillin allergy. Generally viral meningitis tends to be less severe, and treatment is directed towards symptoms and with a recovery being made in 7–14 days.

Table 5.4 CSF estimations in meningitis diagnosis			
	Normal	Bacterial meningitis	Viral
Appearance	Clear	Cloudy, turbid	Clear/cloudy
Cells	0–5/mm^3	10 000–55 000/mm^3 (polymorphonuclear)	300 mm^3 (mononuclear)
Pressure	80–180 mmH$_2$O	> 180 mmH$_2$O	Varied
Protein	15–45 mg	Increased	Normal/slight increase
Glucose	45–75 mg/100 ml	20 mg/100 ml	Normal
Culture	Negative	Infective organism	No bacteria Special investigations may demonstrate virus

Nursing strategies

One of the main aims in caring for a patient with bacterial meningitis is to prevent the spread of infection, therefore patients are maintained in protective isolation. (This is not necessary in viral meningitis.) A quiet darkened room and the use of adequate analgesia will help lessen headache and photophobia, and also reduce the risk of seizures. The patient should be nursed in bed with all his hygiene needs; bathing, turning, positioning, toileting provided. Poor appetite caused by nausea may prevent the patient eating, therefore, fluids should be encouraged especially if excessive sweating from fever is present.

Antipyretic drugs may also be prescribed and the use of fanning may help lower elevated temperature. Frequent mouth care for dry mouth from fever and dehydration should be provided. Since the potential for increased ICP is present the nurse should monitor neurological signs frequently and report changes, also reporting the presence of rashes/petechiae. If the patient is unconscious see Nursing Care Plan 5.1.

Encephalitis

Bacteria and virus can also cause diffuse swelling and inflammation of brain tissue which unfortunately has a high morbidity and mortality rate. Onset is often rapid and once coma occurs, treatment is often ineffective.

Brain abscess

These are usually secondary to infection elsewhere, for example ear, mastoid sinus, lung. A brain abscess is a collection of pus encapsulated by a thick wall. This then acts as a space-occupying lesion producing similar features to those of brain tumour (Table 5.2). As it expands it mimics an expanding lesion inhibiting CSF flow and increasing ICP.

Therapeutic management

Management is a combination of surgery and drug therapy. The abscess requires to be drained, the care being the same as that for any craniotomy (see pp. 161–162) and antibiotics will be given to combat the infection.

Guillain–Barré syndrome (polyneuropathy)

Epidemiology and aetiology

This is relatively uncommon, affecting 1.7 per 100 000 population, with similar incidence in both sexes. The aetiology is also unknown but around 50% of patients recall a respiratory/gastrointestinal infection 1–3 weeks before the onset of symptoms. Inflammation of the peripheral nervous system leads to demyelination.

Common symptoms

The onset is rapid, characterized by transient paraesthesia, muscle pain and paresis/plegia in selected muscles which is often symmetrical, and most often ascending: – legs – trunk – arms – cranial nerves.

Investigations

This is made from history of recent infection and physical/neurological examination. Although the CSF may demonstrate elevated protein and increased WBC, this only develops days to weeks later.

Therapeutic management

There is no known medical treatment. Occasionally steroids are prescribed, but their use remains controversial and indeed may be harmful. Treatment is therefore supportive.

Nursing strategies

In severe cases, respiratory muscle and bulbar palsy may occur, resulting in the need for tracheostomy and artificial ventilation (see Ch. 6). The standards of nursing care are a particularly important determinant of a successful outcome. Few disorders offer such a challenge to the nurse as the management of the severely disabled patient, dependent on ventilatory support, but at the same time totally aware of his surroundings, able to hear and understand. The physiotherapist also has an important role at this time, both in respiratory management and in prevention of contractures, the nurse continuing care in her absence. Recovery may be slow and in some cases neurological disability may persist.

CEREBROVASCULAR DISEASE
Epidemiology and aetiology

In developed countries stroke is third in mortality rates, behind heart disease and cancer, vascular disease being one of the commonest causes of admission to hospital.

The elderly are most often affected and although

drug abuse and some congenital problems may contribute to cerebrovascular disorders, the actual cause may be unknown. However, certain predisposing factors are known: hypertension, existing cardiac disease (rheumatic heart disease), diabetes mellitus, smoking, heredity (diabetes and hypertension showing heredity traits), age, sex and race. Recognition of people at risk is therefore likely to reduce death and disability from strokes.

Type of disorder

Cerebrovascular disease encompasses all forms of vascular disease affecting the brain, which may result in a **stroke** (synonymous with **cerebrovascular accident**, CVA), which produces a localized loss of body function, or a transient ischaemic attack (TIA), the same as a stroke but function returns within 24 hours. Excluding trauma, strokes can be classified as thrombotic, embolic or haemorrhagic, all of which alter cerebral blood supply causing nervous tissue damage by oxygen depletion.

Cerebral thrombosis

Here atheromatous changes associated with atherosclerosis occur within the cerebral circulation (see Ch. 12), eventually causing complete blockage of the vessel lumen. This depletes the oxygen supply to the part of the brain supplied by the diseased vessel. Death of the tissue, or infarction, may occur.

The clinical features vary depending on:

1. The site of infarction.
2. The extent of vessel blockage.

CVA from thrombosis is most commonly a disease of the elderly. Gradual occlusion, presented as TIAs, causes a progressive deterioration in the patient's condition, clinical features occurring and diminishing with no lasting effect, but recurring at intervals. Eventually, when the blockage becomes complete, deficits become permanent. Occlusion may affect any of the vessels of the circle of Willis, but most commonly the internal cartoid and middle cerebral arteries. These supply the motor and sensory areas and internal capsule within the temporal and frontal lobes, the presenting feature usually being a hemiplegia. If the dominant hemisphere is affected (containing the speech pathways), the patient may also have speech problems, such as a dysphasia.

Embolism

An embolus may also block cerebral blood vessels. In this case obstruction occurs suddenly, the embolus having broken off from vegetations around diseased heart valves, such as those which occur in subacute bacterial endocarditis, or occasionally a fat or septic emboli may be the cause. Sometimes a thrombus may give off multiple emboli.

Haemorrhage

Haemorrhagic stroke can result from:

An intracerebral haemorrhage This is associated with atherosclerosis and hypertension, causing bleeding into an area of brain from a ruptured intracerebral vessel.

Subarachnoid haemorrhage which may be due to rupture of an aneurysm (weakness in an artery wall, which may be congenital, acquired from atherosclerosis/infective processes), occurring often at the bifurcation of vessels within the circle of Willis or to a congenital arteriovenous malformation (AVM). This is an abnormal blood vessel collection fed by one or more major cerebral arteries, drained by dilated veins, the latter rupturing. Both bleed into the subarachnoid space, although both can also rupture into the cerebral tissue.

Common symptoms

The clinical features will obviously depend on the underlying cause, location of the bleed or clot within the brain. Many patients who have had TIAs may go on to have a major thrombotic stroke which may develop over several hours or days presenting with some of the following depending on the area of the brain involved:

- motor disorders, hemiplegia, dysphagia
- sensory disorders – spatial-perceptual deficits
- visual field defects
- language problems dysphasia
- altered consciousness.

In haemorrhagic stroke all age groups can be affected, the signs and symptoms occurring very suddenly and again may be similar to those mentioned, dependent on the area of brain affected. In addition the patient complains of intense headache, vomiting, photophobia and neck stiffness.

In all three types if loss of consciousness extends over 48 hours the prognosis may be poor.

Investigations

CT scan/MRI

This is often the first choice since the location of the

damage can be identified, as can structural changes due to oedema, clot and/or hydrocephalus.

Lumbar puncture

In areas where scanning facilities are not available this may be performed to obtain a CSF specimen, which may appear blood stained. The doctor may not perform this investigation because of the risk of inducing brain herniation if the patient is suspected of associated increased ICP from the haemorrhage.

Cerebral angiography

Angiography is necessary to visualize the neck and cerebral vessels, to assist the doctor in diagnosing cerebrovascular disease and to determine the need for medical and/or surgical intervention. Since this is an invasive procedure its need or timing is based on careful consideration of the benefit and risk of further damage to the patient.

Doppler scan

This is a non-invasive diagnostic procedure. An ultrasound probe detects alterations in frequency of sound that is produced by changes in the speed of blood flow due to stenosis/occlusion of the internal or external arteries.

Other investigations, clotting screen, electrocardiogram, may be performed to eliminate other systemic disorders.

Therapeutic management

The way in which the patient is managed either medically or surgically is dependent on the cause or condition of the patient.

Medical management

Initially this will be directed at the prevention of further progression of the stroke, infarct and may also be dependent on the doctor's preferences. Anticoagulants may be prescribed to prolong clotting time and prevent thrombus formation, for example for patients with atrial fibrillation or antiplatelet/aggregation drugs (aspirin or dipyridamole) given to those suffering from TIAs. However, in other patients who have had a stroke such drugs may not be prescribed since they can increase the risk of intracerebral haemorrhage. Patients who suffer from hypertension may be treated with antihypertensives. Nursing the patient in the acute phase, especially if consciousness is altered, is directed at recognizing and preventing deteriorating consciousness as well as caring for the unconscious patient (Nursing Care Plan 5.1). Rehabilitating the patient begins as soon as possible (Nursing Care Plan 5.2). It is also an important part of medical therapy to try to minimize the risk factors, for example dietary indiscretions, cigarette smoking.

Medical management following subarachnoid haemorrhage

Following a subarachnoid haemorrhage (SAH) vasospasm may occur which precludes angiographic investigations and therefore surgery. In order to try to avoid vasospasm the doctor may prescribe a calcium channel blocker, for example nifedipine, which prevents the calcium from gaining entry into vascular smooth muscle, thus avoiding vasoconstriction, decreased blood flow and further ischaemia. Other medication used to relieve ICP may be the use of corticosteroids and osmotic diuretics (see p. 157). Ideally following SAH the patient is nursed in bed, in a quiet environment, avoiding elevations in blood pressure and preventing activities that may increase ICP (see p. 156–157) and the possibility of another bleed. The headache can be reduced by administration of prescribed codeine phosphate.

Surgical management

Once the aneurysm/AVM has been angiographically identified surgery may be offered to the patient – the affected vessel may be clipped to avoid further rebleed. Controversy continues over the exact timing of operation, as the earlier it is carried out the greater the morbidity and mortality. Occasionally surgery may have to be performed very early following AVM, aneurysmal rupture which has resulted in deteriorating consciousness from an associated intracerebral haematoma and/or hydrocephalus.

Following surgery the care given is as for any other craniotomy patient (see pp. 161–162). It should be noted that damage already incurred at the time of rupture may not resolve and therefore the subsequent care problems may be similar to medical rehabilitation.

DEGENERATIVE DISORDERS

According to the *Concise Oxford Dictionary* degeneration is 'a deterioration in tissue or a change in struc-

Nursing Care Plan 5.2	Nursing care of patient with hemiplegia: problem-solving approach		
Problem	**Goal**	**Nursing action**	**Rationale**
A. MOBILIZATION			
1. Loss of motor power/tone on affected side **Potential therefore to develop spasticity**	Increase strength on affected side	❏ Careful positioning at all times. Assist with passive/active exercises. Avoid positioning pillow under foot first or foam role in affected hand. Never pull on affected arm (Figs 5.15–5.17)	Interruption of cortical influences to anterior horn cell causes flaccid paralysis but with return of reflex activity, hypertonicity results affecting especially antigravity muscles, e.g. shoulder, hip, causing spasticity. Careful positioning to oppose the developing spasticity should be adopted from the acute stage Exercise prevents contractures which may inhibit rehabilitation Excessive stimulation increases spasticity When an arm is flaccid gravitational pull stretches joint/muscle with potential for malalignment and subluxation if pulled
2. Sensory disturbance	Increase patients awareness. Give maximum input to affected side	❏ Approach patient from affected side. Place locker/side table on affected side. Protect patient from hot/cold liquids/heat pads	This enables cross-facilitation, e.g. the sound side crosses the midline to initiate bilateral activity. Sensory disturbance, especially diminished sensation, may cause accidental burning
3. Specific sensory loss/disturbances related to left-sided hemiparesis: proprioceptive loss, visuospatial, disordered body image	Minimize any perceptual disability	❏ Encourage sensory stimulation, e.g. touch the affected side. Discourage use of right/left Recognize that inability to execute a learned movement without muscle weakness (apraxia) is a sensory impairment ❏ Position limbs within patients field of vision. Avoid moving patient's position in ward.	The R and L parietal lobe functions differently; the dominant side (i.e. 75% L side) is concerned with communication, the non-dominant interpreting what is happening to the body and its environment. Damage therefore to R hemisphere can cause failure to recognize what is seen as well as disregarding/denying the affected side; patient neglects that side/half of his environment.
4. Loss of balance		❏ Re-educate patient's postural control mechanism by: • encouraging patient to roll from side to side when turning • bridge trunk, i.e. lift trunk off bed • support himself on affected side • ensuring patient can maintain balance at side of bed	Without normal muscle tone, postural control is lost so great difficulty in maintaining balance occurs. Once trunk control has been achieved in bed the natural progression is to regain equilibrium standing and walking in parallel bars
B. MAINTAINING A SAFE ENVIRONMENT			
1. Visual disturbance Field defect	To ensure patient safety	❏ Encourage patient to recognize/accept problem Promote compensation by making full use of intact visual field, e.g. encourage patient to turn head from side to side. Arrange to be seen by optician if necessary Orientate to any new environment	Visual field defect occurs due to interruption of optic nerve fibres en route to occipital lobe in and around temperoparietal region producing an homonymous hemianopia, e.g. patients with damage in R hemisphere have loss of vision in left side of both eyes

Nursing Care Plan 5.2 (*cont'd*)

Problem	Goal	Nursing action	Rationale
2. Visual neglect		❏ Increase stimulation to affected side	Sensory perceptual problem as in 1–4 above
3. Mobility impairment		❏ Alter environment to suit patient Ensure furniture is safe Teach safe lifting practice/transfer skills (Fig. 5.18) to nurses and significant others	
C. EATING AND DRINKING **1. Swallowing difficulty especially associated with dysarthria** **Potential risk of developing aspiration pneumonia**	Eat and drink safely, maintaining weight and fluid balance	❏ Check patient environment, e.g. airway/suction equipment Position patient upright if possible with head slightly forward Note likes/dislikes, arrange semisolids if necessary Weigh patient weekly and record Maintain accurate fluid balance Arrange/provide special equipment necessary for eating and drinking	This may be required in the initial stages when choking and aspiration potential may be a problem, the correct eating position may avoid this It is easier for patients with swallowing difficulties to swallow semisolids more safely than fluids Non-slip mats/special cutlery will enable patient to be more independent
2. Incomplete emptying of mouth		❏ Remind patient to chew on the unaffected side Inspect inside of mouth/gums for food collection Give frequent oral hygiene	
D. COMMUNICATION **1. Communication difficulty, e.g. dysphasia, impaired cognition**	Find a method of communication suitable to patient Avoid frustration	❏ Check patient can hear and language used by patient Check if dentures are worn and if they fit well Face patient, speak clearly and slowly Ask only one question at a time Avoid use of negatives and non-verbal communication Use communication aids where appropriate in discussion with speech therapist Avoid fatigue Do not allow patient to become frustrated/isolated	Speech centre and its connections are situated in dominant hemisphere Although damaged the patient's ability to think rationally should not necessarily be affected and patients should not be treated other than an intelligent adult A code for yes/no established early will help reduce frustration

ture', which applies to a diverse group of progressive neurological disorders. The most common disorders, Parkinson's disease, multiple sclerosis, motor neurone disease and myaesthenia gravis, will be discussed.

Parkinson's disease

Parkinson's disease is a movement disorder affecting voluntary learned actions.

Epidemiology and aetiology

Parkinson's disease affects 1–2 per 1000 of the population, the onset occurring usually between 55 and 65 years of age, affecting both sexes equally and is one of the commonest disabling disorders after stroke. It may be seen to be increasing in prevalence but this is probably due to an increased ageing population

The actual cause of Parkinson's disease remains

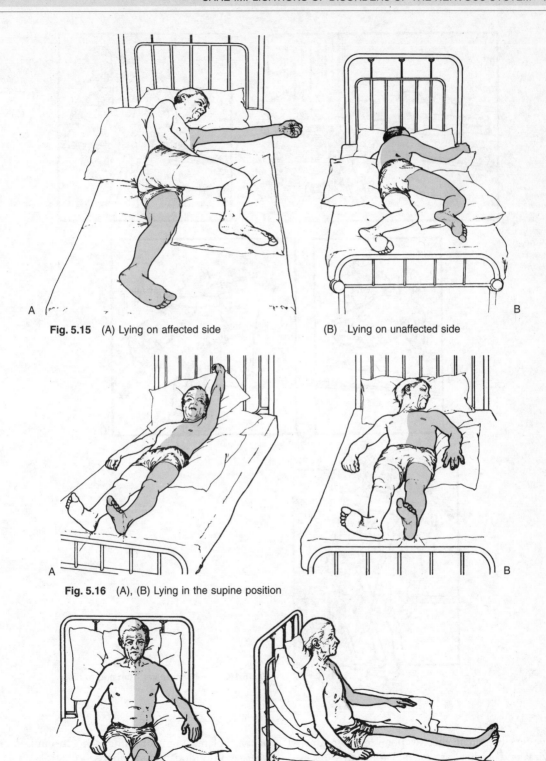

Fig. 5.15   (A) Lying on affected side   (B)   Lying on unaffected side

Fig. 5.16   (A), (B) Lying in the supine position

Fig. 5.17   (A), (B) Sitting up in bed

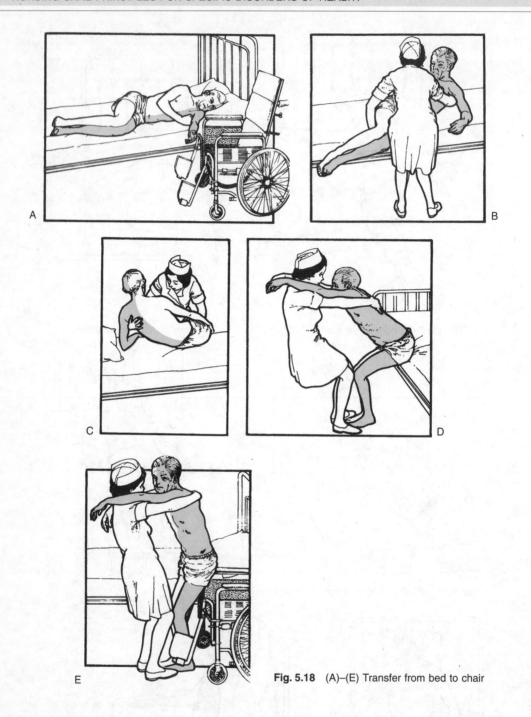

Fig. 5.18 (A)–(E) Transfer from bed to chair

elusive but three main theories point to environmental, viral and ageing factors. In Parkinson's disease there appears to be a marked reduction in the neurotransmitter dopamine within the basal ganglia and of the melanin pigment within the substantia nigra. The action of dopamine is opposed by acetylcholine, another neurotransmitter, the correct balance of each being necessary for voluntary skilled movement.

Common symptoms

The disease has an insidious onset, progressing slowly until activities of living are affected. There are three main features:

1. Poverty in movement (bradykinesia)   This is an early feature but often the most disabling. Bradykinesia interferes with the initiation of movement; starting to walk and other automatic movements disappear, like swinging the arms when walking, causing the distinctive stooped posture and shuffling foot steps. The face also tends to be 'mask like' with reduced blinking and eye movement. Swallowing becomes slow so that saliva tends to drool from the half-open mouth and speech is quiet, slurred and monotonous.

2. Tremor   This is usually seen in the hands or arms occurring mainly at rest, abolished with movement, disappearing during sleep. At rest it is a fairly course tremor involving particularly the thumb and forefinger giving rise to the 'pill rolling' description.

3. Rigidity   This gives rise to the flexed posture, with the muscles often working in opposite directions. If a limb is bent it may be stiff throughout; likened to a lead pipe, hence 'lead pipe rigidity!'. Where a tremor is also present bending of the limb produces a 'cog wheel' rigidity. Gradually everyday tasks take longer and longer.

Investigation

The above three classical features tend to be diagnostic of Parkinson's disease, although it may be necessary to exclude atherosclerotic causes (i.e. multiple small strokes) or repeated trauma (e.g. the 'punch drunk state' associated with boxers). The disorder can also be drug induced, in which case it is referred to as parkinsonism (see Ch. 9).

Therapeutic management

This can be achieved mainly by drug therapy, with the aim of restoring the balance between the dopamine and acetylcholine neurotransmitters. Since dopamine is reduced the balance can be achieved by increasing dopamine or reducing acetylcholine levels.

Levodopa preparations   Since dopamine is unable to cross the blood–brain barrier the precursor levodopa is given which is useful in relieving the rigidity and bradykinesia. Levodopa given alone unfortu-

nately can cause postural hypotension and cardiac arrhythmias, so it is usually given in combination, for example, levodopa and benserazide (Madopar), levodopa and carbidopa (Sinemet), the added drugs preventing the systemic side-effects.

Unfortunately a bizarre feature is the 'on/off' phenomenon, an adverse side-effect that some patients may develop after receiving levodopa therapy. During the 'off' period, which may last 5–60 minutes but increasing in time, the patient has no response to drug therapy, the 'on' period occurring when drugs are effective. Drug therapy may be more beneficial if the same dose is prescribed more frequently in smaller doses.

Anticholinergic drugs such as benhexol (Artane), procyclidine (Kemadrin) and orphenadrine (Disipal) block the acetylcholine receptor sites. They are particularly useful in controlling the tremor, reducing salivation and decreasing rigidity. However, anticholinergic drugs are not without their side-effects, namely dry mouth, blurred vision, constipation and occasionally confusion and loss of memory.

Other drugs

Dopamine agonists such as bromocriptine (Parlodel) which mimic the action of dopamine may be given but their use has not been as successful as might have been hoped.

Amantadine hydrochloride (Symmetral), an antiviral drug, may be given to help rigidity although its actual action remains unknown.

Selegiline prolongs the action of levadopa and may be useful when levadopa wears off quickly, however since it is a mild stimulant it can cause insomnia and psychiatric disturbances and therefore should be taken in the morning.

Patients with Parkinson's disease should be admitted to hospital to have their drug therapy established or altered since each patient's needs are different and the amount or type of drug should be tailored to meet these individual needs. It may be that only some and not all the features of the disease will be abolished.

Nursing strategies

As well as stabilization of drug therapy, nursing strategies in consultation with the multidisciplinary team involve helping the patient and significant others to maintain maximum independence.

Eating and drinking   This tends to be a slow process

requiring patience and understanding, the nurse may occasionally be required to cut the patient's food. The occupational therapist can provide suitable adapted crockery, cutlery and non-slip mats. Patients with swallowing difficulties may find that a liquid and puréed diet are most suitable, although the nurse should be aware that some patients unknowingly aspirate liquid into their lungs increasing the risk of aspiration pneumonia.

Eliminating   Accidental urinary incontinence is often a problem. Due to immobility and rigidity the patient may be unable to reach the toilet in time. The use of zips/velcro instead of buttons may help to ease the problem. In addition, inability to initiate micturition can add to the patient's frustrations. Constipation is also common and can be helped by advising that fibre and fluid be increased in the diet. Patients with urinary incontinence may however be sceptical regarding a fluid increase.

Maintaining a safe environment   A common problem many patients with Parkinson's disease experience is falling. Accident prevention must identify factors in hospital and at home that might contribute, so that effort can be taken to alleviate them, for example ward layout, poor lighting, loose rugs.

Communicating   Facial expression and body language is an important part of communication but for patients with Parkinson's disease their immobility, rigidity and mask-like facial appearance suggest a lack of understanding. The nurse should listen and watch the patient's face and mouth carefully and should never talk loudly at him/her. Speech therapy, reading aloud, singing and raising the voice may be beneficial.

Personal cleansing and dressing   The patient may require assistance with personal hygiene, extra care being required to remove perspiration and oil from the skin and hair which tends to be greasier. Mouth care may require to be increased, as drooling of saliva may cause the chin to become quite moist with a risk of breakdown. Some drugs may however cause excessive dryness.

Mobilization   Maintaining normality for as long as possible is important and patients should be advised to remain active and independent. Physiotherapy exercises designed to improve the efficiency of muscles and prevent deformities should be encouraged. Using a wide-based gait, humming a marching tune maintains balance and improves walking. Should the patient be bed-bound, reduced immobility increases the risk of skin breakdown, therefore 2-hourly turning should be employed which will also prevent pulmonary complications. Passive limb exercises will prevent stiffness and contractures.

It is worth noting that when patients with Parkinson's disease are admitted to hospital for treatment of other disorders, drug administration times may not suit their carefully established medication times. Administration times should therefore not be altered to suit the ward, since this may cause the Parkinson's disease to become out of control.

Surgical therapy   Surgical treatment occasionally is performed to abolish a persistent incapacitating tremor. This involves stereotactic surgery whereby a lesion is made in the ventrolateral nucleus of the thalamus by means of the insertion of a thin probe to freeze the appropriate tissue.

Patients and significant others can be encouraged to obtain further information, advice and support from the Parkinson's Disease Society, a voluntary organization, with branches and local contacts throughout the country (Head Office, 22 Upper Woburn Place, London WC1H, 0RA; tel: 071 383 3513).

Ethical dilemma

Recently it has been demonstrated that the implantation of fetal dopamine producing cells into the basal ganglia of patients with Parkinson's disease may be beneficial. This has however raised many moral and ethical issues. The BMA has issued guidelines for such operations in an effort to alleviate such issues.

Multiple sclerosis

Epidemiology and aetiology

Multiple sclerosis affects young adults between 20 and 45 years, usually women more commonly than men in a ratio of 3 : 2. Its prevalence appears to increase in northern climates, urban areas and those in higher socioeconomic groups. The aetiology remains unknown although it is thought it may be an autoimmune disorder or be triggered by an infection or virus, or indeed may be multifactorial.

Common symptoms

The disease is characterized by a slow often chronic progressive course. Inflammation of the myelin sheath around nerve fibres occurs, followed by demyelination and gliosis. This demyelination occurs randomly hindering the impulse conduction throughout the

> **Box 5.2   Clinical manifestations of multiple sclerosis**
>
> **Sensory symptoms**
> Numbness, paraesthesia
>
> **Motor symptoms**
> Weakness, paralysis, sphincter disturbances,
> e.g. loss of bladder control or bowel function
>
> **Brain stem**
> Diplopia
>
> **Cerebellar symptoms**
> Reduced co-ordination, ataxia, intention tremor,
> slurred speech
>
> **Other features**
> Optic neuritis: loss of vision, blurring of vision,
> fatigue, mood alterations, e.g. depression/euphoria
> fatigue

body. As the disease progresses, the affected nerve fibres degenerate, increasing deficits, some becoming permanent. These lesions can form anywhere within the CNS but tend to be restricted to brain stem, optic nerves and spinal cord.

Symptoms vary greatly, depending upon demyelination sites. Clinical manifestations are included in Box 5.2.

Multiple sclerosis is characterized by periods of **exacerbation** (relapse) whereby dysfunction occurs in the area supplied by the affected nerve, followed by complete recovery, **remission**. Over time various combinations of nerve dysfunction occur with each relapse, or a cumulative effect from repeated attacks to the same site may cause progressive deterioration.

In the young adult the disease tends to follow a relapsing–remitting course, many years separating exacerbations without significant disability occurring, the average life expectancy being approximately 25 years after initial onset. A more progressive form of the disease may be encountered when the onset of the disease occurs in middle age.

Patient implications

The patient may have suffered vague transient symptoms over many months, such early features easily being mistaken for hysteria, so possibly the initial diagnosis is a great relief. Then the patient and significant others must come to terms with the disorder. Most people wrongly associate multiple sclerosis sufferers with a wheelchair, yet less than one in ten will be confined to this.

Investigations

One of the main difficulties with multiple sclerosis is that no reliable diagnostic test exists, the diagnosis is often made on the pattern of clinical features which has occurred over time. Some laboratory tests may aid in establishing the diagnosis, for example CSF may reveal an increase in immunoglobulins as well as elevated protein. Neurophysiological tests, electromyeography (EMG) and visual evoked potentials may show abnormal recordings. Nuclear magnetic imaging (NMR) can demonstrate areas of demyelination. Diagnosis however is often made by excluding all other neurological disorders which present similar features.

Therapeutic management

There is as yet no curative treatment. Drug therapy as in other degenerative conditions helps to control specific symptoms during exacerbations or relieves complications of some symptoms.

Steroid therapy Adrenocorticotrophic hormone (ACTH), given to reduce the inflammation, may increase the rate of recovery from a relapse of multiple sclerosis. Neurologists may differ in their approach in administration of ACTH.

Antispasmodics Diazepam, dantrolene or baclofen, given singly or in combination, may be required to control muscle spasms. When bladder spasticity is problematical resulting in frequency, distigmine bromide (Ubretid) or emepronium bromide (Cetriprim) can be prescribed.

Diet Therapy with linoleic acid, gluten free and low cholesterol diets have all been advocated at times. Their effects are debatable.

Hyperbaric oxygen Interest in this has increased over the past few years as a means of delivering oxygen to tissue. For a number of people using this therapy (the decision is made by the patient), some of the features of multiple sclerosis show that such reported cases of improvement may only be a reflection of the relapsing and remitting course.

Surgical treatment

Some patients have severe spasticity and pain in the lower limbs, thus intrathecal phenol injections may be given to damage selective nerve roots without affecting the bladder.

Nursing strategies

As the disease advances impaired motor and sensory

skills and poor co-ordination may require similar care as in the hemiplegic patient (Nursing Care Plan 5.2). For those with bladder dysfunction and paraparesis, the care is similar to that of a paraplegic person (Nursing Care Plan 5.10). It is important however to encourage the patient to achieve independence for as long as possible.

Motor neurone disease

Epidemiology and aetiology

This disorder usually occurs in middle age, affecting men more commonly than females. The aetiology is unknown.

Common symptoms

Motor neurone disease (MND) is a disorder affecting various structures within the motor system, resulting in progressive weakness and wasting. Various levels within the motor system can degenerate, and clinical features depend on the level or combination of levels affected, varying from paralysis, muscle spasticity/flaccidity, reduced muscle power, wasting to atrophy.

When the motor nuclei of the cranial nerves or corticobulbar pathways are damaged, ie. bulbar palsy, the patient may develop dysarthria and dysphagia from involvement of muscles involved in swallowing, chewing and speaking. The tongue also atrophies.

Patient implications

This is a very incapacitating and distressing illness to patients and significant others. Patients presenting bulbar features may only survive 2–3 years, dying from exhaustion, aspiration pneumonia and cachexia. Those with anterior horn cell involvement resulting in progressive muscular atrophy may survive more than 10 years until progression leads also to bulbar palsy.

Investigations

The clinical features tend to be diagnostic of motor neurone disease, although occasionally they may resemble a peripheral neuropathy. Needle electrodes may be introduced into skeletal muscles to study the electrical potential of the muscles and nerves by electromyography (EMG). In MND this demonstrates denervation with fasciculations (muscle twitching).

Therapeutic management

There is no drug therapy known to halt the disorder, treatment being symptomatic and supportive; for example, a gastrostomy may be performed if chewing and swallowing become difficult. Antispasmodics, such as dantrolene sodium, may be prescribed to relieve spasticity in affected limbs, or aperients may be necessary for constipation.

Nursing strategies

Nursing care must be aimed at assisting the patient to be as independent and comfortable as possible by managing symptoms. As muscles become weaker then the introduction of appliances, splints, walking sticks, may prove helpful. It is also important to prevent accidents and to ensure that the patient does not become overtired.

Communication can be extremely difficult, especially if the patient lives alone and needs to summon urgent help. Advice regarding communication aids can be given by the speech therapist and pretaped telephone messages can be made.

For those patients with chewing and swallowing difficulties a deficit in fluid balance and nutrition can occur. Drooling saliva and choking can cause the patient great embarrassment and the patient in hospital or at home may wish to eat alone. Suction should however, be available. A choking episode can be very frightening and often patients do not like being alone at night, since they may be unable to summon help. Initially frequent puréed meals should be given, however, as swallowing becomes more difficult various alternative feeding methods may need to be employed.

At the terminal stages the patient experiences respiratory insufficiency, managing secretions becomes difficult and often eye contact is the only means of communication. The patient should not be left alone, but allowed to die peacefully and with dignity.

Myasthenia gravis

Epidemiology and aetiology

This is an uncommon disease affecting one per 100 000 primarily females under 40 years, although the incidence is equal in both sexes over 40 years. The cause is thought to be autoimmune, the accepted theory being that the defect blocks, renders inactive or destroys the postsynaptic acetylcholine (ACh) receptor site. Occasionally thymus abnormalities, for example thymoma, may produce antibodies to voluntary muscle.

Common symptoms

The clinical features may vary from muscle weakness

to fatigue, depending on the involvement of all or selective muscles. The various manifestations become worse with repeated exertion, or as the day progresses.

Patient implications

The ocular muscles, either unilaterally or bilaterally, are often affected first giving rise to ptosis and/or diplopia. Involvement of the muscles controlling mastication, swallowing, neck and facial movements follows, so that dysarthria and dysphagia occur. The patient's head may fall forward, the jaw propped closed with his hand, and speech fades to a whisper. These features may become more apparent as the patient continues to talk, or as a meal progresses.

Loss of power accompanied by fatigue may also be apparent in muscles of the shoulder girdle or hip joint. Involvement of the respiratory muscles (intercostals and/or diaphragm) may result in respiratory insufficiency and can be potentially fatal from respiratory arrest.

Investigation

The patient's history and clinical features with pattern of muscle weakness may aid the diagnosis. Acetylcholine receptor antibodies are often detected in such patients as are thymic antibodies. Nerve conduction studies (EMG) will assess the fatiguability of a motor nerve when repeatedly stimulated. A pharmacological test using an anticholinesterase drug is used to confirm the diagnosis; for example, edrophonium (Tensilon) injected intravenously will give a brief remission of symptoms.

Therapeutic management

Anticholinesterase drugs (e.g. neostigmine, pyridostigmine) are effective in controlling myasthenia gravis but are not curative. They act to improve neuromuscular transmission by preventing the action of acetylcholinesterase so that acetylcholine may be prolonged. The dosage and timings are individually determined and self-medication even in hospital should be facilitated, since timing is often critical, the patient recognizing through experience when medication is required.

The patient also should be aware that gastrointestinal upsets, cramps, diarrhoea and excessive salivation may occur, but can be relieved by atropine. Increasing weakness, increased secretions (may be

unnoticed if atropine is prescribed) and increasing respiratory difficulty may auger a 'crisis' situation. This may be due to exacerbation of original features, as in a 'myasthenic crisis' indicating the need to increase medication, or caused by overdosage of anticholinesterase drugs, a 'cholinergic crisis'. It may be difficult to initially determine the cause, and therefore anticholinergic drugs should be omitted and the patient artificially ventilated until the cause is established. Edrophonium (Tensilon) may be needed to determine the type of crisis since it improves those in myasthenic crisis but temporarily worsens patients in cholinergic crisis.

Steroid therapy may be beneficial in severe generalized myasthenia, although deterioration may occur prior to improvement and the administration therapy protocol remains controversial. The anti-immunological drug azathioprine may be given concurrently with anticholinesterases or replace steroid therapy when the disease proves resistant to such treatment. In time when immunological control has been achieved and the patient maintains a remission anticholinesterase therapy may cease.

Plasmapharesis is one of the newer treatments and is a process of plasma exchange whereby the circulating antibodies that interfere with acetylcholine receptors are removed. Since it gives only short-term improvement, its use may be more effective in crisis situations.

Surgical treatment

A thymectomy may give complete remission/improvement especially in patients with myasthenia who have thymomas or hyperplasia of the thymus gland.

Nursing strategies

The main aim of the nurse is to help the patient and significant others to adjust to the constraints imposed upon him by the disease process. Initially both psychological and emotional support will be important. The patients should become knowledgeable about the actual disease process and they should be aware of the reason for drug therapy, the dosage, the time and the importance of maintaining accuracy and punctuality. Also they and significant others should be able to recognize side-effects and overdosage/crisis features and the action required.

The nurse will need to indicate factors that may exacerbate symptoms, extremes in temperature, infections, physical and emotional stress, so that they can be avoided. Adjustments to life-style may be required. Mealtimes should coincide with the peak effect of anticholinesterase (30 minutes after medication) so that maximal strength is present in the muscles for chewing and swallowing.

It is important that the patient pace him/herself, planning well ahead, providing adequate rest periods to minimize weakness. The patient should also be aware of the need to avoid the use of non-prescriptive medications since many interact with anticholinesterase therapy. It may also be beneficial to the patients to wear a medical alert bracelet/necklace, identifying the disease, drug therapy and physician treating him.

SPINAL DISORDERS

Spinal lesions result from intrinsic pathology within the cord, or within or without the meninges – extrinsic. The causes of spinal lesions are varied (Table 5.5). This text will concentrate on the most common causes of spinal lesions, injuries and degenerative lumbar disc prolapse.

Table 5.5 Cause of spinal disorders

Cause	Example
Congenital	Spinal dysraphism
	Syringomyelia
	Canal stenosis
Acquired	
1. Traumatic	Fractures
	Dislocations
	Gunshot/stab wounds
2. Vascular	AVM
	Haematoma
	Infarction
3. Neoplastic	
a. Intradural intramedullary	Astrocytoma
	Ependymoma
b. Intradural extramedullary	Meningioma
c. Extradural	Metastases
	Myeloma
	Neurofibroma
	Lymphoma
4. Infective	
a. Acute	Abscess
b. Chronic	Poliomyelitis
	Neurosyphilis
5. Degenerative	Rheumatoid arthritis
	Cervical spondylosis
	Disc prolapse
	Canal stenosis

Trauma

Epidemiology and aetiology

Between 15 and 20 new spinal injuries/million population occur yearly. Of these, 75% occur in those under 40 years, with 25% in those below 20 years of age. Nearly half occur as a result of vehicular accidents, the rest from sports injuries, assaults and falls. Fracture-dislocation of the verebral column has the potential to damage the spinal cord, at the time of injury or later. Damage depends on various factors related to the injury, type, force and direction of impact (Fig. 5.19).

Common symptoms

The features depend on the level and severity of damage but all functions of the cord, motor, sensory and autonomic, are affected to a greater or lesser degree so that, initially, there may be below the level of the lesion:

1. flaccid paralysis of skeletal muscle
2. loss of spinal reflexes
3. loss of sensation
4. loss of vasomotor tone
5. loss of the ability to perspire
6. loss of bladder and bowel function
   (Note: 4 and 5 occur especially in cervical lesions.)

A thoracic or lumbar lesion results in **paraplegia**, lower limb paralysis; a cervical lesion, **tetraplegia**, paralysis in all four limbs. The prognosis for recovery depends on the completeness of the lesion, complete transection indicating very minimal/no recovery. Damage to the high cervical cord results in respiratory paralysis, many patients not surviving the accident but those who do may be ventilator dependent.

The most important implication to the patient is to prevent any further cord damage occuring post-injury, therefore all patients who have sustained trauma, those who complain of neck pain, paraesthesia, limb weakness and all unconscious patients must be suspected of having a spinal injury until proven otherwise. At the scene of the accident the patient should be immobilized on a spinal board or in a cervical collar with the head and neck maintained in a neutral position to prevent further damage.

Investigation

As far as possible, the patient should not be moved, especially unsupervised, since this may further damage the cord. Neurological examination should

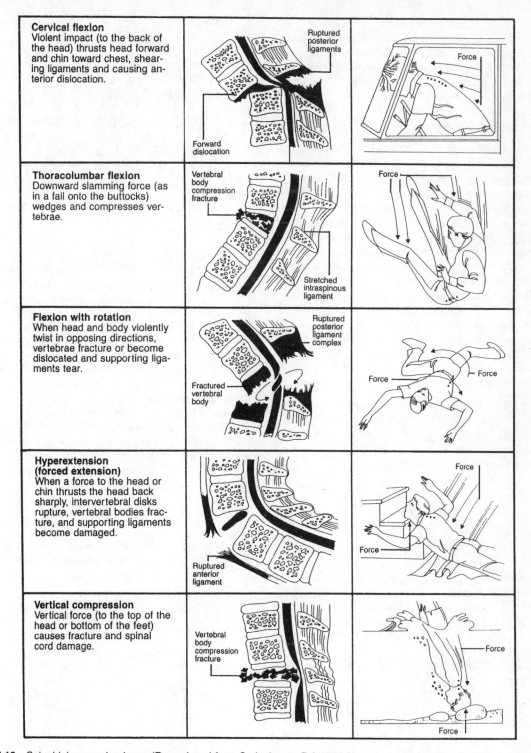

Cervical flexion
Violent impact (to the back of the head) thrusts head forward and chin toward chest, shearing ligaments and causing anterior dislocation.

Thoracolumbar flexion
Downward slamming force (as in a fall onto the buttocks) wedges and compresses vertebrae.

Flexion with rotation
When head and body violently twist in opposing directions, vertebrae fracture or become dislocated and supporting ligaments tear.

Hyperextension (forced extension)
When a force to the head or chin thrusts the head back sharply, intervertebral disks rupture, vertebral bodies fracture, and supporting ligaments become damaged.

Vertical compression
Vertical force (to the top of the head or bottom of the feet) causes fracture and spinal cord damage.

Fig. 5.19 Spinal injury mechanisms. (Reproduced from Springhouse P A 1987 Neurological Problems. Springhouse Group.)

elicit, motor, sensory and automatic loss. A plain spinal X-ray to visualize the whole spine to assess fracture-dislocation and stability should be done. A CT scan and/or MRI will demonstrate vertebrae, canal and cord, and myelography may be carried out to exclude cord compression.

Therapeutic management

Conservative treatment is used in the majority of patients, the aim being to preserve as much cord function as possible in patients with unstable fractures and neurological impairment, skull traction may be applied to achieve optimum alignment. The patient is nursed in a wedge turning frame, or Stoke Egerton bed for several weeks to allow fractures to heal. Surgery may be necessary and to minimize further cord impairment if neurological symptoms deteriorate to remove an associated disc protusion or to stabilize C1/C2 fractures using a Ransford Loop technique (Fig. 5.20). Patients with unstable cervical injuries without neurological deficits may be nursed in a Halo frame allowing self-care and early discharge (Fig. 5.21).

Nursing strategies

The care of the spinal-injured patient is presented using Orem's Model of Care (Nursing Care Plan 5.3). Excluding the care required in the acute stages of spinal injury, the plan could be adapted to care for a patient with multiple sclerosis.

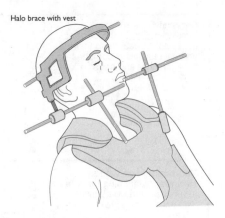

Halo brace with vest

Fig. 5.21 Halo frame

Degenerative spinal disorders

Epidemiology and aetiology

Back pain affects all socioeconomic groups and is associated with repeated trauma, accidents and poor body mechanics; poor posture/lifting techniques place strain and stresses on intervertebral bodies/disc/ligaments, which allowing the disc to protrude and compress the spinal nerve leaving the intervertebral foramen below. Therefore, a disc protusion between L5 and S1 compresses the first sacral nerve. The lumbar region – L4/5, L5/S1 – carrying the total body weight plus any object the person may carry, is the site most commonly affected. The mean age is around 35 years, the incidence in males being slightly higher (Fig. 5.22).

Common symptoms

The patient may have had backache or sciatic pain on and off for years due to increasing pressure on the

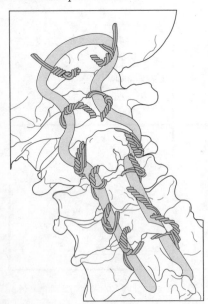

Fig. 5.20 Cervical fixation using a Ransford Loop

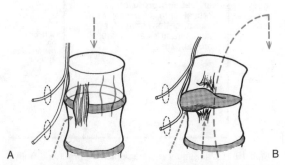

A   B

Fig. 5.22 (A) Normal lumbar vertebrae and intervertebral discs (B) Prolapsed lumbar intervertebral disc

Nursing Care Plan 5.3 Orem's Self-care Model in spinal injury/damage				
		Intervention		
Problem*	**Goal**	**Wholly compensatory**	**Partially compensatory**	**Rationale**
Respiratory muscle paralysis (actual in cervical damage)	Maintain O$_2$ perfusion Prevention of atelectasis	❐ Assess respiratory function ❐ Frequently record/report observations ❐ Monitor O$_2$ saturation, maintain level according to instructions ❐ Administer humidified O$_2$ if required ❐ Give oral/tracheal suction if necessary ❐ Assist in intermittent positive pressure breathing (IPPB) via Bennet according to instructions ❐ Assist patient to expectorate/cough especially following cervical damage ❐ If tracheostomy and/or ventilator required, nurse accordingly	❐ Assess as per wholly compensatory ❐ Continue O$_2$ therapy as required ❐ Encourage deep breathing and expectorating ❐ Nurse/patient will report any respiratory change ❐ Nurse will reinforce understanding of respiratory care to patient and significant others	Following cervical damage all intercostal muscles are paralysed. If phrenic nerve is unaffected; leaves cervical cord C3–5 level, then patient will use diaphragm as only muscle of respiration. Patient therefore requires to recognize change/deterioration in respiratory function
Sufficient fluid intake (P) **Dehydration (P)**	Avoid dehydration Maintain electrolyte balance	❐ Reinforce nil fluids orally according to instructions ❐ Assist in administration of prescribed IVI fluids and electrolytes ❐ Give oral fluids, when bowel sounds are present, on doctor's instruction	❐ Encourage patient to drink adequate fluids and teach patient/significant others the importance of maintaining adequate fluid balance	Following cervical damage patient may initially develop an adynamic ileus, therefore nil orally
Inadequate nutritional intake (P) **Unrecognized adynamic ileus (P)**	Prevention of complications of an adynamic ileus Balanced diet achieved	❐ Reinforce nil orally ❐ Initiate gastric intubation, aspirate according to doctor's instructions ❐ Measure, record and report abdominal girths ❐ Listen with stethoscope for peristaltic sounds ❐ Maintain IVI ❐ Give oral fluids (small sips of fluid only to prevent choking) when permitted. Feed patient adequate diet	❐ Encourage oral/fluids diet ❐ Assist patient to eat when they are tetraplegic ❐ Discuss with patient/significant others the need to maintain a balanced diet avoiding weight gain	Potential risk of an adynamic ileus following cervical damage with the added risk of vomiting/inhalation and sudden respiratory arrest Fear of choking in patients with cervical damage

Nursing Care Plan 5.3 (*cont'd*)

Problem*	Goal	Intervention Wholly compensatory	Intervention Partially compensatory	Rationale
Faecal impaction (P)	Achieve adequate bowel evacuation	❏ Assess by manual examination the presence of faeces in rectum and digitally evacuate ❏ Initiate bowel training emptying/regimen as in partially compensatory	❏ Ensure adequate diet/fluids ❏ Teach patient/ significant others the need to establish a bowel training regimen, e.g. bowel check, every 2–3 days administer suppositories monitor results, and digitally evacuate if necessary Teach to recognize need for stool softeners	Following injury bowel is initially atonic, therefore bowel requires manual evacuation. As reflexes return reflex emptying can be achieved
Initially atonic bladder (A)	Prevention of bladder distension/ overflow incontinence	❏ Assessment of urinary output/bladder distension	❏ Assessment of bladder function when reflexes return	
	Prevention of infection	❏ Catheterize according to policy, record output ❏ Institute closed drainage system ❏ Give catheter care	● establish a suitable reflex stimulus, e.g. abdominal tapping to reflexedly empty bladder ● follow this by residual	Impaired nervous supply initially leads to urinary retention, overstretching of bladder leading to potential permanent damage, thus the need for catheterization
	Establish reflex bladder emptying	❏ Recognize that passing of urine may be related to bowel impaction	catheterization to monitor effectiveness of reflex emptying ❏ Educate patient/ significant others to self-catheterize if above is not achieved or to monitor residuals ❏ Discuss with patient/ significant others problems associated with catheterization, i.e. infection trauma ❏ Teach patient and significant others importance of adequate fluid intake	When reflexes return bladder training regimen commences
Forced immobility (A)	Maintain spinal alignment Prevent any further cord damage	**Acute phase** ❏ Nurse according to instructions, e.g. in cervical fracture-dislocation ❏ Nurse patient on Stryker frame or electrical turning bed with skeletal traction via skull tongs (Fig. 5.23A&B)	**Lumbar damage** ❏ Maintain spinal alignment according to instructions ❏ Nurse on electric turning bed ❏ Log roll when moving patients, e.g. inspecting pressure areas	The aim following fracture-dislocation is initially immobilization reduction of fracture stabilization When healing has occurred rehabilitation aims at returning the patient to optimum potential in the community

Nursing Care Plan 5.3 (*cont'd*)

Problem*	Goal	Intervention Wholly compensatory	Intervention Partially compensatory	Rationale
	Prevent contractures	❒ 2-hourly turns to relieve pressure or as directed by doctor ❒ Inspect skin at turns ❒ Observe tong sites for loosening, soakage or infection ❒ Clean and spray tong sites ❒ Evaluate and report any motor and or sensory changes ❒ Position viewing mirrors and encourage use ❒ Encourage patient to take an interest in an activity that is within his capabilities and interest ❒ Passively move joints through a full range of movements daily to prevent stiffness/contractures which may interfere with rehabilitation ❒ Position accordingly ❒ Splint limbs in position of function according to doctor/physiotherapist's instructions	❒ Use 3–4 nurses when log rolling (Fig. 5.24) ❒ Use counter pressure when inserting/withdrawing arms to prevent sideways movement of spine (Fig. 5.25) ❒ Encourage patient to carry out self-care activities within capabilities without altering stabilization and/or causing exhaustion **Rehabilitation** ❒ Encourage patient to participate in rehabilitation programme ❒ Teach patient to become active in his self-care needs including social and psychological ❒ Teach patient and significant others importance of passive limb movements ❒ Demonstrate correct positioning to prevent contractures ❒ Demonstrate use of splints to maintain optimal position of function	No contractures develop that will mitigate against rehabilitation
Sensory deprivation (P)	Prevent sensory deprivation	**Acute phase** ❒ Encourage patient to increase visual stimulation by use of preset mirrors, reading/listening materials ❒ Inform the patient regarding time, ward activities/routines ❒ Teach nurse and significant others that abnormal behaviour, e.g. hallucinations, may relate to sensory deprivation	❒ Reassure patient and encourage discussion regarding body image/sexuality ❒ Answer all questions honestly and/or refer to appropriate person ❒ Teach necessary skills to achieve self-care	Patient during immobilization/stabilization may have very restricted visual environment, e.g. views only perhaps the ceiling and the floor
Loss of body image/sexuality (A)	Increase confidence in self-care	**Rehabilitation stage** ❒ Appreciate patient may experience anxieties/feelings regarding body image/sexuality		If mental welfare is not achieved this affects physical and social well-being

Nursing Care Plan 5.3 (*cont'd*)

Problem*	Goal	Intervention Wholly compensatory	Partially compensatory	Rationale
Social isolation (P)	Encourage social interaction	❐ Answer/discuss patient's feelings regarding body image/sexuality ❐ Offer counselling support, e.g. sexual counsellor ❐ Inform patients of self-help groups, Spinal Injuries Association and/or other counsellors if necessary, psychologist, marriage guidance		Procreation is the normal desire
Fear of being stared at because of disablement (P) Grieving process (P) Lack of motivation (P)	Maintain social interaction Allow to grieve	❐ Accept that the patient will want solitude and will need to grieve his loss (i.e. paralysed body) and is likely to go through various stages of grief, e.g. denial, anger, aggression, depression ❐ Explain to significant others the reason for grieving process ❐ Know when to leave patient alone and when to listen ❐ Support the patient during the various stages, motivating them to attain self-esteem	❐ Provide aids/ equipment to enable social activity ❐ Introduce patient and significant others to societies/self-help groups/sports open to the disabled ❐ Encourage the patient to participate in preaccident activities, e.g. drinking with friends, but to recognize that some modification may be needed, e.g. to avoid overflow incontinence ❐ Continue to motivate and encourage self-esteem/value to society	Patients need to grieve loss of function in order to aid recovery Patients with disability are stigmatized in society and are very sensitive to this
Internal (P) potential to develop: pressure sores; infection; deep venous thrombosis; autonomic; dysreflexia	Prevention of hazards to well-being	❐ Pressure sore: Assess patient's risk using acceptable scale: Norton Waterlow Turn 2 hourly, Stryker frame, electric bed, later ordinary bed Observe any reddening, etc. over pressure areas, take preventive action ❐ Deep venous thrombosis (DVT): Observe calf for swelling/increased warmth/redness. Note: patient will *not* feel pain/tenderness Use antiembolic stockings while immobile Administer prophylactic minihelp if prescribed	❐ Teach patients and significant others to turn 2 hourly ❐ Teach patient the need to relieve pressure by lifting self while sitting Patient will avoid, e.g. hot pipes/hot water bottle Report any broken area ❐ Patient and significant others taught to recognize and report features of DVT	Death is more likely from the complications of hazards to well-being than to spinal cord injury

Nursing Care Plan 5.3 (*cont'd*)

Problem*	Goal	Intervention Wholly compensatory	Partially compensatory	Rationale
		❏ Infection: Note alteration in temperature Note urine output, colour, sedimentation and smell Observe sputum Obtain any relevant specimen for microbiology investigation	Recognize infected urine	Unique to spinal cord-injured patients especially damage above T6 caused by abnormal stimuli which creates an exaggerated response of sympathetic nervous system due to loss of cerebral control. Frequent source of stimuli, bowel impaction, rectal stimulation, UTI, pressure sores
	Identify patients at risk from autonomic dysreflexia Avoidance of stimuli which precipitates symptoms	**Autonomic dysreflexia** ❏ Patient and significant others will be taught the features of autonomic dysreflexia and the emergency it reflects Features: headache, sweating, flushing, bradycardia, hypertension		
External **Wheelchair access** **Mobility** **Housing**	Ensure safe environment Ensure mental well-being	❏ Assessment of patient by multidisciplinary team for wheelchair, applicable to that patient ❏ Teach significant others wheelchair manipulation ❏ Wheelchair access and house modification assessed	❏ Teach patient skill of manipulation of their wheelchair ❏ Patient and significant others help in house modifications	Wheelchair mobility access essential for mental well-being, unless suitable house modifications are provided, patient may not be able to live outside hospital

*Problem: (A) actual; (P) potential.

lumbar or sacral nerves. Acute lumbar disc protusion occurs suddenly; the patient lifts an object awkwardly and feels something 'give' in his back. Initially he may be unable to straighten up and feels a shooting pain down the leg.

This pain is termed sciatica. Scoliosis may develop in an attempt to ease the pain, the spine flexing towards the affected side. Coughing and sneezing increases the pain.

The distribution of pain depends on the affected nerve. In fifth lumbar nerve compression, the pain radiates along the back of the thigh and leg crossing into the foot towards the great toe, whereas pressure on the first sacral nerve causes pain in the lateral aspect of the leg and foot and into the small toe. Since it is the lower neurone lesion there will be mini-mal wasting and motor power loss of the affected muscles.

Patient implications

Low back pain is responsible for tremendous economic loss in industry due to absence at work.

Investigation

1. General examination may reveal a scoliosis/ muscle spasm.

2. Straight-leg raising increases pain due to stretching of the sciatic nerve.

3. Pain can also be induced by pressing the appropriate intervertebral disc space.

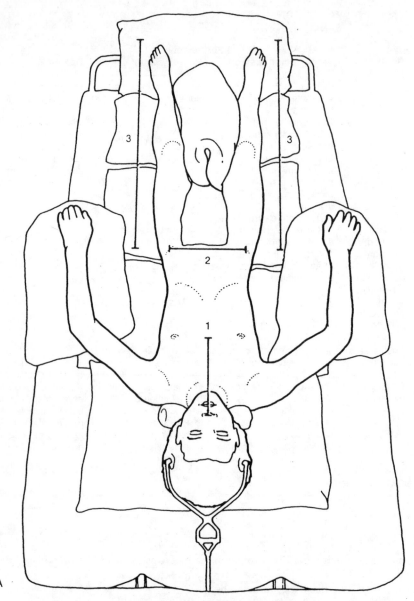

Fig. 5.23 Spinal alignment: (A) supine position; (B) lateral position. (Reproduced from Spinal injuries. Nursing Times 24 February, 1982, p 4)

4. Plain X-rays may show narrowing of the disc spaces and myelography should demonstrate disc protusion.

Therapeutic management

If treated conservatively with bed rest, heat, anti-spasmodics, analgesics and non-steroidal anti-inflam-matory drugs, most lesions resolve. Some, however, require surgical excision if the pain persists or a neurological deficit develops, for example due to compression of the nerves to the bladder and bowel. Until a bladder and bowel deficit resolves, care will be as in Nursing Care Plan 5.3.

Surgery – discetomy – involves removal of muscle attachment, ligament and bone to achieve sufficient

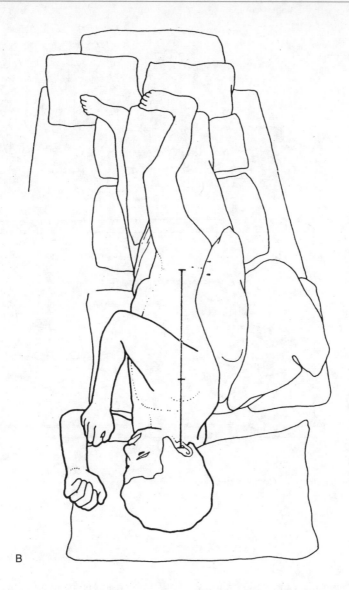

B

exposure to remove the prolapsed disc material. A **microdiscetomy** involves removal of disc material from between the spinous processes of the affected vertebrae, leaving bone intact.

Nursing strategies

Pre- and postoperative general care is the same as for any operation. Specific care is given in Nursing Care Plan 5.4.

Spinal anaesthesia

An anaesthetic agent can be injected at L3/4 level into the epidural space or intrathecal space as a means of alleviating pain, and may be used:

● to control abdominal postoperative pain
● to treat intractable pain, especially from bony metastases.

The intrathecal route is used only when a single injection is required and a quick postoperative period

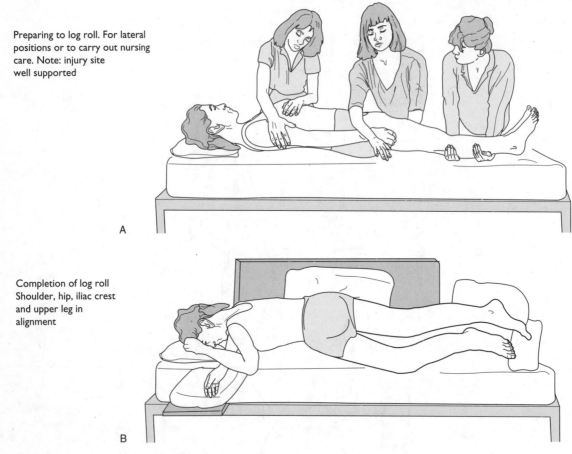

Preparing to log roll. For lateral positions or to carry out nursing care. Note: injury site well supported

A

Completion of log roll Shoulder, hip, iliac crest and upper leg in alignment

B

Fig. 5.24   (A) Log roll preparation. (B) Completion of log roll

is expected, whereas an epidural cannulation allows the excess catheter to be taped to the patient's back for further doses to be added.

Lignocaine, bupivacaine (Marcaine) and morphine are the drugs usually chosen. They act by blocking nerve impulse transmission and their effects depend on the volume and concentration given. Since the thicker sensory fibres are more susceptible, sensory loss occurs.

Sympathetic nerve blockade is also unavoidable, resulting in vasodilatation and thus hypotension and motor fibres can also be blocked intentionally or as a complication. The spread of the analgesia achieved also depends on the patient's position. Morphine however blocks only pain transmission.

Hypotension is the main patient implication, therefore it is important to maintain frequent blood pressure recordings, increasing the frequency following each additional dose. An IVI should be commenced prior to the procedure to enable volume replacement should collapse occur. Respiratory difficulties or respiratory depression occasionally occurs, associated with epidural morphine. This may require reversal using naloxone. The patient may require to be catheterized following an epidural as he will be unable to appreciate when the bladder is full. This may not be necessary following intrathecal anaesthesia since sensation and thus bladder control returns once the anaesthesia wears off.

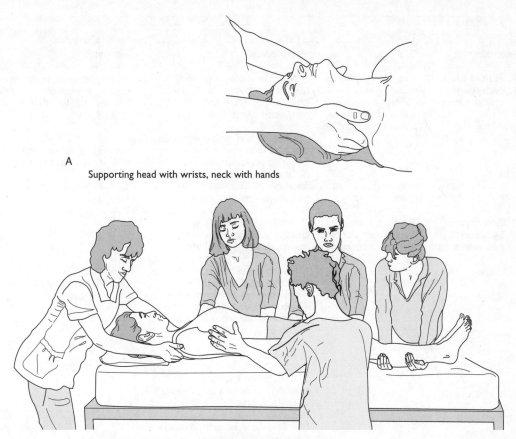

A   Supporting head with wrists, neck with hands

B

Counterpressure to prevent movement of spine. While starting from top, arms are inserted one by one

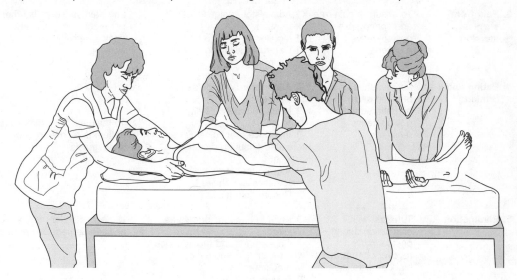

C

Counter pressure applied during withdrawal of arms from beneath patient

Fig. 5.25 (A) Neck support. (B) Counterpressure for insertion of arms. (C) Counterpressure for withdrawal of arms

Nursing Care Plan 5.4   Specific post of care relating to lumbar surgery

Problem	Goal	Intervention	Rationale
1. Patient has undergone spinal surgery	To promote good recovery from general anaesthesia and surgery and to prevent complications	❒ Maintain a patent airway – assess skin colour, respiratory rate, rhythm, effort and administer oxygen therapy as prescribed ❒ Observe and record vital signs and limb function ½–4 hourly for 24 hours postoperatively ❒ Observe and record wound drainage ½–4 hourly for 24 hours postoperatively	Usually takes around 4 hours to excrete anaesthetic drugs O₂ therapy may therefore be given for several hours Diminished power sensation may indicate cord damage compression
2. Bed rest for 24 hours postoperatively	To prevent the complications of bed rest and immobility	❒ Assist patient with regular change of position ensuring maximum support for lumbar wound: • turning via stomach • careful positioning to maintain spinal alignment • avoid overstretching of lumbar area, leg positioned with pillow for maximum comfort ❒ Avoid pressure on wound from lying on back ❒ Ensure (thromboembolic) stockings worn until fully mobile Encourage breathing and limb exercises Use Spenco/sheepskin mattress if available, for comfort	Slight flexion of knees enables back muscles to relax
3. Pain from surgical incision	To ensure a pain-free and comfortable postoperative recovery	❒ Administer analgesia as prescribed ❒ Monitor its effectiveness ❒ Careful positioning to ensure optimum comfort	Leg pain-sensory disturbances may not resolve immediately postoperatively due to inflammation/swelling
4. Eating and drinking	Maintenance of nutrition and hydration during postoperative recovery	❒ Administer IV fluids as prescribed ❒ Maintain safety/sterility of IV cannula ❒ Introduce oral fluids/diet as tolerated ensuring preistalsis present ❒ Administer prescribed antiemetics as required ❒ Record fluid intake	To maintain fluid intake when patient is recovering from anaesthesia
5. Elimination	To assist with elimination during postoperative recovery and prevent bladder distension	❒ Provide bedpans/urinals as required ❒ Observe for and report difficulty with micturition and assist with optimum ❒ Record urine output	Urinary retention may arise due to position/damage to nerve supply
6. Lumbar wound	To promote wound healing and prevent infection	❒ Observe and record lumbar wound soakage ½–4 hourly for 24 hours	

Nursing Care Plan 5.4 (*cont'd*)			
Problem	**Goal**	**Intervention**	**Rationale**
6. (cont'd)		Observe wound drain for patency 1 hourly until drain is removed and record drainage Apply secondary wound dressing if soakage is excessive and inform medical staff if problem persists Clean and redress wound using aseptic technique first day postoperatively Remove sutures 5–7 days postoperatively as directed by medical staff	Excessive serous drainage may indicate CSF leak with resultant risk of postoperative infection

REFERENCES AND FURTHER READING

Allan D 1984 Care of the unconscious patient. The Professional Nurse 2(1): 15–17

Cole K 1988 Is Parkinson's disease preventable? Professional Nurse 4: 1–15

Dawson P 1983 Rehabilitation after cerebrovascular accident. Nursing Times 79(6): 23

Evans R, Lewis J 1989 Motor neurone disease. Nursing 3(33): 9–11

Jenett B 1983 Medical aspect of head injury. Medical International 1(30): 1414–1422

Larson E 1980 Epidemiology of brain tumours. Journal of Neurosurgical Nursing 12: 3,121

Lindsay K W, Bone I, Callender R 1993 Neurology and Neurosurgery Illustrated, 3rd edn. Churchill Livingstone, Edinburgh

Mamdefield H 1993 Making sense of brain stem death. Nursing Times 89(35): 32–34

Matthews B 1985 MS: the facts, 2nd edn. Oxford University Press, Oxford

Newson–Davis J 1987 Myasthenia gravis. Medical International 2(48): 1988–1991

Pritchard A, Mallett J 1992 Royal Marsden Hospital manual of clinical practice. Blackwell, Oxford

Quigley J et al 1989 Neurological investigations. Nursing 13(33): 12–17

Roper N, Logan W, Tierney A 1990 The elements of nursing; a model of nursing based on a model of living, 3rd edn. Churchill Livingstone, Edinburgh

Teasdale G 1975 Acute observation of brain function: 1 Assessing conscious level. Nursing Times 71(24): 914–917

Teasdale G, Galbraith S, Clark K 1975 Acute impairment of brain function: 2 Observation record chart. Nursing Times 71(25): 972–973

Tortora G J, Grabowski S R 1993 Principles of anatomy and physiology, 7th edn. Harper Collins, London

Whitney J L 1987 Assessing your patient for increased intracranial pressure. Nursing 17(6): 34–41

Wilson K J W 1990 Ross & Wilson: anatomy and physiology in health and illness, 7th edn. Churchill Livingstone, Edinburgh

6

Care implications of disorders of the sensory organs

Patricia M. C. Gillies

INTRODUCTION

THE SENSES

The senses are made up of sight, hearing, smell, taste and touch, which enable man to live safely in his environment. Sensory nerve endings located in the eyes, ears, nose, tongue and skin send impulses via the sensory nerve pathway to the cerebral cortex for interpretation. If one or more of the senses deteriorate or fails, other senses may become more acutely developed to compensate. This process is more likely to happen in younger individuals, whereas in the elderly, deterioration in all the senses can occur which leads to an inability to compensate.

Development of the senses commences early in fetal life and is further stimulated through early bonding with the mother which is important for the future emotional and physiological development of the child. Midwifery staff encourage this by lying the baby on the mother's abdomen until the placenta has been delivered and the cord cut, before giving him/her to the mother to cuddle, and put to the breast. At this early stage the baby experiences the gentle touch and smell of his mother, the sound of her voice, as well as seeing her close to and having his sense of taste stimulated by the colostrum from the breast.

Many people maintain a normal life-style despite impairment in one or more senses, with the help of aids such as spectacles or hearing aids. When such a person becomes ill, the nurse must ensure that these aids are properly used to prevent an unnecessary sense of isolation, possible wrong diagnosis, undue morbidity and slow rehabilitation.

Sight

Sight enables a distinction to be made between colours, shades, depth and distance as well as enabling recognition of faces, writing and artwork. If a patient is immobilized or nursed in isolation the nurse should ensure that the patient gets sufficient visual stimulation. A fish tank can provide entertainment as well as having a calming effect on anxious patients. The patient's chair or bed can be moved to enable the patient to look out of the window or have a change of view.

Most patients appreciate their cards being on display, to remind them of caring family and friends. If the patient is to be in hospital for a length of time, personal effects and photographs may be beneficial. For most activities the nurse should ensure there is adequate lighting without glare; however in some disorders, such as meningitis, the patient can be sensitive to light, therefore the room should be darkened by closing the blinds or curtains. To help patients maintain normal body rhythms and sleep patterns, light should be dimmed at night time and the patient disturbed as little as possible. If a patient's sight deteriorates or fails the nurse must be aware of what aids and compensations to use.

Hearing

The ability to hear allows communication with others, and enhances the safety of the environment. As different tones can convey different meanings, the ability to hear is linked with the interpretation of the sounds which take place in the brain. Sound is measured in decibels (dB), normal speech registers at 50 dB, whispering at 20 dB and alarm equipment at 80 dB (Biley 1993).

Certain noises in the environment with which a person is familiar can be blocked out; for example someone living next door to a school might never hear the school bell when it rings, but would be immediately alert to a house alarm. In a strange environment a person is more conscious of the separate features of this 'background noise'. Hospitals too have their own noises, caused by trolleys, infusion pumps, telephones, doors banging, commodes, hot water pipes, fluorescent lights and fans, as well as the hum and talk from staff, patients and visitors. Nurses should take time to explain to the patient what causes the different noises. This is particularly beneficial when the patient is unable to see or move.

As an ill patient's tolerance for sound is often lower than that of a fit person, it is important, especially at night, for nurses to keep the noise level to a minimum, to ensure the patient has sufficient rest and sleep. Noise has been blamed for increasing the patient's perception of pain, delaying wound healing and therefore increasing the patient's stay in hospital.

As hearing is the last sense to go, and the first to return when a patient loses and regains consciousness, nurses and others must be careful what they say in front of patients who appear unconscious.

Smell

The loss of smell (anosmia) makes the environment less safe. Imagine not being able to smell burning, leaking gases or smoke. It has other implications too: smells recall pleasant times, and this can be used in therapy to promote relaxation and relieve psychological distress.

The sense of taste is closely linked to smell, the absence of which is particularly noticed when nasal passages are blocked, for example, when suffering from the common cold (coryza).

Unpleasant smells can cause patients to feel nauseous and they may be less likely to eat. The judicious use of deodorants, air conditioners and charcoal-impregnated dressings can help to eliminate or control unpleasant smells.

Smells can have a different effect on different people; one person may like a certain perfume, whereas another person may find it unpleasant. Nurses should therefore refrain from using strong perfumes or aftershaves which may upset a patient who already feels nauseated. The smell of stale cigarette smoke and the aftermath of last night's meal which contained garlic may also upset patients.

Taste

If a person loses his sense of taste he may eat tainted food. Care must therefore be taken to check the expiry date of food and ensure that all food is stored at the correct temperature and in an appropriate container.

The loss of taste or alteration of taste caused by chemotherapeutic drugs may lead to the patient eating less (anorexia). Poor oral hygiene will also affect the sense of taste and nurses have an important role to play in ensuring that the patient's oral hygiene is not neglected.

Touch

Touch is very important to people, especially when they are feeling vulnerable or ill – young children may say 'kiss it better' when they injure themselves. Older people also appreciate their hand being held during an uncomfortable procedure or a stressful time. If the patient is very upset, a hug can convey more empathy than a thousand words, although care must be taken as some people feel uncomfortable being touched by strangers. As many of the procedures carried out on patients involve intimate contact with sensitive areas, nurses must be as understanding as possible to prevent the patient becoming embarrassed.

Patients in hospital are at risk of sensory imbalance due to either sensory deprivation or sensory overload.

SENSORY DEPRIVATION

Sensory deprivation occurs when there is a partial or complete loss of the sensory stimuli of sight, sound, smell, taste and touch. Patients likely to experience sensory deprivation are those nursed in isolation, in intensive care units, (Barry–Shevlin 1987) those in the terminal stages of their illness and those who have suffered a cerebrovascular accident (Baggerley 1991).

The latter condition causes a lack of mobility which reduces the stimuli the brain receives from the muscles and joints thus resulting in a loss of proprioception.

Sensory deprivation causes a shorter attention span leading to a difficulty in absorbing information regardless of how simple it may be. Other symptoms are restlessness, anxiety, sleep disturbances and the possibility of disorientation to time, place and persons (Moore 1989).

The nurse can minimize the risk of sensory deprivation or overload by providing a calm, quiet atmosphere together with well-planned nursing care, allowing time for adequate rest and sleep.

THE EYE

ANATOMY AND PHYSIOLOGY

The eye is the organ of sight. Light rays pass through the lens onto the retina and are then converted into nerve pulses which are transmitted by the optic nerve to be interpreted by the brain.

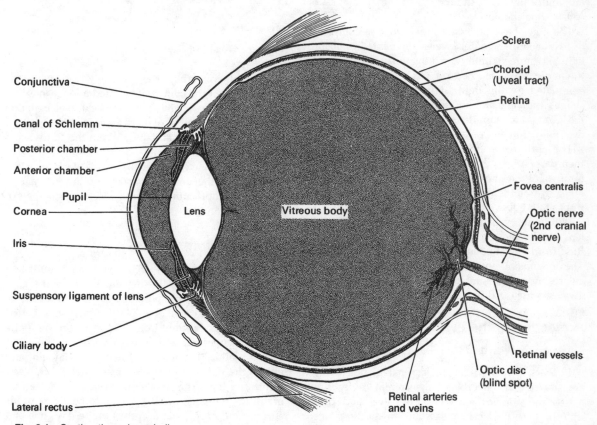

Fig. 6.1 Section through eyeball

Each eyeball is suspended by six muscles in the cranial orbit cushioned on a layer of adipose tissue (Fig. 6.1).

Layers of the eye

The outermost layer is made up of the sclera and cornea. The sclera, forming five-sixths of the surface of the eye, is an opaque white coat composed of connective tissue and collagen fibres. These fibres maintain the shape of the eye and give attachment to the external muscles of the eye.

The cornea, which is transparent with no blood vessels, is positioned in front of the iris, and allows light to pass to the retina. Due to the cornea's greater curvature it protrudes from the sclera.

The middle choroid layer (uveal tract) is composed of the vascular pigmented choroid which prevents reflection of light rays. It is continuous with the ciliary body which manufactures aqueous fluid, and the iris which gives the eye its colour. The iris has an aperture in its centre called the pupil. Control of the muscular iris is by the 3rd cranial nerve which regulates the amount of light entering the eye by either dilating or constricting the pupil.

The inner layer of the eye, the retina, is composed of two layers. The outer layer is pigmented to absorb light and store vitamin A, and the inner layer contains the nerve receptors, the rods and cones. The rods are stimulated in dim light, allowing for perception of shapes, movement and peripheral vision, whereas the cones are stimulated by light for fine visual discrimination and colour perception.

The optic nerve fibre originates in the retina and then passes through the choroid, sclera and the optic foramen of the sphenoid bone to meet the nerve of the other eye at the optic chiasma which is situated in front of and above the pituitary gland (Fig. 6.2).

Within the eyeball, the biconvex transparent flexible lens divides the anterior chamber containing aqueous fluid from the vitreous body in the posterior chamber. The aqueous humour secreted by the ciliary body circulates around the anterior chamber before draining away via the canal of Schlemm.

Protection of the eye

The eye is protected in the following ways:

1. Tears, produced in the lacrimal glands, which are situated in the orbit of the cranial cavity, flow across the anterior surface of the eye, and drain into the nose via lacrimal sacs and ducts. Tears, also known as lacrimal secretions, contain mucus, anti-

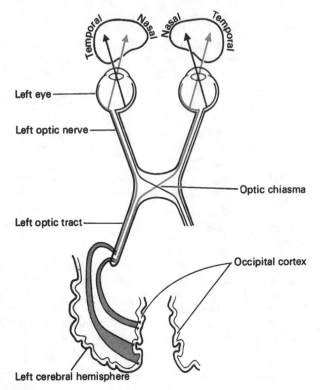

Fig. 6.2 Visual pathways and fields

bodies and an antibacterial enzyme which ensure the eyeball is kept moistened, lubricated and clean.

2. Eyelids protect the eyes from external irritation and can prevent 99% of light entering the eye (but will not prevent retinal damage from the sun when a person lies facing the sun).

3. The conjunctiva lines the inside surface of the eyelids and the anterior surface of the sclera and produces a lubricating mucus which protects the eye from drying out.

Normal vision

Normally the eyes can focus on near and distant objects (Fig. 6.3) by adjusting the shape of the lens. This normal refractive power is termed emmetropia. To be able to see detail of an object clearly, an inverted image must be brought into exact focus on the centre of the macula lutea at the fovea centralis. The cones in and around this area are sensitive to daylight and enable the person to see colour and detail of objects (central vision). The rods situated nearer the periphery of the retina enable the person to be aware of his surroundings (peripheral vision) in the day time and to permit some night time vision.

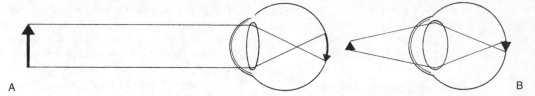

A   B

Fig. 6.3   (A) Normal eye focusing a distant object (over 20 feet away). (B) Normal eye focusing a near object (note alteration in shape of lens)

The pigments in the rods and cones of the retina convert the radiant energy of the light ray into nerve impulses which are transmitted via the optic pathways (Fig. 6.2) to the visual area of the occipital cortex for interpretation as sight. The changes which take place due to the ageing process are described in Table 6.1.

DISORDERS AFFECTING NORMAL VISION

Myopia (short sightedness)

In myopia the length of the eyeball is greater than normal, therefore light rays are brought to a focus at a point which falls short of the retina. The person

Table 6.1	Effects of the ageing process in the eye		
Physiological changes	Effect	Implications	Nursing management
Lens becomes less elastic and more rigid	Decrease in focusing ability of the eye	Inability to focus on nearby objects (presbyopia)	Encourage the over 40s to have their eyes tested yearly, reading glasses may be required, ensure good light for reading and/or close work
Lens discolours or yellows	Amount of light reaching retina is decreased	Affects colour vision	Use metal or clear spoons when giving tablets (white tablets would merge with a white spoon)
Breakdown of normal lens protein and an input of water into the lens	Increase in cloudiness of the lens (cataract)	Increasing age increases the risk of lens opacities, leading to impaired vision	Monitor deterioration in vision, spectacles may be of use in the early stages, but surgery may become necessary Provide a safe environment whilst encouraging independence
Dilator muscles of the iris become less efficient	Restricts size of the pupil	Amount of light reaching retina is decreased, eyes take longer to adjust to changes in light	Ensure adequate lighting Maintain a safe environment, ensuring there is nothing that the patient can trip over
Iris becomes more rigid and the pupil becomes smaller	Restricts visual field	Peripheral vision is decreased, may affect driving	Encourage older people to move their heads to widen their visual field, especially when driving
Decreased absorption of aqueous humour	Raised intraoccular pressure	Increase risk of glaucoma leading to poor eye sight and risk of accidents	Encourage the over 65s to have regular eye checks, especially for eye pressure (6 month–yearly) Ensure patients take their eye drops as prescribed
Decrease in lacrimal secretions	Eyes feel dry and irritable	Eyes may need to be bathed frequently (several times a day)	Bathe eyes with normal saline or use artificial tears, as prescribed

Note: as many as 75% of over 75 year olds have visual problems.

can compensate by holding objects closer to the eyes, but objects at a distance appear blurred. Correction is achieved by wearing spectacles with concave lenses which aid focusing on the retina (Fig. 6.4).

Hypermetropia (long sightedness)

In hypermetropia the length of the eyeball is shorter than normal, therefore light rays are brought to a focus at a point beyond the retina. Objects are seen clearly at a distance but appear blurred close to the eyes. Correction is by wearing spectacles with convex lenses which bring the image forward to the retina (Fig. 6.5).

Astigmatism (uneven curvature of the cornea)

The person with astigmatism is unable to focus horizontal and vertical rays of light on the retina. Correction is achieved by wearing cylindrical lenses.

Strabismus (squint)

Although in strabismus the eye may deviate in any direction, there are two types of squint – concomitant and paralytic.

Concomitant squints are found in young children. By 6 months, a baby's eyes should be parallel when viewing objects at a distance and curving towards the nose when viewing objects close at hand. To prevent double vision the child's brain suppresses the image formed by the uncontrolled or 'wandering' eye, which begins to lose its acuity as a result.

The paralytic squint can be found in any age but is more common in adults. It may be caused by trauma, tumour, aneurysm, endocrine or neurological problems. The person will usually complain of some degree of diplopia (double vision). It may be the first symptom of the underlying pathology, and should be taken seriously.

Therapeutic management

Treatment must be carried out as soon as the diagnosis of squint has been made as the normal and deviant eye alternate on focusing on objects, or the normal eye only is used with the visual cortex ignoring impulses from the deviant eye. The following treatments may be used singly or in combination to treat the squint: spectacles to correct refractive errors, occlusion of the 'good' eye to improve vision of the 'squinting' eye, orthoptic treatment to restore or develop binocular function by special exercises for the eye muscles, or surgery.

INFLAMMATORY CONDITIONS

Inflammatory or infective conditions of the eye, if not treated promptly, may cause permanent damage and subsequent impairment of vision.

Conjunctivitis

Inflammation of the conjunctiva may be caused by viruses such as herpes simplex, herpes zoster and measles; by bacteria such as staphylococci, streptococci, gonococci and pneumococci; from chemicals; or

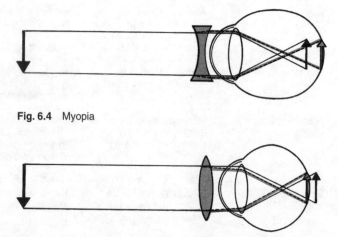

Fig. 6.4 Myopia

Fig. 6.5 Hypermetropia

as an allergic reaction to certain proteins such as pollen or make-up.

Clinical features

The patient will complain of a 'gritty' irritable eye or eyes which appear red and watery. Normally visual acuity is not affected. In gonococcal or pneumococcal infections there is a discharge which may be abundant and purulent.

Therapeutic management

A swab should be taken for bacteriology before commencing treatment. The eyes may be bathed with normal saline before treating with the prescribed antibiotic for bacterial infections, or a steroidal ointment for allergic reactions. Each eye is treated separately to prevent the spread of infection.

Patient implications

Advice needs to be given to patients many of whom will be self caring. See Box 6.1.

Box 6.1   Advice to patients with eye infections

- hand washing before and after treatment
- avoid touching the eyes unnecessarily
- sole use of towel
- care in washing and drying face, not to spread infection from one eye to the other
- instil drops or apply ointment correctly by placing substance as prescribed
- avoiding skin contamination
- use separate bottles or tubes as prescribed for right and left eyes
- importance of completing treatment
- avoid using eye patches or plastic shades unless prescribed
- use dark glasses or dim light if photophobia present
- if allergic reaction, avoid known allergens.

Keratitis

Inflammation of the cornea, usually as a result of a foreign body or superficial injury which has become infected, causes corneal ulceration and scarring. Keratitis may be prevented by prompt removal of foreign bodies and early treatment of injuries and/or infections of the eye. Keratitis may also be prevented in patients who have lost their blink reflex (i.e. unconscious patients) by taping the eyelids shut, thus preventing exposure of the cornea for lengthy periods. If this care is not taken, the patient may develop blindness.

Clinical features

There will be a decrease in visual acuity due to opacity of the cornea. The eye(s) will appear red, with excessive lacrimation and discharge. The patient will complain of pain, irritation and photophobia. If ulcers develop and/or the cornea is perforated, the aqueous humour can escape leading to the collapse of the anterior chamber and intraocular bleeding.

Therapeutic management

The instillation of fluorescein is used to outline ulcerated areas. Prompt treatment is required to prevent visual damage, due to either leakage of aqueous humour, or infection spreading, damaging internal ocular structures.

Treatment involves prescription and administration of topical antiviral drugs for viral infections, topical antibiotics and systemic antibiotics for bacterial infections and mydriatics may be instilled topically to dilate the pupil and prevent iritis.

Pain may be relieved by the use of topical anaesthetics, oral analgesia or hot spoon bathing. Rest is usually required to prevent further damage.

Uveitis

Inflammation of the uveal tract is termed uveitis; when only the iris is involved it is termed iritis; when the iris and ciliary body are involved, it is called iridocyclytis, and when the choroid is affected it is termed choroiditis.

It is caused by trauma, local infections, systemic infections such as gonorrhoea, systemic conditions such as rheumatoid arthritis, ankylosing spondylitis and sarcoidosis, or in many cases the cause is unknown (idiopathic).

It may be acute and clear away quickly, or become chronic with fibrotic replacement of specialized tissue, and adhesions between the iris and the lens. The latter results in disturbed vision or blockage to the flow of aqueous humour, causing a secondary glaucoma or secondary cataract due to impairment of lens nutrition.

Clinical features

The pupil will be small, and if the iritis has been present for several days, it will appear irregular because of adhesions to the underlying lens. There will also be redness at the margin of the cornea. The patient will complain of pain, photophobia and visual impairment.

Therapeutic management

Diagnosis must be confirmed before treatment can be commenced. This will involve the instillation of mydriatic drops which paralyse the ciliary muscle and iris sphincter, giving relief from pain due to spasm, as well as dilating the pupil, and preventing adhesions between the iris and the lens.

Corticosteriods may be prescribed topically to inhibit the inflammatory response, as well as systemically for more serious cases. An eye pad may be used to relieve the photophobia and give comfort to the eye. Topical antibiotics may also be prescribed, as may systemic analgesia for the pain.

TRAUMA

Accidents involving the eye should always be treated promptly and expert help sought.

Foreign bodies

Epidemiology and aetiology

Particles may enter the conjunctival sac and give rise to irritation.

Therapeutic management

If a particle becomes impacted in the conjunctiva of the upper lid, the upper lid should be everted and the foreign body carefully lifted off with a saline-soaked cotton bud. If the foreign body is loose it can be irrigated out.

When a particle lodges in the cornea it will normally be seen, if it lodges in the sclera, it might not be. After a full history and testing the eyes for visual acuity, the doctor will remove the foreign body under a local anaesthetic. After the particle has been removed, flourescein is instilled to ascertain the amount of corneal abrasion caused. An antibiotic and mydriatic might be instilled before the eye is covered with a pad. The patient's eye should be checked by the doctor the following day after the initial inflammation has settled to ensure all particles have been removed.

Perforation

Epidemiology and aetiology

Any sharp instrument or object may perforate the cornea or sclera and damage the structures within the eye.

Therapeutic management

At the scene of the accident the wound may be covered by a sterile dressing, then the patient should be transferred immediately to hospital, keeping the head still. Emergency surgery is required.

Normal preoperative care will be performed (see Ch. 4). The surgery required will depend on the severity of the injury. It may involve cleaning and suturing the injury. However, in some cases removal of the eye (enucleation) is required.

Direct violence

Epidemiology and aetiology

A severe blow, for example by a squash ball, may damage the internal eye. Rupture of small blood vessels of the iris results in blood collecting in the anterior chamber (hyphaema). Complete bed rest is required to allow the blood to be absorbed. Failure to absorb the blood could result in secondary glaucoma. Cataract (see p. 210), retinal detachment and vitreous haemorrhage may also result after this kind of injury.

Patient implications

Following eye trauma there is a tendency for individuals not to seek medical advice. Though a periorbital haematoma (black eye) will usually resolve in about a fortnight, normally leaving no damage to the eye, the patient should still have his eye examined by a doctor.

Burns

Epidemiology and aetiology

Burns may be caused by heat or cold (thermal), ionizing radiation or chemicals. Thermal burns (heat) can also damage other parts of the body, but a firework for example may cause damage mainly to the eyelids which must be considered when carrying out first aid.

Therapeutic management

All patients sustaining burns to the eye should be sent to hospital.

First aid for chemical burns entails copious washouts of the affected eye, allowing the washed-out fluid to drain away from the unaffected eye without causing further damage to the patient and the first aider. Notes should be made of the chemical which has caused the trauma, since this is important in the treatment.

In hospital, the eye(s) will have anaesthetic drops instilled (to relieve pain and reduce spasm of lids) before being irrigated with normal saline or a buffer solution (whichever is most appropriate for the type of chemical involved). Topical antibiotics and systemic analgesia may be required and a pad or eyeshield applied.

A full ophthalmic assessment will be carried out following emergency treatment. This may be required for legal purposes, particularly if the accident occurred at work. Further surgery may be required at a later date to deal with cataract or scarring.

Detachment of the retina

Retinal detachment occurs when the innermost layer of the retina containing the rods and cones becomes separated from the vascular pigment epithelial layer. A breech in the retina allows fluid to accumulate beneath it, causing further separation.

Epidemiology and aetiology

Detachment occurs most frequently in individuals with myopic eyes as the myopic retina becomes especially thin and is liable to develop breaks; it is also common after cataract extraction. It may be secondary to trauma, inflammation or less commonly in the presence of a malignant growth in the choroid. Retinal detachment may appear at any age.

Clinical features

The patient complains of seeing flashing lights as the retina tears, and then a feeling as if a curtain has been pulled across the vision. There is no pain. Serious loss of vision will result if the retina is not returned to and secured in the normal position.

Therapeutic management

Occasionally a patient may be admitted for a period of complete bed rest, with the head positioned to allow the retina to fall back into place, and the sub-retinal fluid to be absorbed. However, normally surgery will be required. If there is a hole or tear with no subretinal fluid present, then light coagulation, laser or cryotherapy may be used to seal the edges of the hole.

COMMON DISORDERS OF THE EYE
Open angle glaucoma

Glaucoma is defined as a rise in intraocular pressure

within the eye. The two main types of glaucoma are closed angle (acute) and open angle (chronic). If left untreated, glaucoma will reduce the blood supply to the optic nerve with the resulting progressive loss of vision.

Epidemiology and aetiology

In open angle glaucoma the onset is symptomless and insidious with the retinal receptors being damaged by the raised pressure and the optic nerve fibres gradually dying. This disorder is often only diagnosed during a routine eye examination.

Patient implications

Open angle glaucoma is most likely to affect those over 50 years. Everyone over this age should have their eyes tested at least every year, or more frequently if there is a history of glaucoma in the family.

Clinical features

The patient may complain of loss of peripheral vision. The intraocular pressure is measured and is usually raised to 30 mmHg or more (normal 20 mmHg). The optic disc is observed for evidence of atrophy or the death of nerve fibres. If the disc is cupped, glaucoma is present.

Therapeutic management

The aim of treatment is to reduce the rising pressure. This is achieved by the administration of pilocarpic eyedrops to constrict the pupil or oral tablets of Diamox, a weak diuretic which has a specific effect on aqueous humour, and surgery or laser treatment for the drainage of aqueous humour to the subconjunctival space.

Closed angle glaucoma

Closed angle glaucoma is an ophthalmic emergency which occurs twice as frequently in females, in the middle to older age groups. The tension must be reduced within hours or the patient could become blind. Therefore all patients with closed angled glaucoma are admitted to hospital as an emergency.

Clinical features

There is a severe pain in the affected eye, associated with redness and blurring of vision. The cornea appears steamy and the pupil is oval, fixed and mid-dilated. Patients may also experience nausea and vomiting.

Therapeutic management

Acetazolamide and/or mannitol are injected intra-venously to diminish the amount of vitreous fluid and decrease the intraocular pressure. Pilocarpine eyedrops can be given 30 minutes after this to con-strict the pupil. Pilocarpine may also be administered prophylactically to the unaffected eye.

Following the initial emergency treatment surgery will be carried out in both eyes. A drainage operation is performed on the affected eye to allow aqueous humour to flow through a permanent fistula to the subconjunctival space.

Later a peripheral iridectomy is performed on the second eye as a prophylactic measure. Laser treat-ment is an alternative to surgery.

Cataract

A cataract is any opacity of the lens.

Epidemiology and aetiology

It may be caused by one of a number of factors:

- Maternal rubella during pregnancy may cause congenital cataracts, although these are now less common as a result of rubella vaccination.
- A penetrating injury which causes rupture of the lense capsule.
- Some endocrine conditions in young to middle age.
- Exposure to radiation.
- Senile cataracts due to degenerative changes of old age are the most common.

Clinical features

Mistiness of vision, with difficulty in reading close work. There is usually a decrease in colour perception.

Therapeutic management

When the patient can no longer see sufficiently well with either eye to continue normal activities, surgical extraction of the lens is carried out. Replacement of the lost focusing power is achieved by a suitable spectacle, contact lens or interocular lens.

INVESTIGATIONS OF EYE DISORDERS

When a patient presents with a damaged or diseased eye, a careful ophthalmic examination and history must be undertaken. The patient's past medical history, age and life-style will also be considered before a diagnosis is made.

The following investigations may be carried out:

- Visual acuity, near vision and distance vision are tested.
- Snellen's chart or E test for non-English speaking or illiterate adults. A graded picture chart is suitable for young children (Fig. 6.6). The patient stands 6 m from the chart and is asked to read as far from the chart as he can. Visual acuity is meas-ured according to the number of lines of letters he can read accurately, this is then expressed as a frac-tion (normal vision = 6/6; ability to see top letters only = 6/60). The patient may be moved closer to the chart = 3/60, or if he is unable to see at that range, the examiner will hold up fingers to be counted, failing this, his perception to light will be ascertained. The person is regarded as totally blind if he is unable to perceive light.
- Opthalmoscopy involves observing the interior of the eye using an opthalmoscope.
- In slit lamp examination the structure of the eye is magnified by a beam of light to facilitate examination.
- A tonometer is used to measure intracoccular pressure. The flow of aqueous humour into and out of the anterior chamber maintains the pressure at 15–20 mmHg in a normal eye.
- A visual field test determines the loss of vision in certain eye conditions.
- Staining the eye involves using a dye such as flourescein sodium in either liquid or strip form (moistened with normal saline). The cornea will stain a bright luminous green if there are corneal abrasions present. Patients should be warned that nasal secretions may be coloured due to the dye (draining down lacrimal ducts to nose).
- Bacterial investigation of lacrimal secretions in-volves a specimen being taken from the conjuncti-val sac preoperatively, to verify the presence and sensitivity of micro-organisms.

For further details see Chawla (1993), and Perry & Tullo (1990).

THE ROLE OF THE NURSE IN THE INVESTIGATION

The nurse should ensure that the patient receives a

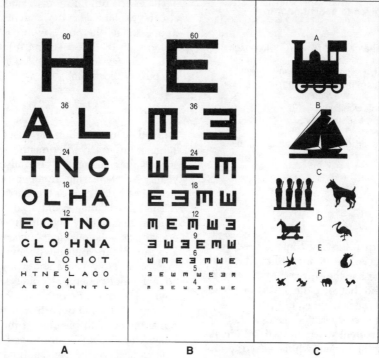

Fig. 6.6 (A) Test type – Snellen. (B) Test type – 'E' test. (C) Test type – recognition of objects

clear and concise explanation of what to expect to occur before, during and after examination. It is imperative that this is given at the patient's level of understanding. The nurse assists the medical staff by ensuring that equipment is in working order and that lighting is appropriate. During and after the examination, the nurse must ensure that the patient is as relaxed as possible, comfortable and that his/her safety is maintained. Any drugs which are given are documented. All investigations performed are noted in the appropriate documentation.

Nursing implications

In addition, the nurse should ensure that where medication is prescribed the following points are adhered to. Medications for different eyes are clearly labelled left eye, right eye. Care should be taken to prevent damage occurring to the cornea by ensuring that forceps or inappropriate dressings are not used. Gloves should not be worn because of the powder in sterile latex gloves and poor tactile feedback.

Before and after surgery the usual pre- and postoperative checks are carried out, as well as the following specific ophthalmic checks:

- Patients are nursed normally on their unaffected side but following an enucleation, they will lie on their affected side.
- Noise is kept to a minimum and the patient is approached from their unaffected side.
- If a pad or shield has been applied the nurse must observe its affect on the patient's unaffected eye. Any problems are promptly reported to the nurse in charge.

Before discharge, the nurse needs to advise patients on the various points given in Box 6.1.

Aids and appliances

The nurse should ensure all patient's spectacles are kept clean and free from scratches. Contact lens must be maintained in optimum condition. The nurse should be able to insert and remove contact lens, ensure storage methods are sterile as well as using appropriate cleaning procedures (Perry and Tullo 1990).

If the patient has had an enucleation, the nurse must ensure that the patient is comfortable handling and wearing his/her artificial eye. The patient will require the nurse's help to begin with when inserting, removing and cleaning the prosthesis.

Box 6.2 Advice given to patient prior to discharge

- Report pain, discharge or other worries to hospital or GP as soon as possible
- Avoid lifting heavy weights or bending forward (check with the surgeon for how long)
- Avoid straining at bowel evacuation
- Take care with hair washing
- Hand-washing and aseptic technique for drops, etc.
- Check who will insert drops – train as appropriate

Therapeutic management

Medications

Most drugs used to treat the eyes come in the form of ointments or drops. Before giving either, the nurse must ensure that she has the correct prescription for the correct patient and that the patient has not already received medication for that date and time.

Since the patient's co-operation is essential, the nurse must tell the patient when she will administer the drop(s). Usually the patient will be asked to look up, allowing the nurse to slightly evert the lower lid to instill the drops in the lower fornix between the middle and outer third (Fig. 6.7).

To apply ointment to the eye, the patient again looks upward and the lower lid is slightly everted, allowing the ointment to be squeezed into the lower fornix from the inner to the outer aspect. The patient is asked to gently close his eye and excess ointment can be removed from the lashes (inner to outer direction). The patient should be informed that ointments may cause blurring of vision for a short time.

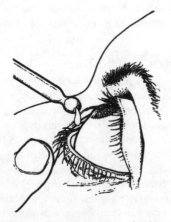

Fig. 6.7 Instillation of drops into lower fornix

The effects of topical medications to the eye should also be explained to the patients. For example, mydriatics dilate the pupil, with consequent blurring of vision with the effect lasting from 14 days (atropine) to 6 hours (cyclopentolate), whereas miotics constrict the pupil (pilocarpine).

Surgery

With the introduction of laser treatment, microsurgery, improved equipment and drugs, ophthalmic surgery has changed drastically over the past few years. An increasing number of patients are now treated as a day case or their hospital stay is short.

This has advantages and disadvantages. The shorter time available may inhibit the development of an empathetic relationship between nurse and patient and thus failure to deal with any anxieties the patient may have. However, a shorter hospital stay has the advantage of patients sleeping in their own bed and having less time off work.

Many wards and departments now use the 'named' nurse policy with pictures of the staff on prominent view. The visually handicapped person may be unable to observe the photographs, so the information will have to be given to them in a different way, for example with the use of auditory tapes. On admission to the ward, the nurse should escort the patient round the ward, with the patient holding the nurses's arm and the nurse leading. This allows the patient to become orientated to the new environment and helps the nurse assess the patient's ability and confidence. To improve his/her mental image of the ward the patient should be allowed to make use of tactile stimulation. The patient should be introduced to fellow patients and other members of the ward team to prevent any feelings of isolation. It is essential to find out as quickly as possible what the patient prefers to be called, as using his/her name enables the patient to know he is being addressed.

No matter which model of care is used, careful assessment of the patient is necessary. Orem's Self-care Model enables the nurse, in a systematic way, to help the patient with his self-care deficits. (Aggleton and Chalmers 1985). On admission, the deficits may be slight, but immediately postoperatively everything will need to be done for the patient. This model also encourages the nurse and patient to plan the care together, setting realistic goals, with behaviour stated to be reliably evaluated. The nurse's role will be to care, guide, support (physically and psychologically) and teach the patient (and family members if appropriate) within an environment which promotes growth and development. This allows rehabilitation to be ongoing from admission, through stay, to discharge to the community. During rehabilitation the nurse will ensure that the patient (and family) has sufficient knowledge and ability to cope in the community.

Communication

It is believed that at least 80% of our perception of our environment is through sight. To compensate for this loss in a visually handicapped person, the other senses must be developed and utilized.

The nurse should approach the blind person in a calm manner and, if there is sight in one eye, the approach should be on the side of vision, calling the person's name to gain his attention. During conversation, the nurse should identify herself, listen to the patient's point of view and, most importantly, tell the person when she is leaving the room. Remember, the tone of voice used can convey different meanings, so take care to prevent misinterpretation. As with any patient nurses are encouraged to explain to the patient what they are going to do and why. This is particularly essential with the blind person in order to maintain their interest and co-operation. Noises on the ward should be explained to the patient, and if possible all extraneous noises should be kept to a minimum.

The sense of touch is important for the blind person. Some patients may ask to feel the nurse's face to get a mental picture. Touch becomes even more important if the patient has both visual and auditory defects.

The sense of smell may be heightened and it has been suggested that this could be utilized by using different smelling pot-pourris in different rooms or areas of the ward to distinguish which room the patient is in.

Patient education

The nurse must ensure that the patient (or someone else at home) has the knowledge and ability to administer prescribed medication correctly. Tablets or drops may be dispensed in individual doses to help the patient. Advice should be given regarding wounds or dressings and the district nurse and/or the social worker should be informed of the patient's discharge to enable them to support the patient in the community. Follow-up appointments with travel arrangements should be confirmed with the patient.

To obtain many benefits, the visually handicapped must be registered as blind with the appropriate form (BP1 in Scotland, BD8 in England) being completed by the ophthalmologist. To qualify 'a person should be so blind as to be unable to perform any work for which the eye sight is essential'. Sometimes the nurse will have to encourage the patient to register, as the patient may feel that his handicap is not too severe, or there is a stigma attached (more details on stigma can be found in Ch. 8).

Responsibility for visually handicapped people is shared among the Health, Education and Social Work Departments in Great Britain.

THE EAR

ANATOMY AND PHYSIOLOGY

The outer ear stretches from the auricle (pinna), along the external auditory canal (lined with a few hairs and ceruminous glands producing wax), to the tympanic membrane (eardrum). The middle ear is an air-filled cavity of the temporal bone extending to the oval window. The air is carried by the auditory tube (eustachian tube) from the nasopharynx to the middle ear. This equalizes the air pressure on both sides of the tympanic membrane. The auditory tube is usually closed, except when yawning or swallowing. The inner ear is made up of a bony outer shell, composed of a cochlea, vestibule and semicircular canals, separated from the membranous lining by perilymph, while the fluid within the membranous cavity is filled with endolymph. (See Fig. 6.8).

The semicircular canals are arranged in three planes and are filled with endolymph with specialized nerve endings projecting into the fluid. Movement of the head causes the endolymph to move in the semicircular canals and this stimulates the nerve endings to send impulses to the brain providing information about the position of the head and body.

Hearing occurs as follows. Sound waves collected by the auricle are passed along the external auditory canal to vibrate the tympanic membrane (slowly at low frequency, quickly at high) before being carried and amplified by the ossicles within the middle ear to the oval window. Because the area of the tympanic membrane is about 20 times greater than that of the oval window, the increased force overcomes the resistance of the cochlea fluid and sends it into waves. These waves stimulate the receptor cells of the organ of Corti before they reach the round window. It is at the organ of Corti that the mechanical aspect of sound is translated to a nerve impulse. This is transmitted via the cochlea nerve to the brain for interpretation.

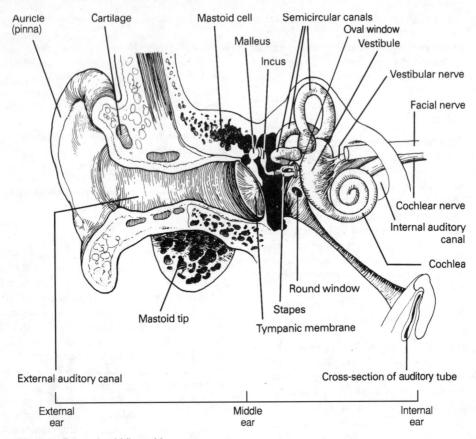

Fig. 6.8 External, middle and inner ear

EPIDEMIOLOGY AND AETIOLOGY

Homeostatic changes in the ear or associated structures may result in hearing loss and/or disturbance in balance. These will affect a person's ability to cope with everyday activities. Disorders of the ear may be divided into:

1. Trauma such as:
   a. foreign objects stuck in the outer ear
   b. head injuries
   c. intense noises, affecting mainly the inner ear.
2. Infections such as:
   a. bacterial, viral or fungal, affecting the outer ear
   b. acute or chronic otitis media affecting predominantly the middle ear arising from respiratory infections, transmitted by the auditory tube.
3. Diseases such as:
   Ménière's disease (overdistension of membranous labyrinths).

As with vision, the ageing process has adverse effects on hearing (Table 6.2).

PATIENT IMPLICATIONS

Young children experiencing deafness may have difficulty with their speech. They may require special help to develop their verbal communication skills. They may also be taught lip reading or sign language. Since communication relies greatly on the spoken word and hearing, the child's social and emotional development may be stunted, and the educational abilities may be affected. It is therefore important when working with the deaf, particularly the young, to use a holistic approach and not just treat the deafness.

Patients who are both blind and deaf require more specialist help. A speaker touching the hand of the 'listener' in various positions is an example of one method used.

Patients with conductive deafness particularly may benefit from a hearing aid, which should be supplied by the NHS. It is important to stress to the patient that hearing aids only amplify the sound. Background noises, such as coughing or laughing, often interfere with the reception of sounds the deaf person is interested in, namely speech. To help the deaf person hear

Table 6.2   Effects of the ageing process on the ears

Physiological changes	Effect	Implications	Nursing management
Atrophy of auditory nerve		Variable degree of deafness	Early recognition and referral to ENT department Hearing aids may be tried, but usually with no great effect
		Patient becomes more isolated	Encourage interaction with others
Deterioration and atrophy of organ of Corti	Nerve impulses following high-pitched sounds are not transmitted to the brain for interpretation	Ability to hear high pitched sound is the first to go, then loss of middle and lower frequencies (presbycusis) (note patient often shouts)	Speak clearly but do not shout Avoid distracting background noises Talk into least impaired ear Ensure facial expression and gestures are sending the right signals
Atrophy or sclerosis of tympanic membrane	Sound waves not passed into middle ear	Deafness	As above
Fusion of ossicles	All frequencies affected	Profound deafness Patient talks quietly	As above
Increase risk of wax build up in external ear	Becomes harder with greater risk of impaction	Patient has difficulty hearing	Warmed almond oil should be inserted the day before the ears are syringed or wax removed
Degeneration of vestibular function due to decreased blood supply and neuronal death	Altered perception of body position causing swaying and/or dizziness	At risk of falling	Ensure patient can use walking aids such as Zimmers Baths, showers, toilet, etc. should have hand rails

best, the space between the talker and the listener should be between 5 and 7 feet (1.50–2.2 m). In the elderly, sounds may become muffled, especially with the consonants; hearing aids will only amplify these distorted sounds, making the use of the hearing aids counter productive.

Aids such as lights attached to doorbells, alarm clocks and timers help to compensate for sounds. Other adaptions on telephones and televisions and individual communicators compensate but do not replace the ability to hear. Many cinemas and theatres and churches have communication links to aid the deaf. Some cinema films and many television programmes now have subtitles which also help the deaf.

NURSING ROLE IN DIFFERENTIAL DIAGNOSIS

Although parents might notice their baby is not responding to noises, it is often the health visitor checking the baby's development who first notices the problem. Between 6 and 8 months a routine hearing test is called out when babies should respond to familiar quiet sounds like voices by turning towards the sound. Each ear is tested, with the nurse being about 1 m just out of vision of the baby. Other factors such as mental retardation or physical disability need to be considered before a diagnosis of deafness is made. At 2 years of age, the test involves asking the child to follow simple commands within the limits of their stage of development. Children also have audiometry tests carried out several times during their school years.

In ear, nose and throat outpatient departments, nurses are involved in carrying out investigations to identify the type of deafness. Nurses in general wards may also come across patients of all ages, but noticeably the older patient, who demonstrate signs of hearing loss that will require a fuller investigation. The occupational health nurse working in industry will know the hazards associated with the work environment and may carry out hearing tests when someone starts a new job and periodically thereafter.

She also ensures that protective ear muffs are used when appropriate in accordance with the Health and Safety at Work Act (1974).

INVESTIGATIONS

Hearing tests involve:

1. **Using the spoken work and a ticking watch**. Each ear is tested separately (with the other ear covered) at a range of 1 m, starting with a quiet whisper and, if necessary, increasing in loudness until the patient hears the sound.
2. **Tuning fork test**, e.g.:
   a. Rinne test
   b. Weber's test – place a tuning fork (512 Hz or 256 Hz) on the vertex of the skull:
      i. if hearing is normal the sound will be heard in the centre of the head
      ii. if there is conductive deafness the sound will be heard better on the affected ear
      iii. if inner ear deafness the sound will be heard better on the unaffected ear.
3. **Audiometric tests**. A method of testing the hearing of children who cannot be tested by conventional means. The test is based on the electroencephalogram being altered by perceived sound without the requirement of behavioural response.
4. **Vestibular function tests**, e.g.:
   a. Rotation test
   b. Caloric test.
5. **X-rays**. Radiology determines mastoiditis

HEARING LOSS

There may be partial or complete hearing loss, which may be conductive, sensorineural or combined conductive/sensorineural

In conductive deafness, sound waves fail to reach the inner ear due to defects in the outer ear, middle ear or the oval window. This can be caused by:

- excess build up of wax in the outer ear
- damage to tympanic membrane (blast, pressure injury, chronic otitis media)
- otosclerosis
- foreign body in outer ear
- acute otitis media.

Otitis media is seen frequently in children, usually following a respiratory infection. Otosclerosis more commonly affects women in the 15–40 year age range and has a familial tendency. Despite intensive campaigns to vaccinate all teenage girls against rubella, congenital deafness as a result of rubella during pregnancy still occurs.

In sensorineual (perceptive or nerve) deafness there is damage in the organ of Corti, or the acoustic nerve, or within the brain. This can be caused by:

- congenital factors (absence of inner ear due to rubella in the mother, anoxia, kernicterus, prematurity or a genetic defect)
- Ménière's disease
- vascular disorders of cochlear vessels
- acoustic neuroma (tumour of 8th cranial nerve)
- infections such as mumps or meningitis
- trauma (head injury, blast, continuous noise)
- drugs (aminoglycosides such as streptomycin or gentamicin)
- presbycusis (degeneration).

Although disorders of the ear are very seldom life-threatening, the quality of the person's life-style may greatly deteriorate due to tinnitus, vertigo or deafness.

Tinnitus (ringing or noises in the ear without auditory stimuli) may be caused by:

- overdose of aspirin
- cochlea nerve degeneration
- inflammatory disorders of the middle or inner ear.

Vertigo (disturbance in balance) results in the sensation of self or environment rotating, with the person feeling dizzy, lightheaded and falling. It is often accompanied by nystagmus, nausea, vomiting or clumsiness.

INFECTIONS
Clinical features

Most infections of the outer ear are caused by bacteria causing pain, with redness, swelling and oedema of the walls of the external auditory canal sometimes with purulent lesions, and a raised temperature.

Infections of the middle ear (otitis media) begin with a dullness of hearing, pyrexia and then pain, severe in many cases, which will ease if the eardrum is ruptured. Before it ruptures, the eardrum looks red and bulging. Once ruptured a discharge may be seen. In children with enlarged adenoids, fluid builds up in the middle ear, causing deafness and discomfort in the ear and, on examination, the eardrum is immobile. Because of the consistency of the fluid, it is often termed 'glue ear'. Chronic otitis media follows several attacks of otitis media, causing a rupture in the tympanic membrane, with a foul-smelling discharge and mild deafness.

Acute labyrinthitis results in vertigo, nausea, vomiting and nystagmus and is usually blamed on a viral infection.

Ménière's disease is characterized by sudden and recurrent attacks of vertigo, nausea, vomiting, tinnitus, hearing impairment and nystagmus which can incapacitate the patient for days.

Therapeutic management

If wax has built up in the ear, it may be removed by syringing with normal saline, tapwater or 1% sodium bicarbonate at 37° C. Prior to syringing, the wax should be softened by inserting almond oil or cerumenolytic agents warmed to body temperature. The same procedure can be used to remove foreign objects from the ear, though if they are vegetable in origin, fluid should not be used (as this will expand the vegetable). Instead a Jobson–Horne probe or angled forceps may be used by the doctor to remove objects which cannot be removed by irrigation. Before carrying out any syringing procedure on the ear, the nurse should check that the patient does not have an acute inflammation of the external or middle ear, or has not previously had a perforation of the tympanic membrane.

If antibiotics are not effective in treating otitis media the surgeon may perform a myringotomy (an incision in the tympanic membrane) to allow the pus to drain outwards. This surgical wound heals with less scarring than if the membrane ruptures, resulting in improved function. In serious otitis media, or 'glue ear', when the ear is filled with tenacious mucinous material, the surgeon will perform a myringotomy and insert a grommet (Fig. 6.9) into the incision to ensure adequate ventilation of the middle ear cavity. The grommet is pushed out by the healing tympanic membrane, but during this time (usually months) normal ventilation and drainage should have been re-established via the internal auditory tube.

Fortunately, due to the use of antibiotics and improved health care, the incidence of chronic otitis media and its complications (such as destruction of the ossicles or chronic mastoiditis due to infection and necrosis) has decreased. Improved surgical techniques using the binocular operating microscope now allow reconstructive surgery to be carried out instead of the radical surgery of the past.

Although a hearing aid may be of benefit in the early stages of otosclerosis, most patients will require a stapedectomy to correct their deafness. Again the use of microscopic surgery allows the surgeon to remove the stapes and fit a prosthesis.

Some specialised centres are now able to offer cochlear transplants to correct sensorineural deafness.

Patients with Ménière's disease may be prescribed antiemetics (such as dimenhydrinate (Dramamine) and sedatives (such as promethazine). As attacks become more acute the membraneous labyrinth is destroyed and they may not respond so readily to medication. Surgery, or ultrasound treatment following a mastoidectomy, may be required.

Nursing strategies

In assessing the patient who is deaf, it is useful to know the type of deafness and how long the patient has been deaf, whether the aids he is using are suitable and in working order, and which methods he uses to communicate – lip reading, sign language.

The patient, family, friends, doctors' letters and any previous notes will all help in familiarizing the nurse with the patient's history. This information enables the nurse to communicate well with the patient and ensures the patient's deafness does not disadvantage him during his hospital stay.

The following guidelines should help the nurse as well as other medical staff, family and friends communicate effectively with the deaf person.

The environment should be well illuminated and

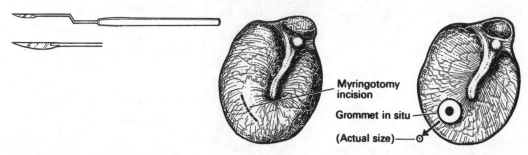

Fig. 6.9   Grommet inserted into tympanic membrane following myringotomy and clearance of secretions

distracting noises eliminated as much as possible. The deaf person should be introduced to other members of the group.

The nurse should position herself so that she is facing the person. Notes should be made whether the patient hears better on one side and the nurse's position should be adapted accordingly. As mentioned previously, the distance between patient and nurse should be 5–7 feet (1.5–2.2 m).

Since the patient's sight is of particular importance, any spectacles worn should be clean and clear.

The nurse must ensure that she attracts the patient's attention prior to speaking and speaks slowly and clearly without exaggerating movements or raising her voice. The nurse should also avoid covering her facial expressions or mouth when communicating.

It is important to check that the patient is understanding the conversation. If there are difficulties, providing props or writing materials may help. The nurse should ensure that if a hearing aid is worn it is in working order. Hearing aids should be cleaned at least weekly to enhance their function. Laughing at any misinterpretations is not appropriate and may destroy any therapeutic relationship which has been developed.

Sometimes people with disabilities such as deafness are avoided as communication may be more difficult or time consuming. An empathic manner and patience will be greatly appreciated, ensuring communication is as effective as possible.

THE NOSE

ANATOMY AND PHYSIOLOGY

The anterior part of the nose, the vestibule, is lined with squamous epithelium. Coarse hairs found here prevent large dust particles and insects from entering

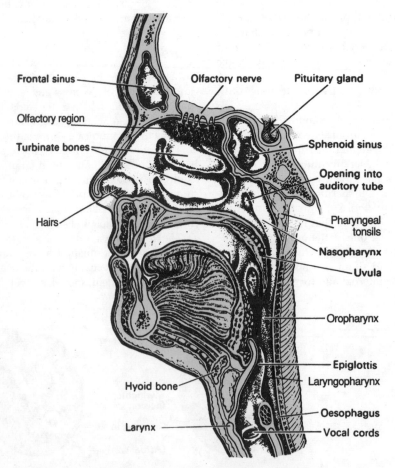

Fig. 6.10 Sagittal section (through nose, nasopharynx and larynx)

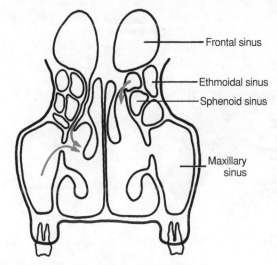

Frontal sinus

Ethmoidal sinus

Sphenoid sinus

Maxillary sinus

Fig. 6.11 Ostia draining paranasal sinuses

the nose. The remainder of the nose is lined with ciliated columnar epithelium and mucous-secreting goblet cells. The mucus traps bacteria and small particles which are then swept away by the cilia and swallowed. The mucus also moistens the incoming air. Due to the structure of the nose, with its various bones projecting into it, the surface area is extremely large with a rich blood supply, which helps to warm the air. (See Fig. 6.10).

The sensory nerve endings for smell (olfactory nerves) protrude into the attic of the nose.

The nasal sinuses (air spaces which lighten the skull) connect with the nasal cavities, giving resonance to the voice. (See Fig. 6.11).

EPIDEMIOLOGY AND AETIOLOGY

The effects of the ageing process on taste and smell are detailed in Table 6.3.

Infections of the upper respiratory tract may be either viral or bacterial in origin. They can occur at any time of the year but are more prevalent during the winter months.

Bleeding noses (epistaxis) in children occur more frequently in boys and may be caused by injury, vigorous nose blowing or nose picking. Epistaxis is less common in middle adult life but in the older patient may be linked with drug therapy (such as aspirin or anticoagulants), a bleeding disorder or possibly hypertension. In most cases, the epistaxis

Table 6.3 Effects of the ageing process on the sense of taste and smell

Physiological changes	Effect	Implications	Nursing management
Number of taste buds decrease	Food loses its taste	Patients may add more salt or sugar to bring out the flavour of food Decrease in appetite	Explain the loss or discourage the elderly from increasing their salt and sugar intake, use more herbs and spices Serve food attractively Offer sherry before meals
Decreased production of saliva	Substances to be tasted must be in solution of saliva	Decreases the person's ability to taste food	Encourage the production of saliva Encourage fluids at meal times
	Salivary amylase is reduced, affecting starch digestion	Starchy foods may cause indigestion	Encourage the production of saliva
	Build up of sordes	Increased risk of oral infection	Clean teeth and gums at least twice daily Attend dentist at least 6 monthly
Decrease the number and efficiency of olfactory receptors	Decreased ability to smell	May not smell smoke, burning or gases	Ensure that smoke detectors are fitted and maintained Ensure the elderly are aware of the dangers When grilling or frying food, never leave the kitchen All electric wires must be well insulated Ensure all gas appliances are well maintained Ensure gas appliances are switched off when not lit
		Decrease in appetite	Ensure food looks attractive

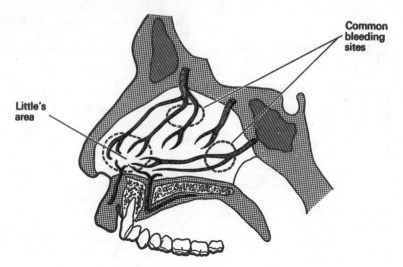

Fig. 6.12 Blood supply to the nose showing common bleeding sites

responds quickly to treatment, but in rare cases it may be life-threatening if the bleeding cannot be stopped. Figure 6.12 shows the common bleeding sites in the nose.

Allergic rhinitis (hay fever) is an antigen–antibody reaction due to an inhaled or ingested allergen. It results in sneezing, watery eyes and rhinorrhoea.

Trauma involving bone injury of the nose may follow sport injuries (such as boxing or rugby), road traffic accidents or, especially in young children, by foreign objects being inserted into the nostrils.

CLINICAL FEATURES

Injury to the upper respiratory tract is usually characterized by oversecretion of mucus. A fracture of the nasal bones may lead not only to pain but also swelling, displacement and bleeding. A purulent discharge may be noted when a foreign object has been inserted into the nostrils and forgotten about.

PATIENT IMPLICATIONS

Infections of the upper respiratory tract, although seldom serious, are easily spread. Soiled tissues should be collected in plastic bags and disposed of as soon as possible, not left lying around allowing the micro-organisms to multiply. As infections such as coryza (common cold), pharyngitis and laryngitis are spread by droplet infection, anyone with these infections should avoid contact with others. This is especially important when dealing with immuno-suppressed patients.

For health purposes all smokers should be en-

couraged to give up smoking; this is particularly important if an infection is present.

Enlarged adenoids in children due to repeated upper respiratory infections will require surgery to prevent a narrow nasal airway.

NURSING ROLE IN DIFFERENTIAL DIAGNOSIS

The patient suffering an epistaxis may give a history of trauma. If the bleeding is severe, the patient may exhibit signs of hypovolaemic shock. Patients with a history of hypertension do not necessarily have an increased risk of epistaxis, but the severity of the epistaxis may be greater than that in people with a normal blood pressure.

By observing the character of the discharge from the nose, the nurse can aid in the diagnosis.

A clear discharge without trauma may be due to a viral infection, an allergic response or vasomotor rhinitis. However, a clear discharge following a history of trauma may be due to leakage of cerebrospinal (CSF) fluid. This is termed rhinorrhea. If this is suspected, the nurse can test the discharge with a multistix. If CSF is present, it will reveal the presence of glucose.

A thick and purulent discharge is usually due to a bacterial infection such as sinusitis, whereas a foul-smelling discharge is usually due to a foreign body being left in situ long term.

INVESTIGATIONS

• Radiological test such as X-rays or CT scans.

- Nasal swabs for culture and sensitivity of micro-organism.
- If allergic rhinitis is suspected, patch testing of the patient may be performed to identify the allergen(s) (see Ch. 13 for more detail).

THERAPEUTIC MANAGEMENT

Viral infections such as coryza (common cold) will normally be allowed to run their course, with drugs such as paracetamol being prescribed for its anti-pyretic properties as well as its analgesic effect. Because of the possible side-effects on the liver, para-cetamol is not prescribed for children under 1 year of age. If sinusitis presents with a purulent discharge, it will be treated with antibiotics following identifi-cation of the causative organism. Analgesics may be prescribed for the intense headache associated with sinusitis as well as nasal decongestant drops or steam inhalations. If the condition does not resolve an antral lavage may be required, or if this is unsuccessful, sur-gery such as a radical antrostomy may be performed.

Most commonly, bleeding from a epistaxis comes from Little's area (Fig. 6.12), especially in children. The onset is usually quite sudden and may be fright-ening for the patient. A calm manner, with a clear explanation of what has happened and the treat-ment to be given, will help relieve the patient's (and family's) anxieties. The patient is advised to sit down with the head slightly forward over a basin, as this position prevents blood running down into the pharynx causing coughing and spluttering. Gentle pressure to the cartilaginous part of the nose should be applied for 10 minutes, with the patient advised to breathe through the mouth. The patient should be instructed not to swallow any blood, but to spit it out into the basin. Swallowing blood causes vomiting which may exacerbate the bleeding. If applied pres-sure does not stop the bleeding, the doctor will conduct an examination after inserting cotton wool soaked in 10% cocaine. Cocaine is a local anaesthetic and vasocontrictor. If possible the damaged blood vessel is cauterized using a silver nitrate stick or trichloroacetic acid. Petroleum jelly may be applied to prevent crusting thus allowing the damaged epi-thelium to thicken and heal. For persistent bleeding, the patient's nose will be packed anteriorly (Fig. 6.13). If this is not successful a posterior pack (Fig. 6.14) or an epistatic balloon such as a Simpson's or a Foley's catheter will be inserted (Fig. 6.15).

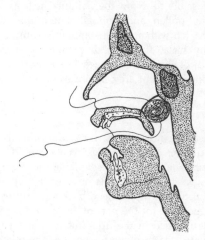

Fig. 6.14 Posterior nasal pack

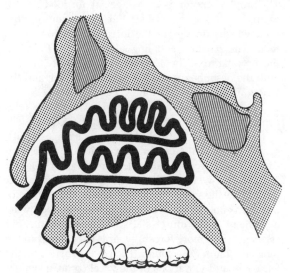

Fig. 6.13 Nasal pack (anterior) in position

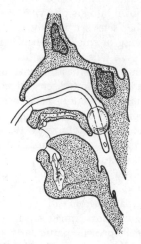

Fig. 6.15 Catheter in situ

If the pack is in situ for more than 24 hours, antibiotics will be prescribed to prevent infection. If the bleeding has been excessive, the patient may well be shocked, and require a blood transfusion. Further investigations will be required if the cause of the epistaxis is not found.

Fracture to the nasal bones causing swelling and bruising often constitutes an emergency. The only first aid should be the application of cold compresses to relieve the pain, reduce swelling and to stop the bleeding. If X-rays demonstrate that the bones are out of alignment, a plaster of Paris splint may be applied for a few days to maintain the bones in correct alignment.

Patients with allergic rhinitis should avoid known allergens. Wearing spectacles may keep pollen out of the eyes, and sunglasses may reduce photophobia. If it is impossible to avoid the irritant (such as house dust mite, pollen and animal skins), the rhinitis may be treated with an antihistamine. Sodium cromoglycate by nasal spray or drops may prevent the occurrence of rhinitis. Decongestants may be used in severe congestion but are best not used continually.

NURSING STRATEGIES

When instilling nose drops, it is important that the surface mucosa of the nose is well exposed to the medication. The procedure is explained to the patient and he is positioned with his head well back and to one side. If extending the head back in a sitting position is impossible for the patient, he should lie down. A drop is instilled in the uppermost nostril and the patient instructed to move his head to the other side so that drops can then be instilled into the other nostril. The patient should spit out any medication that has run down into his pharynx.

As with other senses it is only realized how important the sense of smell is, when it is absent, for example in coryza when the nose feels 'blocked up'. Some disorders, such as head injuries or Korsakoff's syndrome, lead to a distorted sense of smell. To assess a patient's ability to identify smells correctly, a group of scientists from Philadelphia packaged 40 odours on scratch and smell charts (Torrance 1985). These may be used when a person is claiming to have lost his sense of smell due to an accident.

We rely on our sense of smell to determine the flavours of food and drink. Unpleasant smells may discourage the patient from eating and drinking. With this in mind, the nurse must ensure there are no unpleasant smells present, particularly at meal times. Unpleasant smells may be masked by the use of potpourris or air fresheners in the ward, and the use of charcoal in dressings and stoma bags.

The sense of smell and taste deteriorates in old age, therefore it is important to ensure that the elderly patient's appetite is stimulated in other ways, for example by a preprandial sherry or by arranging the food in an attractive manner. Deterioration of smell and taste should be explained to older patients, as many of them try and enhance the flavour of the food by an excess of salt and sugar which should be discouraged.

THE PHARYNX, LARYNX AND TRACHEA

Whilst these organs are not directly linked to the senses, the pathology affecting them may have implications for the integrity of both taste and smell and so are considered here.

ANATOMY AND PHYSIOLOGY

The pharynx is described in three parts, the nasopharynx, oropharynx and laryngopharynx (Fig. 6.10). The nasopharynx lies behind the internal nasal cavity and has two openings to the internal nares, and two openings to the auditory tubes. On its posterior walls are the pharygneal tonsils (often called the adenoids). The nasopharynx is a passageway for air, which is closed off by the soft palate and uvula when food is swallowed. The pseudostratified ciliated epithelium wafts the dust and mucus towards the nasopharynx which has one opening from the mouth, the fauces. The oropharynx forms a passageway for food as well as air, and has a lining of stratified squamous epithelium which copes with the increased friction of the food. The palatine and lingual tonsils are found in the oropharynx. The laryngopharynx is continuous with the oesophagus for the passage of food, and the larynx for the passage of air.

The larynx (also called the voice box; Fig. 6.16) connects the pharynx with the trachea. The walls of the larynx are composed of nine cartilages which give it a rigid structure and prevent it from collapsing easily. The thyroid cartilage (Adam's apple) is larger in men than women. The epiglottis closes the larynx during swallowing. Stretched across the inside of the larynx are the vocal cords which are altered by the movement of the muscles attached to the aryntenoid cartilages. The more forcefully air is expelled from the lungs the louder the sound. The pitch depends on the tenseness and vibrations of the vocal cords, generally the tenser the vocal cords with increased vibrations,

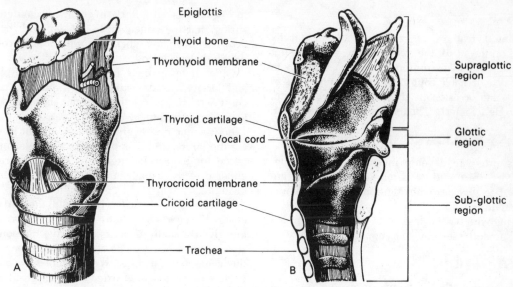

Fig. 6.16   The larynx. (A) Front view. (B) Sagittal section

the higher the pitch. Vocal folds are usually thicker in males, vibrating less and producing a deeper voice than in females. The nerve supply to the larynx and vocal cords is via the recurrent laryngeal nerve and branches of the superior laryngeal nerve.

The trachea (also called the windpipe) is continuous with the larynx and divides into the left and right bronchi. The mucosal lining is of pseudostratifed ciliated columnar epitheliums which wafts the dust upwards to be swallowed, and produces a thick mucus secretion. The tracheal wall is supported by 16–20 C-shaped rings of cartilage. The openings of the 'C' face the oesophagus, enabling the oesophagus to expand towards the trachea during swallowing.

EPIDEMIOLOGY AND AETIOLOGY

In childhood, lymphatic tissue such as the adenoids hypertrophy causing nasal and auditory tube obstruction which leads to pharyngeal infections and ear problems respectively. As adenoids atrophy from the age of 8 years to puberty, adults do not suffer from adenoiditis. Although tonsillitis may affect adults, it is much more common in childhood. Chronic laryngitis is more common in males than females, occurring mainly in people who use their voices a lot, for example teachers, singers, and sergeant majors. It is aggravated by smoking and drinking spirits.

The main causes of trauma to the larynx and trachea are: penetrating wounds such as lacerations to the throat, either accidental or intentional; blunt trauma, especially after road accidents; ingestion of corrosive fluids, or too hot fluids; inhalation of gases or flames and damage caused by endotracheal tubes with inflatable cuffs.

Malignant tumours of the larynx are usually squamous cell carcinomas, with only 2% metastasizing. Carcinoma of the larynx occurs mainly in smokers and is more common in men (approximately 10:1 males to females). It can occur at any age but the age group most commonly affected is 55–70 years.

CLINICAL FEATURES

Infections

Viruses most commonly cause sore throats, and are usually associated with a runny nose, watery eyes and sneezing. In bacterial infections such as acute tonsillitis, the tonsils will appear inflamed and oedematous, with a general feeling of malaise and pyrexia. Though rare, a peritonsillar abscess (quinsy) may complicate acute tonsillitis, with a raised temperature of 40°C, rigors, severe pain, thickened speech and halitosis. It is usually unilateral with the affected tonsil enlarged and covered in pus. Pharyngitis also causes a severe sore throat with pyrexia and dysphagia. Acute laryngitis often follows a cold in the winter months and results in the patient's voice being reduced to a whisper, with a painful croak (dysphonia). Chronic laryngitis results in hoarseness, with a tendency to clear the throat frequently.

Tumours

The clinical features of carcinoma of the larynx depend on the site of the tumour. If the cords are not involved, a vague discomfort in the throat, thickness of the voice, irritable cough, swollen lymph nodes in the neck and occasionally dyspnoea may be present. If the cords are affected, hoarseness is usually present.

PATIENT IMPLICATIONS

Patients prone to develop infections of the upper respiratory tract and/or laryngitis should be encouraged to give up smoking and avoid pollutants in the environment.

Patients who have a history of hoarseness for 2–3 weeks should be seen by a laryngologist.

INVESTIGATIONS

Patients, particularly the young or anxious, may require the assistance of the nurse to calm them down to enable the doctor to examine their throat. A good rapport with the patient needs to be developed, with the nursing staff appearing calm and confident. Sometimes the child's favourite toy or a suitable doll kept in the department may require to be examined first. If a throat swab has to be taken, the nurse must ensure that there is adequate light and the patient is in a comfortable position. After the explanation to the patient, the tongue is depressed using a spatula and the swab is taken quickly over the affected area, ensuring that the patient does not gag and the swab does not touch any other area of the mouth, contaminating the specimen.

Other investigations carried out on the pharynx and larynx include radiological techniques such as chest X-ray, CT scans of the larynx and, if dysphagia is present, a barium swallow.

Endoscopic fibroscopy allows the doctor to visualize the larynx and if appropriate to take samples of tissue for biopsy. Laryngoscopy may be performed either directly, usually under a general anaesthetic, or indirectly, with a mirror and light.

If a local anaesthetic has been used, the nurse must ensure the effects have worn off before fluids or foods are given, usually 4 hours post investigation, with sips of water being given at first. If a general anaesthetic has been required the principles of pre- and postoperative care are carried out (see Ch. 4 for more details).

THERAPEUTIC MANAGEMENT

Infections caused by bacteria, such as a streptococcal tonsillitis, respond well to antibiotics given orally. Quinsy may require the administration of intravenous antibiotics. It must be ensured that the course of antibiotics is completed and taken as prescribed. Paracetamol may be given for its antipyretic effect as well as its analgesic effect.

Steam inhalations are of great benefit in upper respiratory tract infections and laryngitis. Patients with laryngitis should also rest their voices, perhaps for as long as 2 weeks. Fluids should be encouraged to reduce the viscosity of mucus and pyrexia.

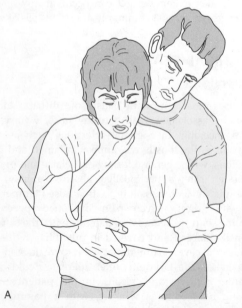
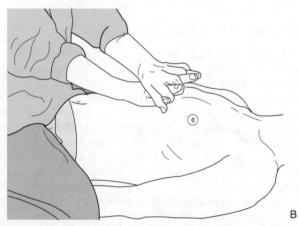

Fig. 6.17 Heimlich manoeuvre. (A) Place the fist between the navel and rib cage and cup fist with the other hand. (B) Reposition victim if original position prevents use of the abdominal thrust.

If a foreign body such as a piece of food becomes stuck in the larynx or trachea, with the person becoming cyanosed and unable to speak, the foreign object may be removed using the Heimlich manoeuvre (Fig. 6.17). If the patient is still standing, the first aider should stand behind the victim, placing his arms around the victim's abdomen with the clenched fist supported by the other hand just below the diaphragm, and give a sharp compression inwards. This should force air under pressure through the airway to dislodge the obstruction. It may also be performed with the patient lying down, the first aider straddling the victim and placing his hands, clasped, one on top of the other below the diaphragm and giving a short, sharp push upwards. If this is unsuccessful, the victim will require immediate hospitalization for endoscopic removal of the foreign body.

Tracheotomies may be performed as an emergency but in most cases this is a planned operation (Box 6.3). A tracheotomy involves an incision into the anterior wall of the trachea with the insertion of a tube, which may be temporary or permanent. The tube may be cuffed, thus allowing a tight seal which prevents aspirate or excess secretions from entering the lungs. It also enables intermittent positive pressure ventilation (IPPV) to be more effective. To prevent necrosis at the site of the cuff, the pressure on the cuff must be regularly released (e.g. 5 minutes every hour). Non-cuffed tubes may be either plastic (Portex and Shiley) or silver (Jackson or Negus), and are used when a cuff is no longer required.

Tonsillectomy and adenoidectomy operations are carried out when these organs, instead of preventing the development of lower respiratory tract infection, become a focus of infection themselves. The indications for surgery are controversial but the following criteria are usually acceptable. The patient experiences three or more attacks of tonsillitis in 1 year, or has enlarged tonsils or adenoids causing middle ear infections, an attack of quinsy or peritonsillar abscess or suffers frequent absences from work or school due to sore throats.

Tumours

Radiotherapy may be carried out for a tumour limited to one vocal cord (5-year survival 80–90%).

Laryngectomies may be either partial or total, depending on the site and size of the tumour. When only the top half of the larynx is removed, the patient has no permanent tracheotomy and has a normal voice. The preferred operation for a total laryngectomy is the Blom and Singer puncture procedure, where a trachea–oesophageal fistula is surgically created to allow the diversion of pulmonary air into the vocal tract enabling speech to occur. The trachea–oesophageal fistula allows a catheter to be inserted from the trachea through the oesophagus into the stomach, through which the patient is fed for 10–14 days postoperatively. If there is no evidence of leaking of saliva or inflammation, the catheter will be replaced with a silicone prosthesis; this has a valve with a retention collar and flange which can be taped above the stoma, to prevent dislodgement. The proximal end of the prosthesis has a slit which permits respiratory air into the oesophagus for vocalization, but prevents aspiration of fluid into the trachea. A small airflow port on the undersurface of the tube allows respiratory air to be diverted through the prosthesis when the stoma is occluded by the patient's thumb while exhaling. A tracheostome valve may be fitted, which opens for normal breathing but closes for speaking.

NURSING STRATEGIES

Inflammatory conditions

The aim of the nursing management of patients with tonsillitis, pharyngitis and acute laryngitis is to

---

Box 6.3   Reasons for tracheostomy

- To provide and maintain an adequate airway
- To bypass obstruction in the airway caused by:
  - oedema, e.g. following radiation or burns
  - tumours, e.g. of tongue, pharynx or larynx
  - inhaled foreign bodies
- To bypass damage to mouth and pharynx caused by:
  - burns or scalds
  - traumatic wounds
- To allow the removal of tracheobronchial secretions, especially if frequent and long-term suction is required
- To assist lung ventilation
- Following surgery, e.g.:
  - post laryngectomy
  - extensive head and neck surgery
- Neurological, e.g. damage to recurrent laryngeal nerve leading to bilateral vocal cord palsy causing stridor
- To provide IPPV to patients with disorders of:
  - respiratory centre following trauma, e.g. a stroke
  - respiratory muscles, e.g. in myasthenia gravis or tetanus
  - nerve pathway, e.g. polyneuritis
- To reduce the amount of dead space by approximately 50% and eliminate the resistance offered by the upper airway

relieve pain, treat the infection and compensate for short-term loss of self-care. The patients will require a decrease in physical activity until their pyrexia has settled. The room should be a comfortable temperature and well ventilated. Natural fibres for night clothes and light bed clothes are beneficial. Adequate fluids should be encouraged and a light diet given. As the patient responds to antibiotics, analgesia and good nursing care, his physical activities can be increased, the patient taking responsibility for his personal and oral hygiene. The nurse must ensure that the antibiotics are taken correctly, and for the prescribed length of time. Any side-effects of the drug therapy should be reported to the medical staff who may wish to discontinue the drug. The nurse will also evaluate if the treatment is effective by monitoring the patient's appearance and vital signs, until they stabilize within normal ranges for the age of the patient.

Surgery

Before an adenoidectomy or tonsillectomy, the patient should show no evidence of infection. If present, the operation will be postponed since it increases the risk of postoperative bleeding. The main aim of postoperative care is to ensure an adequate airway and prevent bleeding. To help prevent obstruction by the tongue or inhalation of blood secretions, the patient will be nursed in the recovery position with the head low until the patient's condition has stabilized. Suction and oxygen should be at hand. To encourage co-operation and aid recovery, adequate analgesia must be given. Due to the possibility of a reactionary haemorrhage (within 24 hours of surgery) the nurse must monitor the patient's condition. A rising pulse, restlessness, frequency of swallowing (even when asleep), pallor, sweating, a fall in blood pressure or vomiting (swallowed blood) would indicate haemorrhage from the tonsillar bed. A return to theatre to control the bleeding and/or a blood transfusion might be required. A secondary haemorrhage (between 7 and 10 days postoperatively) is usually due to infection. To prevent this occurring, the patient must use the pharyngeal muscles for swallowing, thereby inhibiting colonization of bacteria. The nurse can encourage the patient to eat and drink by offering cool drinks and favourite foods. Gargles and mouthwashes given frequently (every 2 hours) may help to relieve the pain and rough feeling of the throat.

The aim of the nursing care of a patient with carcinoma of the larynx is to prepare him/her physically, and with his/her family, psychologically and socially, pre- and postoperatively. Particularly, attention must be paid to pain control, improving the nutritional state and dehydration, and establishing a therapeutic relationship. The diagnosis of cancer may cause a number of anxieties and fears, as may the prospect of the surgery involved. By allowing the patient and his/her loved ones to talk and air their feelings, fears and concerns, progress can be made. They should also be informed of the intensive care facilities and treatment which will be required. For more details see Nursing Care Plan 6.1.

Other members of the health team such as the physiotherapist, speech therapist and dietician will also participate in care and advice.

THE TONGUE

ANATOMY AND PHYSIOLOGY

The tongue lies in the floor of the mouth to which it is attached. It is composed of muscle covered with mucous membrane containing the nerve endings responsible for taste. In addition to being the organ of taste, the tongue is also necessary for chewing, swallowing and speech.

EPIDEMIOLOGY AND AETIOLOGY

As previously mentioned, the sense of taste plays an important part in enabling the individual to appreciate the enjoyment of food, thus any impairment in the sense of taste may adversely effect the appetite and nutrition in general. Taste buds enable the individual to differentiate between bitter, salt, sweet and sour tastes and, as with other senses, are affected by the ageing process. This is particularly noticeable in the elderly who have a tendency to add more salt than is necessary to food.

CLINICAL FEATURES

Infection of the tongue and mouth mainly occurs as a result of other underlying conditions and is commonly seen in the febrile unconscious or terminally ill patient. Other infections can specifically affect the tongue, particularly *Candida albicans* which causes thrush and is characterized by the formation of white patches and ulcers on the mucous membrane.

PATIENT IMPLICATIONS

Untreated infection of the tongue and mouth may

Nursing Care Plan 6.1   Care for a patient undergoing a total laryngectomy

Problem	Goal	Nursing action	Rationale
1. Anxiety a. About disease	Patient is relaxed prior to surgery	❏ Provide a calm atmosphere ❏ Assess level of patient's understanding and knowledge of diagnosis ❏ Encourage patient and family to ask questions ❏ Explain (with the medical staff) pre- and postoperative care and rehabilitation ❏ Clarify any misconceptions ❏ Discuss hospital routine	Encourages effective learning Patients well prepared preoperatively respond better postoperatively
b. About hospitalization	Patient understands hospital routine and treatment	❏ Introduce patient to staff and other patients Orientate patient and close family to ward and intensive care unit Demonstrate unfamiliar equipment, and explain use	Will help calm the patient Will help patient settle into ward Will help reassure patient and family, to decrease fear of the unknown
c. About being unprepared for theatre	Patient prepared psychologically and physically for theatre To be relaxed and well informed prior to surgery	❏ Discuss any fears related to surgery and rehabilitation ❏ Explain pre- and postoperative care in relation to: • communication, introduce speech therapist • drug therapy • altered airway and suction, demonstrate a tracheostomy tube • oxygen therapy, demonstrate masks and fittings • fluid replacement, demonstrate a nasogastric tube • hygiene, oral and personal • physiotherapy, e.g. deep breathing • exercises and mobility as often as required • prepare site for operation just prior to surgery	Stress may: a. delay healing b. increase pain c. delay recovery, prolonging hospitalization Paper and pencil provided, speech therapist should meet patient preoperatively Patient will have a tracheostomy in situ Humidified oxygen given postoperatively Patient may be frightened of intravenous tubes and nasogastric tubes Nurse required to carry out all activities of daily living immediately postoperatively Deep breathing more difficult to learn postoperatively Repetition aids understanding Decreases risk of infection
d. About altered body image	To enable patient and family to cope with the altered body image	❏ Introduce someone who has adjusted well to his/her laryngectomy Explain preoperatively the necessity for a stoma and the care required	Allows patient to see recovery is possible May help to reduce fear of surgery As the patient will require to look after the stoma when he leaves hospital, he must accept the stoma and be able to suction effectively, cough up and remove the secretions, keep the area around stoma clean and choose an effective cover for stoma, e.g. polo neck inserts
2. Loss of normal voice	Patient is able to communicate effectively	❏ Explain the options for developing speech Introduce the speech therapist	The nurse and speech therapist should work together to aid the patient's speech

Nursing Care Plan 6.1 (*cont'd*)

Problem	Goal	Nursing action	Rationale
2. (cont'd)		Encourage visitors not to exclude the patient in conversation When nasogastric tube is removed, speech therapy is commenced	Speech is not the only way to communicate, but others often take more time Patient knows the order of care
3. **Difficulty in breathing:** a. Caused by altered airway b. Caused by ineffective airway clearance c. Caused by oedema of neck	Maintain a clear airway with normal breathing patterns Maintain effective airway clearance To reduce oedema	❒ Monitor rate and depth of respiration quarter hourly, progressing to 4 hourly ❒ Ensure there are no plugs of mucus in the tracheostomy tube Administer oxygen with humidification ❒ Observe neck for inflammation Support head and keep neck slightly flexed when sitting up	An increase in respiratory rate and tachycardia with a wheezing sound indicates a need to suction As the air no longer passes through the nose where it is moistened, filtered and heated, oxygen must be humidified A rapid pulse with restlessness may indicate haemorrhage (or hypoxia) Best position for breathing and healing
4. **Infection of respiratory tract**	To prevent infection of respiratory tract	❒ Using an aseptic technique suction as above Suction catheter inserted with suction off, then withdrawn with suction on Remove and clean inner tracheostomy tube 2–3 hourly Change patient's position 2 hourly Note colour, amount and consistency of secretions Send specimen of sputum to bacteriology	Decreases risk of secretions To avoid damage to tracheal mucosa Prevents secretions crusting and becoming a focal point for infection To decrease the risk of hypostatic pneumonia Blood may indicate trauma, increased mucus secretions may indicate infection For culture and sensitivity
5. **Altered nutritional state**	To ensure an adequate nutritional intake: • to maintain body weight • to aid healing of wounds Patient enjoys food in spite of diminished sense of smell and possible difficulty in swallowing due to surgery	❒ Monitor intravenous fluids until nasogastric feeding commenced Administer nasogastric feeds as per chart Liaise with dietician regarding feeds Remove nasogastric tube (usually 10–14 days postoperatively following methylene blue test) ❒ Inform patient his sense of taste may be impaired initially, due to the loss of the sense of smell ❒ Progress diet through soft to normal	To maintain a fluid intake of at least 1500 ml in 24 hours Nasogastric feeding commenced 24 hours after surgery (if bowel sounds present) Protein and vitamins required for healthy wound healing, carbohydrates required for energy When nasogastric tube removed, speech therapy commenced when patient starts to eat normally As breathing is via the trachea, air does not pass through the nose affecting the olfactory nerve ends, the senses of smell and taste are closely linked Depends on patient's tastes and progress
6. **Inability to communicate normally**	To maintain effective communication	❒ Ensure patient realizes he will not have a natural voice	Patient may either think he will not talk again or does not realize the voice is affected by the surgery

Nursing Care Plan 6.1 (*cont'd*)

Problem	Goal	Nursing action	Rationale
6. (cont'd)		Discuss preoperatively the difficulties and solutions available	Difficulties in communication may frustrate the patient, leading to anger or despair
		Confirm patient can write	Even nowadays some patients are unable to write, use alternatives
		Provide a 'magic' board or pencil and paper (remember writing is slower than speaking, be patient)	Allows the patient to maintain control
		Provide a bell	Patient may be frightened if he/she cannot attract the attention of a nurse
		Liaise with speech therapist and surgeon	Speech programme usually started when patient is eating normally
		Speak normally	The patient is not deaf
		Use touch appropriately	Demonstrates empathy
7. Inability to maintain personal hygiene due to surgery	Patient is able to participate in his care with the nurse compensating for the deficits in the patient's self care as appropriate	❏ Explain prior to all care what you are going to do and why Encourage questions, ensuring privacy and time	Patient will have to carry out his own care at home Make compliance with treatment more acceptable if the patient knows why and how the treatment will be carried out
	Patient feels comfortable and clean	❏ Bed bath first day postoperatively Encourage baths initially	Patient will be tired postoperatively Encourages mobility, showers should only be used below the neck (if showering wear shield over stoma)
8. Impaired skin integrity	Wound around stoma remains clean and heals well	❏ Assess for signs of infection at wound site Monitor vital signs	Inflammation, redness or purulent discharge, a raised temperature and an increase in pulse rate may indicate infection
		Clean wound and change dressing as required (usually when cleaning inner tracheostomy tube 3–5 times daily)	Dressing becomes easily soiled when the patient is coughing up secretions, if not changed would be an excellent breeding ground for micro-organisms
		Observe discharge from drains Remove drains (when discharge is negligible)	May be blood stained
9. Difficulty in maintaining oral hygiene	Maintain integrity of oral mucosa and prevent dental decay	❏ Clean teeth with a soft brush if patient can tolerate it Encourage 2–4 hourly mouthwashes, dentures if worn should be removed and cleaned 2 hourly	Foam sticks are ineffective in removing plaque Aids comfort, cleans the mouth and reduces halitosis Frequency of oral hygiene needs to be increased during oxygen administration and when the patient is not drinking or eating
10. Impaired mobility due to anaesthesia and surgery	To prevent complications of immobility	❏ Preoperatively practice deep breathing and leg exercises Encourage increasing mobility, up to sit in a chair first postoperative day	To prevent complications such as deep venous thrombosis or a pulmonary emboli, active or passive physiotherapy to legs is required
		Administer prescribed analgesia postoperatively (usually not opiates)	Pain relief is most effective if given before it becomes too intense Patient will mobilize better without pain, may decrease respiration

Nursing Care Plan 6.1 *(cont'd)*			
Problem	**Goal**	**Nursing action**	**Rationale**
10. (cont'd)	To maintain adequate neck and shoulder movement	Support head and neck with pillows ❐ Encourage patient to support head and neck when moving	Prevents strain on sutures and tracheostomy Enables patient to participate in care
		Liaise with physiotherapist with regard to head and neck exercises	Physiotherapy will strengthen remaining muscles
11. Anxiety due to discharge	Patient and family are able to cope with patient's discharge home	❐ Evaluate patient and family's understanding of care and treatment	Patient and family's ability to cope will depend on their level of knowledge, facilities and support available in the home and community
		Demonstrate and observe patient in relation to: • replacing dressing around tracheostomy tubes and tapes • correct technique in tracheostomy care • removal of secretions (provide suction catheter and suction machine/or arrange) With dietician, advise on diet With speech therapist, advise on speech	Patient is able to remove and clean tracheostomy tubes (sodium bicarbonate 1 tspn/1 pint will remove encrustation, then tube rinsed in normal saline and dried) May be able to cough up secretions but if not will have to use suction
		Advise on covering stoma and dress as required ❐ Provide information regarding • laryngectomy club	Humidification and filtering of air as nose is bypassed Provides a social and educational function, keeps laryngectomees up to date with developments
		• returning to work and socialising	May return to work and socialize weeks after operation, but avoid smoke and upper respiratory tract infections
		• hobbies	Special aid to cover stoma when swimming

spread to effect other parts of the gastrointestinal or respiratory tract and will also cause extreme localized discomfort, as the mouth is a particularly sensitive area.

THERAPEUTIC MANAGEMENT

Mouthwashes, regular oral hygiene together with specific antifungal therapy (e.g. nystatin), will provide effective treatment.

NURSING STRATEGIES

Infection of the tongue and mouth can usually be avoided by appropriate nursing care. The patient should be encouraged to carry out his/her own oral hygiene wherever possible, using toothbrush and toothpaste with mouthwashes when necessary. In patients who are unable to carry out personal mouth care, the responsibility falls to the nurse to ensure oral hygiene is carried out as frequently as required using appropriate preparatory mouth lotions together with frequent drinks of fluids which will encourage the production of saliva. Where dentures are worn these may have to be removed temporarily until the infection has been successfully treated.

THE SKIN

ANATOMY AND PHYSIOLOGY

The skin is composed of an outer four or five layers of epithelial cells called the epidermis. The main cells

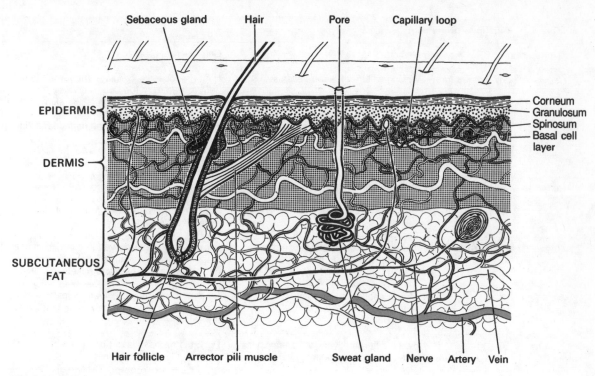

Fig. 6.18 Section through the skin

are the rapidly multiplying keratinocytes producing keratin, which act as a waterproof barrier for the skin and underlying tissues. The older keratinocytes are pushed to the surface by the new cells, lose their nuclei, change shape and die before being shed on the surface. Each cell lasts for about 35–45 days, with the body losing one million cells every 40 minutes. This means that in an adult 20% of the protein intake is used for growth and repair of the skin. Melanocytes producing melanin are found in the basal layer. These give the skin its colour and protect it and the underlying organs from damage by ultraviolet rays. Other cells found in the epidermis are the Langerhans cells associated with immunity and Merkel's cells associated with touch reception. (See Fig. 6.18).

The inner layer of the skin is the dermis, composed of strong elastic connective tissue with collagen. It supports many nerve endings (touch, pressure, pain and temperature) and blood vessels which supply sweat glands, sebaceous glands, hair follicles, the rest of the dermis and epidermis. The blood vessels help regulate the body temperature by contracting and dilating as necessary to maintain the constant core temperature of the body.

Hair follicles extend down into the dermis from the epidermis. At the base of the follicle is a collection of cells called the bulb, which grow to become the hair (the root is below the level of the skin and the shaft protrudes from the skin). Arrector pili muscles controlled by the nervous system keep the hair follicles in an upright position. Fright and low temperature activate them, resulting in the appearance of goose pimples. Sebaceous glands opening into the hair follicles secrete sebum which keeps the hair and skin soft and pliable, as well as inhibiting the growth of certain bacteria.

Sweat glands excrete sodium chloride and water onto the skin surface helping to maintain the body's temperature. In excessive sweating both salt and water require to be replaced. Small amounts of albumin and urea are excreted by the sweat glands when the kidneys and liver are not functioning normally. Lymph vessels drain intersitital fluid and help protect the body from invading pathogens. Beneath the dermis is a layer of loose connective tissue known as the hypodermis, which varies from areolar to adipose tissue, depending on the area. This helps to anchor the skin to underlying organs, acts as a shock absorber and insulates the deeper tissues from heat loss. For functions of the skin see Table 6.4.

Table 6.4 Functions of the skin

Skin function	Method	Comments
Regulates body temperature	Varying calibre of blood vessels	Heat produced by cellular metabolism must be removed from the body's core by the blood vessels taking blood to the skin surface to be cooled by the air
	Activity of sweat glands	As sweat evaporates on the surface, cooling takes place
	Adipose tissue	In a cool environment insulates the body core to retain heat
Removes waste products	Albumen and urea removed by sweat	Used when the kidneys and liver are not working properly
	Sodium chloride lost by sweat	Both salt and water need to be replaced in excessive sweating
Manufactures vitamin D	Absorption of ultraviolet rays convert sterol substances in the skin to vitamin D	Covering up the skin even in sunny climates leads to a loss of vitamin D, resulting in osteomalacia in adults and rickets in children
Absorbs drugs	Topical application of creams, ointments	Smaller doses may be given topically compared with the systemic route leading to fewer side-effects
Waterproof	By the different layers of keratinocytes in the epidermis producing keratin	Prevents excess water absorption and abnormal loss of body fluid
Perceives stimuli	Nerve endings and receptors detect stimuli related to pain, touch, pressure and temperature	Destruction of the dermis results in loss of response to stimuli, whereas loss at the epidermal layer will lead to increased sensitivity to stimuli
Protects against infection	Macrophages in the epidermis destroy bacteria, sebum inhibits growth of acteum bacteria, with the mucous membrane the skin protects the body from invading micro-organisms	Infections are usually caused when there is a break in the skin
Protects against trauma	Intact skin protects underlying tissues	Mechanical pressure or chronic irritation may lead to localized thickening or lichenification

For the effects of the ageing process on the skin see Table 6.5.

Wounds either surgical or non-surgical, pressure sores or burns may all cause trauma to the skin. A wound is defined as a break in the skin and deeper tissues due to accidental lacerations or surgical incisions. Healing takes place in order to restore the intact barrier provided by the skin.

EPIDEMIOLOGY AND AETIOLOGY

Surgical wounds are planned, allowing the edges of the wound to be joined together in opposition using sutures, and healing is by primary (first) intention.

If the wound is deep and wide it may be left open to heal by secondary intention. Thus healing occurs in four identifiable stages, as shown in Box 6.4.

There are many factors which facilitate wound healing. The patient's nutritional state is important; an adequate intake of protein, calories, vitamins, zinc and fluid is necessary. The presence of illness such as cancer or HIV-related illnesses inhibits wound healing. The rate of wound repair is slowed down by the presence of infection, a haematoma or unnecessary interference with the wound, for examples by patients picking at the wound or when the wrong type of dressing is applied. Drugs such as corticosteriods and those used in chemotherapy affect the

Table 6.5 Effects of the ageing process on the skin

Physiological changes	Effects	Implications	Nursing management
Epidermis and dermis thin	Skin appears transparent	Skin at greater risk of damage from trauma, pressure or chemicals	Frequent change of position (at least 2 hourly) Use of pressure-relieving aids Avoid use of local heat appliances
Elastin fibres degenerate, collagen fibres stiffen	Skin appears wrinkled	Skin appears dry and itchy May be hastened by exposure to sun and/or wind	Apply emollients to skin and add to bath water Decrease use of soaps Avoid excessive exposure to wind and sun
Decrease in adipose tissue	Skin sags	Altered body image e.g. breast sag Intolerance to cold	Size and change in style of clothes may be required Require extra layers of clothes or elevation in room temperature More susceptible to hypothermia
Alteration in sites of adipose tissue	Increased fat deposits on hips and ankles	Clothes and shoes may not fit comfortably	Size and style may need to be changed
Decrease in number and efficiency of sebaceous glands	Dry skin	Skin more friable, increased risk of damage	Add emollients to bath and apply to skin Avoid soap products
Increased fragility of blood vessels	More liable to damage	Bruises easily	Handle gently when touching skin
Slowing of response of diameter of blood vessels	Superficial blood vessels less efficient in dilating or constricting	In hot conditions heat dissipation is poor, when exposed to cold conditions body is less able to conserve heat	Keep room at comfortable temperature Avoid going out when the temperature is high Wear layers of natural fibres in cold weather
Nails thicken and become brittle		Nails difficult to cut	Soak feet before cutting nails Arrange chiropody if required
Increase in facial hairs in females		Alters appearance	Cut or shave hairs as often as required Preserve dignity
Loss and thinning of hair from body and scalp (mainly in men)		Increased risk of heat loss	Maintain adequate clothes Encourage the use of hats in cold weather
Decrease in number and efficiency of sweat glands	Decline in efficiency of body's cooling effect Reduction in perspiration	At risk of heat exhaustion	Avoid exposure to excessive heat Encourage fluids in hot weather
Delayed action genes become activated	Hair loses its colour and looks grey and dry	Altered body image	
Decreases in number and efficiency of melanocytes	Skin loses its protection against the sun	Increased risk of skin cancers, especially in fair-skinned people	Patient education regarding dangers of exposure to the sun
Increase in size of some melanocytes	Skin appears pigmented on exposed areas	Increased risk of malignant melanoma	Patient education regarding dangers of exposure to the sun
Decrease in number and efficiency of nerve endings	Decreased ability to feel pain, heat, cold or touch	An increased risk of damage to skin from trauma, pressure chemicals or excess change	Create a safe environment

Box 6.4	The four identifiable stages of healing
Stage 1	Inflammatory phase takes up to 3 days, and results in formation and epithelialization
Stage 2	Destructive phase takes up to 6 days with bacteria and dead tissue being destroyed
Stage 3	Proliferative phase takes up to 24 days, when the epithelial cells have migrated across the wound surface. Collagen is formed and there is an increased growth of blood vessels. This forms the granulation tissue which fills the gaps left by the wound
Stage 4	Maturation phase takes between 24 days and a year or so. The scar tissue becomes less vascular, changing from pink to white. Collage continues to be produced and strengthens the wound. The new tissue regains approximately 80% of its strength by 3 months

inflammatory response, delaying wound healing. It is also important to note that high anxiety may inhibit wound healing and that adequate sleep is necessary for anabolism (tissue renewal).

PATIENT IMPLICATIONS

If clips, staples or sutures are used, wound healing by primary intention leaves minimal scar formation with little or no loss of function of the affected area. In an infected or wide wound, healing requires a greater formation of granulation tissue. In this case, contraction from scar tissue leads to keloidal tissue (overgrowth of scar tissue) and/or decreased function of the affected area. If wounds do not heal naturally (e.g. because of infection) healing by tertiary intention involves debridement of the wound and skin closure by suturing. Some surgical procedures may provoke collections of fluid under the surface which may cause infection to develop. The surgeon may therefore insert a drain as a prophylactic measure.

THERAPEUTIC MANAGEMENT

Wounds, whether surgical or accidentally acquired, form a break in the skin and therefore a break in the body's main defence mechanism. If the wound has been stitched or clipped together, once the initial dressing is removed no further action is required until the stitches or clips are removed. All wounds should be observed for the presence of a discharge, haematoma, swelling, redness, pain or loss of function. This check will be done a quarter to half hourly in the

initial stages, changing to daily if no abnormalities are detected in the first few days. The dressings should not be removed for this purpose. Other signs of infection include a raised temperature, tachycardia, sweating and a feeling of malaise. If there is a discharge, a wound swab will be taken for culture and sensitivity and the dressings changed as often as necessary. The nursing care of patients whose wounds are bleeding postoperatively can be found in Chapter 9.

To be effective, dressings for wounds must fulfil certain criteria. They must be a barrier to microorganisms, allow excess exudate to be released from the wound surface and allow absorption of exudate from wound. They should contain no loose threads or fibres which could enter the wound and be able to be removed from the wound without causing damage (Turner 1985).

Wound dressings should allow gaseous exchange to take place, provide thermal insulation and maintain a moist environment where the wound and dressing meet. They must be sterile and comfortable and not require too frequent changes.

NURSING STRATEGIES

Dressing changes may be performed in specially designated areas. To prevent cross-infection, infected wounds are treated last. All dressings require an aseptic technique and the nurse should have a trolley prepared with the appropriate materials. A clear explanation will be given to the patient regarding his wound care management before his dressings, and prior to discharge. An analgesic may be required and sufficient time allowed for it to exert an effect prior to potentially painful changing of dressings.

To enable the wound to be assessed it is useful that the same person observes the wound each time. This is not always practical, so other means must be used. Charting the size of the wound using clear plastic to draw the outline of the wound, or photographing the wound may be used. To plan the management of the wound the nurse requires an up-to-date knowledge of research into dressings and lotions (Dealey 1983, Leaper 1986, Morison 1989). This will enable the nurse to decide on the most appropriate dressing required and the frequency of changes needed.

When the wound has been cleaned and dressed (and drains removed if required), the nurse must leave the patient in a comfortable position and document the findings. This will enable an evaluation of the care given, and any further changes in care implemented as appropriate.

Box 6.5 Factors which predispose to pressure sores

- Unconsciousness
- Paralysis
- Friction
- Plaster of Paris or other forms of splints
- Traction
- Incontinence
- Nutritional deficiency

PRESSURE SORES

A pressure sore (or decubitus ulcer) is due to a breakdown in the integrity of the skin. It is caused by localized pressure compressing blood vessels in the area, which leads to ischaemia of the skin and underlying tissues.

Epidemiology and aetiology

Factors predisposing to pressure sores are given in Box 6.5. Using the Activities of Living model (Roper et al 1985), care required for patients at risk of pressure sores development is given in Table 6.6.

Clinical features

Due to insufficient oxygen and nutrients reaching the cells, the ischaemia leads to cell death and tissue necrosis. The area at first looks blanched and cool, changing to red and warm, before breaking down or necrosing. During the early stages pain may be felt before the area becomes numb.

Patient implications

If a pressure sore develops, the patient's hospital stay may be prolonged, with the patient suffering increased pain and/or discomfort. An infection may spread from the localized break in the skin to the blood stream causing septicaemia and a general debilitation.

Investigations

Investigations involve taking a swab from the wound for culture and sensitivity to identify the presence of micro-organisms. Thermography may be performed to identify areas of poor skin blood flow. Photographs or tracing charts are used to measure the area of the pressure sore before, during and after treatment to evaluate its effectiveness.

Therapeutic management

Certain precautions should be taken to prevent pressure sores developing. If patients are emaciated or malnourished a well-balanced diet, rich in proteins, vitamins and minerals, will help prevent pressure sores developing, and aid healing. An adequate fluid intake (at least 2–3 litres of fluid daily) should be encouraged. If the patient is obese, a weight reduction diet may be ordered by the dietitian. The nurse can encourage the patient to eat his diet by serving the food attractively and at the correct temperature.

Nursing strategies

To help nurses assess which patients are at particular risk, a nurse may use an assessment tool such as Waterlow (Waterlow 1985) or Norton Scale (Table 6.7). The method in the Table 6.7 consists of assessing the patient on a score of 1–4 on five different aspects of his condition. Patients who score a total of 14 or less are considered 'at risk' and require intensive measures to prevent pressure sores developing. In planning the prevention and, if necessary, the treatment of pressure sores the nurse should be aware of the up-to-date research relating to aids and dressings available (Morison 1992).

The patient's position must be changed at least 2 hourly to prevent skin damage. This is necessary whether the patient is in bed or in a chair. Whenever possible the patient is encouraged to move himself, and mobility is encouraged as soon as is possible. Patients who are in a wheelchair and catheterized are at particular risk as they will not be taken to the toilet very often. Taking the patient to the toilet encourages mobility and decreases incontinence. Patients who are incontinent or perspiring heavily should be washed and dried promptly. If possible, the cause of the incontinence should be investigated and treated appropriately.

Nurses must ensure there are no foreign objects, such as scissors, or wrinkles in the undersheets of the bed. Nurses must also keep their nails short, and wear no jewellery on hands and arms, as these can cause trauma to the patient's skin (see also care of the plaster in Ch. 11).

The treatment of pressure sores is detailed in Table 6.8.

BURNS

Burns may be: thermal due to fires, steam or hot liquids; chemical due to caustic agents, either acid or alkali; electrical due to domestic supply, power-lines

Table 6.6   Groups at risk of pressure sore development (using Roper, Tierney and Logan Model)

Activity	At-risk factor	Cause	Management
Breathing	Breathless patient Oxygen mask	Sitting upright Elastic too tight	Change position or mobilize at least 2 hourly Ensure correct fit
Communicating	Unconscious patient Speech problems	Unable to explain Pain or numbness	Change position 2 hourly/as necessary Spend time with patient, develop other forms of communication
Mobility	Unconscious patient Paralysed patient Patient very weak Very obese patient	Lack of mobility Lack of mobility Lack of mobility Lack of mobility	Change position 2 hourly/as necessary Encourage 2-hourly relief of pressure Encourage nutrition, care as required Reduction diet, encourage exercise
Safe environment	Plaster cast Crumbs, scissors, etc. Wrinkles, holes in sheet Pressure from bedclothes Finger nails Jewellery Shearing force Bed cradles	Too tight, loose plaster Irritation, pressure Irritation, pressure Bedclothes too tight Scratches Scratches Poor lifting technique Patient sticking to bedpan Unrelieved pressure	See care of plaster (Ch. 11) Ensure no foreign objects in bed Ensure sheets are free of holes and wrinkles Ensure bedclothes loose, especially at toes Nurse's nails short, well cut Use fob watch, no jewellery on duty Ensure correct lifting technique Lift patient carefully off bedpan Ensure bed appliances are not directly next to patient's skin
Controlling body temperature	Pyrexial patient Hypothermia Patient with circulatory problems	$\uparrow$ Metabolic rate leading to restlessness and sweating Constricted blood vessels in skin Ischaemia and/or hypoxia	Bed rest, help with activities of living Gradually increase patient's temperature, special care when handling patient Administer oxygen as prescribed, treat underlying problem
Eating and drinking	Obese patient Poor nutrition Underweight Dehydration	Sustained pressure Lack vitamin C – poor wound healing Negative nitrogen balance Bony prominences at risk Diarrhoea	Change postion 2 hourly/as necessary Vitamin C supplement $\uparrow$ Protein $\uparrow$ vitamins Dietician Small appetizing meals Encourage a well-balanced diet, encourage drinks and change position Treat underlying cause, replace fluids orally/intravenously
Elimination	Incontinence Urinary Faecal Excessive sweating	Maceration of skin Maceration of skin Pyrexia	Monitor incontinence Treat underlying cause, use barrier cream Minimal bed covers, rest, use fans, tepid sponges, natural fibres in night clothes
Personal hygiene and dressing	Incontinent patient Not washed and dried Use of soap Excessive sweating with pendulous breasts	Maceration of skin Maceration of skin Dried skin Two moist skin surfaces together	Keep patient clean and dry Change bedlinen as necessary Use barrier creams, avoid using soap if possible Keep skin surfaces apart, use supporting bra (cotton)
Sleeping	Lack of movement	Heavy sedation	Change position 2-hourly for those 'at risk' or as necessary

Table 6.6 (*cont'd*)

Activity	At-risk factor	Cause	Management
Sexuality	Nylon nightdress Catheter	Static → sweating Pressure	Use cotton nightdress Use correct type of catheter Observe positioning of catheter and drainage bags
Dying	Malignancy Shock Elderly	Increased malignancy leading to hypoxia Peripheral circulatory failure Dry inelastic skin ↑ Risk of incontinence Lack of mobility	Encourage good nutrition, change position as necessary Administer drugs as prescribed to improve circulation and hypoxia Use emollients, good nutrition Monitor and treat underlying cause Encourage exercise

Table 6.7   Assessment of a patient's risk of forming pressure sores*

Physical condition		Mental condition		Activity		Mobility		Incontinence	
Good	4	Alert	4	Ambulant	4	Full	4	Not incontinent	4
Fair	3	Apathetic	3	Walks with help	3	Slightly limited	3	Occasionally incontinent	3
Poor	2	Confused	2	Chairbound	2	Very limited	2	Usually – urine	2
Bad	1	Stuporous	1	Bed-fast	1	Immobile	1	Doubly incontinent	1

*Reproduced from Exton-Smith et al 1962.

Table 6.8   Treatment of pressure sore according to grade

Grade	Definition	Treatment
1	Redness of skin surface	Keep skin clear and dry Barrier cream may be applied
2	Break in skin surface with no damage to subcutaneous tissue	Clean with 0.9% saline and leave area exposed
3	Break in skin surface with some loss of subcutaneous tissue	Clean with 0.9% saline and cover with sterile occlusive dressing
4	Necrosis of skin and underlying tissues	Treat with desloughing agent and cover with non-adherent occlusive dressing

In addition to the specific treatment, regular pressure relief of the effected areas at least every 2 hours.

or lightning; or radiation due to exposure to sun, X-rays or nuclear energy.

The damage caused is related to the length of exposure and the intensity of the burning agent.

Epidemiology and aetiology

Those particularly at risk are the elderly, the young, patients who have hypoglycaemia due to diabetes, patients with neurological problems resulting in fits or falls or people under the influence of excessive alcohol or drugs.

Clinical features

A superficial burn destroys the epidermis, and appears red and dry. Pain is due to damage to the cutaneous nerve endings.

A partial thickness burn destroys the epidermis and part of the dermis and appears red and blistered. It causes pain due to the exposure of the nerve endings to the air.

A full thickness burn destroys the dermis and may be extended to the subcutaneous tissue, muscle or bone. The skin may appear white, brown or black and leathery. Often there is no pain present as the nerve endings have been destroyed.

Patient implications

The patient who has been burned is 'at risk' of developing dehydration, infection, pain, anxiety and respiratory problems.

Nursing role in differential diagnosis

The area of the burn may be calculated using Wallace's 'Rule of Nine' (Fig. 6.19). The difference in percentage due to age must be emphasized, for example a young child's head is 18% of the total body surface area whereas in an adult, the head equals only 9%. The depth of the burn will also be calculated before treatment is commenced. However it should be remembered that if the burn is electrical, the surface damage may appear small, but the damage to underlying tissues may be very severe.

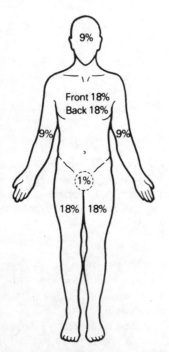

9%

Front 18%
Back 18%

9%   9%

1%

18%   18%

Fig. 6.19 Wallace's 'Rule of Nine' (Reproduced with permission from Colmer M R (ed) 1986)

Therapeutic management

First aid

If electricity is involved, the power should be switched off prior to any intervention. If the person's clothes have caught fire the flames should be smothered, ensuring the first aider remains safe. As in all emergency situations, ensure the airway is clear, the victim is breathing and his circulation is adequate. The burned or scalded area should be submerged in a container of cold water or put under running cold water for at least 10 minutes (**DO NOT APPLY ICE**). The wound may then be covered in a clean cloth or cling film before taking the victim to hospital.

Nursing strategies

On admission, the patient will require opiates to relieve the pain and anxiety, and fluids will be given to replace those lost. The volume of fluid to be replaced is calculated using a specific formula.

The nurse will assess the condition of the patient, taking particular note of respiratory function (respiratory rate, depth and ease of breathing), circulatory function (blood pressure and pulse; colour of the skin; the amount of fluid lost and urine output), the extent of the area and depth of the burn and the psychological state and conscious level.

The aim of the treatment is to relieve pain and discomfort, prevent complications such as shock, infection, renal failure, respiratory failure, cardiac failure, drastic weight loss and/or contractures, help the patient and family adjust to his altered body image and commence rehabilitation as soon as possible (Nursing Care Plan 6.2).

As most cases of burn injuries are preventable, community staff, such as district nurses and health visitors, may observe hazards in the home and have a duty to prevent accidents by educating their clients to the hazards.

Patient education

Prevention of accidents and first aid should be included as part of the curriculum of all school children. Regular advertising via television, magazines, newspapers and billboards should also highlight potential hazards and how to deal with them.

INFECTIONS

Infections of the skin may be caused by bacteria, viruses, fungi, parasites and mites.

Nursing Care Plan 6.2 Care plan for a patient with burns			
Problem	**Goal**	**Nursing action**	**Rationale**
1. Difficulty with breathing	Maintain an adequate airway Arterial blood gases within normal limits Breathing sounds clear	❐ Observe respirations Check smell of breath ❐ Administer humidified oxygen if prescribed Care of endotracheal tube if in place ❐ Suction if required Encourage expectoration Check pulse Assist with activities of daily living	Impairment of respiration due to inhalation of smoke, fumes or flames Hypoxia as a result of decrease in RBCs, hypotension, pain or shock Oedema of face or neck may lead to obstruction of respiration May require intermittent positive pressure ventilation Severe chest burns may lead to restriction of chest movement due to eschar Hypoxia causes tachycardia (due to hypovolaemia)
2. Impaired communication	To improve communication	❐ Ask simple, closed questions Adapt a code (one hand squeezed for yes, two for no) Include the family Provide paper or a 'magic' pad for patient to write on	If patient is unable to talk, e.g. due to an endotracheal tube in situ, patient can still understand what is happening Care will be improved if you have the co-operation of the patient and his family Allows patient to express his feelings and maintain independence
3. Alteration in fluid balance	To maintain an adequate fluid intake	❐ Assess dehydration Maintain and monitor intravenous fluids (usually via a central line) As per formula (from time of accident) Weigh patient daily Monitor vital signs	Fluid is lost: • from circulating blood volume • by an increased permeability and dilatation of capillaries, shifting fluid into the interstitial spaces • as plasma protein seep into tissues there is a reduction in intravascular colloidal osmotic pressure resulting in generalised oedema Amount of fluid adjusted according to haematocrit levels and urine output Body weight is more accurate for assessing fluid status than intake and output As circulating volume decreases BP ↓ and cardiac output is reduced
4. Alteration in electrolyte balance	To maintain an adequate electrolyte balance	❐ Maintain intravenous fluids (containing sodium chloride and potassium as prescribed)	Damaged tissues release potassium Loss of fluids through wound and oedema lose electrolytes Sodium retention and potassium loss in urine due to stress
5. Alteration in urinary output a. Caused by decrease in urinary volume b. Caused by increase in urinary output	To maintain an adequate output To maintain an adequate output	❐ Monitor hourly urine volumes (per catheter) ❐ Observe output	Urinary output decreased due to: • hypovolaemia and hypotension • renal tubular damage may result in shock phase • increased protein breakdown from damaged tissues, especially muscle, results in renal failure 2–3 days after injury fluid is no longer lost in tissues Too much fluid will lead to overload (see cardiac failure)

Nursing Care Plan 6.2 (cont'd)

Problem	Goal	Nursing action	Rationale
6. Nausea, vomiting and gastric distension	To relieve nausea, vomiting and gastric distension	❏ If necessary, pass nasogastric tube, aspirate 4 hourly or as required	Gastrointestinal peristalsis is greatly decreased, leading to paralytic ileus
7. Alteration in nutrition due to loss of plasma proteins	To improve and maintain nutritional state	❏ Give 100 ml of fluid hourly if tolerated Remove nasogastric tube ❏ Increase intake from fluids through soft foods to normal diet, rich in proteins, carbohydrates, iron and vitamins; given as small, frequent meals, with protein supplements	Thirst is a common complaint with burned patients, but oral fluids and food may be restricted for 24–48 hours for patients with severe burns When bowel sounds have returned and clear fluid is tolerated Protein necessary for tissue repair, e.g. plasma proteins, skin and blood cells, carbohydrates for energy, iron to help RBC formation, vitamin C is necessary for synthesis of corticosteriods and tissue repair Malnutrition increases risk of complications
8. Difficulty with eating	To encourage and enable patient to feed himself	❏ Provide adapted equipment Provide privacy if desired	To maintain self-esteem Patient may be embarrassed if they have difficulties
9. Loss of appetite	To regain normal appetite	❏ Find out patient's likes and dislikes Give mouth washes or clean teeth before and after meals Present food attractively and at the correct temperature Use charcoal and deodorizers to mask unpleasant smells	More likely to eat food he likes A dirty mouth discourages eating Food at the wrong temperature is unappetizing Obnoxious smells can affect the appetite
10. Impaired mobility caused by decreased strength	To maintain body alignment	❏ Explain procedure to patient Support limbs, use splints and aids appropriately Change position 2–3 hourly	Co-operation of patient necessary as correct alignment may be uncomfortable To prevent contractures and promote healing Patient unable to move himself
11. Contractures	Prevent contractures and restore normal function of limbs To decrease oedema of burnt extremities	❏ Encourage range of movement (ROM) exercises ❏ Elevate limb Use aids appropriately Ambulate as soon as possible	Position of comfort may encourage contractures Encourages lymphatic and venous drainage Inappropriate equipment may cause further damage and be expensive Lack of mobility causes: • boredom • constipation • urinary problems • increased risk of pressure sores • muscle atrophy • loss of calcium from bones

Nursing Care Plan 6.2 (cont'd)

Problem	Goal	Nursing action	Rationale
12. Potential for infection a. Skin	Suppress the growth of bacteria	❏ Good handwashing technique by all staff and visitors	Prevents cross-infection
		Expose the burnt area to the air	Allows observation of wound Speeds up drying process (bacteria thrive on moisture) Coagulation of serum prevents heat loss
	Promote separation of dead tissue and new growth		Speeding up tissue regeneration and limits degree of scar tissue formation
		❏ Gentle cleaning of wound for dirt and sloughing skin	Avoid damage of viable tissue against infection
		Maintain room temperature at 28–34°C	
		Nurse on sterile sheet and use cradle to support top sheets and blankets	Patient's immune system depressed
		Nurse in protective isolation Clean perianal area well, especially after bowel movements	Patient's own intestinal flora may be main cause of infection (wound and urinary tract infections UTI)
b. Urinary tract infection	To prevent development of urinary tract infection	❏ Use strict aseptic technique if catheterizing	Catheterization is a major cause of UTI
		Maintain fluid intake to 3 litres in 24 hours	Prevents urinary stasis
		Administer prescribed antibiotics, and monitor effects	Nurse should be aware of potential side-effects of antibiotics
13. Shock	To prevent shock	❏ Establish baseline observations of temperature, pulse, respiration and blood pressure Observe vital signs as per chart Observe skin colour Observe conscious level, restlessness/anxiety Observe urinary output	In early stages pulse will be rapid and thready; blood pressure normal to begin with but will fall if shock progresses; respiratory rate faster and shallower; temperature falls (may also be due to loss of skin surface causing hypothermia) or rises due to infection (In the state of irreversible shock blood pressure, pulse, temperature and respiration and urinary output will all fall)
14. Anxiety a. About hospitalization	To reduce emotional distress Patient accepts hospitalization and understands the aims of treatment and rehabilitation	❏ Assess patient's level of knowledge Explain routine, drugs, procedures, therapy and rehabilitation	Lack of knowledge may increase anxiety The co-operation of the patient is necessary as the length of hospitalization may be long and the treatment painful/uncomfortable
b. About potential disfigurement	To accept disfigurement To compensate for disfigurement	❏ Encourage patient to look at and touch scars	Patient and relatives will accept disfigurement more easily if the staff explain that the scars will look better as time goes on
c. About loss of control	Patient maintains his dignity	❏ Encourage patient and family to discuss problems All treatments discussed with patient Encourage patient to carry out activities of daily living with help as required from staff or family	Most people have never been in hospital before and look to the staff for guidance In early stages the patient might be disinclined to do much for himself and rely on the staff for decision making, they must encourage the patient to maintain control of his treatment

Nursing Care Plan 6.2 (*cont'd*)

Problem	Goal	Nursing action	Rationale
d. About pain	To relieve pain	❑ Administer prescribed analgesics Discuss pain and how it will be controlled	Only partial and superficial burns will cause pain, full thickness burns destroy nerve endings but patients may expect pain and therefore will feel it
e. About discharge from hospital	Patient demonstrates a positive attitude to rehabilitation	❑ Explain exercises, diet and community resources	Discharge should be planned with the patient, family and community support as well as the hospital staff

Bacterial infections

Epidemiology and aetiology

Debilitated patients, diabetics and anyone who has a cut or laceration is at greater risk of developing bacterial infections of the skin. Staphylococci may cause boils (furuncles), carbuncles, impetigo and cellulitis. Impetigo may occur when hygiene is poor. Cellulitis is a complication of skin ulcers, wounds or dermatitis. Streptococci may also be responsible for cellulitis or impetigo as well as erysipelas.

Clinical features

A boil is a common infection of hair follicles, appearing as a hard, red, painful nodule which ruptures and discharges pus. It then becomes necrotic before healing and becoming a purple macule. Boils may appear on the face, hands, neck or buttocks. A carbuncle involves a group of hair follicles, and appears as a large, red, painful nodule which discharges pus. The area between the hair follicles becomes necrotic and a layer of slough develops. This area, when discharged, may leave a deep, purulent ulcer, with the patient developing a high fever, malaise and toxaemia.

Impetigo is an itchy, contagious condition characterized by erythematous macules; they become discharging vessels which can be seen on the face, arms and legs of children and teenagers. It is caused by a streptococcal infection.

Erysipelas is caused by Group A streptococcus. The face and around the ears appear bright red and tender with a sharply defined, bordered plaque which may develop into vesicles or bullae. It is usually found in the very young and elderly and may last 2–3 weeks.

Cellulitis is a widespread inflammatory condition caused by gram-negative bacteria. The patient has an extensive erythema which is very tender and oedematous, malaise, fever and enlarged lymph nodes.

Patient implications

Approximately 5% of patients with streptococcal impetigo are at risk of developing post streptococcal glomerular nephritis (see Ch. 17). To prevent this complication it is essential that antibiotics are taken as prescribed and that the whole course is taken.

When a person has a history of frequent outbreaks of boils, they should have their blood and urine tested for sugar, as diabetics are prone to boils.

Nursing role in differential diagnosis

The nurse should pay particular attention to any previous history of skin infection in the patient and close friends or relatives. The patient's living conditions may also be relevant.

The nurse will take swabs from the affected areas and send them to the laboratories for culture and sensitivity before antibiotics are commenced. Blood cultures may also be taken.

Therapeutic management

Antibiotics, either oral or parenteral, will be prescribed for most bacterial infections.

Boils and carbuncles may be treated by moist heat locally applied, for example a kaolin poultice, to draw and drain the pus out, thus relieving the pressure and consequent discomfort. A cool, wet dressing will give relief. The crusts of impetigo may be removed with a warm saline solution and erythromycin soaks applied as prescribed.

Viral infections

Viruses produce local lesions, and may cause a widespread reaction to infection. The common viral infections include warts (verrucae), herpes simplex (cold sores) and herpes zoster (shingles).

Epidemiology and aetiology

Warts, especially of the hands and feet, are a common occurrence in children. Many warts are self limiting to weeks, months or years because of spontaneous evolution. Plantar warts (verruca on soles of feet) are spread by people using communal changing rooms and showers in recreational facilities. Genital warts are spread by sexual contact.

Herpes simplex may recur following reactivation by heat, cold, stress, sunlight or menstruation.

Herpes zoster occurs in people who have been initially infected with the varicella virus (chickenpox). The virus lies dormant in the dorsal root of the cranial or spinal ganglia, with 50% of patients having ophthalmic involvement. The dormant virus may be triggered by stress.

Clinical features

Warts of hands and feet appear as plaques of hyperkeratinized tissue, and may be single or clustered. Genital warts look flat or cauliflower like and occur in the anogenital area.

Herpes simplex appear as small, painful blisters which become pustular before crusting. They occur frequently around the mouth, and last between five and eight days.

In herpes zoster, the pain along the nerve pathway frequently precedes the appearance of the vesicles which also become pustular and crust. The most frequent nerves affected are the ophthalmic division of the trigeminal nerve and the thoracic nerves (T5–T10).

Investigations

Scrapings from lesions may be taken for culture and sensitivity, but history and careful physical examination are usually sufficient.

Patient implications

People using communal changing rooms and showers should be encouraged to dry their feet well to prevent the spread of verrucae. Those with verrucae should wear waterproof footwear in swimming pool areas.

Patients with genital warts should attend a genitourinary outpatient department for treatment as other sexually transmitted diseases may be present.

Immunosuppressed patients should have no contact with patients with herpes simplex or zoster as in their case it could be fatal.

Therapeutic management

Warts on hands and feet may be painted with salicyclic acid or cryosurgery may be carried out. The lesions of herpes simplex may be kept dry by 70% alcohol solution. If herpes viruses are diagnosed early enough, acyclovir will be prescribed for all patients with good effect. In immunosuppressed patients who develop herpes, they will require acyclovir, interferon and zoster immune globulin. Analgesics may be given to all patients with herpes zoster. Carbamazepine may be used to treat trigeminal neuralgia following herpes zoster infection.

Nursing strategies

Patients will be assessed to determine who can be treated in the ward/department and which patients should be referred to other departments for treatment. For example, the ophthalmic clinic will treat lesions affecting the eye, the genitourinary clinic for genital herpes simplex and warts, the pain clinic for intractable pain due to herpes zoster.

The aim of the treatment of the patient with herpes zoster is: to relieve pain by analgesics and calamine; prevent secondary infections, cross-infections for example to the eye; provide rest; nourishing diets, and ensure that patients have natural fibres next to their skin and light bedclothes are used.

Fungal infections

The superficial fungal infections are caused by the yeast fungus candida (monilia or thrush) or by dermatophyte fungi (tinea or ringworm).

Epidemiology and aetiology

Certain factors increase the risk of a patient acquiring fungal infections: a hot, humid environment; macerated skin from occlusive dressings or clothing; drugs such as antibiotics, corticosteriods or contraceptives; hormonal changes due to diabetes; Cushing's syndrome; pregnancy, or poor general health. The presence of leukaemia, cytotoxic therapy, HIV-related illnesses and other disorders which cause immuno-suppression greatly increase the risk of a patient developing fungal infections of the skin and mucous membranes.

Clinical features

Candida, mainly *Candida albicans*, affects the mouth, female genital area, skin folds and areas of skin around the nails. In the mouth, white patches appear which can be easily scraped off. In the vagina, there is a creamy discharge with acute pruritus. The skin folds appear as bright red, well-defined patches with a scaly edge, sometimes moist and weeping.

Ringworm infections affect all parts of the body and appear as scaly plaques with erythema. In tinea pedis (athletes' foot) there is scaling, maceration and fissures at the toe web. When ringworm affects the scalp or beard there may be hair loss.

Patient implications

Anyone who has their hands frequently in water is advised to wear gloves to prevent maceration of their skin.

Shoes and clothing should be kept aerated, and the use of cotton and other natural fibres encouraged. Sensitive areas such as under the breasts, genital areas and the feet should be carefully dried after washing.

Therapeutic management

Fungal infections may be treated with nystatin, clo-trimazole (Canestan) or miconazole (Daktarin) locally or griseofulvin orally. Drug compliance is vital, therefore the patient should have a good knowledge of the effects of the drugs and for how long they will have to be taken.

Nursing strategies

Since fungal infections may be prevented, the role of the nurse is to assess which patients are at risk and carry out preventative measures (see above). Good hygiene is essential in prevention and care of fungal infections.

Skin infestations

Infestations of the skin include mites such as the scabies mite (*Acarus scabei*) and pediculosis (head, body and pubic lice).

Epidemiology and aetiology

Scabies and head lice occur frequently in children whose hands and head come in close contact with other children. Scabies and body lice are associated with crowded and/or poor living conditions, whereas head lice favour clean hair, females more than males. The louse lives on blood which it obtains four to five times a day. Body lice lay their eggs in the seams of clothing. Pubic lice are mainly spread through sexual contact.

Clinical features

Scabies produce characteristic burrows which appear as thread-like lines on the wrists, hands, axillary folds, elbows and feet, resulting in an intense itch and rash.

In head infestations, the female louse lays six to eight eggs a day which are glued to the base of the hairs and appear pearly white. The eggs leave the shells (nits) and darken in colour (according to hair colour), reaching adulthood in about 10 days. They live up to 30 days. Intense itching, especially around the ears, will draw attention to the lice and nits. Body lice also cause intense scratching, mainly in the area of clothing seams as the louse mainly goes to the body only to eat, preferring to live in the clothes. The pubic louse is found in pubic hair or other hairs of the body, causing itching and scratching.

Patient implications

As all members of the family and close contacts may be affected with scabies or pediculosis, they will all have to be treated. In body lice, the clothes need to be treated (by drying in a tumble dryer for at least 15 minutes, fumigation, washing in very hot water or dry cleaning). As the bites from the louse result in the deposition of foreign protein, and eventual sensitization, rashes and secondary infections such as impetigo may occur. Early diagnosis and treatment is important to prevent progressive illness.

Therapeutic management

Benzyl benzoate or benzene hexachloride (Lorexane) is applied all over (from the neck down) for a period of 8–12 hours, after which the patient has a bath. This procedure is usually repeated a week later. Calamine lotion may be applied to sooth the itch.

As head lice may become resistant to treatment, many areas (public health officers) recommend a programme which rotates the treatment annually (or every 3 years) while others will use one of the treatments until resistance occurs. The two main treatments are malathion (Prioderm, Dermac) and carbaryl (Carylderm). The lotion is applied to the hair and scalp to kill the lice and eggs (but will not remove the nits). The hair can be combed out the next day with a fine tooth comb.

Nursing strategies

In assessing infestations the nurse must be aware of the areas affected and the most appropriate treatment necessary. The patient and family's co-operation is necessary for treatment and eradication, therefore the nurse must explain the diagnosis and treatment in a sympathetic manner, taking great care not to destroy the person's self-respect.

In implementing care the nurse must ensure she is not at risk of catching the infestation herself.

Patient education

Campaigns to decrease the incidence of head pediculosis need to involve the whole community, especially schools, nurseries and playgroups. The full co-operation of the teachers as well as the parents is necessary.

Health education should help to remove the stigma and misconceptions from pediculosis and scabies, encouraging good hygiene and allowing an open discussion regarding the disease and its treatment.

Eczema/dermatitis

Eczema and dermatitis are synonymous, but some of the conditions seem more closely associated with one name.

Epidemiology and aetiology

Atopic eczema occurs in young children, and is more common in families where there is a history of asthma or hay fever. Seborrhoeic dermatitis in babies is called cradle cap and while it can occur at any age, it most commonly effects teenagers and may resolve spontaneously at maturation.

Varicose dermatitis is seen in the older population.

Clinical features

In the early stages of dermatitis, the skin appears red and inflamed, before developing minute blisters which may swell and burst. The patient may complain of intense itching, which may also be painful.

Atopic eczema affects the face before spreading to other parts of the body. The skin is dry and itchy, progressing to red, weeping patches which are susceptible to infection. Flexures may thicken and, because of the itch and scratching, become lichenified. The symptoms tend to improve gradually but may reappear in adolescence.

Seborrhoeic dermatitis is found in the face, scalp, upper trunk or between two skin surfaces or areas where sebaceous glands are concentrated. It appears as macules and papules which may be dry or greasy, giving the area an erythematous appearance, which may be itchy.

Contact dermatitis may be either primary irritant or allergic. In primary contact dermatitis, an inflammatory reaction is seen immediately on the skin when it comes in contact with the irritant. In allergic contact dermatitis, at last one previous contact with the allergen is required before the host develops a sensitivity. The skin eruptions appear within 12–48 hours, depending on the strength of the allergen, timespan or exposure and development of immunity. In both, the skin appears erythematous with papules developing into vesicles which burst or dry up and crust.

Varicose dermatitis is associated with venous stasis, when the skin around the ankles becomes fragile, reddish in colour, developing a speckled appearance due to small blood vessels bursting. The skin is very itchy, and is at great risk of breaking down. A varicose ulcer may quickly follow varicose dermatitis.

Investigations

Patch testing may be carried out to identify allergies.

Therapeutic management

Topical applications are required for dermatitis. Emulsifying ointments and aqueous creams are used to treat dryness, whilst topical steroids of different strengths may be required for active areas.

Oral preparations, such as trimetheniramine (Vallergan), may be used for their antipruritic effects, with the added benefit if used at night of sedating the patient.

If there is a secondary infection, local antibiotics may be applied, with oral preparations being used occasionally.

Psoriasis

Psoriasis may be due to a reduced control of epidermal cell division by the hypothalamus, resulting in a greatly increased cell division of epidermal cells. These cells may be replaced every 6 days or so instead of every 35–45 days. Psoriasis may go into remission, relapsing when a trigger such as stress, trauma or an infection occurs.

Epidemiology and aetiology

Approximately 2% of the population may be affected with psoriasis at some time in their life. Between 5% and 10% of patients with psoriasis have an associated arthritic condition.

Psoriasis can occur at any age but usually presents at adolescence, with equal prevalence in males and females. Although not a hereditary condition, there is a familial tendency.

Clinical features

Psoriasis commonly presents as sharply defined plaques with silvery scales. The lesions may be singular, groups or spread all over the body.

There are four main types of psoriasis:

1. Guttate mainly affects children and young adults following a streptococcal infection. The lesions are a few millimetres in diameter and spread all over the body.
2. Plaque is the commonest type with coin-like lesions spreading all over the body.
3. Flexural appears in areas where two skin surfaces are in contact, and is characterized by an erythematous reaction with no scales.
4. Pustular is a rare form, affecting mainly the soles of the feet. Lesions appear pustular, containing sterile pus.

Psoriasis may affect the nails in 50% of patients, when the nail appears thick and porous, and may become detached from the nail bed.

Patient implications

As with all skin disorders, psoriasis may affect the patient's whole life. Due to its appearance, some children can become very embarrassed and be loath to take part in sporting activities. Holidays may be affected with some hotels being less than sympathetic to people with the condition. Hairdressers may prove difficult if the scalp is affected. The choice of jobs may be limited, especially in the catering business. Periods of hospitalization can also have an effect on job prospects.

Special clothes should be kept for when the creams are applied. Patient compliance may be difficult due to the unpleasant treatments.

Therapeutic management

Treatment may be topical and/or systemic, depending on the severity of the condition.

Topical treatments include: tar baths; tar with salicylic acid; tar shampoo for scalps; dithranol which is applied to lesions and the remaining skin protected by talc or petroleum jelly. Dithranol is usually applied for periods of 20 minutes to an hour, or a weaker solution may be applied for 12–24 hours. Ultraviolet light can be also used with psoralens (PUVA). Psoralens such as methoxsalen are used 2 hours prior to ultraviolet therapy. Corticosteroids with or without polythene occlusions may occasionally be used. Natural sunlight improves psoriasis in most patients.

Systemic treatments include methotrexate which inhibits formation of new epithelium. It may be given orally, intramuscularly or intravenously (British National Formulary 1994). Etretinate is given for severe psoriasis, but is only used in hospitals or prescribed by a consultant dermatologist because of the side-effects.

Nursing strategies

Only when the lesions are severe or the patient's general condition warrants it, is the patient with psoriasis admitted to hospital. In some units, the patients may be treated daily in the outpatient department or admitted during the day or night (allowing the patient to continue working or studying), whilst others may have their dressings done by the community team.

In assessing the choice of treatment, the doctor, nurse and patient are involved. The patient's involvement increases compliance, as many of the treatments are uncomfortable and/or messy. Orem's Self-care Model would be suitable as it allows the nurse (with the family) to compensate for any deficit in the patient's self-care, and encourages the patient to have control over his own treatment. It is important to explain to the patient why you are wearing gloves to carry out the treatment (nurses are using many different ointments and creams throughout the day, and gloves help prevent sensitization). During the dressing, the nurse is able to listen to the patient and discuss problems if they arise. In evaluating the treatment the nurse should observe for improvement or deterioration in the lesions, and the patient's general condition.

Patient education

It must be stressed to the patient, family and general public that psoriasis is not contagious, infectious or dirty. The treatment should be explained to the patient. If using dithranol it must be explained that the dark staining on the skin will disappear in a few weeks but clothes may be permanently stained.

Acne

Acne is characterized by an increased production of sebum, with a blockage in the pilosebaceous follicles and a plug of keratinized skin which results in blackheads (comedones).

Epidemiology and aetiology

Acne is less common in sunny climates. It mainly affects teenagers. The condition may be due to an increase in androgens, which results in an increased number of sebaceous glands, and therefore an increase in sebum production. Drugs such as androgens, corticosteroids and phenytoin may induce acne, as may chemicals (chlorinated naphthalenes) used in the rubber industry.

Clinical features

Acne mainly affects the face, neck, upper back and chest. Early on, blackheads (coloured by melanin, not dirt) appear due to blockage of the hair follicles by dried sebum and keratin. Superficial papules follow (due to sebaceous glands distending), which may become infected causing pain and nodular formation.

Patient implications

The media and advertisements portray most people with no imperfections – beautiful skin, hair and body. Most people are susceptible to this advertising and teenagers are no exception. Those who develop acne or suffer from other skin complaints may become self-conscious and become reluctant to socialize. The nurse can encourage a positive self-image, and remind the client that beauty is only skin deep, and encourage him/her to emphasize their positive attributes.

Therapeutic management

Treatment is aimed at preventing more acne from developing, by preventing the formation of plugs and preventing the growth of pathogenic bacteria. In mild acne, skin detergents, for example cetrimides, antiseptics, keratolytics (peeling agents) and topical antibiotics, may be used. In moderate to severe acne, oral antibiotics such as erythromycin, as well as benzoyl peroxide or tretinonin, may be used. These treatments may have to be given for many months and this must be carefully explained to the patient.

Diet (including chocolate and fatty foods) does not seem to influence acne.

Nursing management

As few patients are admitted to hospital with acne, the nurse's role is limited. The nurse can explain the causes, and treatments required, and help the patient adjust to an alteration in body image and boost his self-esteem.

SKIN TUMOURS

These may be either benign, premalignant or malignant.

Epidemiology and aetiology

Malignant tumours, notably malignant melanoma, are on the increase. This may be due to the increased number of people taking holidays in sunny climates, wearing minimal clothing and the increased use of sunbeds.

Malignant melanomas are caused by short blasts of exposure to the sun, while other malignancies seem to be caused by continued sun exposure, such as those found in farmers, outdoor workers and sailors. Caucasians are ten times more likely to develop skin malignancies than dark-skinned persons, with those with fair hair at greatest risk. In the UK approximately five in 100 000 are affected while in Australia 40 in 100 000 are affected by malignant melanoma, with the survival rate after 5 years following surgery being 68%.

Irritation may also lead to a malignancy; for example, tumour of the lip as found in pipe smokers. Tumours of the skin, while found in all age ranges, are more frequently seen in the older patient, especially in seborrhoeic warts (non-malignant), and squamous cell and basal cell carcinomas.

Clinical features

In seborrhoeic warts (basal cell papilloma) the lesions are raised and palpable, either single or multiple, and mainly found on the trunk and face.

Basal cell carcinomas (rodent ulcers) are the most frequent cancer of the skin, appearing on the face and trunk. They begin as a nodule, spreading outwards, giving a central depression and looking 'pearly'. They do not normally metastasize and may be singular or multiple.

Squamous cell carcinomas appear as papules or nodules with an irregular border and may be either single or multiple. Malignant melanomas may start off as a mole or appear spontaneously. Squamous cell carcinomas and malignant melanomas may metastasize.

Investigations

Skin scrapings for cytology may be taken, or the tumour may be removed without prior biopsy.

Therapeutic management

Surgery by curettage or the use of liquid nitrogen may be used for benign tumours. Surgery or radiotherapy, depending on number and size, will be used for basal and squamous cell carcinomas. Malignant melanomas require a large area to be excised with/without radiotherapy.

Nursing strategies

Preoperative treatment and postoperative care will be given by the nurse. The nurse's main role will be in educating the public about preventing the development of malignant skin conditions and advising the individual patient on health care and follow-up. Because of the mortality rate in malignant melanomas, nurses will be required to assess the patient's emotional state as well as his physical state. In planning the patient's care the nurse and patient will be aware of the difficulties associated with mutilation, recurrence of the disease and its effect on the patient's life-style. This thoughtful approach will enable the nurse to carry out the necessary care using a holistic approach.

Patient education

Everyone should be aware of the dangers of sunlight. Whilst on holiday in hot climates, exposure to the sun should be limited to 15 minutes on the first day, gradually increasing exposure, depending on skin colouring. Avoid exposure to the sun between 11.00 a.m. and 3.00 p.m.

Advice which is given to the Australians includes: slip on a top, slap on a hat and slop on a sunscreen!

To decrease the mortality of malignant melanomas, it is essential to start treatment early. If patients recognize changes in size, colour or shape of moles, or if they are itchy, bleed or crust, they should seek medical guidance promptly. If three or more changes are present a dermatologist's appointment should be speedily arranged. Material on preventing and recognizing aspects of skin malignancies should be freely available to the general public using posters, magazine articles and leaflets readily available in GP surgeries or at travel agents.

COMPLEMENTARY THERAPIES

Nurses are taught that the holistic approach to care is best for the patient. Recently there has been an increased awareness of the use of complementary therapies which also believe in the holistic approach. Among the wide varieties of complementary therapies available, nurses appear particularly interested in aromatherapy, massage and reflexology. These have a close relationship with our senses. Aromatherapy uses essential oils in a variety of ways, with different oils used to treat different complaints (e.g. camomile for inflamed skin, eucalyptus for influenza and lavender for suppressed physical immunity). The essential oils are well diluted in a vegetable oil and massaged into the skin, allowing the oils to penetrate the skin and be inhaled; the patient benefits from the touch and smell. As the smell seems to be an important factor the oils sprayed around the patient or put in the bath are also beneficial.

Massage can be of benefit in relaxing the patient or relieving areas of swelling. The use of stroking, kneading or striking will depend on the effect wanted, as well as choice of speed and depth of massage.

Reflexology (or reflex zone therapy) helps reduce stress in the body, working with the body's own healing processes to achieve a state of well-being by using pressure on certain parts of the feet (and hands). In reflexology the body is divided into ten longitudinal zones, with an energy link between all parts of the body, and the appropriate zone found in the foot. By applying pressure to the appropriate part of the foot, the equivalent zone may have its energy flow restored to the correct balance.

With all forms of complementary therapy, the nurse must be aware not only when they can be of benefit but, as importantly, when it would be dangerous to use these therapies. For example, massage should

---

Suggested assignments

Ethical dilemmas

1. It is not a statutory requirement for practitioners of complementary therapies to hold a recognized qualification. Discuss the implications for the health care professionals whose patient is receiving treatment which may be harmful.

2. As the nurse allocated to care for a young child suffering from severe scalds, you overhear the parents discussing the accident which makes you think it wasn't an accident. How will you deal with this?

3. Many eye injuries are a result of participation in amateur sports.
   Should it be compulsory in sports such as squash for participants to wear head and eye protection? How could such a regulation be enforced?

4. The number of cases of skin cancer is on the increase. The people at greatest risk are those with fair skins, particularly if they have been exposed to strong sunlight as a child.
   Should skin protection creams and lotions be provided on the NHS? What would be the implications of such a decision?

5. Identify the key issues for an education programme needed to enable a person who becomes blind or deaf to maintain an active, independent lifestyle in safety. Outline how this programme might be implemented.

---

not be used in active inflammation, cancer, bleeding or infections. Before using any treatment, the practitioner should have a good knowledge of the therapy and possess a recognized qualification. Such a qualification, acquired following a period of registered nursing or midwifery practice, could be a valuable adjunct to the skills which can be offered to many patients and their families, as nurses extend their role, and care becomes increasingly a matter of partnership between client and carers.

REFERENCES AND FURTHER READING

Aggleton P, Chalmers H 1985 Orem's self care model. Nursing Times 81(1): 36–39

Aggleton P, Chalmers H 1986 Nursing models and the nursing process. Macmillan, London

Baggerly J 1991 Sensory perceptual problems following stroke. Nursing Clinics of North America 26(4): 997–1005

Barry-Shevlin 1987 Maintaining sensory balance for the critically ill patient. Nursing April 3(16): 597–601

Biley F C 1993 Impact of noise on surgical wards. Surgical Nurse 6(1): 15–17

Bowie I 1990 Wounds to the eye. Nursing 4(15): 24–27

British Medical Association and Royal Pharmaceutical Society of Great Britain 1994 British national formulary. BMA/RPSGB, London

Chawla H B 1993 Ophthalmology, 2nd edn. Churchill Livingstone, Edinburgh

Colmer M J (ed) 1986 Moroney's surgery for nurses. Churchill Livingstone, Edinburgh

Davis P 1989 Aromatherapy an A–Z Daniel, Essex C W

Dealey C 1993 Role of hydrocolloids in wound management. British Journal of Nursing 2(7): 358–365

Exton-Smith et al 1962 An investigation of geriatric nursing problems in hospital. National Corporation for the Care of Old People. Churchill Livingstone, Edinburgh

Forrest A P M, Carter D C, MacLeod I B 1991 Principles and practices of surgery, 2nd edn. Churchill Livingstone, Edinburgh

Laurence D R, Bennett P N 1992 Clinical pharmacology, 7th edn. Churchill Livingstone, Edinburgh

Leaper D 1986 Leg ulcers: antiseptics and their effects on healing tissue. Nursing Times 82(22): 45–47

Marieb E 1989 Human anatomy and physiology. Benjamin/Cummings, Redwood City

Marquardt H 1983 Reflex zone therapy of the feet. Thorsons, London

Maxwell-Hudson C 1988 The complete book of massage. Dorling Kindesley, London

Moore T 1989 Sensory deprivation in the ICU. Nursing 3(36): 44–47

Morgan D 1992 Formulary of wound management products: a guide for health care staff, 5th edn. Media Medica, Chichester

Morison M 1987 Priorities in wound management Part 2. Professional Nurse 2(12): 402–411

Morison M 1992 A colour guide to the nursing management of wounds. Wolfe, London, pp. 33–55

Perry J P, Tullo A B (eds) 1990 Care of the ophthalmic patient: a guide for nurses and health professionals. Chapman & Hall, London

Pritchard A, David J 1988 Royal Marsden Hospital manual of clinical nursing policies and procedures. Harper and Row, London

Ramsden R 1992 Cochlear implantation (Update) 44(11): 1038–1048

Roper N, Logan W W, Tierney A J 1985 The elements of nursing, 2nd edn. Churchill Livingstone, Edinburgh

Saint John Ambulance Association and Brigade & Saint Andrew's Ambulance Association 1992 First aid manual. Dorling Kindersley, London

Tisserand R 1988 Aromatherapy for everyone. Penguin, London

Torrance C, Milligan S 1985 Olfactory disorders: on the scent. Nursing Times 81(28) p. 45

Tortora G, Anagnostakos N 1987 Principles of anatomy and physiology. Harper and Row, London

Turner T et al 1985 Advances in wound management. Wiley, Chichester

Waterlow J 1985 A risk assessment card. Nursing Times 81(48): 49–55

7

Care implications of disorders of learning

John Davidson

INTRODUCTION

This chapter provides an outline of mental handicaps, now called learning difficulties, and their implications in nursing care. It is not intended to be all inclusive or exhaustive but merely to provide an insight so that interest may be stimulated to encourage further reading in the subject.

Care for people with learning difficulties is given in a variety of settings, ranging from care in the family home, care in community units such as hostels to care in hospitals. Today there is much emphasis on the discharge of residents from hospital units to community units. Many larger hospitals are decreasing in size therefore more individuals with learning difficulties are being rehabilitated back into the community. Hospitals now tend to offer more specialized care and the need for skilled community staff is increasing.

It is possible that someone with a learning difficulty may require medical or surgical care in an acute set-up. This chapter provides the non-specialist nurse with guidelines on the adaptation of care to take account of the patient's particular needs. Some of the skills required in the care of people with learning difficulties may be relevant and adapted to care for other client groups.

HISTORY OF MENTAL HANDICAP CARE

Until the industrial revolution and the increase in technology, the birth of a child with limited learning capacity was of minor significance. The wide social divide enabled wealthy families to support these 'weak-minded' members out of the public eye. The vast amount of unskilled work required enabled those from poorer families that grew to adulthood to earn their share of a family's income. In those days, many of today's causes of mental handicap, infection and trauma in particular would have led to early death (Heaton Ward 1984).

As literacy and more technical employment increased in society the development of the middle classes with a limited ability to hide their less able members led to the creation of asylums, usually outside towns and with varying degrees of concern for the welfare of occupants and quality of care provided.

By the turn of the century it was believed that people with learning disabilities deserved more than a life of confinement, regimentation and idleness, and that they should be provided with education and training to enable them to develop some functional skills and contribute in part to society, even if in a controlled environment.

Many attempts were made to bring legislation before parliament which would control asylums and lay down rules and regulations. Most failed and it wasn't until 1890 that the Lunacy Act, after years of activity by pressure groups, successfully arrived on the statute book. Prior to this, individuals with learning difficulties were treated as less than human. The act, however, proved to be long winded and a disappointment. It concerned itself with matters of detention, care and release from care, and had little scope for development. Unfortunately, it made no distinction between the mentally ill and the mentally retarded.

In 1899 the Elementary Education Act (Defective and Epileptic Children) empowered local authorities to set up special schools for these children and raised the school leaving age to 16. As these provisions were only recommendations local authorities chose to ignore them even in the face of powerful advocates for total care.

The Royal Commission on the Care of the Feeble-Minded (1904–08) was given the task of looking at the needs of defectives. They recommended the formation of a central board to work in conjunction with the powerful local authorities

Following the recommendations of the Royal Commission, the Mental Deficiency Bill was formulated and became the Mental Deficiency Act in 1913. There were a number of categories on a rising scale, beginning at the lower end with idiots, then imbeciles and lastly the feeble minded. In 1927 a fourth category was added, that of moral defective. This differed from the others in kind, not degree. It allowed for the individual who showed some permanent mental defect coupled with strong vicious or criminal propensities, in which punishment had little or no effect, to be locked up in an institution for mental defectives.

Many young women were placed in institutions under this moral defective category because they had given birth to illegitimate children. The 1913 Act was supposed to be a milestone in the care of mental defectives but became a cumbersome millstone. The act was in force until 1959 when a new Mental Health Act was placed on the statute book in England and Wales, with similar legislation coming into force in Scotland in 1960.

Later, the Mental Health Act (1983) was passed; this concentrated upon much the same details as the 1959 Act. The term mental deficiency changed to mental handicap; part of this was again due to the influence of pressure groups to change the name because 'mental handicap' was thought to be less demeaning than 'mental defective' and could be perceived in ways similar to physical handicaps. Today, as a result of the work of pressure groups such as Barnardos and MENCAP, the title 'learning difficulties' is becoming more acceptable than the term 'mental handicap'.

The Royal Medico Psychological Association (RMPA) awarded certificates recognizing training for care of mentally handicapped persons. In 1919 the General Nursing Councils for England and Wales, Scotland and Northern Ireland were created by statute and a specialist branch of nurse training was established in 1924; in Scotland Registered Nurse for Mental Defectives (RNMD); in England and Wales Registered Nurse for Mental Sub-normality (RNMS). The RMPA certificate was amalgamated into the GNC certificate at this time. In 1929 the Local Authorities Act brought these asylums under the responsibility of local authorities and at the inception of the NHS in 1948 the care of these institutions was transferred into the medical domain.

In 1954 a Royal Commission on law relating to mental illness and mental deficiency recognised the need to distinguish between social welfare and care needs of the clients, and the joint functions which institutions had to fulfil which the welfare state had otherwise separated out. Social workers were to be employed to cater for welfare needs and nurses for physical and educational needs, the medical profession retaining overall responsibility.

The Commission concluded that there was a great need to change the approach to mental handicap nurse training to reflect an increased emphasis on community care, on education and training. The syllabus was to continue to emphasize the development of nursing skills, underlining the medicalization of the problems clients faced. Hospital services were also to raise the standards of existing services to improve the quality of life of those who continued to require institutionalized care. Smaller units were to be created within hospitals and skilled nurses were to be trained to provide family-centred care in community mental handicap teams.

From the late 1960s new training programmes were implemented to develop appropriately skilled practitioners and community mental handicap nursing courses were developed to meet the needs of the expanded role in community care settings.

As nurses are now working in more independent ways outwith institutions, the knowledge and skills developed must reflect this increased autonomy and consequent accountability. The development of philosophies of care and models of nursing by colleagues in general care areas have been utilized and adapted to meet the needs of people with learning disabilities. A systematic approach to care planning, the nursing process, enables individual patient needs to be identified and met in any setting.

The special needs of people with learning disabilities and their families are met through an understanding of physiology, psychology and sociology applied to skills in behaviourism, education, recreation and family-centred care.

LEARNING ABILITY AND DISABILITY

The capacity to learn from experience is fundamental to survival. Creatures can learn from personal experience – touch something hot, it burns, don't do it again – from observing others and practising the same skills – nest building, hunting for food. This innate capacity is called intelligence and in the so-called higher animals can extend into conceptual and abstract thought processes which enable previous knowledge to be applied to different situations and new experiences.

Innate intellectual capacity also depends on the capacity to recall the previous experience and learning ability is measured in terms of the time it takes for an individual to acquire new skills or knowledge. Thus all individuals can learn, but may have a learning disability if the speed and nature of their learning is inadequate to allow them to develop a level of autonomy and independence within their society.

Some kinds of ability, such as creativity, are distinct from learning ability, though their expression may be linked to other skills which require learning. Testing for learning ability or intelligence is the purpose of intelligence tests. However, because there is inevitably some cultural influence in the tests contents, an individual who has not had the opportunity to learn specific things may score low, which does not reflect his true learning ability. Similarly, physical disabilities such as deafness, visual impairment or co-ordination difficulties may impair learning and thus test results may be misleading.

Motivation to learn is also an important factor. Environmental factors which threaten physical survival are strong motivators, but in complex social and emotional environments there may be competing influences which affect learning. Thus the general ability reflected in an intelligence test may not match academic achievement or social or personal success within a given cultural environment.

INTELLIGENCE TESTING

In Western Europe, regular schooling for all began to show the differences in ability in populations previously masked by very varied backgrounds and expectations. It became clear that to enable all individuals to achieve their maximum potential, identification of 'backward' children would be helpful.

Around 1900, the French psychologist Binet began intelligence testing. He tried to find backward children in schools by creating a standardized test used under controlled conditions. His idea was taken up in America by the revision of the Binet test at Stanford University in 1916. This was known as the Stanford/ Binet test. The essential feature of intelligence testing is that it is comparative. Intelligence test scores are made in relation to other people in the same and other age groups on the same test. The Stanford/Binet test was revised in 1937 and is now usually known as the Terman Merrill test. By this time it was used to identify the highly intelligent as well as backward child. In Britain, the results determined the nature of secondary education to be offered. The comparative nature of intelligence testing led to the ideas of mental age (MA) and of the intelligence quotient.

Intelligence quotient

The intelligence quotient, or IQ, expresses intelligence as a ratio of mental age to chronological age:

$$IQ = \frac{\text{Mental age (MA)}}{\text{Chronological age (CA)}} \times 100$$

100 is used as a multiplier to remove the decimal point, also to make the IQ have a value of 100 when MA equals CA. If the MA lags behind the CA the resulting IQ will be less than 100, but if the MA is above the CA the IQ will be above 100. Binet devised a scale of units of MA, this scales intelligence with the kind of change that normally comes with growing older. A bright child's MA is above his/her CA; a dull child's MA is below his/her CA.

How far is intelligence universal and absolute? There are several important factors here:

1. **Age**. Intelligence increases with age up to 25 then declines. The IQ is a measurement related to age group; this will not change. This decline is in part due to declining cognitive structures or brain cell death and reflects difficulties in adult testing which are not sufficiently discriminating once a wide range of different knowledge and skills become part of an individual's functioning.

2. **Socioeconomic factors**. High IQ usually leads to a good job. Higher IQ types will thus tend to be in the higher social classes and vice versa. This does not mean that being in a lower social class will necessarily involve only low IQ individuals but might relate to attitudes to learning or experiences resulting in a lower IQ.

3. **Race and culture**. No IQ test is culture free. Most tests are based on physically normal, white, Christian, urban social groups with full opportunities. The only group such a test is valid for is that group alone. IQ testing until very recently was a very popular form of assessment. IQ testing was based on the concepts that:

a. intelligence can be measured like height, weight and can vary in amount or in rate of growth but is essentially stable

b. intelligence is determined by genes, like height, colour of hair, etc. Environmental influences were not considered important.

Initially, test scores were used to determine educational needs. Those scoring below 70 were considered mentally handicapped, and deemed to require special education provision.

Different terminology, mild, moderate, severe or profound retardation, was used to reflect the degree of impairment, the most severe assuming the individual to be uneducable. However, it has become evident that IQ test scores are an insufficient basis for classifying individuals and determining the education strategies to measure their future functioning in society.

The role of the environment and social conditions are now being given more importance in an effort to distinguish between normal, dull and subnormal functioning. The level of an individual's social competence – what he can do in his environment – is of greater significance. For example, a farm worker who is unable to finish school but can live independently as a hired hand is normal in his environment even though he may be recognizably dull. The same man might find it difficult to cope successfully in the city. Thus the distinction between dull, normal and subnormal is a complexity of the social conditions under which independence must be maintained. By changing the social criteria and/or moving from one place to another, individuals might change their classification. Psychological assessment based on an individual's behaviour and level of social competence was first introduced in 1959 with the concept of an individual's ability to adapt to environmental demands in a particular type of assessment which determines what an individual can and cannot do in his present environment. There are now various assessment procedures which utilize this concept; the best known are the Adaptive Behaviour Scales (ABS) and Progress Assessment Charts (PAC). Both these tools fulfil several functions:

1. They provide a profile of behaviour, skills level and coping strategies.

2. They provide a basis for diagnosis and classification of the underlying disorder.

3. They identify the individual's needs, enabling appropriate programme planning, training and behaviour modification.

4. They create a framework within which programme evaluation and individual progress may be assessed.

The Adaptive Behaviour Scale has items that cover personal care habits, eating skills, cleanliness, appearance, travel experiences, money handling and shopping skills. Such skills are essential for independent, socially acceptable functioning in the community. Maladaptive behaviours, for example violence, destructiveness or antisocial tendencies that may result in rejection by others, can be identified. These scales are most suitable for use with adults.

Progress Assessment Charts are available in different forms for children and adults. These were developed by Gunsberg between 1966 and 1977. There are six designed for client assessment to provide a data base for individual programme planning. For example, the Progress Assessment Chart 1 (PAC-1) was developed to assess the social development of children with learning difficulties between the ages of 6 and 16 years and provide a basis for programme planning and evaluation. The PAC-1 has four domains: communication, self-help, socialization and occupation. The first three domains have 40 items, the fourth has 20 items. The items mainly require a yes/no answer and can be represented in a chart of concentric circles, each circle representing a higher level of skill, the innermost circle being the very basic level. Someone familiar with the client's behaviour collects the information. The Progress Assessment Chart gives a fairly comprehensive picture of social functioning by assessing the presence or absence of selected social skills and social information, most of which can be taught to the client with learning difficulties. Unfortunately, a test score tends only too easily to become a permanent label used to explain and excuse inadequate functioning. The assessment should serve primarily as a base for organized attempts to improve the situation.

DIAGNOSIS OF LEARNING DISABILITY

It is unwise during the first 6 months of life to make the diagnosis of learning difficulties; however, there are a few exceptions, for example in Down's syndrome when the characteristic appearances are present at birth. Although the diagnosis of learning difficulties is ultimately a psychiatric responsibility, it is one to which parents, nurses, general practitioners, paediatricians, school medical officers, psychologists and social workers can contribute. Recent years have seen the establishment of assessment clinics where children who are seen to be having problems, or are suspected cases of learning difficulty, may be referred for diagnosis and advice concerning treatment and training. The time when parents are told of the diagnosis of the child having learning difficulties must be carefully chosen with regard to the parents' personalities and stability. It is important that the information about the child is given by someone with sufficient knowledge to give authoritative answers to the inevitable questions which will follow. Telling the parents should not be delayed for too long.

Learning difficulties manifest themselves in the developing child as delay in the various stages of development towards independent living. The normal milestones of development against which delays will be assessed are shown in Figure 7.1. Many children with learning difficulties are often not diagnosed until they reach school age. It is when they attend school that the teachers become aware that these children are having problems in learning. Once the diagnosis of learning difficulties is made in the child, parents often ask the inevitable questions about the occurrence of the condition in other siblings. In the past, much of the advice which was given was ill founded and was based on limited knowledge and information. Now such advice should only be given after the most careful consideration of all the relevant aspects, and if possible by a specialist in genetics. These people are the best equipped to give statistical, accurate forecasts of the probabilities of the condi-

tion reappearing in subsequent siblings. The parents should be helped to be honest, first with themselves and later with other people, about the true nature of their child's disability. The assessment of learning difficulties should not be a once and for all exercise as it has been so often in the past. These children continually need help to develop and, like normal children, they will develop although at a much slower pace. Therefore, these children should be reviewed regularly to establish progress and to identify their level of functioning. Programmes should be carefully decided on that will enable these children to progress, and develop into productive fulfilled adults.

Investigations

There are a range of investigations available which can be used to diagnose the possibility of a child being born with learning difficulties. These include amniocentesis, genetic screening and counselling and metabolic screening. It is also important to be aware of mothers who may be at risk through previous births resulting in an individual born with learning difficulties or because of the mother's age which can make her more susceptible. It is then necessary to offer advice and support so that an informed decision can be made regarding the pregnancy.

PHILOSOPHY OF CARE

Individuals with learning difficulties have the ability to learn and to develop, although this may be slower than in the general population, providing proper education and training is given at an early stage in life and is continued throughout the developmental period. Carers must be able to meet the individual's physical, psychological and social needs, so that the person develops as a whole person and not as component parts of a person.

Teaching cannot and should not be carried out in isolation, but should be relevant to everyday living and to the social and self-help skills that the individual will need at that stage of development (Whelan and Speake 1979). The individual with learning difficulties is a human being, with not only the right to life, but also the right to a quality of life in keeping with human dignity. Individuals with learning difficulties have the same rights as their peers in society, which, if they are unable to exercise them themselves, must be protected by the advocacy of the carers including the nurse.

The nurse's role is to support and encourage individuals with learning difficulties and their families and must be carried out with this important principle

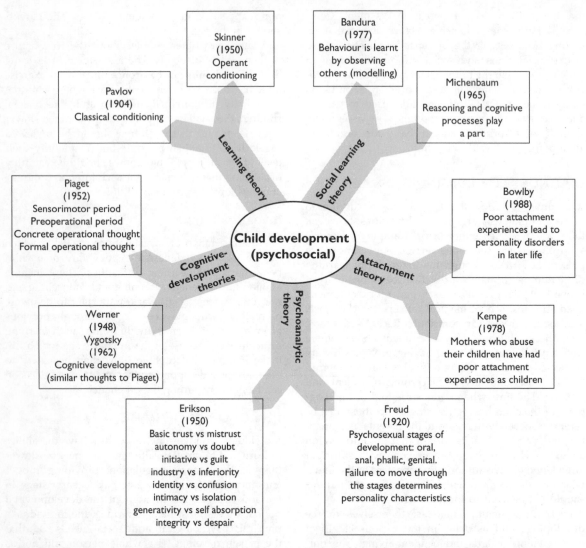

Fig. 7.1 Theories of normal milestones of child development against which delays can be assessed

in mind. An understanding of the causes of the disability and awareness of the social implications will facilitate an appropriate nursing response.

CAUSES OF LEARNING DIFFICULTIES

The causes of learning difficulties are many and varied, as illustrated in Figure 7.2.

There are implications of establishing a differential and specific diagnosis for both the individual's management and that of the family. Therefore, an understanding of the causes is important for all groups involved in the care of an individual with learning difficulties.

Hereditary factors

Hereditary factors are considered as being either chromosomal or genetic. Each chromosome is a strand made up of thousands of genes.

Each gene is responsible for a specific hereditary characteristic such as skin, hair or eye colour or the production of a particular protein.

In humans each cell contains 46 chromosomes grouped in pairs, 22 pairs are referred to as autosomes and one pair as sex chromosomes. The 22 pairs of autosomes are matched. The female has matched sex chromosomes referred to as XX. In the male they are unmatched and referred to as XY. For identification

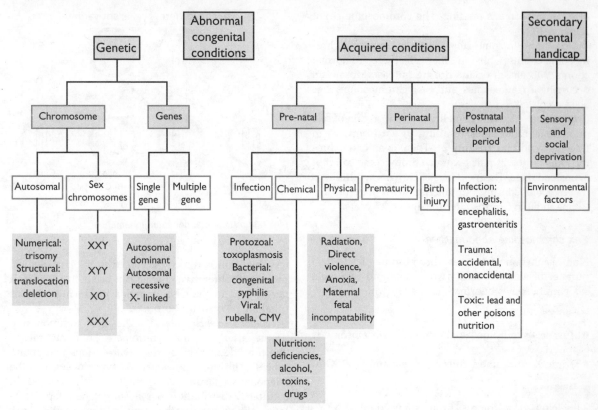

Fig. 7.2 Framework showing causes of learning difficulties

purposes chromosomes are numbered from 1 to 23. The largest pair number 1 and are arranged by size to the smallest. This facilitates the description of normal and abnormal chromosomes.

Human cells, other than sex cells, reproduce by the process of *mitosis*. In this process a cell divides in order to multiply. One cell divides to form two cells. Each of the two new cells formed by mitosis contains a complete set of genes identical to those in its parent cell. The function of mitosis then is to reproduce its own kind; it is the mechanisms of heredity for cells.

Meiosis is the type of cell division that occurs in the sex cells. As a result of meiosis primitive sex cells become mature sex cells called gametes. Male gametes are named sperm; female gametes are named ovum. During meiosis the diploid (meaning two or pairs) chromosome number (46) is reduced to 23 in the gametes. The fusion of the two gametes at conception forms the zygote which has 46 chromosomes, 23 chromosomes being contributed by each parent to the new offspring. As the chromosomes in the gametes pair up, the genes responsible for specific characteristics come together. Certain features are dominant – that is the characteristic will occur in the child if present on only one gamete (e.g. brown eyes) – but the individual may pass on a recessive gene from the other gamete to a child who, if that was paired with another recessive gene for blue eyes from the other parent, would be blue eyed. About 50 chromosomal abnormalities have been found, although most are rare.

Autosomal abnormalities

Both male and female sufferers will be found when abnormalities occur in the autosomes. There are two main types of autosomal abnormalities, structural and numerical.

Structural

Translocation The transfer of all or part of a chromosome during mitosis to a chromosome of another pair is called translocation. The chromosome count remains 46. The translocation can occur between any two pairs of chromosomes and usually results in learning difficulties.

Deletion This produces an abnormality when part

of a chromosome is missing. The chromosome count remains 46.

Mosaicism In some cells there are abnormal chromosome counts, whilst in other cells there are normal counts. Mosaicism occurs during mitosis. Mosaicism occurring in autosomes and sex chromosomes has been recorded.

Numerical This abnormality is a loss or gain of one or more chromosomes resulting in a trisomy, as in Down's syndrome trisomy 21. There is an extra chromosome on the 21 pair giving a chromosome count of 47 instead of 46. The incidence of Down's syndrome is one in 600 live births, but this rises with maternal age to one in 50 live births after the age of 25 years.

Sex chromosome abnormalities

Non-disjunction of the sex chromosomes leads to a number of abnormalities. Two female and two male sex chromosome abnormalities are known.

Female

- Turner's syndrome – only one sex chromosome is found X0.
- Triple X syndrome – chromosome count is 47 XXX.

Male

Klinefelter's syndrome – chromosome count 47 XXY.

Because the chromosomes each contain numerous genes affecting a wide range of physical and mental characteristics, there are likely to be adverse effects on a wide range of attributes associated with any chromosomal abnormality, some of which are incompatible with life.

Genes

Conditions which have a genetic inheritance can be considered in three ways:

- autosomal dominant inheritance
- autosomal recessive inheritance
- sex-linked (X-linked) inheritance.

Autosomal dominant inheritance (Fig. 7.3) Symptoms of the particular genetic abnormality will be present to a greater or lesser degree in all cases where the abnormal gene has been inherited. There is a constant risk of 1 in 2 that the condition will be passed on. Either sex can suffer from the condition. Examples of autosomal dominant conditions are tuberous sclerosis (epiloia) and neurofibromatosis.

Neurofibromatosis (Von Recklinghausen's disease) Affected people usually have normal intelligence un-

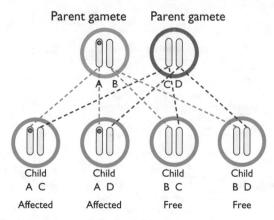

Fig. 7.3 Autosomal dominant inheritance

less the brain is directly involved in the pathological process. Proliferative change can occur in peripheral nerves and in the CNS or retina producing nodules (phakomas) or neurofibromas.

Tuberous sclerosis (epiloia) The most common syndrome after Down's syndrome. The name means 'brain hardening' or 'fibrosis with lesions like potato tubers'. The skin shows several types of lesions: the adenoma sebaceum rash spreads over the face first in a butterfly distribution; *café au lait* patches; depigmentation 'Shagreen' patches (raised areas of the skin). Life expectancy in severe cases is reduced.

Autosomal recessive inheritance In this mode of inheritance illustrated in Figure 7.4 both parents must carry the defective gene, but they do not suffer from the condition. Either sex can suffer from the condition. There is a constant risk that one in four of the offspring will have the recessive condition. There is a risk that one in two of the resulting offspring will be

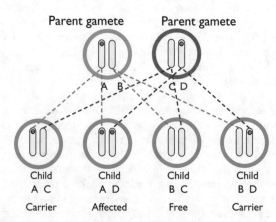

Fig. 7.4 Autosomal recessive inheritance

carriers without showing the condition. Examples of autosomal recessive inheritance are phenylketonuria (PKU), galactosaemia and Tay–Sachs disease. A large number of autosonal recessive conditions exist but most are rare.

Phenylketonuria (PKU) This has an incidence of one in 12 000 live births. The condition gives rise to a failure to metabolize phenylalanine to tyrosine and then to melanin, producing high levels of phenylalanine and its end-product in the blood and urine. The enzymes phenylalanine hydroxylase is absent. If left untreated almost all individuals have severe learning difficulties. If treated, subjects may be normal mentally and physically or have only mild learning difficulties. Diagnosis is by the Guthrie test within 7 days of birth followed by biochemical estimation of phenylalanine level in capillary blood. The diagnosis is confirmed by finding more than 20 mg/dl phenylalanine in capillary blood, and phenylpyruvic acid and other metabolites in the urine. Both these criteria must be fulfilled before starting treatment.

Sex-linked (X-linked) inheritance In this mode of inheritance males are affected when they inherit the defective gene on their X chromosome. The risk is one in two for the male of a carrier mother with the condition. Females carry the condition but are not affected by it. Again there is a constant one in two risk. All female children from affected males will carry the affected gene. Male children of affected males will be neither sufferers nor carriers. This is illustrated in Figure 7.5. Examples of sex-limited inheritance are fragile X syndrome, Lesch–Nyhan syndrome and a rare form of hydrocephalus.

1. **X (sex) linked limited hydrocephalus with aqueduct stenosis.**

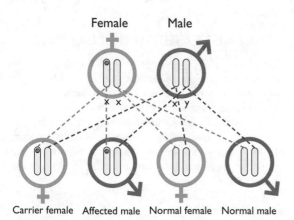

Female   Male

Carrier female   Affected male   Normal female   Normal male

Fig. 7.5 Sex-linked (X-linked) inheritance

2. **Fragile X syndrome.** Fragile site on the X chromosome detectable in the laboratory. Characteristics are large forehead, ears and jaw and, following the onset of puberty, macro-orchidism (enlarged testicles). A number of behavioural characteristics are reported such as autism, hyperactivity and self-injurious behaviours. Learning difficulties can be severe, although most would be said to be moderate. Whilst both sexes may inherit this type of chromosome, the effects are only seen in males, as they do not have another normal X chromosome to compensate. Learning disability resulting from defective genes on the short Y chromosome rarely occurs.

Acquired conditions

During pregnancy a number of causes of learning difficulties operate. Although the causative factors are not as clear as in genetic inheritance, nevertheless a knowledge of these factors in learning difficulties is important in its prevention.

Infections

Examples of maternal infections that have caused learning difficulties can be considered under the headings:

- bacterial
- viral
- protozoal.

Bacterial Congenital syphilis, resulting from maternal infection, was at one time common in mental handicap but is now rare. With improved antenatal care and the use of antibiotics the number of individuals born with congenital syphilis has reduced.

Viral Rubella (German measles) is the best known maternal infection that can be a cause of learning difficulties. Infections during the first trimester are particularly significant, as the earlier the infection strikes, the more severe will be the damage in affected cases, with a greater degree of learning difficulty.

Other viral infections implicated in the causation of learning difficulties causing damage to the developing fetus are: chickenpox, poliomyelitis, mumps, cytomegalovirus, toxoplasmosis.

Protozoal This presents a danger between the second and sixth month of pregnancy. Spontaneous abortion or stillbirth occurs in about 10% of cases where there has been an infection during pregnancy. A small proportion born with the infection have severe learning difficulties.

Chemical

Maternal nutrition The child in the womb is totally dependent on its mother. If there is an interruption to the supply of nutrients, including oxygen, the developing fetus will be affected. Factors such as intra-uterine deprivation, severe maternal malnutrition and placental insufficiency are of significance.

Rhesus incompatibility (kernicterus) Rhesus (Rh) factor incompatibility can result in brain damage. When a woman does not have the Rh factor in her blood, she is said to be Rh negative. If the child inherits the Rh factor from the father the child is Rh positive. There is a high risk of Rh positive blood from the child entering the mother's bloodstream and antibodies developing. These offer no risk to the mother, but could affect the fetus if this happens during pregnancy, or a subsequent Rh positive fetus if it occurs in labour. The Rh factor exchange transfusion can be carried out in utero or immediately after birth. If the child is left untreated severe learning difficulties will result.

Toxic agents Toxic agents can injure the developing fetus. Some commonly available agents are alcohol, drugs and smoking. In the prenatal period toxic substances can damage the developing brain. At one time lead poisoning was fairly common when water supply pipes and the base for white paint contained lead. These have now been recognized as dangerous and have been reduced or eliminated in many areas. Other areas which are causing concern are leaded petrol and fumes from motor vehicles exhaust pipes. The use of unleaded petrol is being encouraged to help eliminate the amount of lead in the atmosphere.

Physical factors

Radiation of the fetus can cause damage, especially if exposure is early in the pregnancy. Direct violence to the developing fetus can lead to brain damage. If the brain is deprived of oxygen for a period of time irreversible changes occur in the brain. There are a number of causes of oxygen deprivation in the perinatal period including:

- eclamptic fit
- prolonged labour
- umbilical cord around the neck of the child during delivery.

Other possible causes of birth injury include:

- forceps delivery
- fetal distress
- prolonged labour and difficult birth.

In the period immediately after birth:

- severe dehydration, usually from diarrhoea and vomiting, may lead to hypocalcaemia
- hypoglycaemia which may cause learning difficulties.

Monitoring the fetus during labour is essential to enable early signs of fetal distress and potential danger to the fetus to be detected.

In the postnatal period damage can occur due to:

- Infection – gastroenteritis, meningitis, encephalitis can all put the child at risk of severe brain damage.
- Trauma – severe injury to the head in an accident can cause brain damage, e.g. road traffic accidents, child abuse, cerebral haemorrhage.

The classification of learning difficulties can be organized in various ways, none of which is wholly satisfactory, as there are anomalies and overlaps in all systems. Whatever system is used the classification should not be the most important or overriding factor for parents or carers. This should only be used as a means of improving care and quality of life.

Following birth, it is important that the environment for the child is correct so that he can be stimulated and can develop the necessary skills. However, this causes problems for some individuals because although it has nothing to do with abnormality in the individual, the environment has a great deal to do with the individual's learning and the way that the child is reared. A lack of stimulation in the child's environment where the child is not played with, not spoken to or encouraged to explore his environment, means that opportunities for learning are decreased thus rendering the child susceptible to learning difficulties.

GENERAL FEATURES OF LEARNING DIFFICULTIES

Although the causes of learning difficulties have been described previously there are some common factors that the nurse may observe. Nowadays, there is less emphasis on clinical syndromes and greater emphasis is placed on the ability of the individual to learn. Nevertheless there are some general features which are commonly found and are relevant to the care that an individual requires.

Physical features

Poor muscle co-ordination often results in awkwardness of hand movement, grasping and reaching which can cause problems in development. The inability for fine finger movement can result in an individual using gross hand activity (the whole hand) to pick up objects where only the thumb and two fingers may be needed. This gives the action a very clumsy appearance and often causes frustration for the individual. Many individuals also have problems in hand/eye co-ordination and lack the ability to coordinate the hand/eye movements. When reaching for objects they tend to overshoot the object, resulting in them being unable to pick it up.

Psychological features

Depending upon the degree of learning difficulty, individuals may lack the ability to think or formulate ideas for themselves, coupled with a short attention span. This makes it difficult for the individual to select for attention one of several presenting stimuli and therefore he tries to pay attention to them all at one time. This often leads to a lack of ability to concentrate and distraction from the main task. Individuals with learning difficulties often fail to maintain eye-to-eye contact, therefore it can be difficult to encourage the development of concentration to task. Eye contact may only be maintained for a few seconds to a minute. It is therefore important to develop in the individual the ability to look at objects and to concentrate on them by developing programmes which encourage him to look at one presenting stimulus at a time.

Social features

Social behaviour in the normal individual begins almost at birth as a baby begins to respond to individuals around him. He begins to recognize familiar faces, especially that of the mother. The baby will respond to the mother's touch or voice. As the child begins to grow, he starts to learn behaviours which will help him to adapt and become an acceptable individual in society. The child begins to learn right and wrong and to differentiate what is acceptable behaviour and what is not. He learns from the family and peer groups in a number of ways by imitation, by observation and by tone of voice. For the child with learning difficulties, social maturity is delayed, as are all aspects of learning. The individual may find it difficult to differentiate between right and wrong. He may find it difficult to learn from past experiences and be unable to use the knowledge appropriately so that the same type of behaviour is repeated over and

over again. This is not conducive to learning. Similarly, because an individual with learning difficulties has reduced inhibitions and a lack of ability to respond to normal social cues, behaviour which might be accepted in an institutional setting is not accepted in the wider community. There is no role model that he can learn from, as the ability to mix with peers who have normal social behaviours is reduced in the institutional setting (Alaszewski 1990).

Behavioural features

An individual with learning difficulties may show behavioural features such as hyperactivity, aggressiveness, unawareness, destructiveness and distractibility. Also present may be repetitive and obsessional behaviour. Behaviours like these may set the individual apart from others in his peer group and may hinder his development. It is therefore important to deal effectively with these behavioural problems so that the individual can begin to start learning. It may be necessary to implement some form of behavioural modification programme to correct these. Much thought should be given to this and discussion with the multidisciplinary team including the psychologist should take place to agree what the problems are before any programme is implemented to change an individual's behaviour. The parents will also need to be involved in the discussion and consulted so that they may co-operate with any programme.

ASSOCIATED CONDITIONS

Other conditions are often associated with learning difficulties and many individuals may have multiple handicaps. Associated conditions can arise from damage to the brain which leaves the individual with physical disabilities that exacerbate the learning difficulties. Conditions such as epilepsy, cerebral palsy, autism, mental illness, and physical disabilities such as visual and hearing impairments, may arise.

MANAGEMENT OF THE PERSON WITH LEARNING DIFFICULTIES

There are various features to be considered when managing a person with learning difficulties:

1. The aim of treatment must be to provide each individual with a good quality of life by providing appropriate services to meet his needs.

2. The planning of a therapeutic programme must

take account of the individual's needs and circumstances, including the wishes and abilities of family members and professional carers.

3. Whilst many people suffering from learning difficulties will demonstrate a couple of the features described, specific management strategies need to be devised to address each of them within the context of an individual patient profile (IPP).

4. The recognition of individual differences in people with learning difficulties, as for all other individuals, has replaced a previously held attitude which grouped all such persons into problem categories leading to standardized patterns of care.

5. The shift from institutional to community-based care has underlined the need for individual management strategies, which are recommended on the IPP.

6. The treatment regimen must take account of individual strengths and weaknesses, cultural and ethical considerations and any known wishes of the person or his family.

7. The systematic approach to developing the plan requires team assessment, a written plan incorporating clearly defined goals to be achieved, agreed achievement dates, how the therapy is to be implemented including rewards, positive or negative reinforcement strategies and assessment criteria.

8. Using an appropriate model, e.g. Roper, Logan, Tierney Activities of Living or Orem's Model in Action, a holistic approach to care planning, identifying needs and carers' roles in relation to desired goals can be achieved.

9. A key worker, who will probably be a nurse, will need to be identified to co-ordinate the whole process from data collection to evaluation of the effectiveness of the plan.

10. The effectiveness of the plan will be reviewed by the whole team, including family members and the individual if possible, at regular intervals.

The specific features described above may respond to particular strategies as discussed below:

- Physical difficulties compounded by intellectual impairment need to be overcome by a deliberate educational programme, because the normal learning mode of imitation fails due to the lack of concentration. For many individuals skills that most take for granted need to be taught. In the teaching of either simple or more complicated skills, there are some basic principles to be followed (Box 7.1).
- The task to be learned must be analysed, demonstrated, practised and repeated until competency is achieved. An example of the analysis of the skill of eating is shown in Box 7.2.

Box 7.1 Principles of skill teaching

1. The skill to be taught should be defined and an assessment of the individual made to see if he/she is ready to learn this skill
2. The skill is then analysed and broken down into small steps
3. Each step is taught using the same pattern at each performance
4. As each step is taught, the step should be demonstrated by the carer and the person given verbal prompting to perform this skill him/herself
5. The person must be able to see clearly the demonstration from his/her own perspective. In some cases, it may be necessary to take the individual's hand and perform the steps with him/her. Where necessary, as the individual performs the steps, corrections should be made
6. In all skills teaching, practice must continue until it becomes a habit
7. Once this skill has been mastered, it is then necessary to observe that the skills are being maintained. As the individual starts to master the skill, prompting and rewarding is gradually faded out so that they no longer need to be rewarded and prompted to perform the skill. Competence in the skill becomes its own reward

---

Box 7.2 Analysis of skill of eating

To sit at a table, pick up a piece of cake and take it to the mouth, the individual needs:

1. A base from which to start, that is sitting and head control
2. Balance – the ability to make immediate, small and accurate alterations with the trunk muscles to compensate for the arm movements
3. The ability to stretch the arm in the right direction
4. The ability to stretch the arm for the right distance
5. Complex movements – close the fingers with an arm stretched
6. Control of strength so that the fingers close enough to pick up the cake but do not crush it
7. Control of speed – so that the cake doesn't smash into the face
8. Body image sense – the hand comes accurately to the mouth
9. Absence of the reflex which allows the arm to bend when the face is turned away (asymmetric tonic reflex)
10. Duration – keeping the contraction up for long enough

- The individual must be motivated to continue to try to achieve, often in the face of disappointment and frequent failure. Success is a valuable motivator – it may be useful to encourage the person to complete a task as his first step in learning, for example to zip up his jacket at the end of dressing, rather than start with putting on a vest which might take a long time during which he will get cold which is a disincentive. This is a technique known as backward chaining. As soon as this part of the skill is learned, the immediate preceding action is practised until the person has mastered the whole task.

- Starting at the beginning of a task (forward chaining) may be motivating provided the supervisor takes over before failure leads to disillusionment and refusal to practise.
- The degree of difficulty, the complexity of the task and the individual's abilities will determine the chain of actions which make up the skill. The nurse's role is to carry out this analysis taking account of these factors, implement the planned programme of training to an agreed time-scale and evaluate progress.
- Psychological features, e.g. lack of concentration, poor attention span and failure to co-ordinate, can be addressed using play and other activities to encourage more eye-to-eye contact and develop co-ordination skills.
- Social training involves creating opportunities for the individual to participate in a wide range of activities with normal peers, discouraging unacceptable behaviour and clarifying and rewarding desirable activities (Keele 1983).

DEALING WITH BEHAVIOURAL PROBLEMS

The presence of a behavioural problem is not always a clear-cut matter. Many individuals in their normal environment have been acting in a particular way for a considerable time before someone decides that it is a problem that needs to be dealt with. Before attempting to change the behaviour of someone, it is important to consider whether the behaviour is a problem for the individual or whether it is a problem for the setting in which he finds himself. This is an important question to ask because it may not be the individual that needs to change but rather the routine and practices that take place in an individual's environment. A behaviour may be regarded as a problem if it:

1. is inappropriate given the person's age and level of development
2. is dangerous to him/herself or others
3. interferes with the learning of a new skill

4. causes disruption and stress to those who live or work with the individual and impairs their quality of life
5. goes against social norms.

If it is clear that the behaviour is causing a problem then provided that consultation with either the individual or the representative takes place, ways need to be found to help him/her over the problem.

Difficult behaviour presents a continuing challenge to those who work with individuals with learning difficulties. Some of the behaviour problems will be found in the general population, for example tantrums, but there are other problems less commonly found in the general population, for example self-injurious behaviour. In dealing with behaviour problems there are no ready-made solutions. They cannot be isolated but need to be understood in the context of the individual and the society in which he/she lives. Before deciding on the appropriate interventions to deal with the problem behaviour, a full assessment needs to be made to see how frequently the behaviour occurs and in what situations; to see if any particular event triggers the behaviour and how those around the individual react to the problem. Unacceptable behaviour may be because of the actions of those around. For example, if someone with learning difficulties is asked to perform a task but wants to be left alone he/she may start to shout. If the carer then leaves him alone, the shouting has been rewarded and will be repeated whenever the person is asked to perform the task.

In most cases the undesired behaviour carries a useful function for the individual. Merely removing it will not provide a long-term solution as the need it served has not been met. Something which is equally satisfying but more acceptable must be put in its place.

The four stages of the nursing process provide a framework for the implementation of a behaviour modification programme.

1. assessment
2. planning
3. intervention
4. evaluation.

Observation and recording of behaviour are carried out during all stages. There are several techniques for observing and recording behaviour.

The observations which are made during the assessment period comprise the baseline record. It is so called because a knowledge of the natural frequency of the behaviour which is to be changed provides a base against which to assess the effects of the treatment procedures employed during the intervention period. A decision to attempt to change behaviour should always come from direct observation and recording of that behaviour in the setting in which it usually occurs.

Accurate baseline recording depends upon the definition of behavioural and environmental events in objective terms. In defining behavioural and environmental events, it is helpful to make use of the A, B, C model (Antecedent, Behaviour and Consequence, Box 7.3).

Defining behavioural events

The biggest problem in defining behavioural events is in establishing clear criteria so that one or more observers can agree on when a behaviour has occurred. For example, if it is desired to record the number of times a child hits other children, the criteria of a hitting response must be clearly given so that the observer can discriminate hitting from patting or shoving responses (Presland 1989).

Defining environmental events

Environmental events must be as precisely defined as the behaviour of the patient who is under observation. The baseline record should provide a stable measurement of the problem behaviour in relation to environmental events. Recording of behaviour should continue until a stable baseline is achieved, that is one in which no marked ascending or descending trends are evident in the behaviour under study. If a baseline record is ascending or descending, the application of behaviour modification procedures will be difficult to evaluate unless they are implemented to reverse the trend.

The complex environment in which an individual lives may be further complicated in a hostel or hospital setting by a wide range of different carers and other disabled individuals. Each disabled person may be permitted to behave to a different standard according to the individual treatment plan. Each carer may respond differently from others, or even be inconsistent from day to day.

People with learning difficulties are all different and need different responses. The individual needs to know what to expect so the boundaries of acceptable behaviour must be clearly agreed by all carers, the reinforcement sanctions understood and applied consistently by all carers.

Inevitably the limits will be tested, as will the ability or will of the carers to enforce the agreed limits. Difficulties arise because exceptions are made and further behavioural problems may result. When this occurs, the caring team must analyse what went wrong, and why, and appropriate steps should be taken by the team leader to ensure that consistent patterns of care are delivered.

People with learning difficulties need order to their lives tempered with freedom. They need to grow in an environment rich with rewarding behaviour. Carers need to concentrate on the appropriate behaviours the individual already exhibits, which should be reinforced and from which further appropriate behaviours can be developed.

EPILEPSY

Epilepsy is not a disorder of learning difficulties. Many individuals suffer from epilepsy but would not be considered as having learning difficulties. The condition is discussed here because it is seen quite commonly in individuals with learning difficulties.

The word epilepsy is derived from the Greek word for seizure. It occurs when there is an abnormal electrical discharge in the grey matter of the brain. This develops suddenly, ceases spontaneously and is likely to recur. Epilepsy is not a disease in itself but is generally regarded as a symptom of some underlying cause; in some cases a lesion of the brain plays a part in causation. A person with epilepsy only experiences the symptoms of epilepsy during a seizure, otherwise the individual is healthy. All individuals have a threshold beyond which fits may occur if a stimulus of sufficient intensity is supplied.

Although epilepsy is symptomatic of an underlying cause, in almost half of the patients, despite investigation, the cause is never found and the disorder is described as idiopathic.

Classification of seizures

The classification of the International League Against Epilepsy (Box 7.4) has been generally adopted and supported in publications over the past decade,

Box 7.3		
A	**B**	**C**
Antecedent Event (may act as an eliciting stimulus for the behaviour in question)	Response of Patient	Consequent Event (may serve as reinforcement for the behaviour)

Box 7.4   The International Classification of Epileptic Seizures by the International League against Epilepsy

Partial seizures
These begin in a local area of the brain
1. *Simple partial seizures:*
   Consciousness is not impaired with symptoms appropriate to the function of the discharging area of the brain: motor, sensory, autonomic, psychic or any combination of these
2. *Complex partial seizures:*
   a. simple partial features followed by brief clouding of consciousness or more prolonged automatism
   b. impaired consciousness at onset –
      i.   clouding of consciousness only
      ii. automatism
3. *Partial seizures, evolving to secondary generalized seizures (tonic-clonic, tonic or clonic):*
   a. simple partial seizures evolving to generalized seizures
   b. complex seizures evolving to generalized seizures
   c. simple partial seizures progressing to complex partial seizures and the generalized seizures

Generalized seizures (convulsive or non-convulsive)
1. *Absence (petit mal) seizures*
2. *Myoclonic*
3. *Clonic*
4. *Tonic*
5. *Tonic-clonic (grand mal) seizures*
6. *Atonic*

Unclassified

---

although other classifications continue to be devised and find varying degrees of support.

Partial seizures

Partial seizures occur locally in the brain, and the manifestation of effects will depend on the part of the brain affected. If the disturbance arises in the motor cortex, movements of muscle groups normally controlled by the motor cortex will be affected. This may ultimately trigger a generalized seizure. If the area affected is sensory, as in temporal lobe epilepsy, the individual may have internal experiences ranging from a dream or nightmare, with a host of sensations affecting the senses of sight, touch, taste, smell with chewing movements of the mouth and tongue.

Generalized seizures

Absence (petit mal) seizures   These brief periods when the individual is unaware of his/her surroundings occur mainly in children and young adults. They are not always recognized as seizures, the child often being accused of day dreaming. The child has in fact missed a part of the lesson and this affects both that and subsequent learning. He may be considered a slow learner or dull as a result.

Myoclonic seizures   These are sudden spasmodic contractions of muscle most commonly found in infants.

Tonic or clonic seizures   Major generalized seizures in which either the tonic or clonic phase is absent.

Tonic-clonic (grand mal) seizures   The tonic-clonic seizure follows a typical pattern, as shown in Box 7.5.

Atonic or akinetic seizures   These seizures are characterized by a sudden total loss of consciousness and postural control which leads to the individual falling.

Box 7.5   Typical pattern of a tonic-clonic seizure

Prodromal period	The seizure may be preceded by vague symptoms affecting taste or smell; behavioural changes may also be common. The nurse with knowledge of the individual would be aware of these changes indicating that a seizure is imminent. The individual who is normally quiet may become quite robust; the robust individual may become quiet. This can go on for a period as long as 24 hours
Aura	As the seizure commences the individual may experience some physical or psychological sensations which often are highly unpleasant. This signals the onset of the epileptic seizure and the individual may cry out
Tonic phase	During this phase the individual rapidly becomes unconscious. All body muscles contract leading to constriction of respiratory movement and the individual becomes cyanosed. Tightening of the abdominal muscles may lead to urinary and faecal incontinence. This phase can last up to 1 minute
Clonic phase	This phase consists of repetitive jerking of the body, sometimes accompanied by frothing at the mouth, with gasping attempts for air. Once the seizure has subsided there is often a phase of deep sleep of varying duration. On waking the individual may show signs of confusion and carry out actions which he/she is not aware of. This is known as postictal automatism

Almost immediately consciousness is regained. Frequently, as a result of falling, injuries to the head or face are sustained.

Unclassified seizures These, as the category indicates, are seizures that do not easily fit into the categories described and a precise description is of more benefit than a diagnostic label.

Status epilepticus The most common form of status epilepticus is seen in the tonic-clonic seizure in which the clonic phase will immediately be followed by a tonic phase without interruption. The individual is in a continuous convulsive state. Status epilepticus is a serious medical emergency and can be life threatening, because of the recurring periods of apnoea.

Consecutive, uninterrupted seizures can also occur in other forms of epilepsy, particularly absence – status absence. These prolonged absences make the person vulnerable to injury and, whilst not in themselves life threatening, need to be recognized and treated.

Management of epilepsy

Since epilepsy is in itself a symptom the main aim of the investigation is to determine the underlying pathology. It is important that the doctor obtains a detailed family medical history of the patient, noting any particular history of birth trauma, febrile convulsions, head injury, past history of meningitis and encephalitis, drug/alcohol abuse, or any previous seizures experienced by the patient or any family member. If the patient has experienced a seizure in the presence of witnesses, a relative, friend or nurse, a detailed description and assessment of the attack is vital since an objective account may help the doctor to arrive at a precise diagnosis. Many seizures occur spontaneously but some factors can be identified in individual cases. Observations should include the type of attack, the frequency in relation to any previous attacks, any activities the patient was engaged in prior to the attack, sudden loud noises or flashing lights that may have been associated with its commencement.

In the case of some female patients, there may also be a relationship between the onset of the attack and the onset of menstruation. In general, the diagnosis will be made on the basis of the patient's history and on the account of any witness to any attacks. Other investigations are aimed at determining whether there are any identifiable causes for the epilepsy, which may or may not require specific treatment. Skull X-ray and electroencephalogram may be performed to exclude any fractures or focal areas which may indicate the possibility of the presence of an underlying structural lesion.

In general, patients who have had more than one seizure would be prescribed anticonvulsant drugs. The anticonvulsant chosen depends on the type of epilepsy. Because of the long-term need for treatment with anticonvulsants, it is important that the correct drugs should be prescribed and the minimum number of drugs used to control seizures. Now that blood levels of anticonvulsants can be readily obtained the aim is to use the smallest number of drugs prescribed at the correct dosages to control the seizures without toxic side-effects. (Levitts 1982).

CEREBRAL PALSY

The term is used to describe a number of disorders of posture and movement. Cerebral palsy is not itself a disorder of learning difficulties but is often associated with it. If intellectual impairment, epilepsy, disorders of hearing, speech or emotional problems co-exist, the management will be more difficult (Levitt 1982).

The most common cause of damage is that brain cells are deprived of oxygen during a difficult delivery; however, rhesus incompatibility and infant jaundice may also cause destruction of brain cells. As brain cells do not regenerate, the damage is permanent and cannot be cured; on the other hand, it does not increase as in degenerative diseases.

Because of the complexity of the brain no two cases are identical and this, with the many other factors affecting the child such as personality and the standard of care, make it virtually impossible and certainly very dangerous to give an accurate prognosis of the degree of disability in adulthood.

The description of cerebral palsy is by type:

1. **Spasticity.** There is damage to the motor cortex affecting the motor centre. This is the most common form of cerebral palsy with approximately 75% showing this type. The extent and parts of the body affected vary (Box 7.6).

Box 7.6 **Parts of the body affected in spasticity**	
Monoplegia	only one limb is affected
Hemiplegia	one arm and one leg are affected
Paraplegia	both legs are affected
Quadriplegia	all four limbs are affected
Diplegia	all four limbs affected, with the legs more than the arms.
Triplegia	involvement of three limbs

2. **Athetosis.** In athetosis there is damage to the basal ganglia which causes frequent involuntary movements interfering with normal body movements. Body movements are unreliable and are often described as writhing. The involuntary movements are increased by excitement, and the effort to make a voluntary movement becomes more difficult. Approximately 40% of individuals have hearing defects. Approximately 10% of cerebral-palsied individuals show athetosis.

3. **Ataxia.** Damage to the cerebellum shows in a loss of muscular co-ordination. This condition is comparatively rare.

4. **Mixed types.** Approximately 10% of cerebral-palsied individuals present a mixed form of the three types. The management of this condition depends on careful assessment to identify the range of problems which must be overcome and selected strategies which should be employed to overcome them (Levitt 1982).

BODY IMAGE

This is one defect which is often difficult to understand and which sometimes accompanies brain damage. The individual fails to appreciate the size, shape or position of his body in relation to his environment or parts of his body in relation to other parts.

The affected person may not perceive the similarity between a glove and his hand, and therefore not put on the glove correctly. Similarly, a person may not negotiate his way around a room without knocking into objects causing himself injury, or may fail to wash a leg which is not recognized as part of self.

These problems will impair a person's ability to perform expected tasks and this must be differentiated from a refusal to co-operate in an open training programme. Careful observation to identify and discriminate between these is important to the successful outcome.

AUTISM

The autistic child has problems with communication, often remaining mute, has unacceptable behaviour and social isolation.

Management of autism

At the centre of any approach to help autistic people must be the realization that autistic behaviour is potentially stressful, both for the autistic person and for the care worker. This can be one of the reasons why staff in non-specialized settings only involve themselves with the autistic person when it is absolutely necessary and for most of the time leave him alone (Wing 1976). Some of the problems for carers are outlined in Box 7.7.

Anyone who has experience of an autistic person in a professional setting will have identified that they are not the easiest of people to work with. It is hard not to be put off by some of the idiosyncratic and sometimes frankly bizarre behaviours which are demonstrated. The carer has to cultivate comparative unshockability, meet some of the more spectacular behavioural excesses with calmness and try to use the situation to positive effect. An important facet in the care and education of autistic people is positive intervention. There has to be a deliberate planned intrusion into the autistic person's solitariness to develop positive responses and facilitate social development.

Management or treatment of the autistic person should be educationally based; interventionist, perhaps obtrusive; demanding; designed for the individual; dynamic rather than static; systematic and consistent; recorded and updated (Wing 1976).

There is still some biological and psychological research to be done into the precise nature of autism and also into the best method of intervention. It is important that such knowledge and expertise as do currently exist are fully utilized and that those who

---

Box 7.7 Problems for carers in managing the autistic child

1. Unpredictable aggression
2. Being unable to identify what the autistic person really wants
3. Handling obsessive or ritualistic behaviour and the strong resistance to changing it
4. Trying to find a way into the autistic person's isolation
5. Trying to motivate the autistic person to use a skill which he has learned but does not utilize unless he is prompted
6. Having to adhere to highly structured ritualized routines, imposed by the individual
7. Coping with the lack of freedom, putting a great deal into relationships and getting very little in return
8. Having to maintain a high level of concentration to monitor and control behaviour
9. Handling bizarre and unacceptable behaviours
10. Having to settle for very slow progress
11. Realizing that to be really effective, teaching can only be done on a one-to-one basis
12. Finding it almost impossible to get the autistic person to engage in any group activities

are responsible for autistic individuals in any setting are able to identify their special needs and respond appropriately.

MENTAL ILLNESS

Mental illness (see Chs 8–10) may be superimposed on disorders of learning and this requires specialized psychiatric nursing care.

PHYSICAL ILLNESS

Individuals with learning difficulties are not immune from physical illness. These can range from minor to major illnesses requiring specialized nursing care in a general hospital. The illnesses are discussed in other chapters in this book.

It is important to recognize that a diagnosis of physical illness is complicated in persons with learning difficulties because of:

1. difficulties in building up relationships
2. difficulties in communication.

The transfer to general hospital for specialist treatment may result in management difficulties. The distress and confusion may cause a regression in the individual's behaviour and the staff generally lack the knowledge and expertise to help a person with learning difficulties. For these reasons, a return to his/her normal environment as rapidly as possible should be planned.

MULTIDISCIPLINARY APPROACH TO CARE

People with learning difficulties need to be fully assessed in order to determine their capabilities now and in the future. It is the responsibility of the multidiscplinary team to provide specialist knowledge and skills which enable the planning of a programme in conjunction with the individual and carers to promote achievement of maximum potential. Assessment should not be a one-off exercise but needs to be a continuous process. The individual with learning difficulties has a life-long handicap. In most cases, there is no cure. Therefore planning needs to take place to ensure that the individual is given the best opportunities for development. Once the assessment takes place the multidisciplinary team, along with the relatives and individuals themselves, meet together to discuss where the best help can come from. No one person has the prerogative to help and each member of the team has specialist knowledge available for the person.

The nurse is an important member of the team because of the specialist skills he/she has in assessment, observation, communication, planning and delivering care. Physical problems may be dealt with by the paediatrician or the orthopaedic surgeon. Psychological problems can be dealt with by the clinical or educational psychologists; psychiatric problems by the psychiatrist. Speech therapists, physiotherapists, teachers and occupational therapists all have expertise which is invaluable in assessment. Social workers too are important in the team as they would take a full family history to identify family problems and where help may be needed in the family. Early identification of the handicap, planning services to deal with the handicap and intervention are important roles of the multidisciplinary team.

COMMUNICATION THROUGH THERAPY

In this section, a number of therapies will be described which are used with people with learning difficulties and which have been shown to be beneficial in some instances.

Play therapy

Individuals with learning difficulties do not tend to play spontaneously. Nevertheless, play is an important form of learning. Play helps to develop hand/eye co-ordination, communication, imagination, body image and motor development. Often the lead in play is taken by an adult to encourage and develop skills in the individual. The nurse, along with the play therapist, is in an ideal position to stimulate play and to arouse the curiosity of her charges. Careful thought must be given to the objects of play so that the chosen game is neither too difficult nor too easy for the individual leading to boredom and disinterest. Play sessions need to have some organization but should not be so organized that there is little room for manoeuvre. Play, as well as being a learning experience, must be pleasurable for the people taking part (McCarthy 1992).

Carers often devalue the importance that play has in the development of the individual. Frequently, there is too much concern with other things to give value and importance to play sessions. Everybody, whether they are young or old, needs to relate through play and leisure activities which may take many forms (Keele 1983). Individuals with learning difficulties need to be encouraged to take part in a range of play activities such as sand and water play, climbing, rough and tumble play, and also be allowed to sit and observe others. Appropriate leisure activities must be devised as individuals mature and age.

Music therapy

People with learning difficulties can be isolated from society, especially if they have problems in communication and self-expression. They often become frustrated because of their inability to explain their wishes and desires and this can be expressed in socially unacceptable behaviour. Because of this behaviour they become even more rejected and isolated by society. Music can be seen as a means of communication as it has unique qualities which makes it an ideal medium for therapy. Music is a form of language which is universally accepted and individuals can gain pleasure and respond to it. Music is present in our everyday life; it appeals to all; it is present in all cultures.

From birth, an infant is surrounded by music in one form or another and as he grows there is a response to the music either by movement, listening or accompanying it. Music can also express emotional feelings and how individuals react to situations that they may find themselves in. A music therapist responds to the individual's moods by using improvised music and tries to awaken a musical response from the individual on an instrument. Many sessions may be required before the person responds but once the response is made the therapist can provide support and aid development, so that as the sessions develop they become a more shared creative experience. Withdrawn individuals have blossomed through music therapy and have become active, alive people. Music therapy takes place with individuals or groups where each can gain something for themselves which is valued. The music therapist plays an important part in the assessment of the individual, as he can often give information which helps towards a more complete understanding of the person.

Drama therapy

Drama therapy, like music, helps individuals to express themselves where there may be difficulties in communication and expression. Drama therapy can help to express innermost thoughts and desires. People with learning difficulties often have difficulty in expression and making others understand what their needs are. Through mime, dance and drama they can enact their thoughts and feelings without embarrassment.

Drama therapy, as with music therapy, has helped individuals to blossom because they are seen as important and worthwhile and that the contribution that they make, no matter how small, is valued. It helps them to relate to others and to themselves.

Art therapy

Art therapy is another form of communication. Individuals who have difficulty in communicating can use paints, crayons and pencils to express how they feel about themselves in drawings and paintings. The art therapist can gain an insight into the individual, although it must be remembered that art can be pleasurable in itself without having any hidden meaning. Art therapy also allows individuals to work on their own or in groups to develop skills in sharing, working together, giving and taking and to become valued in the group. The physical activities involved may also improve co-ordination and concentration skills.

Complementary therapies

These are seen as valuable for people with learning difficulties and complement the work of nurses, physiotherapists and other forms of therapy.

Aromatherapy

Aromatherapy is a technique whereby essential oils can be used with massage to develop bonds with the individual. The oils used will depend on the needs of the individual. There are many oils available with differing properties, some being used to relax, some to stimulate. An important point to note is that the individual benefits from this not just because of the effects of the oils but also from the one-to-one relationship that takes place during the massage. Trust and friendship is built up between the individual and the therapist. Essential oils can also be used in vaporizers to enhance the individual's well-being.

Massage

Massage is a form of non-verbal communication. It helps the development of interactions in a non-threatening way. When performing massage a degree of trust is built up between the masseur and the individual, often because of the intimate nature of the task. It can help people develop relationships with each other.

Massage is valued as it relaxes, calms and soothes. On its own it can help to counteract the stresses of everyday life. For the individual with learning difficulties, massage can help to reduce anxiety, be calming and relax them. Often massage is used with aromatherapy.

COMMUNITY NURSE MENTAL HANDICAP

The role of the community nurse mental handicap (CNMH) has developed over the years, and the functions that are being undertaken by these nurses have increased. The CNMH is centrally involved in the assessment, planning and implementation of programmes based on an individual's needs, and is heavily involved in working with families and individuals in the community. He/she is able to offer advice and support and provide services to the family to help them overcome difficulties and problems that they may experience with learning difficulties at home. The CNMH can be a lifeline for many families and can devise programmes to help make life easier for the individual with learning difficulties and family members. He/she may be the first point of contact for families with social services and other agencies. He/she has the authority to refer to psychiatrists when a problem may warrant psychiatric help. The CNMH may need to be a listening ear for the family if they perhaps feel overwhelmed by the problems of caring for someone with learning difficulties at home. The CNMH role is becoming more important in the community today as more and more individuals are being discharged from institutional settings.

COUNSELLING AND SUPPORT TO THE FAMILIES

Families with an individual with learning difficulties require specialist support. When the child is born with an obvious disability the parents are often stunned and shocked to realize that the child they thought was normal is now different. Families react differently to the way that they accept the news. Many of these families grieve for the normal child that they never had and this grieving process can take quite a long time. The mother still has to manage to care for the handicapped child and to cope with her own grief. The midwife who is present at the birth will help in giving support to the mother. How that is dealt with can often affect the way the mother will react to the baby. The mother can go through many experiences of emotion from guilt to repulsion. Initially, she may not believe that the child is hers and may deny the child. It can be quite difficult for families to come to terms with the fact that their lives will have to change and alterations will have to be made to accommodate the child with learning difficulties.

Brothers and sisters can also experience profound changes in their lives after the birth of the individual with learning difficulties and may suffer because of the amount of attention required for many years by the handicapped family member.

Quite often after birth, the parents will look for reasons for the child to have been born with these problems. They may start to blame each other or other members of the family and this can have serious adverse effects on relationships. The mother may be so overwhelmed with guilt that she may devote all her life and all her time to looking after the disabled child to the detriment of her husband and other children. Other families may settle down easier, accept the problem and try to cope and deal with the situation. No matter how much a family may be coping, support should and must, be available to the family as and when they need it. Support should come right at the start when the parents are told that their child is handicapped in some way. Time should be given for the parents to take in what has been said and then another counselling session is arranged so that the parents can ask questions and clear up any points that are confusing them. It may be necessary to explain again to parents the problems the child has or which may develop. Genetic counselling should be available to the parents to help them to come to a better understanding of the possible causes and implications for future pregnancies. If the condition is inherited, siblings will want to know the risks they run so genetic counselling should be available to them at an appropriate time. As is natural through a child's developing years, the parents will want the best for their child and it is important that the services are geared to this. The child should be closely monitored by the health visitor from birth and by the CNMH who will give advice so that the specialist help and services required can then be obtained.

COMMUNITY CARE AND NURSES

Community care for individuals with learning difficulties is increasing. It is seen as the right of individuals to be cared for in the community. Large institutions have been reduced in size and patients placed in the community either in group homes or in hostels, with a few returning to the family home. However, the care that is provided in the community must be demonstrably better than the care provided previously. Society's attitudes to people with learning difficulties are beginning to change and they are becoming more tolerant. However, there are still a great many problems to overcome. An attitudinal change will only come through education of the public. Community care must provide a network of support that will help the individual to maintain his independence in society. The care must be appropriate for the needs of the individual and must be available when it is required. Most problems experienced by living in the community that warrant re-admission to a hospital unit arise from trying to fit the individual into a service rather than to fit the service around the individual. The planning that takes place in relation to community care must be mindful of this point and the recipients of the care must be consulted about how they can best be helped. Preparing people who live in institutional care for community life is equally important. They must be able to learn the skills for community living in appropriate places. They must also be involved in the decisions about with whom they will live (Alaszewski 1990).

The transition for the individual from living in an institution to living in the community where many options are available to them, for example staffed and unstaffed houses, group homes/hostels, living with families, should take place smoothly. The key worker, who would normally be a nurse, is appointed to the individual as the link person between them and the community. The nurse as key worker would then have responsibility to assess or to arrange for assessments to be made, to initiate and monitor any planned care or movements for the individual and to co-ordinate the services. As a first point of contact for the family, the key worker has an important role in this area. It is important to consider the compatibility of the key worker with the individual as the key worker will be representing the individual and they will often be the point of contact with other agencies. As the individual with learning difficulties gains more confidence and the ability to solve more problems for himself, key worker activities should be reviewed to see if less help is needed by the individual.

SEXUALITY AND THE PERSON WITH LEARNING DIFFICULTIES

The child with learning difficulties may achieve physical maturity but not intellectual or emotional levels to match. This creates problems for some parents who fail to recognize their child's adult status, providing inappropriate styles of dress and restricting independence and access to adult activities.

The expression of sexuality for individuals with learning difficulties is an area which has always caused concern for care staff and parents alike. In recent years there has been a shift of emphasis concerning the control of the sexual behaviour of individuals with learning difficulties. Until the 1970s the subject was seen as taboo and very rarely discussed.

Any writings emphasized the negative consequences of sexual activity of those deemed to have learning difficulties. Since the early 1970s authors have begun to view this subject in a much more positive way in that carers and parents should be helping the individual with learning difficulties to live sexually satisfying lives.

Traditionally, the experience of sexuality by people with learning difficulties was feared by those who made the rules governing western societies. In many instances, where there was recognition that sexual needs arose, there were very rigid rules laid down to prevent these members of society, who were deemed unfit, from procreating.

The development of services in the past two decades which have influenced the policy of giving individuals with learning difficulties the same opportunities as someone else of their chronological age group, have pointed to the need for sex education and counselling for these individuals. Programmes have been and are being developed which emphasize the need for individuals to have a basic understanding of their own bodies and how their body functions. They also stress the need for individuals to be taught how to say 'no' to protect themselves from exploitation; to stress the need for interpersonal and appropriate sexual behaviours, helping the individual towards a more positive life-style closer to that experienced by non-handicapped peers.

The majority of individuals with learning difficulties will develop normal secondary sexual characteristics and may experience the same confusions about these body changes as their normal counterparts. However, because of their learning difficulties, they need more help to understand, not less than the normal adult. Often in the past they were given no knowledge.

The aim of sexual education and counselling should be to focus on enabling and empowering people with learning difficulties to take responsibility through full knowledge and understanding, to enable them to make choices for themselves. Behaviour must be taught that will encourage their participation in community-based life-styles and activities and reduce the risk of exploitation (Craft and Craft 1993).

As sex education packages have been developed for individuals with learning difficulties there has been a growing awareness of the training needs of staff and carers. Many staff have been ill equipped in their initial training to deal effectively with this important area of life. A number of staff training packages have been developed under various organizations like the Family Planning Association and

British Institute of Learning Disabilities. These packages have examined topics such as:

1. staff attitudes
2. expansion of staff knowledge and skills
3. communication skills
4. counselling skills
5. programme design for implementing sex education
6. case studies
7. use of resource packs and other instructional material.

The main objectives of these courses is to encourage staff to meet the needs that individuals with learning difficulties have in sexual and relationship matters. Staff can only do this when they have the opportunity to explore, examine and clarify their own feelings and attitudes. They help staff to acquire skills which can develop comfort and confidence in the subject area by diffusing the sensitivity of the issues and by recognition of the value of individuals.

Sex education and counselling, which began in a selective manner as individuals were being prepared for discharge, or for crisis intervention, is now more widely available. Assessment tools to determine the sexual knowledge an individual has are available. From the baselines derived, a training programme can be tailored to the needs of the individual. Much still requires to be done to change staff attitudes and in the education of individuals before people with learning difficulties can exercise their right to fulfil their sexual and emotional needs to the same extent as other people in society.

In the 1990s two new areas of concern have emerged which will influence the development of sex education in the future:

1. The growing awareness of AIDS and HIV-related conditions. This has had a marked effect on the impetus to teach appropriate sexual behaviour.
2. Growing awareness of problems of sexual abuse in the field of child care. This has significant implications for both children and adults in the field of learning difficulties.

Sexual abuse

The incidence of sexual abuse within the sector of learning difficulties is relatively unknown. It is suggested that individuals with learning difficulties may be more vulnerable to increased risk of sexual abuse because of their own characteristics and their inability to say 'no'.

The individual who has learning difficulties may be seen as a 'safe victim', someone who is eager to please; may be overly responsive to attention and affection; may be seen as adult, but will not make adult demands on a relationship; who possesses limited or no communication skills which makes disclosure difficult and has little or no sex education; they may live in large settings, such as hospitals, where supervision may be difficult; or who may require intimate procedures which would lower the boundaries of personal space. This may be supervised by staff who have limited training and knowledge, unaware of the risks involved. The early advances made in sex education during the 1970s and 1980s have provided a framework which in the future may begin to address this issue of sexual abuse.

There is much still to be understood and all carers and members of the multidisciplinary team need to be aware of the reality of the problem. Further research is required to establish the extent of the problem and identify appropriate management strategies to ensure prevention or early diagnosis.

ETHICAL CONSIDERATIONS

Ethical problems in any setting arise when one member of society has a need which may, if met, conflict with the fulfilment of needs of others or impinge on their rights. In the case of individuals with a learning disability the decisions about many matters have to be taken by third parties, which in themselves may infringe on the rights of the disabled person. In enabling an individual to exercise his rights, the well-being of the general society in which he is placed may be adversely affected.

INTEGRATION WITHIN THE COMMUNITY

If members of the public are asked to express how they feel about supporting individuals with learning difficulties in the community, it would generally be found that the vast majority of the public support such policies. The problem arises when it comes to having individuals with learning difficulties living next door. The responses are more mixed, usually couched in terms of 'would they be happy here', 'they'll miss their friends'. Most people have the choice about where they live and with whom, but often this choice is not extended to individuals with learning difficulties.

Suggested assignments

Discussion points

1. In the light of the Community Care Act 1990, consider how the community as a whole will deal with people with learning difficulties being discharged into the community.

2. Deciding whether severely handicapped babies should be allowed to die naturally is a moral dilemma.

   Discuss.

3. Individuals with learning difficulties should be involved in decisions made about their lives as far as possible.

   How can you as a nurse help in this decision-making process?

4. It is necessary for individuals with learning difficulties to be able to behave appropriately to be acceptable in society.

   Discuss how far nurses have the right to change behaviour.

REFERENCES AND FURTHER READING

Alaszewski A 1990 Normalisation in practice. Routledge, London

Brechin A, Welmsley J 1989 Making connections. Hodder and Stoughton, London

Cavanagh S J 1991 Orem's model in action. McMillan, Basingstoke

Clarke D 1986 Mentally handicapped people: living & learning. Baillière-Tindall, London

Craft A, Craft M 1983 Sex education and counselling for mentally handicapped people. Costello, Tunbridge Wells

Fraser W I et al 1991 Hallas' caring for people with mental handicap, 8th edn. Butterworth-Heinemann, Oxford

Heaton Ward W A 1984 Mental handicap, 5th edn. Wright, Bristol

Keele D 1983 The developmentally disabled child. Medical Economic Books. Oradell N J

Levitt S 1982 Treatment of cerebral palsy and motor delay, 2nd edn. Blackwell Scientific Publications, Oxford

McCarthy G T 1992 Physical disability in childhood. Churchill Livingstone, Edinburgh

Presland J L 1989 Overcoming difficult behaviour. BIMH Publications, Kidderminster

Roper N 1990 The elements of nursing, 3rd edn. Churchill Livingstone, Edinburgh

Shanley E, Starrs T 1993 Learning disabilities – a handbook for care, 2nd edn. Churchill Livingstone, Edinburgh

Tierney A J 1983 Nurses and the mentally handicapped. Wiley, Chichester

Tinbergen N 1985 Autistic children: new hope for a cure. Allen & Unwin, London

Weihs T J 1971 Children in need of special care. Souvenir, London

Whelan E, Speake B 1979 Learning to cope. Souvenir, London

Wiedemann H R, Grosse K R, Dibbern H 1985 An atlas of characteristic syndromes – a visual aid to diagnosis, 2nd edn. Wolfe, London

Wing L 1976 Early childhood autism, 2nd edn. Pergamon, Oxford

8

Care implications of disorders of mood, emotions and sleep

Janis Greig

This chapter has three main sections. The first deals with disorders of mood with particular emphasis on depression, one of the most commonly occurring mental health problems which causes untold misery to sufferers. The second section covers anxiety, a universal experience which ranges from mild tension associated with day-to-day living to severe, disabling episodes of panic. The last section emphasizes nursing strategies for sleep disturbance, experienced by most people at some time in their life.

CARE IMPLICATIONS FOR MOOD DISORDERS

INTRODUCTION

Mood refers to an emotional or feeling state which influences an individual's total personality, thinking, activity and behaviour. Variations in mood are normal and necessary to help an individual adapt and respond to changing situations, events and environments. It can be seen from Figure 8.1 that the normal mood range seems relatively narrow and all individuals occasionally experience highs, lows or mood swings outside this range. Therefore, to distinguish between normal and abnormal mood changes, the severity, intensity and duration of the change must be assessed.

When the mood becomes relatively fixed and persistent, not necessarily related to external events, and interferes with the individual's ability to perform activities of living, it is known as a mood disorder and is very different from normal feelings of sadness or happiness. The two extremes of the mood continuum are depression and mania.

In lay usage, 'depressed' is often taken to mean the

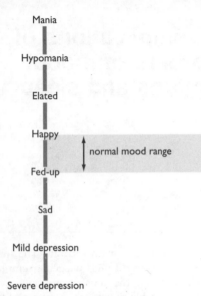

Fig. 8.1 Concept of a mood continuum

same as 'fed-up' but to mental health workers, depression means depressive illness or clinical depression – a syndrome of discrete symptoms requiring intervention and ranging from mild moderate states to severe states with psychotic features. Mania is the much less common polar extreme of depression while hypomania is similar to mania but much less severe.

EPIDEMIOLOGY

Between 20% and 30% of the population may suffer from a depressive episode at some time in their life. Mania is much more rare, affecting 1–2% of the population. Prevalence rates for depression greatly outnumber those of mania and this is found worldwide. When mania is seen, it usually presents as manic-depressive (or bipolar) disorder where episodes of mania alternate with episodes of depression. From 50% to 80% of all suicides and up to 75% of admissions to acute psychiatric units can be attributed to depression. After respiratory complaints, emotional problems like depression and anxiety may be the most common reason for consulting general practitioners and accompany up to 35% of major medical illness (Wilson & Kneisl 1988).

Depression is twice as common in females and the risk rises with increasing age to a peak in the 55–60 years age group. The elderly are at high risk for depression and suicide. In mania, however, the peak age of onset is below age 30 and no obvious gender differences are noted (Stuart & Sundeen 1983). Social

class gradients occur, with the rate of depressive illness at its height in social class 5 (unskilled manual workers), more than twice that of social class 1.

AETIOLOGY

Theories of cause in mood disorders can be summarized in four groups of factors (Box 8.1), often occurring in combination.

Genetic and biochemical factors

Strong evidence exists for the genetic inheritance of mood disorders, especially manic-depressive illness. Increased mood disorder rates are found within and between generations of an affected family when compared with the general population rates. A greater concordance rate for mood disorder is noted in identical rather than non-identical twins. Biochemical changes are also observed, particularly in depression, but it is unclear if these chemical changes cause depression or occur as a result of being depressed.

Studies concentrate on electrolyte, endocrine and neurotransmitter disturbance. The high rate of depression in women has generated much research into the role of female sex hormones in mood disorders associated with the menstrual cycle, the menopause and following childbirth or hysterectomy. No single hormone has been identified as responsible and the evidence remains inconclusive. Monoamine neurotransmitter disturbance has also been widely researched, leading to the monoamine theory of affective disorders. Monoamines are the group of neurotransmitters which include dopamine, noradrenaline and serotonin (5-hydroxytryptamine – 5HT). This theory states that depression is due to a relative decrease in monoamines, particularly noradrenaline and 5HT, while mania is due to a relative increase (Silverstone & Turner 1988). The treatment therefore of depression is to increase and for mania to decrease monoamine levels.

Psychological factors

The theories of Bowlby, Spitz and Robertson highlight the link between the childhood loss of a loved one by death or separation and the predisposition to depression in adult life. This traumatic loss may affect personality development in childhood and act as a precipitating factor in later years.

Freud also described loss of a loved object in childhood and the feelings of anger and guilt that resulted. However, Freud considered these angry feelings were turned inwards towards the self, resulting in self-destructive acts of suicide.

The cognitive model of Beck et al (1979) suggests that depression is caused by faulty thinking developed in the course of the person's up-bringing and early experiences, leaving him vulnerable to depression. This depressive-prone person has a negative view of himself, the world and even the future. These negative thoughts affect self-esteem and lower the mood, leading to more negative thoughts and so on in a 'vicious circle'.

Seligman's learned helplessness theory also emphasizes low self-esteem, lack of control and feelings of hopelessness engendered in childhood as being contributory to depression in adult life.

Physiological factors

Mood disorders (see Ch. 16) can occur secondary to physical illness or to drugs, where interference to neurotransmitters, hormones or brain structure results in mental health problems. Depression is associated with viral infections, endocrine disorders like hypothyroidism or Cushing's syndrome, vitamin B_{12} deficiencies and multiple sclerosis. Drug-induced depression occurs with oral contraceptives, steroids, antihypertensive agents like methyldopa as well as abused substances like alcohol, barbiturates and amphetamines. Mania also occurs secondary to viral infections, brain tumours, epilepsy and metabolic disturbances as well as to drugs like antidepressants and certain antiparkinsonian agents.

Psychosocial factors

Parkes (1976) demonstrates that any change or transition in life is accompanied by disturbance of emotions and that depression is the mood most likely to be associated with loss. (See Ch. 2). The transition may be from being single to being married, from being in a high status job to retiring or from being healthy to being a patient. Parkes suggests that bereavement,

amputation and even loss of home are stressful in similar ways and result in a grieving process. This occurs even when the loss is threatened or potential rather than actual.

Holmes & Rahe (1967) devised a Social Re-adjustment Rating Scale (see Ch. 2) which attempts to quantify the amount of major life changes occurring within a year. A major life change is defined as an alteration to relationships, health, role, status, property or financial situation. The risk of mental illness, especially anxiety and depression, seems to be greatly increased if there is a 'clustering' of change or loss in a relatively short period of time, which overwhelms a person's ability to cope. Brown & Harris (1978) studied the relationship between psychosocial stress and depression in working class women. They found that depression was highly related to childhood losses (especially of mother), three or more children under 14 years of age living at home, lack of employment outside the home and lack of a supportive, intimate partner.

The four groups of causation theories summarized above have expanded the understanding of mood disorders, particularly depression, but although some of the evidence seems strong, the aetiology of mood disorders is not explained by a single theory. The most helpful view might be to take a holistic approach, accepting that mood disorders have multiple causes involving an interplay between biological and psychosocial factors.

COMMON SYMPTOMS

The core features of depression and mania are summarized in Table 8.1.

TYPES OF DISORDERS (Box 8.2)

Grief reaction or brief depression reaction is a low mood state in which the core depressive symptoms mentioned in Table 8.1 are closely related in time and content to a specific stressful event like a bereavement or mastectomy. This condition usually resolves with time and family support and treatment is not normally required unless the grief reaction is delayed, prolonged, exaggerated or absent.

Premenstrual syndrome is a recurring complex symptom beginning up to 2 weeks prior to menstruation (see Ch. 17). A variety of physical symptoms may be accompanied by depression, anxiety, mood swings and irritability.

Baby blues is a common, transient state of tearfulness and irritability occurring in women shortly after

Table 8.1 Common symptoms of depression and mania

	Depression	Mania
Mood	Persistently low, feeling sad Risk of suicide	Persistently elated, sometimes irritable
Activity level	Restless, tense or anxious. May be socially withdrawn. In severe depression, movements and vital signs might be slowed up	Overactive, energetic and restless Movements speeded-up and vital signs raised Risk of physical exhaustion, dehydration or accidents
Thoughts and speech	Low self-esteem. Impaired concentration Gloomy, pessimistic thoughts Worries about health Thoughts and speech very slow in severe depression and delusions about sin, poverty and disease occur	Thoughts and speech are speeded up and may be jumbled. Cheerful, grandiose thoughts and delusions often of a religious or sexual nature Short attention-span, easily distracted Lack of insight
Appearance and non-verbal behaviour	Slumped posture. Poor eye contact. May be tearful or unresponsive. May perform nervous mannerisms. May be unkempt due to apathy	Erratic, bizarre and impulsive behaviour May be verbally aggressive. Sometimes bizarre clothing and usually unkempt due to overactivity
Sleep disturbance	Difficulty in getting off to sleep despite feeling very tired In severe depression, early morning wakening	In extreme cases, total insomnia Difficulty in getting off to sleep May only sleep 2–4 hours a night
Sexuality	Loss of libido Impotence/frigidity Menstrual changes	Libido increased Sometimes sexual content noticeable in speech, behaviour or clothing
Appetite	Anorexia or overeating In severe depression, anorexia and weight loss. Constipation	Variable. Often overactivity prevents an adequate dietary intake Risk of dehydration due to overactivity and sweating

---

Box 8.2 Types of mood disorder

- Grief reaction
- Premenstrual syndrome
- Baby blues
- Neurotic depression
- Postnatal depression
- Affective psychoses
- Puerperal psychoses

childbirth. This condition resolves without treatment and the symptoms are not enough to be classified as a true illness.

Neurotic or reactive depression is a low mood state with core symptoms as described in Table 8.1. It is sometimes also accompanied by anxiety and is often related to a past distressing event, although the depression arising may seem disproportionate. It often requires treatment by the family doctor but patients may need hospital care if there is a risk of suicide.

Postnatal depression is a low mood state occurring in women weeks or months following childbirth and is similar to neurotic depression.

Affective psychoses are severe disturbances of mood with core symptoms as in Table 8.1. They are often recurrent and accompanied by some or all of the following: disorders of the speed and content of thinking, disorders of motor activity and perceptual disturbance (see Ch. 9). Three main subtypes are observed:

- Psychotic depression is a profoundly low mood state with delusions, hallucinations (sometimes) and slowing of physiological and cognitive activity. There is a high risk of suicide and these patients commonly require hospital care. (A rare condition similar to this, but arising in women shortly after childbirth, is peurperal psychosis – depressed type.)

- Mania or hypomania where the mood is persistently elated accompanied by motor excitement, speeded-up thought processes, delusions and occasionally hallucinations. (A rare condition similar to mania, but arising in women shortly after childbirth, is puerperal psychosis – manic type.)
- Manic-depressive psychosis where periods of psychotic depression alternate with periods of mania.

The conditions above centre on the mood level being too high or too low. In some disorders, the mood level is neither high nor low but flat or blunt with a lack of responsiveness or incongruity to circumstance. This flattening of mood occurs in schizophrenia or hysteria where it is known as '*la belle indifferènce*'.

PATIENT IMPLICATIONS

The experience of depression

As seen in Table 8.1, a depressed person (for simplicity, the person will be male in this description) feels sad, hopeless and worthless. He cannot be 'cheered up' and nothing seems to interest or motivate him. He finds it difficult to concentrate or make decisions and work inevitably suffers. Depression makes everyday tasks difficult, leading to poor hygiene of self and home, problems such as debts or arrears in mortgage payments and even neglect of children or pets.

Marital or sexual relationships become strained and sufferers sometimes try to console themselves with alcohol, prescribed or non-prescribed drugs. The misery and suffering experienced leads the depressed person to see suicide as the only or even desired option and the risk of self-harm or actual suicide is high.

The experience of mania

A manic person (for simplicity, the person will be male in this description) feels cheerful, full of energy, talented and perhaps wealthy. His thoughts race and his speech is bizarre and jumbled as he changes the subject every few minutes. He may believe utterly that he is a talented opera singer, despite being tone deaf. He may talk rapidly and continually about Satan, occasionally bursting into a rude sea shanty. He may not have slept at all for 3 days but denies tiredness and claims that he's never felt better. He may dress in a flamboyant manner. He may make sexual overtures to complete strangers and become involved with the police. Work, relationships, self-care skills and home life may deteriorate to the point of re-

quiring hospital care. Impulsive and erratic behaviour increases the risk of self-harm through accidents or aggressive outbursts.

DIFFERENTIAL DIAGNOSIS AND INVESTIGATIONS

The slowing of movements and speech, concentration problems and difficulty with self-care skills found in severe depression may look like early dementia in an elderly persons.

If dementia is wrongly diagnosed, active treatment of the depression will not be given, the elderly person perhaps ending up in a continuing care setting. Unfortunately, psychometric tests like IQ tests are unhelpful in distinguishing between these two conditions but electroencephalogram recording, computerized tomography (CT and CAT scan) and magnetic resonance imaging (MRI) are increasingly used to gain information about the structure and function of the brain, identifying or eliminating dementia as the causative agent.

Two recent investigations, the tyramine challenge test and the dexamethasone suppression test, seek to confirm the diagnosis of depression using biochemical analysis of blood or urine. Although a major breakthrough, the reliability of these tests remains unclear (Rees 1988).

Medical staff are responsible for carrying out a thorough physical examination (especially of the central nervous system), a careful study of family history of physical or psychiatric problems as well as past or present medical history and current medication. Routine analysis of blood and urine is also carried out. In this way secondary mood disorders due to drugs or physical illness can be eliminated and genetic factors noted to aid diagnosis. It should be emphasized that the family is an important source of information, especially when the patient is an unreliable historian.

Assessment of mood is carried out during structured interview sessions by nurses and doctors and more informally by observation of the behaviour of the patient. Most of the latter is done by nursing staff, who, as a result of being with the patients most often, tend to have a closer relationship. Doctors and nurses may also use formal assessment tools such as Beck's Depressive Inventory (Barker 1985), where the patient is asked to read through a list of statements and circle those which most accurately described how he currently feels. A typical inventory statement is shown in Box 8.3.

The inventory statements are related to the main

features of depression and cover feelings of blame, guilt, sadness as well as physical matters such as sleeping and appetite. By totalling scores allocated to patients replies, staff can grade if the patient is depressed and whether it is a mild, moderate or severe depression. This type of assessment can be done on admission to aid diagnosis and help plan care or repeated at regular intervals to evaluate response to treatment.

THERAPEUTIC MANAGEMENT OF MOOD DISORDERS

The main treatment approaches in mood disorders are summarized in Table 8.2, where it can be seen that the affective psychoses (severe depression and mania) tend to be dealt with in a heavily physical way when compared to mild/moderate depression (neurotic depression, postnatal depression, grief reactions).

Counselling is a supportive, problem-solving relationship and is indicated when depression is related to social problems, life changes or particular events such as rape, bereavement or unemployment. To benefit fully from counselling, the patient should have relatively unimpaired insight and be able to converse without the disabling effects of delusions (see Ch. 9).

Behavioural approaches include relaxation exercises, which are particularly suitable when agitation

Table 8.2   Main treatment approaches in mood disorders

Mild/moderate depression	Severe depression	Mania
Counselling	Antidepressants	Antipsychotic drugs
Cognitive-behavioural approaches	ECT	Mood-stabilizing drugs
Antidepressants		

or anxiety accompany the low mood state or when difficulty in getting to sleep is a predominant feature. Another type of behavioural approach is social skills training which seeks to improve self-esteem and social functioning by allowing patients to practise and increase social skills such as eye contact or meeting strangers.

The cognitive-behavioural approach arises from the cognitive model of depression which suggests that negative thinking (also called dysfunctional thinking), developed in the course of a person's upbringing and early experiences, leads to depression. The treatment according to Beck et al (1979) is cognitive therapy which helps the patient recognize and correct these negative thoughts and thereby raise their low mood. Cognitive therapy can be carried out on an inpatient or outpatient basis, either on its own or as part of a combined treatment approach with antidepressant drugs. A major feature of this therapy is the full participation of the patient, not only during the sessions but also between sessions in the form of home assignments such as keeping a diary. Cognitive therapy can be done by psychologists, psychiatrists or, increasingly, nurse therapists where it proves to be equivalent or superior in efficacy to drug treatment. Other than in depression, this therapy can be used in a wide range of mental health problems such as anxiety, panic attacks, agoraphobia, eating disorders, drug abuse and relationship difficulties.

Electroconvulsive therapy (ECT)

ECT is a controversial treatment which may still be considered the treatment of choice for selected patients. The indications for use are psychotic depression where the following predominate: psychomotor retardation (physiological and psychological slowing), delusions of guilt/unworthiness, suicidal ideation and failure of response to antidepressants. A course of ECT consists of up to 12 treatments, usually given twice a week, but the number varies with each individual. ECT is the passage, for therapeutic reasons, of a controlled amount of electricity through the brain. The mood-lifting effect of ECT is unexplained although it is thought to raise monoamine levels, low in severe depression. To reduce distress to patients, ECT is given under general anaesthetic with a short-acting, intravenous barbiturate such as thiopentone and convulsions are modified by a muscle relaxant, like succinylcholine, to minimize the risk of bone injury. Contraindications for ECT would therefore centre on fitness for anaesthetic and include cardiovascular and respiratory problems.

Nurse's role in physical and psychological preparation for ECT

The nurse is the patient's main support during physical examination to ascertain fitness for anaesthetic, where she may also act as chaperone. Much of the information and explanation to allow the patient to give informed consent to treatment is provided by nurses, after the initial introduction by medical staff.

Patients are reassured to know that they will feel no pain and that a familiar nurse will accompany them throughout the procedure. Many of the patients' concerns centre around what will actually happen to them and this 'fear of the unknown' can be greatly allayed by an explanation of the procedure that is simple and jargon free. Emotive terms like 'shock treatment' are to be avoided. Honesty is important when discussing unwanted effects of ECT such as post-treatment headache and disorientation.

Physical preparation for ECT is very similar in principle to preparation for general anaesthetic (see Ch. 4) and includes signing a consent form, fasting for 6 hours and emptying the bladder immediately prior to treatment. Ordinary day clothes are worn and these should not be tight fitting. Prostheses like metal hairpins should be removed, although the nurse should not remove dentures until the last minute to help the patient preserve dignity. Valuables may be taken into short-term storage during the time the patient is out of the ward.

Nurses' role during and after treatment

The known nurse should stay near and in view of the patient, holding his hand if appropriate and making supportive remarks during venepuncture. Dentures, if worn, are removed at this point. This is the only role of the escorting nurse during ECT; the rest of the procedure is carried out by the attendant psychiatrist and anaesthetist.

Once the patient has the cannula inserted and anaesthetic agent administered, electrodes are placed usually bilaterally on the temples which have been wiped with saline to promote conductivity.

Teeth and tongue are protected by the insertion of a rubber or plastic mouth gag. A preset amount of electricity is then administered, causing immediate contraction of all the voluntary muscles equivalent to the tonic phase of a generalized epileptic seizure. After several seconds, rhythmic contractions begin alternating with relaxations, equivalent to the clonic phase of a generalized seizure.

The whole convulsion or seizure should not last longer than 60 seconds since the patient is not breathing due to the effects of the muscle relaxant drug given at the time of the anaesthetic. Individual responses are very variable and sometimes the seizure, modified by the muscle relaxant, is barely perceptible, seen only by concurrent electroencephalogram monitoring. The anaesthetist oxygenates the patient until he is breathing spontaneously, removes the mouth gag and inserts an airway, after which the patient is placed in the recovery position.

The main role of the nurse at this point is care of the unconscious patient. Vital sign measurement by the nurse continues with special emphasis on pulse, respiration and colour. The patient should be allowed to regain consciousness slowly and gradually with the nurse adopting a quiet approach and avoiding loud noises. This seems to help minimize patient distress or disorientation.

When appropriate, the airway and cannula are removed and during these procedures, the nurse should be making reorientating remarks in a soft, calm voice. The content of these reorientating comments includes using the patient's name (first name and full name with title), reminding the patient of the nurse's name, where the patient is and that the treatment is over. After about half an hour, most patients are ready to get up.

Outpatients return home, usually with a member of the family as escort, while inpatients return to their ward. Here they may require paracetamol for post-treatment headache, food and fluids to 'break their fast' and perhaps further rest or sleep on top of their bed. Staff observation should continue at an increased level following ECT as this treatment sometimes causes the retardation to lift before the mood itself lifts, making the patient at greater than ever risk of suicide.

Antidepressant drugs

These can be considered in three main groups:

1. Tricyclic antidepressants, drugs similar in chemical structure to chlorpromazine, have a sedative as well as mood-lifting effect. Examples of this group include amitriptyline and imipramine which are of special use when the depression is associated with anxiety or agitation. Therefore one drug can be used instead of administering an antidepressant and a sedative. The whole daily amount of around 150 mg can safely be given in a single dose, usually at night. This helps with the sleep disturbance pronounced in depression and minimizes sedation or drowsiness during the day.

2. Newer generation antidepressants like mianserin or trazodone are also mood-lifting but are not so sedative. When depression is accompanied by retardation or apathy, further sedation would be undesirable and therefore this group of antidepressants would be prescribed in preference to tricyclics. Although these drugs have side-effects similar to tricyclics, they are not so pronounced and consequently are more suitable for elderly people. For the same reason as above, the whole daily amount can safely be given in a single dose.

3. Monoamine oxidise inhibitors (MAOI) Like antidepressants in the other two groups, MAOI drugs may take up to 3 weeks to produce the mood-lifting effect and all three groups cause similar side-effects to different degrees. These include dry mouth, constipation, dizziness or hypertension, blurred vision, urinary retention, drowsiness and cardiac arrhythmias. Examples of this group include phenelzine and tranylcypromine. MAOI drugs are not usually the first choice in treatment because of an additional problem; a serious interaction between the MAOI drug and tyramine, found in many foodstuffs and beverages. This interaction causes intense headache, hypertension and in very severe cases subarachnoid haemorrhage. If a patient must have a MAOI drug, usually because their depression has resisted ECT or tricyclic antidepressants, it follows then that they must adhere to a diet which restricts the intake of tyramine-rich substances like cheese, meat, yeast extracts and alcohol. MAOI drugs potentiate the action of sedatives and narcotics and interact badly with other antidepressants, as well as many 'over-the-counter' cold preparations. It can be seen therefore that patient education to ensure understanding is essential (Box 8.4). Any complaints of dizziness or headache should be taken very seriously by nursing staff, who should monitor blood pressure and contact medical staff.

Mood-stabilizing drugs

Lithium is a naturally occurring metal of the same group as sodium and potassium. It is usually prescribed as the carbonate (Camcolit, Priadel) for the patients with manic-depressive (bipolar) illness where it acts as a mood stabilizer, dampening down extreme mood swings. It is administered either when the mood is high or low and patients may be maintained on lithium for several years if necessary. Lithium is toxic in small amounts and tends to accumulate in the body, so for these reasons a thorough screening is carried out prior to starting the drug. Serum lithium

---

Box 8.4 Advice for patients having MAOI antidepressants

While taking this medicine and for 14 days after your treatment finishes you must observe the following simple instructions:

1. Do not eat CHEESE, PICKLED HERRING OR BROAD BEAN PODS
2. Do not eat or drink BOVRIL, OXO, MARMITE or SIMILAR MEAT OR YEAST EXTRACT
3. Eat only FRESH foods and avoid food that you suspect could be stale or 'going off'. This is especially important with meat, fish, poultry or offal. Avoid game
4. Do not take any other MEDICINES (including tablets, capsules, nose drops, inhalations or suppositories) whether purchased by you or previously prescribed by your doctor, without first consulting your doctor or your pharmacist.
   Note: Treatment for coughs and colds, pain relievers, tonics and laxatives are medicines
5. Avoid alcoholic drinks and de-alcoholized (low alcohol) drinks

Keep a careful note of any food or drink that disagrees with you, avoid it and tell your doctor

Report any unusual or severe symptoms to your doctor and follow any other advice given by him

---

levels are checked as they will be for the whole time that the patient takes lithium. Screening may also include ECG to check cardiac fitness, blood tests to check liver function and creatinine clearance to check kidney function as well as physical examination. In this way, medical staff ascertain if the patient can detoxify and excrete lithium sufficiently to avoid toxicity. Side-effects of lithium include loose stools, thirst, polydipsia, polyuria, metallic taste in the mouth, 'heavy' arms and legs and nausea. Although troublesome to the patient, these are considered harmless, almost expected side-effects which diminish after a week or two. Signs of toxicity include slurred speech, tremor, vomiting, confusion, restlessness and convulsions. These are serious, requiring checking of serum lithium levels and review of dosage by medical staff. The next due dose of lithium may be withheld by nurses until this has been achieved.

Nurses should ensure that the patient has sufficient intake of fluids and salt as any dehydration or electrolyte imbalance would precipitate lithium toxicity. As with MAOI drugs, the patient needs a high level of explanation and education to ensure safe drug compliance. Carbamazepine, perhaps better known as an anticonvulsant, is sometimes used as a mood stabilizer either by itself or as an adjunct to lithium.

Antipsychotic drugs

Drugs like chlorpromazine and haloperidol are often used to help control overactivity and restlessness in mania as well as promoting rest and sleep (see Ch. 9).

NURSING STRATEGIES

The depressed patient

The activities of living model (Roper et al 1990) can be used as a framework to assess and plan the nursing care needed. Under each activity heading are examples of the likely assessment questions.

1. Maintaining a safe environment

Is the patient suicidal?, if yes, *how* suicidal is he? Does he make direct statements of intent or indirect statements (the future looks black to me)? Is it only thoughts of suicide or is there evidence of actual planning such as giving away possessions or hoarding medicine? Has the patient resorted to self-harm in the past? Has there been a recent attempt? If yes, was it a serious attempt rather than a gesture?

Judge the seriousness of an attempt by assessing the following: lethality of chosen method, definite and detailed plan, strategies to avoid being rescued and patient's expectations of death (Hagerty 1984).

Is the patient willing to comply with treatment or is he trying to leave the ward? Does the patient have sharp objects or medicines amongst his possessions? As a result of the above, does the patient require increased levels of observation, especially in potentially dangerous areas like the bathroom?

2. Communicating

Is the content of the patient's speech morbid, pessimistic, preoccupied with self-harm, death or health worries? Is the rate of speech (and hence the thoughts) slow, hesitant or full of long pauses? Is the patient's speech so slow that he is answering in short sentences only? Is he monosyllabic or mute? Is the speech content bizarre, reflecting delusional beliefs about sin, guilt, unworthiness or poverty? (see Ch. 9). Does the speech content reflect low self-esteem or negative thinking, such as 'I'm a complete failure'? Does the speech content reflect the patient's worries about social problems or major life changes such as bereavement or relationship problems?

Does the patient spontaneously initiate conversation or only respond when directly addressed? Is his posture slumped, does he give eye contact? Is there evidence of agitation such as wringing of the hands?

Does the patient mix with other patients, with staff, with the same sex or the opposite sex? What is the communication like between the patient and his family or friends? Does the patient have insight and understanding of his problems, situation or treatment? As a result of the above, what level of nursing help is required to minimize this patient's communication problems?

3. Resting and sleeping

See assessment of 'Care implications for disorders of sleep' (p. 298).

4. Eating and drinking

What is the patient's usual consumption, habits and preference? Has his appetite changed recently? Is there evidence of weight loss or dehydration? Will charting of weight, food or fluid intake be required? Does the patient have any special dietary needs such as MAOI restriction, cultural/religious requirements or personal preferences such as vegetarianism? Is the patient deterred from eating by the presence of other people or by delusional beliefs about the food? Is there evidence of alcohol or drug abuse? If the patient is very slowed up in movements, is this affecting food and fluid intake?

As a result of assessment of the above, what level of nursing help is required to minimize this patient's problems with eating and drinking?

5. Cleansing and dressing

Is the patient's grooming affected by apathy or slowing of movements? Is the patient neat and groomed or unkempt, smelling of body odour? Does the patient spontaneously attend to hygiene or is it only when prompted? How does the patient react to prompting? Does he show any interest in his appearance? Is he safe to be in the bathroom by himself? Overall, what level of nursing help (if any) does the patient need to maintain hygiene and appearance?

6. Elimination

What is the patient's usual bowel habit? Is the patient constipated? If yes, is it compounded by dehydration or side-effects of antidepressant drugs? Is a fluid balance chart indicated?

7. Working, playing and mobilizing

Does the patient spend much of his time in bed or withdrawn from other people? Is he slow and relatively inactive or restless and pacing? What were the patient's hobbies and interests prior to the illness?

Can these previous interests be used in planning therapeutic activities for the patient? Could this patient benefit from social/recreational therapy? Are relatives keen to be involved? Is the patient employed/unemployed? Is social work involvement needed to help with benefits, work or financial situation?

8. Expressing sexuality

Does the patient have body image problems? If appropriate, is there evidence of menstrual change? Is the patient's relationship affected by impotence/frigidity/loss of libido?

Following assessment, the nurses should have an accurate picture of this patient's particular needs. This individualized approach is essential since depressed patients are very variable in the levels of nursing help needed, with some independent and others requiring full assistance with activity of living skills. It may seem obvious but, at the same time as patient problems or needs are being assessed, patient *strengths* should also be noted.

Barrowclough & Fleming (1986) describe three types of strengths:

- what the patient can already do
- what the patient likes to do
- people willing to be involved.

Examples of strengths might be; uses public transport safely, enjoys a game of cards or brother visits every day and is keen to take patient home for the weekend. Considering strengths instead of just focusing on problems offers a more positive view of the patient and allows a more accurate and holistic assessment.

The main objectives of nursing care for the depressed patient are:

- provide a safe environment and protect from self-harm
- establish healthy communication and relationship forming
- establish and maintain adequate eating and drinking
- establish and maintain a reasonable sleep pattern
- establish and maintain adequate hygiene

- establish adequate elimination
- establish and maintain a constructive level of activity.

See Nursing Care Plan 8.1

Provide a safe environment and protect from self-harm

Following assessment of suicide potential, an increased level of observation may be prescribed to ensure the patient's safety. A newly admitted patient is an 'unknown quantity', so sometimes a higher level of observation is maintained for a few days until staff can assess and determine suicide risk. There are two main levels of increased observation – close and special.

Special observation is carried out for patients assessed as being at high risk of suicide and involves constant supervision on a one-to-one basis by a designated nurse. This may continue even when the patient appears to be sleeping and also when in the bathroom. A rota is usually devised so that the designated nurse is changed hourly. It is impossible to carry this out discreetly since the nurse must accompany the patient wherever he goes within the ward and therefore a careful explanation is given to the patient of the nature and purpose of the special observation, using supportive phrases like 'keep you safe'. It is important to be honest about the reasons for increased observation to allay possible feelings of suspicion and anxiety it may otherwise cause to patients.

Close observation is carried out for patients assessed as being at lesser risk of self-harm and involves careful monitoring by a designated nurse of where the patient is and what they are doing at all times. The nurse, however, does not need constant one-to-one contact with the patient but, as in special observation, leaving the ward is strongly discouraged unless the patient is escorted. Some patients on close observation move up to special observation temporarily for at-risk times or places, usually times of lower staff numbers like meal breaks, night duty or handovers or places of special danger, for example while bathing or shaving.

Occasionally a contractual agreement is made between the staff and patient where the patient abides by negotiated 'rules' like not leaving the ward without telling a member of staff.

Environmental precautions centre on staff's alertness to potentially dangerous items in the patient's possession or surroundings. Patients at high risk of suicide may try to use common objects to harm

Nursing Care Plan 8.1 Care for the depressed patient		
Problem	**Objective**	**Nursing action**
1. **Self-harm risk**	Provide a safe environment and protect from self-harm	❐ Increase observation levels Remove environmental hazards
2. **Communication impaired because of:** a. Irritation or morbid speech content b. Low self-esteem c. Slow thoughts and speech	Establish healthy communication and relationship forming	❐ Divert/distract from bizarre speech Give adult praise and provide opportunities to succeed ❐ Allow time for response
3. **Inadequate food/fluid intake**	Establish and maintain adequate eating and drinking	❐ Check weight regularly Cater for needs/preferences Allow time if slowed up Minimize the effects of delusions on food
4. **Sleep disturbance**	Establish and maintain reasonable sleep pattern	❐ Activity throughout the day Discourage napping Behavioural strategies
5. **Impaired cleansing and dressing**	Establish and maintain adequate hygiene	❐ Prompting to carry out routine of self-caring
6. **Constipation**	Establish adequate elimination	❐ Encourage hydration and exercise Administer suppositories, if prescribed Observe fibre content of diet
7. **Withdrawn, apathy, slowed up**	Establish and maintain constructive levels of activity	❐ Be available to patient on a one-to-one basis Encourage social/recreational activities Involve relatives

themselves. Part of the nurse's role during increased observation is to remain alert to the potential hazards of everyday items such as matches, plastic bags or glass ornaments. As mentioned above, sharp objects and medicines may be removed from the patient's belongings. Special care is required to prevent access to drug cupboards, lotion cupboards, treatment rooms and perhaps bathrooms where even innocuous items like shampoo and cleaning materials can prove to be dangerous to an actively suicidal patient. Male patients may be asked to use an electric shaver rather than have a wet shave with a disposable razor and care should be taken when the patient is using scissors for cutting nails or during group activity sessions.

While it is impossible to make the whole ward completely hazard free, it is feasible, at least, to keep the immediate surroundings of the patient safe. Apart from increased observation, the main way to achieve this is to allocate the patient to a single room if possible which is centrally located and near the duty room or nurses' station.

Co-operation is sought after explanation to avoid patients obtaining medicines or other dangerous objects from visitors or other patients. Liquid drugs are sometimes prescribed instead of tablets to minimize the chance of patients spitting out and hoarding drugs to use in a future self-harm attempt.

Establish healthy communication and relationship forming

After physical safety, the next priority is communication since it is essential in meeting all the other needs of the patient. After all, how is the patient's understanding and co-operation with regard to eating, hygiene, etc. to be gained without it? The main approach should be friendly with the nurse conveying interest to the patient both verbally and non-verbally by spending time with or making herself available to the patient. Open questions should encourage the patients to express their feelings and concern, allowing a ventilation rather than a 'bottling up' of emotions. The nurse should speak slowly and clearly in short, jargon-free sentences which may need to be repeated if the patient is having concentration problems. This is especially important if the patient suffers from psychomotor retardation, taking longer to comprehend and needing longer to make a response to the nurse's question. In very severely retarded patients, the nurse may have to resort to closed questions to merely obtain a yes/no response from almost mute patients.

The nurse sometimes has to work hard to avoid feelings of frustration engendered by the patient's pauses, silences or hesitations and by the need to repeat things. The emphasis is on active listening and toleration of silence where the physical presence of the nurse and the use of touch may be more comforting to the patient than 'bombarding' with questions. If the patient is silent or says 'I don't feel like talking', the nurse may remain quietly with the patient or say 'I'll come back later'. Either of these responses conveys interest and caring; being sensitive to the patient's need for silence without rejection. It is important that the nurse does not take any silence as personal and learns to feel comfortable during long gaps in conservation. Some depressed patients may wish to talk frequently about death, past suicide attempts or other pessimistic topics such as physical health worries. It may be considered as non-therapeutic and even reinforcing to ruminate on such matters to the exclusion of more positive topics. The nurse should never joke or make insensitive remarks like 'it can't be as bad as all that' but at the same time, convey to the patient that it is unhelpful to dwell on negative topics, perhaps saying something like 'I think we've spoken enough about that just now' or 'can we talk about something else?' In this way, the patients can be diverted or distracted by suggesting another topic of conversation or an activity.

Other depressed patients are psychotic, making irrational or bizarre statements which they believe utterly. Response to delusional remarks is covered in Chapter 9 and briefly summarized in Box 8.5.

Establish and maintain adequate eating and drinking

Assessment may be continuing in the form of a weight chart and, in some cases, a fluid balance chart. Individual preferences should be catered for and the dietitian involved to provide the patient with food similar to their normal diet. The patient should be able to choose from a selection on a menu card and may need nursing help to do so if severely depressed. Small portions, attractively presented may encourage the patient to eat even a little. Relatives can be involved and encouraged to bring in 'treats' to tempt the patient but this involvement may be influenced by

---

> **Box 8.5 Advice on responses to delusional remarks**
>
> **DON'T**
> - Joke or laugh at the bizarre remarks – this is insensitive since the patient truly believes these thoughts. Trust in the nurse–patient relationship may be severely damaged by uncaring acts on the part of the nurse
> - Nod, 'go along with' or 'humour' a patient making bizarre remarks – this can be interpreted by the patient as agreement and reinforce or strengthen the false beliefs
> - Argue or try to convince the patient that the belief is false – false beliefs are not logical and delusional patients have poor insight so arguments may reinforce the belief and even provoke an aggressive response from patients
>
> **DO**
> - Guard facial expression and other non-verbal behaviours during the bizarre remarks and make no response whatsoever
> - Say 'I'm sorry, I don't know what you mean' or 'I don't understand you' – this is usually true and gives feedback to the patient
> - Divert or distract from bizarre topics, perhaps saying something like 'these worrying thoughts upset you, let's talk about something else' – dwelling on delusions is reinforcing and hence non-therapeutic
> - Use activity to divert or distract – suggest a walk or a board game
> - Give lots of attention, positive non-verbal behaviours (smiling, nodding) and adult praise if the conversation topic is rational or optimistic – by reinforcing rational or positive statements, bizarre remarks can be reduced and self-esteem raised

---

hospital policies on food handling and storage. Fluids are a priority and the patient should have a minimum of 2 litres a day; the bulk of this should not be tea or coffee – these are stimulants and may further deter sleep in an already sleep-impaired patient. In severely depressed patients, a designated nurse may be assigned to approach the patient hourly offering a glass of iced water or orange juice. Sometimes proprietary supplements are used, where a pleasant-tasting drink may provide a source of protein and carbohydrate for the patient. In patients suffering from psychomotor retardation, the nurse should allow lots of time for these slow patients to finish their meal and avoid 'hovering' near the patient to remove their tray. All the courses of the meal should not be served at the same time to such slow patients as cold food is very unappetizing and may further deter them from eating. Facilities should be available for keeping food warm or reheating, again according to local food handling regulations. Very slowed up patients may require nurse supervision throughout the meal to give assistance or prompt the patient to continue eating.

Delusional beliefs sometimes affect the patient's dietary intake. Patients who have beliefs about guilt or sin sometimes eat better in private rather than being in a busy dining area. Other delusion types like poverty or persecution (the food is poisoned) are dealt with in Chapter 9.

Establish and maintain a reasonable sleep pattern

This is dealt with under 'Care implications for disorders of sleep' (p. 298).

Establish and maintain adequate hygiene

Perhaps of all the activities of living, this is the most variable in terms of the amount of nursing help needed. Some patients are independently self-caring while others need very full nursing intervention. The main approach is to maintain a normal routine of hygiene and assessment will have shown whether the patient needs no help or whether reminding, prompting and persuasion is required. In very slowed-up patients, assistance may be needed for bathing, washing hair or clothes. Adult praise and extra attention is given for any positive action; for example, if a patient combs his hair without staff prompting, the nurse might say 'it's good to see you taking an interest in yourself'. It is important when giving praise to remember that the patient is an intelligent adult, despite their temporary dependence. Care should be taken to avoid babyish or patronizing comments. As mentioned in maintaining a safe environment, increased observation may be required while the patient is attending to his hygiene needs such as shaving, bathing or cutting fingernails.

Establish adequate elimination

Following assessment, the patient's normal bowel habit will be known.

Constipation, common in depressed people, can be helped by ensuring adequate hydration and intake of food. Increased mobility, activity and exercise can help stimulate peristalsis. The fibre content of the diet may be increased. In some cases, enemas or suppositories may be prescribed.

Depressed patients often interpret the feelings associated with constipation such as wind, bloating and abdominal discomfort as symptoms of physical illness. The nurse can help by relating these feelings to being depressed or to the side-effects of anti-depressant drugs.

Establish and maintain a constructive level of activity

Many depressed patients, withdrawn and experiencing communication problems, are best related to on an individual basis rather than in groups, especially in the acute phase of their illness. Placing such a patient in a group activity may be overwhelming for them and reduce their self-esteem instead of improving it. Ensuring success and thereby raising the self-esteem of a depressed patient is the main approach and this cannot be achieved by involving them in activities which, at that time, are too much for them. Later on, group activities can be considered such as current affairs/newspaper groups, relaxation activities, community meetings, social skills groups, health and fitness activities, outings and other social/recreational pursuits.

While a depressed patient is deemed unsafe to leave the ward or unable to benefit from groups, activities should be planned on a one-to-one basis. These may be low key and centre on escorted walks and self-care activities as well as interactions with the designated nurse. Care should be taken if the activity involves potentially dangerous items, as in using scissors in an art session. Relaxation techniques to reduce tension and promote sleep can be introduced at this stage and followed up in group sessions when the patient is ready.

Involvement of the family is important to maintain contact with the outside world and keep in touch with family news. If considered safe, the family can be full participants in providing social-recreational activities for patient, such as a trip in the car or a visit home for the day.

Evaluation

Monitoring a patient's progress should be carried out on a daily basis and care modified accordingly. Formal evaluation of mood would include redoing the original assessment and noting changes in the patient's level of functioning. Careful written records should include note of the following indicators of recovery in a depressed patient:

- reduced frequency of suicidal or bizarre speech
- reduced tension or tearfulness
- increased eye contact, smiling or positive statements
- longer length of sleep

- more interest in appearance or activities
- better appetite.

Evaluation is crucial to ensure that the patient receives the care he needs for as long as he needs it, without fostering dependency on the nursing staff. Whenever the patient is ready and able to cope with his own activities of living, the nurses' role is to pull back and allow this to happen.

The manic patient

The activities of living model (Roper et al 1990) will be used as a framework to assess the nursing care needed. Under each activity heading are examples of the likely assessment questions asked or considered by the nurse.

1. Maintaining a safe environment

Is the patient at risk of accident because of overactivity or impulsive behaviour? Is the patient irritable or verbally aggressive to staff or fellow patients? Does the patient cause friction with others due to interrupting or noisy behaviour? Is the patient willing to stay or trying to leave the ward?

2. Communicating

Is the patient's speech (and hence thoughts) speeded up? Is his speech content bizarre, sexual or religious in nature? Does the patient talk about grandiose plans, spending sprees or have an inflated self-image? Is the patient rude, condescending, irritable or easily distracted when talking to others? Does he have a short attention span or decreased concentration in conversation or activity? Does the patient jump from one topic of conversation to another without logical association? Is the patient's speech content jumbled or incoherent? Is his ability to relate to others affected by problems of physical overactivity?

3. Eating and drinking

Is the patient's fluid balance compromised by physical overactivity or sweating? If yes, is fluid balance charting indicated? Is his food intake affected by physical overactivity or distractibility? Do grandiose delusions about food affect his diet? What are this patient's food preferences or special dietary needs? Does the patient overeat or appear 'greedy'? Has there been recent weight loss or gain? If yes, is a weight chart indicated?

4. Sleeping

Assessment of sleep follows under 'Care implications of sleep disorders' (p. 298).

5. Cleansing and dressing

Is the patient unkempt, sweating and smelling of body odour? Is he dressed appropriately for the climate? Is he dressed in a bizarre, flamboyant or seductive manner? Is he prone to removing clothing, leading to public displays of nudity? Does the patient have an interest in his appearance, attend to personal hygiene needs spontaneously or only when prompted? How does the patient react to prompting?

6. Elimination

What is the patient's usual bowel habit? Does the patient suffer from urinary retention or constipation due to his overactivity? Is dehydration a potential risk due to overactivity? If yes, is fluid balance charting indicated? Does the patient urinate in inappropriate places due to overactivity and disinhibition?

7. Working, playing and mobilizing

Does the patient show increased responsiveness to environmental stimuli such as an 'audience' of fellow patients, the television or music? Is he even more stimulated to overactivity by attention, noise or social/recreational activities? Does the patient dominate, interrupt or prove disruptive in group sessions? What is the frequency, intensity and duration of his restlessness? What were the patient's hobbies and interests prior to the illness?

8. Expressing sexuality

Is the patient flirtatious, seductive, rude or overtly sexual in speech, clothing or behaviour? Does he have an increased libido? If yes, is it directed at staff, fellow-patients or visitors? Is the patient disinhibited in terms of nudity or masturbation?

Following assessment, the nurse will have an accurate picture of the patient's strengths and needs from which to plan care strategies, tailored to the individual. Manic patients are very variable in their needs; some are physically overactive, while others are speeded up only in thoughts and speech, some are very sexually disinhibited while others are not and some are easily irritated while others are cheerful and gregarious.

Nursing Care Plan 8.2 summarizes the nursing strategies for a manic patient. The main objectives of nursing care might be as follows:

- maintain a safe environment and protect other patients
- establish healthy communication and relationship forming
- establish a reasonable sleep pattern
- establish adequate eating and drinking
- establish adequate hygiene
- establish adequate elimination
- establish constructive levels of activity
- establish appropriate expression of sexuality.

Maintain a safe environment and protect other patients

Like the depressed patient, the manic patient may require an increased level of supervision to ensure his safety. However, in this care, suicidal intent is not the issue but the danger of accidents such as tripping or falling due to physical overactivity. Very restless patients in this state sometimes jog, run and even dance around, paying no regard to potential hazards like rugs and furniture. Nurses may have to temporarily remove or reposition coffee tables and chair legs to prevent falls.

Close or special observation by a designated nurse on a rota basis should also prevent the manic patient carrying out impulsive or dangerous behaviour; for example, inserting a pen into an electric socket or flushing money down the toilet. The safety of the patient's possessions is sometimes a factor and the nurse may have to intervene to prevent the manic patient giving away money and personal effects to fellow patients or visitors.

Irritability, aggression and sexual disinhibition can combine to make this patient compromise the safety of other patients and become a target for retaliation. For example, the manic patient can be aggressive, insulting or rude, placing a fellow patient in potential

Nursing Care Plan 8.2 Care for the manic patient		
Problem	**Objective**	**Nursing action**
1. Risk of aggression or accidents	Provide a safe environment	❐ Increase observation levels Reduce environmental stimuli Protect other patients

2. Communication impaired due to:
  a. Irrational, grandiose speech content
  b. Speeded up thoughts and speech
	Establish healthy communication and relationship forming	❐ Reduce reinforcement of bizarre speech
		Divert/distract from bizarre speech
		Limit set on sexual speech content

3. Sleep disturbance	Establish reasonable sleep pattern	❐ Single room Non-stimulating environment
4. Inadequate food/fluid intake	Establish adequate eating and drinking	❐ Check weight weekly Cater for needs/preferences Flexible approach
5. Impaired cleansing and dressing	Establish adequate hygiene	❐ Supervision and prompting Use a clothing checklist Limit setting to protect dignity
6. Constipation/urinary retention	Establish adequate elimination	❐ Encourage hydration Gentle prompting
7. Overactivity	Establish constructive levels of activity	❐ Reduce environmental stimuli Encourage non-competitive activities Protect other patients
8. Increased libido and disinhibition	Establish appropriate expression of sexuality	❐ Increased supervision Protect other patients Limit setting

danger or, as a result of his annoying behaviour, the manic patient can attract aggression from others. It is the role of the nurse during increased observation to predict, defuse and prevent such incidents. The distractibility which is such a pronounced feature of mania can be used to the nurse's advantage in defusing potentially dangerous incidents and often a single remark like 'would you like to come for a walk?' is all that is required. See Chapter 10 for more strategies to deal with the aggressive patient.

Establish healthy communication and relationship forming

The whole approach of the nurse should be calm and quiet to prevent stimulation of the manic patient. A nurse who is loud, joking and overly cheerful can be 'infectious' to a manic patient, inspiring further elated comments or behaviour in an almost competitive manner. Slow, jargon-free speech, avoiding double meanings, should be adopted by the nurse. Care should be taken to guard non-verbal behaviour like facial expression and the nurse must avoid smiling and laughing at the sometimes truly hilarious comments or antics of the manic patient. Sometimes these patients mean to be funny and seek response from staff but other times the comments or behaviour result from delusions which the patient utterly believes. It would therefore be either reinforcing or uncaring but certainly non-therapeutic to laugh along or 'humour' these patients.

When a manic patient says, for example, 'I have the powers of telepathy' or 'I am on a mission from God', similar rationale and guidelines apply as were summarized earlier in this chapter for response to bizarre or delusional remarks (see Ch. 9). The aim of the nurse is to reduce reinforcement of bizarre speech and actions, distract or divert from bizarre behaviour and increase reinforcement of rational behaviour.

When a manic patient is unable to set limits on his own speech and behaviour due to the effects of the illness, the nurse may take over this function temporarily. This approach is known as limit setting and involves giving clear firm messages and feedback to patients to prevent further stimulation, increase their personal control and reduce inappropriateness. To achieve limit setting, the nurse must firmly register disapproval of speech content or action both verbally and non-verbally, while avoiding being authoritarian, as this could provoke an aggressive response from the patient. Nurses should remind themselves that consistency is crucial and that this approach is for therapeutic rather than punitive reasons. Examples of limit-setting responses might be: 'I'm going now, I'll come back when you've settled down', or 'That kind of talk is unacceptable, can we change the subject?'. The aim of the nurse during limit setting is similar in principle to concepts previously discussed such as withdrawing reinforcement from bizarre and unacceptable topics by ignoring or not responding, by giving clear messages of disapproval and by distracting/diverting and reinforcing appropriate behaviour.

Establish a reasonable sleep pattern

See under 'Care implications for disorders of sleep' for strategies to minimize sleep disturbance.

Establish adequate eating and drinking

The nurse should again consider the basic principles of encouraging a reasonable intake of food and fluids by catering to the patient's preferences or special needs, giving attention to choice and presentation.

Very restless patients are at risk of dehydration and may need 4 or more litres of fluid in a day to counteract increased sweating, associated with physical overactivity and increased metabolic rate. Ongoing fluid balance charting may be required to monitor intake and output, although gaining the co-operation of the manic patient may be extremely difficult. Fluids may need to be offered hourly by a designated nurse and the bulk of these should not be tea or coffee to avoid any further stimulating effect.

Weekly weight charting may be proposed to check for weight loss, the dietitian consulted and supplementary feeding considered if poor food intake due to overactivity is pronounced. The key approach of the nurse should be flexibility with regard to set meal times; for instance, if the patient declines lunch at 1 p.m. and asks for something to eat at 3 p.m., it would be ideal if food could then be offered at that time. Local food handling and storage policies may make it difficult to offer a full meal but sandwiches or fruit could be provided.

Some manic patients are overstimulated by the presence of an 'audience' of other patients in a busy or crowded dining area and respond by becoming noisy, more overactive or disruptive, which further deters them from eating. Again flexibility on the part of the nurse could allow the patient to be served on their own, in a quiet part of the ward. Gentle persuasion and limit setting is the overall approach to avoid provoking an irritable or even aggressive response from the manic patient.

A few manic patients may have grandiose delusions associated with food (Box 8.5 provides principles of response to bizarre/delusional remarks).

Establish adequate hygiene

Excessive sweating may lead to body odour requiring the nurse to gently prompt the manic patient to have a daily shower or bath. Clothing made from natural fibres (i.e. cotton) may be preferable to man-made fibres if sweating is a prominent feature. The patient's distractibility can again be used to the nurse's advantage if a request for the patient to bathe is met with hostility. Instead of 'nagging' the patient and provoking an aggressive response, the nurse can say 'I'll leave you now and ask you later when you are more calm'. If sexual disinhibition is complicating the patient's hygiene needs, increased supervision may be required during dressing, undressing or bathing to prevent episodes of nudity or exhibitionism upsetting other patients. Sometimes a clothing checklist is used in a limit-setting way to ensure that the manic patient does not emerge from bedroom or bathroom in a state of undress. For example, the nurse might closely observe the patient during the bath and then, using the checklist, ensure that zips are done up and clothes tucked in before the patient leaves the privacy of the bathroom and enters the full glare of public scrutiny. By so-doing the nurse is protecting the dignity of the manic patient as well as protecting other patients from upset.

If the patient dresses flamboyantly in clashing colours or bizarre styles, the nurse can try gently prompting, persuasion and offering alternatives – 'what about this one instead?' Whereas there is no negotiation about 'decency', some leeway must be allowed for adequately covered yet bizarre clothing styles.

Establish adequate elimination

Often there is no problem in this area but, for a few patients, extreme overactivity leads to urinary retention or constipation. In this case, a designated nurse may need to prompt the patient hourly or 2 hourly to visit the toilet. Adequate hydration and an increased intake of food will also help the patient to resolve constipation problems and fluid balance charting may continue if urinary retention is a prominent feature.

Occasionally some patients urinate in inappropriate places like the waste-paper bin in the dayroom. Increased supervision and a limit-setting approach by nursing staff should prevent this, as well as protect fellow patients.

Establish constructive levels of activity

Since the likely patient problem in this area is overactivity, the role of the nurse is to *reduce* the overall level of activity and increase the amount of purposeful rather than aimless or bizarre activity. This approach is sometimes described as providing a non-stimulating environment, where nurses are calm and quiet, noise from television or radios is kept to a minimum and the manic patient is deterred from joining group sessions. Entering a busy dining area or joining in a current affairs group means that the manic patient has an 'audience' to entertain and may be stimulated to further elated and outlandish behaviour by the attention and comments from others. This is therapeutic neither for the manic patient nor others and therefore a subtle 'seclusion' may occur where the manic patient is dealt with on a one-to-one basis by the designated nurse.

At some time in this patient's recovery, he will be introduced to group activities and discussions but this should be a gradual process, based on the individual's ability to cope. One-to-one constructive activities suitable for this patient would include: self-care tasks like washing clothes, escorted walks, drawing and painting, some sports and board games. Choice of activities would be aided by a knowledge of the patient's strengths gained in assessment.

Care should be taken either to avoid competitive sports and games or to play them without keeping score, thus avoiding argument or irritability. Sports like table tennis may help the patient expend some of his boundless energy and promote sleep but excessive exercise should be avoided as this can increase elation in the manic patient.

Evaluation

Manic patients are very variable in their needs and an individual can fluctuate greatly in the course of a day, therefore evaluation must be ongoing to ensure the correct level of nursing help is provided. Formal evaluation might involve a repeat assessment, similar to the one carried out on admission, and some likely areas considered by the nurse to be indicators of recovery might include:

- lower levels of physical activity
- slower speech (and hence thoughts)
- fewer changes of topic and greater coherence

- reduced bizarre, sexual or religious talk or actions
- increased rational talk
- longer length of unbroken sleep
- increased appetite
- spontaneous attempts at self-caring.

Patients with mood disorders are found in many settings *other* than in mental health units. For instance, the depressed person could be a post-mastectomy patient in a surgical department or be admitted to an accident and emergency unit following an episode of self-harm; the manic person could be a newly delivered woman in a maternity ward.

When caring for depressed or manic patients in non-mental health settings, a few of the nursing strategies proposed may not be feasible. Going for walks, organized outings or therapeutic activities may be impossible. However, the majority of patients' needs can be addressed, regardless of the setting, especially with regard to safety and communication.

CARE IMPLICATIONS FOR THE ANXIOUS PATIENT

All of us have experienced anxiety, one of a group of emotional states which also includes anger, frustration and jealousy. Anxiety is part of modern life and tends to be experienced in relation to external stresses such as work, pain, relationships, examinations and job interviews. It can also be generated by internal stresses, for example fear of failure, perfectionism, self-imposed deadlines and impossible targets, trying to live up to overly high standards, lack of assertiveness and trying to compete with others. Internal and external stresses may of course be related; for example, when a heavy workload (external stress) leads to doubts about personal abilities or knowledge (internal stress).

Like the other emotions, anxiety is not directly observable and is expressed by the sufferer in words, in behaviour and in somatic symptoms. Thus, anxiety can be defined as a physiological, psychological and behavioural response to an actual or threatened fear-provoking stimulus, whether internally or externally generated. In various books the word stress is used in different ways, either to mean the **cause** of anxiety (the stress of unemployment leads to anxiety) or as synonymous with anxiety itself (unemployment caused him/her stress). For the purpose of this chapter, stress will be used to mean the same as stressor – physical problems, personal difficulties or life events which cause anxiety.

Anxiety has been described as a flight or fight response, beneficial in helping individuals to adapt and survive, allowing increased attention and quicker reactions. Peplau (1963) defined four levels of anxiety: mild, moderate, severe and panic. Increased arousal in mild/moderate anxiety allows people to run faster, lift heavier objects and generally improve performance in problem solving and decision making, with heightened awareness and perception.

In severe anxiety, however, the arousal level is such that perception is narrowed, learning and problem solving are impaired and the overall performance is poor. Panic is the most extreme form of anxiety where the individual is disorganized, hyperactive or unable to move, even proving dangerous to himself due to erratic behaviour.

Differentiating between normal, adaptive anxiety and abnormal anxiety centres on the severity, intensity and duration of the response, 'relatedness' of the response to actual or real stressors and, perhaps most important of all, the degree of impairment caused to daily life and functioning. Disorders of anxiety are known as anxiety states or anxiety neuroses.

Box 8.6 shows just some of the very real anxieties which an inpatient may have; many of which centre on a fear of the unknown and may be compounded by lack of information from staff.

The physiology of anxiety

This is also discussed in Chapters 5 and 16.

The internal homeostasis of the body is maintained by the autonomic nervous system and the endocrine system. During an emotional experience, the sympathetic division of the autonomic nervous system is

---

Box 8.6   Possible patient anxieties

The illness
Nature of
Implications of

Nursing/medical procedures/tests
? Painful
? Embarrassing

Wife/husband/children
Effects on them
Ability to cope without him/her

Employment
Will job be 'safe' during absence
Ability to return after discharge

Financial worries
Loss of salary
Keeping up payments

activated, giving rise to symptoms such as increased heart rate. This is part of the preparation for emergency action like fight or flight. Sympathetic stimulation of the adrenal medulla causes release of the hormones adrenaline and noradrenaline which act to release energy stores and to increase metabolism. Adrenaline mimics sympathetic stimulation, causing the reticular-activating system to induce further adrenaline release by the adrenal glands. In this way, emotional arousal is maintained. Noradrenaline, detected by the hypothalamus, causes the pituitary gland to release adrenocorticotrophic hormones which travel in the bloodstream to cause steroid hormone release from the adrenal cortex. An emotionally

aroused person therefore experiences symptoms from three sources – sympathetic symptoms, effects of adrenaline and noradrenaline, and steroid hormone symptoms (Fig. 8.2).

Once the stressful event is over, the parasympathetic division of the autonomic system acts to restore the internal balance of the body (Brown & Wallace 1980). Selye (1976) described an exhaustion stage, when stress is long lasting or chronic and adrenocortical hormones do not return to normal levels. Physical health problems such as lowered resistance to infection, peptic ulceration, hypertension, colitis, headaches and asthma may be the result of chronic stress.

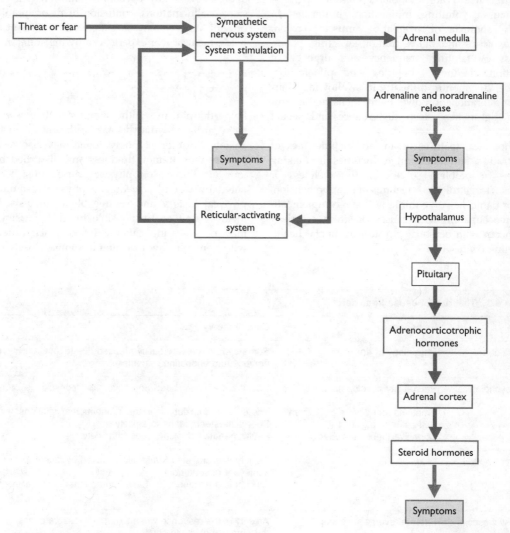

Fig. 8.2   The physiology of anxiety

EPIDEMIOLOGY AND AETIOLOGY

Although all of us experience anxiety from time to time, the prevalence rates for sufferers of anxiety states vary between 20 and 47 per 1000 of the population, making this the most common of all mental health problems. The average age of onset is 20–25 years of age and women outnumber men by two to one (Richards & McDonald 1990).

The main theories of cause are summarized in Table 8.3.

COMMON SYMPTOMATOLOGY

Physiological features of anxiety include: increased respiration, heart rate and blood pressure, palpitations, nausea, vomiting, indigestion, 'butterflies' in stomach, anorexia or overeating, muscle tension, muscular aches and pains, tremor, sweating, pallor, dizziness or fainting, frequency and urgency of micturition, tiredness, shivering and piloerection, headache, dry mouth, difficulty in swallowing, diarrhoea or alterations in bowel habit, menstrual irregularities, nightmares, sleep disturbance and sexual dysfunction.

Psychological features of anxiety include: lack of concentration and attention, difficulties in making decisions or problem solving, feeling helpless or hopeless, forgetfulness, feelings of apprehension, dread or panic, negative thinking (I'm a complete failure), preoccupation with causes of stress, worries/overconcern with personal physical or mental health and feeling confused.

Behavioural manifestations of anxiety include; overactivity or inertia, excessive talking or withdrawal, increased alcohol or tobacco consumption, tense facial expression and posture, nervous mannerisms, stuttering, clumsiness, accident proneness, lack of co-ordination and use of prescribed or non-prescribed drugs.

These features are the core of anxiety states and also predominate in the following conditions: phobias, obsessive-compulsive disorders, reactive depression, acute stress reactions and post-traumatic stress disorder.

Anxiety may also accompany up to 35% of major medical illness and present as another feature of mental health problems such as eating disorders and depression. In any psychotic condition where delusions, hallucinations, confusion or disorientation are present, anxiety may be generated as a result of bewilderment or fear experienced by the sufferer.

DIFFERENTIAL DIAGNOSIS AND INVESTIGATIONS

Hyperthyroidism, with symptoms like sweating, tachycardia and diarrhoea, may be mistaken for an anxiety disorder. Hypoglycaemia may also resemble anxiety with tremor, tiredness and disturbed behaviour. For this reason, physical causes must be eliminated by careful screening – physical examination, physical history and routine blood analysis. While medical staff are responsible for this, nursing staff may be assessing caffeine intake since caffeinism, with tremor, tachycardia and insomnia, closely resem-

---

Table 8.3 Theories of cause in anxiety

Theory	Emphasis	Core of theory
1. Biological	Physiology of anxiety	Some people are very easily aroused due to 'overactivity' of nervous and endocrine systems
2. Psychological	Personality development, e.g. Freud Emotional bonding, e.g. Sullivan Self-esteem, e.g. Will Cognitive theory, e.g. Beck	Unconscious conflict between drives and 'conscience' causes anxiety The origins of anxiety lie in the infant–mother relationship Poor self-esteem leads to anxiety Faulty, negative thinking leads to anxiety
3. Behavioural	Learning theory	Anxiety is a product of frustration caused by failure to achieve a desired goal Anxiety is a learned drive based on an innate drive to avoid pain
4. Psychosocial	External events/stressors	Anxiety is the response when external stressors overwhelm the person's ability to cope

bles an anxiety state. Richards & McDonald (1990) advise that the powerful stimulant effect of caffeine may cause a rise in basal metabolic rate of 10% and that an intake of 500–750 mg daily (five to seven mugs of coffee) may be considered excessive, either causing or contributing to anxiety. It is important to remember that it is not just coffee which is a rich source of caffeine but also tea, cola drinks and non-prescribed analgesics and 'cold remedies' bought from chemists. As with all mental health problems, information is collated from interview, observation and formal assessment tools, either self or staff rated. An example of the latter is the Hamilton Rating Scale for anxiety states. Many other assessment tools measure negative thinking, assertiveness, phobias and self-esteem (Hagerty 1984). Patients may be asked to keep a diary, checklist or a self-rated anxiety scale to help in definition of the problem or in exploring trigger factors for anxiety. An example of a self-rated anxiety scale is seen in Figure 8.3.

THERAPEUTIC MANAGEMENT

Since anxious patients retain insight and tend to have unimpaired communication, talking therapies are very useful in treatment. Psychotherapy or counselling may be indicated, especially if the anxiety state is related to a specific event like bereavement. Many patients benefit from group work and there has been a recent upsurge in self-help groups of different types. Groups may involve discussion or activities like social skills/assertiveness training. Lachman (1983) equates

assertiveness with stress reduction and increased self-esteem; the functions of assertiveness being standing up for personal rights, refusing unreasonable requests from others, making reasonable requests of others, changing the behaviour of others, avoiding unnecessary conflicts and openly communicating wishes or opinions in a clear fashion. Since a lot of stress comes from external sources such as other people, being more assertive with others may be very helpful indeed.

Complementary approaches tend to be behavioural and may include yoga, meditation, physical exercise, aromatherapy, massage, biofeedback, guided imagery, breathing exercises and muscle relaxation. Specific techniques for phobias and obsessional-compulsive disorders are described in Richards & McDonald's book *Behavioural Psychotherapy* (1990). Any one or a combination of these methods would allow stress reduction and therefore anxiety management.

Burnard's book *Coping with Stress in the Health Professions* (1991) offers a good source of these behavioural approaches and gives examples of exercises to be practised. It is important to point out that these anxiety management techniques are not just for patients. As the title of Burnard's book suggests, nurses may use these techniques to reduce their own stress. Like depression, cognitive therapy can be used to correct faulty thinking, increase self-esteem and thereby reduce stress (Beck et al 1985).

Drug treatment may involve the use of anti-anxiety or hypnotic agents, often from the benzodiazepine family. Members of this group of drugs include diazepam, chlordiazepoxide, temazepam, lorazepam, nitrazepam and many others. Apart from relieving tension and promoting sleep, benzodiazepines also have an anticonvulsant effect, muscle-relaxant properties and can be used as premedication or to cover withdrawal from alcohol. Possible adverse effects which are related to their sedative properties include daytime drowsiness, dizziness, slowing of reaction time, headache, forgetfulness and confusion. Driving and operating machinery may be contraindicated if drowsiness is prominent. The patient should be advised to avoid alcohol as it increases the sedative effects of benzodiazepines. Sedation and confusion are especially pronounced in the elderly, for whom reduced doses may be necessary.

If these drugs are taken in high doses over a long period of time, dependence may occur so careful monitoring is required, especially with repeat prescriptions for community-based patients. Cessation of the drug should be gradual to prevent epileptic fits and other withdrawal symptoms (Rees 1988).

Instructions

Place a cross on the scale to signify your current level of

anxiety. You can use the numbers to summarise your anxiety

level, for example 'how anxious are you?' - '5'

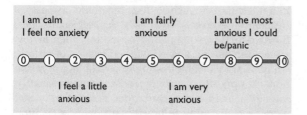

Fig. 8.3 Self-rated anxiety scale

NURSING STRATEGIES FOR THE ANXIOUS PATIENT

Assessment centres on the presence of the physiological, psychological and behavioural features of anxiety summarized earlier. Severity, intensity and duration of the symptoms are noted as well as trigger factors and social stressors. The patient's usual coping strategies are explored – some of which may be negative as in the use of alcohol/tobacco use or positive like using relaxation techniques.

The *effects* of anxiety symptoms on activities of living (Roper et al 1990) is the other focus of assessment.

Maintaining a safe environment

Extreme anxiety may increase the risk of self-harm. Assess as for suicide in the depressed patient. If panic attacks are a feature of the anxiety state, the patient may accidentally injure himself due to erratic and disorganized behaviour, or faint due to hyperventilation, as rapid and shallow breathing may lead to excessive loss of carbon dioxide.

Communication and relationship-forming

The anxious patient may make statements that reflect negative thinking, preoccupation with health or disease and low self-esteem. In severe anxiety or panic, the patient sometimes expresses a feeling of impending dread, doom or even death.

Mobilizing

Anxiety may cause withdrawn behaviour or restless, aimless activity, such as pacing.

Working and playing

Social settings may act as trigger factors to increase anxiety and concentration and attention impairment may lead to difficulties in understanding or retaining information. Problems at work may follow.

Sleeping

See under 'Care implications for disorders of sleep' (p. 298).

Eating and drinking

Anxiety features like nausea can lead to anorexia and overuse of alcohol or caffeine.

Elimination

The anxious patient may suffer from diarrhoea and frequency of micturition.

Expressing sexuality

Sexual dysfunction and menstrual problems can be caused by anxiety.

NURSING CARE OF THE ANXIOUS PATIENT

Anxiety symptoms can affect all of the activities of living; the main approach is therefore to help the patient to reduce his anxiety level so that all other activities like sleeping and eating are enhanced. The objectives for an anxious patient might be:

1. Feel calm and secure in a safe environment.
2. Establish healthy communication and relationship forming.
3. As a result of 1 and 2, establish healthy functioning in other activities of living, by reduction of anxiety symptoms.

See Nursing Care Plan 8.3 for a summary care plan for the anxious patient.

Feel calm and secure in a safe environment

In severe anxiety, there may be an increased risk of self-harm due to the feelings of terror experienced by the sufferer. Following assessment of suicidal intent, nursing care would be given to maintain a safe environment as described for the depressed patient earlier in this chapter. Highly anxious patients tend to feel even more anxious if left alone and for this reason, and to prevent panic attacks, increased nurse supervision may be required.

The anxious patient should be strongly encouraged to identify rising anxiety in himself and tell a member of staff so that panic can be defused and prevented by relatively simple means, such as physical presence and touch, listening and talking, or cognitive/behavioural techniques, such as deep breathing or massage. Relaxation exercises (Richards & McDonald 1990, Burnard 1991) are many and varied but often involve systematic tensing and relaxing of groups of muscles – muscular relaxation leading to psychological relaxation, the opposite of anxiety. These techniques involve following instructions read from a script by a staff member or listening to taped instructions sometimes accompanied by soft music. Relaxation exercises

Nursing Care Plan 8.3 Care for the anxious patient		
Problem	**Objective**	**Nursing action**
1. **Self-harm risk** **Anxiety symptoms/panic attacks**	Feel calm and secure in a safe environment	❒ Assess and care as for self-harm, depressed patient Increased observation Minimize trigger factors Teach anxiety management techniques
2. **Impaired communication**	Establish healthy communication and relationship forming	❒ Calm approach Physical presence/contact Constructive activities as diversion Adult praise Provide opportunities to succeed

3. **Withdrawn/restless**
   Insomnia
   Anorexia
   Diarrhoea/frequency of micturition
   Sexual dysfunction/menstrual problems
   Other physiological and behavioural manifestations of anxiety
	Establish healthy functioning by reduction of anxiety symptoms	As for 1 and 2

are beneficial when rising anxiety is identified and especially prior to bedtime when they may prove more helpful than antianxiety or hypnotic drugs (Childs-Clarke 1990). By teaching anxiety management, the nurse enables the patient to regain control over symptoms and therefore improve self-esteem and functioning in all activities of living; the ultimate aim is independence from staff.

If a panic attack does occur, therapeutic holding (resembling a very firm 'cuddle') can be used to help the patient regain self-control and prevent injury due to erratic behaviour. At the same time, as the patient is being held, the nurse should be continually talking to the patient, using his name, prompting him to take deep breaths in through the nose and out through the mouth and using phrases like 'you're alright, you're safe'.

Hyperventilation or overbreathing commonly accompanies severe anxiety or panic and will cause the patient to feel faint or dizzy, which in turn compounds the already present sensations of impending death or collapse. The treatment of hyperventilation is to restore the excessive loss of carbon dioxide by asking the patient to rebreathe using a paper bag, which the patient holds himself over his nose and mouth. Rebreathing like this should take only a few minutes and reduce feelings of gasping for breath and fainting.

To further make the patient feel safe, the nurse may have to limit contact with other patients or identified trigger factors like social settings, similar to the non-stimulating environment described for the manic patient, at least until the anxious patient develops some control over the troublesome symptoms.

Establish healthy communication and relationship forming

During panic attacks, and indeed throughout her dealings with the anxious patient, the nurse must remain calm, acting as a kind of role model for the patient. This can be difficult since anxiety seems to be 'contagious' and can be communicated from and to staff or other patients.

In the short term, the patient should be strongly encouraged to approach staff when rising anxiety is experienced. The nurse must, therefore, prove herself to be caring, approachable, available and interested by demonstrating good non-verbal behaviour and active listening. Poor concentration and a narrow perceptual field in the anxious patient can lead to difficulties in understanding unless the nurse speaks slowly and calmly, in simple sentences without jargon. Repetition of the message and getting feedback from the patient should help the nurse to ensure that the patient has understood correctly. Imagine a very anxious patient being told by a nurse that he is to have an ECG – the nurse then leaves, thinking the correct message has been passed, but the patient believes he is to have ECT and therefore panics.

Complaints of physical anxiety symptoms or health worries should not be dismissed. Instead, the patient needs clear and simple explanations of the symptoms – 'these palpitations you feel are anxiety symptoms, but it doesn't mean that something is wrong with your heart', or 'if you did some deep breathing you would be able to stop that symptom'. It is important not to dwell unduly on physical symptoms but rather, by using open questions, focus on the underlying feelings or triggers for the symptoms.

By making observations and giving feedback about his anxious behaviour, the nurse can help the patient make the link between trigger factors and anxiety symptoms and thus begin to recognize the early signs of rising anxiety: 'I noticed that you were a bit shaky when your visitors came in – how were you feeling at that time?' The longer term goal would be that the patient learns to do this himself and take appropriate stress reduction measures. For instance, if the patient recognizes that a group meeting increases his anxiety he might carry out a relaxation exercise immediately prior to joining it, cope better in the meeting and therefore feel more confident.

The nurse should dwell on any achievements made by the patient, however small, emphasizing improvement and giving adult praise – 'you stayed in the meeting for the whole hour, that's a big step forward!'

Opportunities for the patient to succeed should be provided in the form of constructive activity or discussion, tailored to the patient's strengths and abilities, including social skills and assertiveness training, art and music groups and outings.

Once the patient learns to have some control over anxiety symptoms, he will also have improved functioning in other activities of living like eating, sleeping and sexual function. The latter causes immense worry to patients who should be advised that these problems are temporary and will resolve when anxiety is reduced.

Evaluation

As in other mental health problems, evaluation comes not only from nursing and medical staff but also from the patient himself. Formal assessment tools such as rating scales can be used to compare current with previous levels of functioning, with indicators of improvement noted. Likely signs of recovery would include:

- fewer or no panic attacks
- reduced frequency, intensity or duration of anxiety symptoms
- increased appetite, longer lengths of sleep

- improved concentration and decision making
- decreased preoccupation with self, with health
- increased interest in appearance, activities or other people
- heightened self-esteem
- increased ability to recognize and manage symptoms

CARE IMPLICATIONS FOR DISORDERS OF SLEEP

INTRODUCTION

Adults spend up to one-third of their lives sleeping and human physiology is greatly influenced by biorhythms – cyclic variations in behaviour and metabolism, running as if to an 'internal clock'. The menstrual cycle of 28 days is an example of this internal clock while the most obvious circadian (daily) rhythm is the sleep–wake cycle. In normal health there is a continuum between sleep, drowsiness, alertness and excitement (Fig. 8.4).

Arousal is mediated by the ascending reticular-activating system and the neurotransmitter serotonin (5HT) is implicated in the sleep–wake cycle (see Ch. 5). Drugs which increase arousal are central nervous system (CNS) stimulants, for example amphetamines, cocaine, caffeine and nicotine, while CNS depressants, for example alcohol and benzodiazepines, have the opposite effect.

THE NATURE AND PURPOSE OF SLEEP

Sleep is characterized by closed eyes, inactivity and muscular relaxation with suspension of conscious-

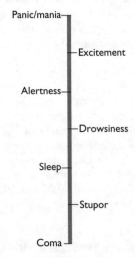

Fig. 8.4 Continuum of arousal

ness. It is not the same however as being unconscious, since the sleeper can readily be roused to alertness.

The purpose of sleep is unclear, with some theories describing it as a device to conserve energy and others as a primitive survival strategy to avoid dangerous night predators. The most widely held belief is that sleep serves a restorative function, and indeed there is evidence to show that growth hormone is increased, protein synthesis is enhanced and cortisol inhibited during sleep. Epidermal and bone marrow cells proliferate due to increased cell division at night, leading to faster tissue repair (Torrance 1990).

Two types of sleep are described, occurring in 90 minute cycles, four to six times a night:

REM (rapid eye movement) sleep – also called paradoxical sleep, accounting for 20% of total sleep time. It is during REM that dreaming occurs.
NON-REM or orthodox sleep, accounting for 80% of total sleep time.

Oswald (1980) suggests that the dreaming part of sleep is 'brain restorative' while the non-dreaming part is 'body restorative'. Dream sleep is implicated in learning and memory as shown by sleep deprivation studies, while Freud referred to this part of sleeping as 'dream work' – dreams having a symbolic content derived from the events of the preceding day or from the person's life (Meddis 1977).

Factors affecting sleep

Two broad groups of factors affect sleep (Figure 8.8).

Intrinsic factors may have physical or psychological origins; extrinsic factors may be classified in environmental or behavioural terms.

Types of sleep disturbance

About 17% of patients visiting their family doctor complain of sleeping problems but the estimated figure for sleep disturbance in the general population might be 30–40% (Oswald 1980).

The most common complaint is insomnia, a subjective dissatisfaction with the quantity or quality of sleep which may be transient or persistent and is most often reported by the elderly, females and lower social classes. People tend to complain of insomnia if their total sleep time falls below 5 hours a night or if it takes longer than 90 minutes to fall asleep (Meddis 1977). Difficulties in initiating sleep can also be called sleep-onset or early insomnia and may be compounded by difficulties in maintaining sleep (intermittent or intermediate insomnia), caused by any of the factors summarized in Figure 8.5. Late insomnia or early morning wakening is less common and frequently accompanies severe depressive illness.

Hypersomnia is excessive somnolence and can be persistent when associated with depression, eating disorders, postviral conditions, brain injury, premenstrual syndrome or disruptions of the sleep–wake cycle caused by sleep apnoea, sleep walking, jet lag or shift work. Overuse of sedatives or alcohol may also contribute to this condition (Rees 1988).

Sleep apnoea, multiple and transient cessations of

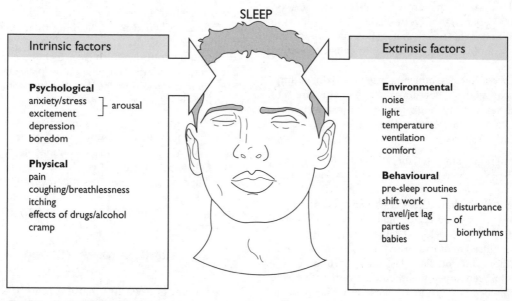

Fig. 8.5 Factors affecting sleep

respiration, is sometimes called sleep-induced ventilatory impairment and is estimated to be extremely common in infants up to 3 months old, when it may be a cause of cot death. It is much less common in adults, occurring in association with obesity, snoring, high alcohol intake and sleeping flat on the back (Closs 1990). Sleep apnoea may arise from central dysfunction in the brain stem or from physical obstruction of the airway by soft tissue.

Other disorders associated with sleep are sleep walking, nightmares, night terrors and bruxism (teeth grinding). These disorders tend to be transient, relate to situational stress and are more common in children where they usually resolve without treatment (Rees 1988).

Assessment of sleep

This would involve comparing the patient's usual quantity and quality of sleep with the current sleeping pattern, taking the following into account:

1. Usual/preferred environment with regard to noise, light and temperature. Does the patient prefer blankets or a duvet? If blankets, how many? How many pillows?
2. Usual/preferred presleep behaviours including time of retiring, time of rising, use of hypnotic drugs, caffeine levels, daytime exercise levels and usual sleep pattern – length of time to fall asleep, intermittent wakening, nocturia, daytime naps and shift work.
3. Patient's subjective assessment of usual sleep quality – does the patient consider himself a good or bad sleeper? Is he refreshed or not following sleep? What are his usual strategies if sleeping is difficult – alcohol, reading, listening to music, sleeping pills?
4. Current factors affecting sleep – pain, cramp, dyspnoea, anxiety, boredom, noise, disturbance of biorhythms, e.g. by hourly vital sign measurement in an intensive care setting. See Figure 8.5 for other factors affecting sleep.

Information gathered from the patient interview would be augmented by nursing observation and the use of more formal assessment methods such as keeping a sleep chart. Closs (1990) advised that open questions to patients about their sleeping behaviour will aid nursing assessment rather than leading, ritualized or closed enquiries. She gives the example that asking 'how did you sleep last night?' will allow the patient to mention any difficulties, rather than the 'did you sleep well?' type of question which is likely to elicit a 'fine' answer, even when the sleep was far from 'fine'.

Therapeutic management of insomnia

Insomnia is commonly treated with benzodiazepine drugs such as temazepam or less commonly with chloral derivatives and barbiturates. For all of these drugs, there is a risk of physical dependence and adverse side-effects. Patients who have taken hypnotic drugs for months or years find that the drugs lose their effectiveness and they are of little benefit in assisting them in falling or staying asleep.

Oswald (1980) demonstrates that long-term use of these drugs may reduce or abolish dream (paradoxical) sleep leading to further daytime difficulties like irritability, feeling 'unrefreshed' by sleep, concentration problems and perhaps even learning and memory impairment. It seems then that hypnotic drugs may only be suitable for short time-limited courses and may not be helpful for a patient with chronic sleep difficulties.

Behavioural techniques can be used when patients experience sleep-onset insomnia – difficulty in getting off to sleep. Childs-Clarke (1990) summarizes three main behavioural approaches:

1. Systematic relaxation using deep breathing and muscle group relaxation when overarousal is keeping the patient awake. Overarousal refers to anxiety, excitement, tension or worry.
2. Paradoxical intention where it is considered that the 'fight' to get to sleep and the worry about not sleeping inhibits the sleep process. The patient is therefore instructed to give up the 'fight' and just lie still in a darkened room, keeping their eyes open for as long as possible.
3. Stimulus control which is a technique derived from operant conditioning where sleep becomes the reinforcement for falling asleep – the two considered as separate behaviours.

The aim is that bed becomes associated with sleep, and behaviours imcompatible with sleep are removed. Many people with insomnia stay in bed reading, listening to music or the television, eating or drinking coffee. Simple instructions are given to patients such as go to bed only when tired, if not sleeping after 15 minutes, get up and only return to bed when sleepy.

Nursing strategies for the patient with insomnia

The main aim is to ensure that the prerequisites for

sleep are present and that factors interfering with sleep are minimized. As far as possible, the patient's usual presleep routine should be followed. For instance, a person who normally retires at 11 p.m. will probably not be able to sleep at 9.30 p.m. Some flexibility is required to offer the patient the chance of watching television in a dayroom until his usual time for going to bed. Someone who usually listens to music before sleeping can use a personal hi-fi, continuing his usual routine but not disturbing other patients. Closs (1990) suggests flexibility in the time at which patients are roused in the morning. Some ward routines seem structured more for staff convenience with patients wakened at 6 or 7 am, whether or not they require treatment. The nurse should aim to strike a balance between the demands of treatment, such as routine insulin administration, and individual patient preference.

It is the usual routine for many people to have a snack and/or a hot drink prior to retiring. Ideally, hospital patients could continue this practice since many hours have elapsed since their evening meal and sleep would be inhibited by hunger pangs and disturbance to presleep routine. Hot drinks could also be provided during the night for a patient unable to sleep and a dayroom made available so that the patient could continue his normal strategies for dealing with insomnia, like reading. Noise, particularly at night, is a frequently reported reason for sleep disturbance in hospital. Noise problems can be minimized in small bay wards rather than long 'Nightingale' wards (Closs 1990), by wearing rubber-soled shoes and by routine maintenance of equipment to avoid, for example, the squeaking of trolleys.

Interruptions of sleep for vital sign measurement should be minimized and only carried out when essential. Night duty staff should try to ensure darkness as much as possible and take care when using their torches to avoid patient disturbance.

The opportunity should be available for patients to modify their bedding or number of pillows – to ask for another blanket or duvet, to have one pillow instead of two – and thus approximate more closely their usual sleeping requirements. While some patients are disturbed by feeling cold, a greater number are disturbed by feeling too hot. The environmental temperature, plastic covers on mattresses and postoperative pyrexia may be to blame, perhaps in combination. Nursing strategies to reduce pyrexia are summarized in Chapter 4 and, apart from making the patient feel more comfortable, may also help to minimize sleep-onset problems or intermittent wakening.

If sleep difficulties are related to specific physical or psychological factors then the nursing strategies to promote sleep centre on removing or reducing the factor (Table 8.4). Patients deterred from sleep by overarousal benefit from a nursing approach similar to the care of the anxious patient, described earlier in this chapter. The nurse should encourage the patient to voice and discuss his worries and offer clear explanations to take away the 'fear of the unknown' or any misapprehensions. A warm bath and relaxation exercises in the evening followed by a hot drink and a snack will help to provide the correct prerequisites for sleep in an anxious patient. It may seem that the nursing strategies to promote sleep are 'commonsense' or not very highly technical but it is worth remembering that the factors which prevent sleep in hospitals are very much the same as those which prevent sleep anywhere. It also follows that the strategies for patients are also strategies for nursing staff on shift work or indeed anyone who has sleep disturbance, whether occasionally or frequently. Some of the strategies proposed may not be feasible – such as fresh air and exercise for a bored but bed-

Table 8.4   Nursing actions to promote sleep

Cause of sleep problem	Nursing action to promote sleep
Pyrexia	Adjust bedding/clothing Tepid sponging Antipyrexial drugs Fan
Pain	Positioning Heat application if appropriate Massage if appropriate Correct timing, dose and type of analgesia
Anxiety/fear	Information/explanations Clear honest messages Relaxation exercises Massage Behavioural techniques Caring/listening approach Warm bath
Dyspnoea	Positioning Sufficient pillows Correct timing of drugs Oxygen if prescribed
Boredom	Fresh air Physical activity Mental activity, e.g. puzzles Reduce daytime napping

bound patient – but the key point in minimizing sleep disturbance is that the nurse should select from a large repertoire those specific strategies most suitable for an individual patient, taking into account his current situation.

ETHICAL ISSUES

Mental health nursing abounds with ethical issues. Dilemmas arise mainly surrounding the issue of patient's rights, such as the right to explanation on which to base informed consent, the right to withold consent to treatment and the right to leave hospital. Patients' rights have to be balanced with patients' needs and in mental health problems, where insight and judgement may be impaired, the power exists in law to detain people in hospital or give treatment against their will. Sometimes the nurse feels very torn between the traditional caring role and a more custodial role. A few nurses find it hard to justify the use of powerful drugs or controversial ECT, given the potentially serious adverse effects such as dependence or memory problems. It might be difficult for these nurses to fully reassure and support a patient undergoing such courses of treatment. The dilemma remains for all nurses regarding the amount of explanation needed for informed consent – too little and it cannot be called 'informed' consent; too much and the patient may not understand or, in fact, be actively dissuaded from consenting because of fear of serious but uncommon adverse effects.

Suggested assignments

Discussion points
1. Do people have the right to commit suicide?
2. ECT research is inconclusive.
   Researchers seem unsure if ECT works, or of how it works and disagree over the severity and duration of memory problems produced.

   Given the above, can the use of ECT be justified?
3. How much do patients need to know about the adverse effects of a drug or treatment?

REFERENCES AND FURTHER READING

Barrowclough C, Fleming I 1986 Goal planning with elderly people. Manchester University Press, Manchester

Barker P 1985 Patient assessment in psychiatric nursing. Croom Helm, London

Beck A T, Rush A J, Emery G 1979 Cognitive therapy of depression. The Guildford Press, New York

Beck A T, Emery G, Greenberg R L 1985 Anxiety disorders and phobias – a cognitive perspective. Basic Books, New York

Blackie F 1990 Mental health: a guide to the law in Scotland. Butterworth, Glasgow

Brooking J I (ed) 1992 A textbook of psychiatric and mental health nursing. Churchill Livingstone, Edinburgh

Brown G W, Harris T 1978 Social origins of depression. Tavistock, London

Brown T S, Wallace P M 1980 Physiological psychology. Academic, New York

Burnard P 1991 Coping with stress in the health professions. Chapman and Hall, London

Childs-Clarke 1990 Stimulus control techniques. Nursing Times 86(35): 29 August

Closs Jose S 1990 Influences on patients' sleep on surgical wards. Surgical Nurse 3(2): 12–14

Cormack D F S, Reynolds W 1990 Psychiatric and mental health nursing. Chapman & Hall, London

Hagerty B K 1984 Psychiatric-mental health assessment. CV Mosby, St Louis

Holmes J H, Rahe R H 1967 The social readjustment rating scale. J Psychosom. 11: 213–218

Lachman V D 1983 Stress management: a manual for nurses. Grune and Stratton, Orlando, Florida

Meddis R 1977 The sleep instinct. Routledge and Kegan Paul, London

Oswald I 1980 Sleep, 4th edn. Penguin, London

Parkes C M 1976 The psychological reaction to loss of a limb. In: Howells J G (ed) Modern perception in the psychiatric aspects of surgery. MacMillan, London, pp 515–533

Peplau H 1963 A working definition of anxiety. In: Burd S, Marshall M (eds) Some clinical approaches to psychiatric nursing. MacMillan, New York

Rees L 1988 A new short textbook of psychiatry. Edward Arnold, London

Richards D, McDonald R 1990 Behavioural psychotherapy. Butterworth-Heinemann, Oxford

Roper N, Logan W W, Tierney A J 1990 The elements of nursing. Churchill Livingstone, Edinburgh

Selye H 1976 The stress of life, 2nd edn. McGraw-Hill, New York

Silverstone T, Turner P 1988 Drug treatment in psychiatry, 4th edn. Routledge, London

Stuart G, Sundeen S 1983 Principles and practice of psychiatric nursing, 2nd edn. CV Mosby, St Louis

Torrance C 1990 Sleep and wound healing. Surgical Nurse 3(3): 16–20

Ward M F 1992 The nursing process in psychiatry, 2nd edn. Churchill Livingstone, Edinburgh

Wilson H S, Kniesl C R 1988 Psychiatric nursing, 3rd edn. Addison-Wesley, California

9

Care implications of disorders of thought and perception

David J. Tait

Thoughts and sensory experiences are, even when centred on common objects of attention, felt to be individually unique. Constructed and elaborated by subjective internal processes, stored and re-examined according to personal need and inclination, they form the essence of human beings, and profoundly influence personalities, emotions and behaviour. It is small wonder then that abnormalities of thought and perception create fear and bewilderment in the individual concerned and those around him, and may render the person unrecognizable to himself and others.

In order to understand the effects of such phenomena and to develop appropriate caring responses, an outline of common disorders in this realm is necessary, followed by a detailed consideration of the major conditions to which they relate.

DISORDERS OF THOUGHT

These include abnormalities of:

Speed (tempo) – this may be markedly increased as in mania or slowed down, as often found in severely depressed or demented patients.

Association – thoughts need to be related to permit logical connections and the ability to reason. They may however become disjointed as in the indirect 'knight's move' thinking characteristic of schizophrenia.

Continuity – normally, allowing for lapses in concentration, progress of thought is not subject to internal interruption. In some mental illnesses however, thinking may be disconcertingly 'blocked', or the necessary pauses and divisions between topics fail to occur.

Possession – generally, no one would deny that his thought processes belong entirely to him. Schizophrenic episodes may involve the conviction that others are stealing the person's thoughts or interposing foreign ones.

Miscellaneous nature – schizophrenia in particular is liable to cause clients to invent and use new words or 'neologisms' (as small children do naturally), and think in a symbolic, concrete or disorganized manner.

Content – delusions are false beliefs held with full force of conviction, immune to reasoned argument or contrary evidence, and which are inexplicable by reference to circumstance. Common forms are grandiose (concerning self-importance) and paranoid (persecutory), each typical of several conditions.

DISORDERS OF PERCEPTION

Common among these are:

Sensory distortions – exaggerations of the normal range of perceptual ability, resulting in either heightened or diminished environmental awareness (the former in anxiety, the latter in confusional states, for example).

Illusions – misinterpretations of environmental stimuli. Classically these are a feature of delirium, although they can occur in health, especially under stress and when perceptual cues are reduced (e.g. mistaking nocturnal shadows for lurking attackers).

Hallucinations – false perceptions, in that they are not produced by any environmental stimulus, being entirely (albeit vivid) products of the mind. They can affect any of the sensory modalities: hearing (auditory), sight (visual), touch (tactile), taste (gustatory) and smell (olfactory), the first being the commonest.

Abnormal 'sense of self'

- Distorted body image (particularly in anorexia nervosa – see below).
- Depersonalization (a strange feeling that the person's body, or parts of it, are foreign, or have materially ceased to exist).
- Derealization (a sensation that the environment is strange, and somehow no longer genuine, like an optical illusion). As with depersonalization, this may occur after severe emotional shock, as well as in schizophrenia.

Various forms of mental illness can be grouped for convenience as disorders of thought and perception: schizophrenia, organic states and anorexia nervosa.

SCHIZOPHRENIA

Introduction: what is schizophrenia?

This commonly encountered term conveys to the layman images of individuals suffering **split** or even multiple personalities, just as Robert Louis Stevenson's respectable character Dr Jeckyll relinquished control of his body to the saturnine Mr Hyde after surgery hours. In reality, such a transformation accords more with psychopathic dissemblance (see Ch. 10), or in benign instances with hysteria (see Ch. 10), although some disruption of personality is characteristic of schizophrenic illness.

The term 'schizophrenia' (literally from the Greek = 'split mind') was first coined by the Swiss psychiatrist Eugen Bleuler in 1911. He believed the basis of the condition to be the splitting apart of the mind's normally integrated functions. Thus the sufferer experienced a dislocation of his thoughts from his feelings (hence inappropriate affect), of his thoughts from reality (the essence of delusions) or lacked connections to link his thoughts together (undermining coherent communication). He might even feel that his body (or parts of it) did not belong to him (depersonalization) and no longer obeyed his commands (resulting in passivity and even stupor).

Bleuler's contemporary in Munich, Emil Kraepelin, distinguished four types of schizophrenic presentation, which persist in today's terminology (Table 9.1).

By the 1960s, lack of reliability in diagnosis (patients were up to ten times as likely to be diagnosed as schizophrenic in New York compared with London) together with the apparent ease with which psychiatric experts could be deceived by researchers simulating symptoms (e.g. Rosenhan 1973) fuelled the so-called Anti-Psychiatry movement. Its adherents, notably Thomas Szasz and R. D. Laing, contended that schizophrenia did not exist as a pathological entity, comprising a large part of the 'myth' of mental illness. This school of thought contended that the label 'schizophrenic' represented at worst the medical contribution to an establishment conspiracy intent on justifying the enforced detention and medication of those members of a society rebelling against corporate norms of behaviour.

At best, the label symbolized the prevailing failure to acknowledge the schizophrenic's critical perception and subsequent rejection of the alienating, stressful and futile nature of modern social reality, in favour of equally valid psychedelic experiences.

Instead, such non-conformist behaviour is treated, as are most forms of deviance, with the communal distrust, disfavour and even outright hostility which forms the common experience and expectations of those who suffer social stigma.

Although these alternative perspectives tended to underestimate the suffering inherent in the schizophrenic experience, they did force self-appraisal

Table 9.1   Kraepelin's classification of schizophrenia

Type	Usual onset	Typical features	Current prognosis
Simple	Early (teens)	Apathy; withdrawal; personal neglect	Poor-lifelong vagrant or recluse
Hebephrenic	Late teens/early twenties	Inappropriate emotional displays; incoherent speech	Improvement (if any) limited
Catatonic	Mid twenties onwards	Trance-like immobility and posturing alternates with unpredictable overactivity	? Preventable with prompt therapy
Paranoid	Mature (mid thirties)	Preoccupation with persecutory delusions and hallucinations	Often well controlled or cured by medication

upon mainstream psychiatry, which resulted in fundamental reviews of methods of not only diagnosis, but also treatment and rehabilitation methods.

Common symptomatology and patient implications

For the sake of convenient organization, common symptoms of schizophrenia can be discussed under the headings below.

Disordered thought and speech

Delusions are characteristic of paranoid schizophrenia. Primary delusions seem to emerge independently and fully formed from the patient's mind, 'out of the blue' as it were. These are often grandiose in nature; for example, the person believes he is the new Messiah. Secondary delusions appear later and reinforce or make sense of a primary delusion, often carrying persecutory overtones; for example, people who ridicule the Messiah notion belong to rival religious groups with malicious intent.

Every day sensory events can be interpreted as carrying intense yet bizarre personal meaning; for example, the audible click of the timer in a parking ticket dispenser may be attributed to a monitoring device or a harmful emission of radiation. This unique phenomenon is termed delusional perception. Obviously such delusions, frequently constructed (or systematized) into elaborate conspiratorial systems, profoundly influence the individual's criteria of a safe environment.

Diminished possession of thought involves experiencing thoughts being 'inserted' into or 'withdrawn' from the sufferer's head, or even 'broadcast' so that his innermost private thoughts become common knowledge. Such passivity feelings are regarded as restricted to schizophrenia, and greatly inhibit the patient's ability to communicate.

Schizophrenic thought has been described as over-inclusive (riddled with irrelevancies), circumstantial (tangential), symbolic (replete with allusions), concrete (showing inability to interpret abstractly) and negative (perversely contradictory), even prone to neologisms, all of which undermine coherent communication. Ultimately, speech could become an apparently meaningless jumble termed word-salad (for an example see Lyttle 1986, p. 239).

Disordered perception

Hallucinations may affect any sensory modality in schizophrenia, but certain auditory forms are unique to it.

These include hearing one's thoughts spoken out loud, before having the chance to think them (**gedankenlautwerden**), being commented upon or argued over in the third person (i.e. referred to by name, or as 'she' or 'he' or worse). Such alien voices can either be abusive, informative or amusing in nature.

Visual hallucinations may involve clear, terrifying images or vague disruptions of the field of view.

Tactile experiences are often sexual in nature, such as genital interference, arousal or even transformation into those of the opposite gender.

Olfactory and gustatory hallucinations most commonly reinforce persecutory delusions; for example, smelling poisonous gas and tasting imagined contaminants in food (i.e. poison or medication).

Disturbed emotion

Typically this takes two main forms.

Schizophrenic affect may be inappropriate (incongruous), serious topics (or silence) eliciting childish giggling (hebephrenia literally translates as 'young mind'), while levity meets with a serious response. Such contradictions may arise from hallucinatory input.

Alternatively mood may be flat or blunt, lack of emotional response precluding any social rapport (sometimes giving the impression of a metaphorical pane of glass surrounding the patient).

However, this is not to say that schizophrenics are never intense, elated or depressed in mood – quite the contrary.

Perplexity arising from their symptoms is sometimes experienced by schizophrenics.

All of the above oddities tend to interfere with the ability to communicate or to enjoy life.

Disturbed motor function

Characteristic oddities in this domain range from extreme hyperactivity to mute stuporous states, enabling the patient to be moulded into and to sustain bizarre postures. Gross catatonic passivity has become increasingly rare in western psychiatry, suggesting that its historical prominence may have resulted from stultifying institutional regimens or the absence of effective treatment. However, manneristic, repetitive and negativistic behaviours are still frequently exhibited (grimaces, rocking and resistance to nursing assistance are respective examples of each).

Paranoid patients may sense that their actions are controlled by others, as if they were robots (so-called **somatic passivity**).

Such symptoms erode the patient's performance in a range of activities (washing and dressing, feeding and even eliminating).

Disturbed motivation

A salient feature of many schizophrenic patients is their loss of drive. Apathy, especially when the illness commences in adolescence, results in loss of previous ambition and outside interests, often extending to self-neglect (e.g. of hygiene, appearance, nutrition) and general idleness. Employment difficulties usually follow, compounded by inattentiveness and unreliable attendance.

Consequently, the schizophrenic with this **simple** pattern of illness may drift insidiously into vagrancy, with possible recourse to petty theft or prostitution.

Disturbed social function

The cumulative effect of the functional handicaps which accompany schizophrenia is to create social isolation. Incoherent or bizarre speech, preoccupation with continuous hallucinations, peculiar emotional responses, ridiculous or frightening behaviour, and personal disinclination to seek company can all contribute to lack of successful interaction and the pursuit of a reclusive, almost **autistic**, lifestyle.

Embarrassed relatives may actively conceal the sufferer from the outside world. Others tend to shun the victim of this stigmatizing label, fearing (often unnecessarily) they will be exposed to unacceptable behaviour (particularly verbal or physical abuse). Schizophrenia sufferers have a significantly lowered rate of marriage, while those who wed are at high risk of divorce. For such reasons, schizophrenics have been described as probably the loneliest people in the world.

Relevant epidemiology and aetiology

Slightly fewer than one person in every 100 of the general population (around seven to nine per 1000) will be diagnosed as schizophrenic at some time in their lives. This incidence seems remarkably constant throughout the world, although in certain regions, such as rural Eire and Arctic Scandinavia, it is as high as 2.8%, possibly because of the particular economic or cultural conditions.

Evidence suggests that individual risk of developing schizophrenia is substantially increased where there is a family history of the condition (Table 9.2). Figures vary between research studies, but hereditary factors seem likely to play a major causative role, a suggestion supported by studies of the children of schizophrenics raised in adoptive homes (who have been found to show the expected familial prevalence

Table 9.2 Probability of developing schizophrenia (prevalence) depending on family relationship	
Relationship to a schizophrenic	Prevalence %
Parent	5
Sibling/dizygotic twin	10–15
Child	14
Child of two schizophrenic parents	46
Monozygotic (identical) twin	50–70
Adapted from Bird & Harrison 1987, p. 27	

despite environmental separation from their natural parents).

Efforts have also been directed towards identifying possible social causes, as genetic factors cannot entirely explain the source of schizophrenia.

Consistent research findings since the 1930s showing that schizophrenics were concentrated in decaying urban areas invited the conclusion that the illness resulted from living in poverty and squalor. However, it is now deemed more likely that such hardships are the consequence of the impaired employment prospects and limited material aspirations which *follow* schizophrenia.

In the 1950s and 1960s abnormalities in family communication were proposed as developmentally crucial, in particular conflicting emotional messages (the so-called **double-bind**), lack of warmth, diminished listening and interparental warfare. It was contended that the resultant flaws in the person's maternal relationship precluded warm and trusting adult relationships.

Such theories have been much criticized as lacking scientific basis and practical usefulness, as well as imposing a burden of guilt on patients' relatives, often those who provide the schizophrenic's main source of support. What clearly emerged from such sociological studies was that following recovery, schizophrenics were more likely to relapse if exposed to an overcritical or smotheringly caring family atmosphere (one of high expressed emotion). Such findings stimulated family education programmes, as well as rehabilitative accommodation projects.

Although research has remained inconclusive, frequent links have been made between chemical imbalances in the brain and schizophrenia, in particular excessive influence of the neurotransmitter dopamine in the limbic system (see Ch. 5). Evidence for this derives from post-mortem studies, reinforced by pharmacological observations. Certain drugs (such as amphetamines and dopa preparations which raise dopamine levels, and hallucinogens like LSD and mescaline which chemically resemble dopamine) are capable of inducing psychotic states indistinguishable from or modelling schizophrenia. Moreover antipsychotic drugs are believed to exert their effects by blockading dopamine-sensitive neurone receptors. This would also explain the symptoms of Parkinson's disease (known to result from underactivity of dopamine pathways in the basal ganglia) which commonly accompany long-term use of such medication. Of course, such biochemical abnormalities, just like domestic tensions, are equally likely to be the result rather than the cause of a psychological illness. As

Warner (1985) comments, 'that there *are* biochemical differences in schizophrenia is certain – just as certain as that there are biochemical correlates in the brain to rage, anxiety and learning Spanish.'

The wide range of hypotheses concerning the genesis of this condition (an article in the British Medical Journal attributed it with conviction to intrauterine exposure to the influenza virus) reflects the inadequacy of any single theory. Most likely the development and cause of schizophrenia in any instance may be influenced by manifold factors. This is reflected in the schematic model, illustrated in Figure 9.1.

Thus an inherited predisposition to the illness could develop into a vulnerable adult personality (perhaps the withdrawn, hypersensitive schizoid

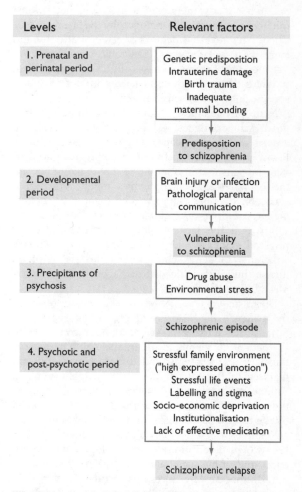

Fig. 9.1 Interactional model of factors influencing the onset and course of schizophrenia. (After Warner 1985)

type characteristic of around a half of premorbid schizophrenics). An identifiable schizophrenic breakdown might then follow experimentation with LSD, or a dramatic change in personal circumstances (becoming unemployed or even getting married). Following recovery, subsequent relapses would be anticipated if the patient returned to a tense home atmosphere, a vagrant existence or failed to take prescribed medication.

What does appear clear is that chronic deterioration can be avoided in the vast majority of patients by prompt treatment and the provision of comprehensive, humane rehabilitation services.

Range of investigations

No scientific tests can be relied upon to establish a diagnosis of schizophrenia. Aside from the metabolic research already mentioned concerning neurotransmitters, computerized tomography (CT) scans (see Ch. 5) have revealed degrees of cerebral atrophy and ventricular enlargement (generally found only in degenerative organic diseases) in 25–40% of schizophrenics. These anatomical changes are not related to specific subtypes of schizophrenia.

Neurophysiological studies have suggested that most schizophrenics exhibit abnormal levels of arousal and responsiveness to environmental stimuli. Possibly this reflects a reduced ability to ignore irrelevant sensory information, so that to avoid becoming overstressed, schizophrenics might retreat into a cocoon of inner isolation. The theoretical interest of such findings as yet far exceeds their practical utility. It is this lack of conclusive cause and effect physical evidence which inspired the antipsychiatry adherents to deny schizophrenia the status of an illness (hence the title of Szasz's book *The Myth of Mental Illness* (Szasz 1972)).

Diagnosis remains largely based on appraisal of the patient's life-history and presenting symptoms. Because the nursing team has 24-hour contact with the patient, its members are uniquely able to observe the patient's behaviour and to report all significant features to the rest of the multidisciplinary team. Salient indicators are the characteristic disorders of thought and perception described earlier, reinforced by the typical disturbances of daily living activities.

Relatives can often usefully supplement the patient's own description of his developmental experiences and of his social and occupational functioning in adulthood. Any recent stressful life-events or family history of mental illness may be of additional therapeutic significance.

Depending on the diagnostic criteria applied, schizophrenia may overlap considerably with other recognized mental illnesses. For example, schizophrenics may demonstrate marked apathy and retarded responses, grandiose delusions, anxiety or emotional detachment. These features are also respectively characteristic of depressive illness, mania, neurotic states and personality disorder (Fig. 9.2).

As the most effective treatments and prognoses for these conditions are generally held to differ considerably, establishing accurate diagnosis through observation and report is essential whenever possible.

Therapeutic management

Well into the current century, success was claimed for a wide range of unlikely physical treatments of schizophrenia. These included 'stimulation' by cold showers and the induction of malarial fever, hypoglycaemic coma and grand-mal epilepsy. Only the last of those retains any therapeutic credibility; although its major application is in depressive illness (see Ch. 8), it is occasionally of benefit in treating resistant catatonic states.

Pharmacological agents were restricted to powerful sedatives such as barbiturates and (the highly unpalatable) paraldehyde, until in the early 1950s chlorpromazine was discovered to have antipsychotic properties in doses creating only mild sedation. Thus

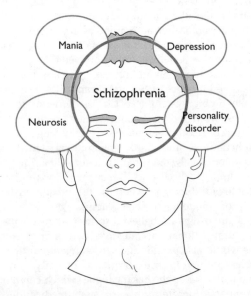

Fig. 9.2 Potential behavioural overlap between schizophrenia and other functional mental disorders. (Reproduced with permission from Gottesman & Shields 1982, figure 1.1)

for the first time patients with active psychoses could receive respite from intense delusions and hallucinations without severe impairment of normal physical and mental activity.

The development of depot preparations was of particular significance. These are antipsychotic drugs concentrated in oil which, once administered by deep intramuscular injection, are gradually released into the circulation over a period of 1–4 weeks (just like goods from a distribution depot). Depots eliminate the disadvantages of both fluctuating blood medication levels and adherence to sometimes inconvenient oral intake regimens. The latter benefit is especially significant, since patient compliance with psychiatric medication is notoriously low. This is due to a myriad of possible factors, including forgetfulness, lack of insight and symptom remission (just as with antibiotics, patients may fail to persist with a course of drugs on feeling better), but probably the chief cause is the appearance of the often unpleasant side-effects of antipsychotic medication.

Short-term anticholinergic effects (disrupting autonomic functioning – see Ch. 5) include dry mouth, blurred vision, constipation, perspiration, insensitivity to cold and postural hypotension. In addition to providing reassuring information on the origin of these effects, the nurse must protect the patient from temperature extremes and from initial fainting attacks.

Jaundice and reduced resistance to infection are potentially dangerous complications, so that yellow discoloration or persistent sore throats require prompt medical attention.

Allergic responses include skin rashes and ultra-violet sensitivity; patients are vulnerable to unpleasant sunburn unless protective clothing and sun tan lotions are worn outside in summer.

As mentioned previously, symptoms of Parkinson's disease frequently accompany use of such drugs (extrapyramidal effects – see Ch. 5). These are generally well-controlled by oral anti-parkinsonian medication such as procyclidine (Kemadrin). Occasionally this has to be administered by injection to rapidly reverse acute distressing muscle spasms in the back, jaw or extrinsic eye muscles (dystonic reactions). Unfortunately, procyclidine and its alternatives increase the risk of tardive dyskinaesia, the often irreversible appearance of disfiguring orofacial contortions and choreiform limb movements. Unhappily this condition not infrequently follows reduction or discontinuation of long-term antipsychotic medications, as well as (paradoxically) their prolonged administration.

General restlessness (akathisia) is another possible side-effect, but unlike psychotic agitation, this responds to dose reduction rather than increase!

Common antipsychotic drugs, dosages and uses are show in Table 9.3.

Non-physical interventions

Although medication has made the specific treatment of psychotic symptoms possible, and is regarded by many psychiatrists as essential to maintenance of recovery (relapse is frequently noted to follow discontinuation), it is no substitute for other forms of therapeutic support.

While a calm, unstressful environment may be beneficial during acute illness, prolonged lack of

Table 9.3 Common antipsychotic drugs used to treat schizophrenia

Pharmacological group and name	Proprietary title	Typical dosage	Comments
Phenothiazines			
Chlorpromazine	Largactil	50–200 mg q.i.d.	Staple agent, sedative in high dosage
Thioridazine	Melleril	25–100 mg q.i.d.	Milder side-effects, high doses can impair sight, not available as injection
Fluphenazine	Modecate	12.5–25 mg every month	Depot preparation; sedative – may induce depression
Butyrophenones			
Haloperidol	Haldol Serenace	5–20 mg q.i.d.	Extrapyramidal side-effects likely
Droperidol	Droleptan	10 mg q.i.d.	Useful in curbing aggressive impulses
Thioxanthenes			
Flupenthixol	Depixol	20–40 mg every 1–3 weeks	Has antidepressant properties
Clopenthixol	Clopixol	200 mg every 2–4 weeks	May inhibit aggression (both are depots)

stimulation invariably undermines progress. Russell Barton (1959), in his seminal book on the topic, noted the predisposition of schizophrenic patients to institutionalization, a condition of apathetic stagnation induced in confined settings as disparate as prisons, monasteries and long-stay psychiatric wards. Moreover, Barton identified oversedation as a key cause of such 'mental bedsores'.

Largely to avoid this problem, recent emphasis has been placed on early discharge back to community residence, ideally via halfway houses and hostels where, initially, at least, some professional supervision is provided. Even those patients returning to family accommodation ought to have support available in the form of community psychiatric nursing and day hospital services.

It is equally important to encourage patients to engage in purposeful activity, initially engaging in ward-based occupational therapy, perhaps progressing through industrial retraining centres to full-time remunerative outside employment. Sheltered workshops and subsidized enclaves within commercial organizations offer people with all forms of disability (including psychiatric) useful paid work in intentionally undemanding conditions, although it must be conceded that economic recession places great pressure on such opportunities.

Tragically, the closure of defunct asylum wards seems not yet to have been matched by a corresponding expansion of community facilities, resulting in horror stories (in the USA as well as the UK) of aimlessly unemployed former psychiatric patients enduring substandard accommodation, malnutrition and financial exploitation. Given such circumstances, it can hardly be surprising if patients who avoid the penal system return to hospital promptly as if through a revolving door.

Because of patients' established vulnerability to stress, their relatives must be helped to accept the limitations which schizophrenia often imposes on occupational and social attainment.

For some patients attaining independence in very basic self-care and communication may be the sole feasible target. For this purpose, the psychological technique of behaviour modification has claimed some success. For example, patients may be selectively rewarded for desirable, if mundane, achievements such as rising at a reasonable hour, attending to personal hygiene or participating in communal activities. Reward may take the form of tokens which can be exchanged for commodities or privileges chosen by the patient (e.g. cigarettes or an outing) – the basis of **token economy systems**.

Social skills can be developed either by nurses

modelling such attainments (teaching by example) or again through providing **social reinforcement** in the form of interest and verbal praise when the patient communicates appropriately. To be effective, such measures must be applied consistently during regular interactions between nurse and patient.

Nursing strategies

Nursing Care Plan 9.1 summarizes the following discussion. Owing to the wide range of possible clinical features, planning nursing care for a schizophrenic patient, even more than in most illnesses, must be based on careful assessment of his individual needs. With reference to the Activities of Living Model, it is possible to outline the common behavioural problems, along with appropriate nursing interventions.

Maintaining a safe environment

Paranoid delusions and hallucinations fill the world with threat, malignant purpose frequently being attributed to benign people and objects.

If the patient is willing to share such private experiences, the nurse should take the opportunity to understand the patient's fears, demonstrate empathy and support, and then take measures to remove the patient's misperceived sources of threat or otherwise protect him from them.

Any precipitants of such thoughts and sensations should be identified, along with coping strategies helpful in minimizing their effect (various intellectual, social or physical activities may provide beneficial diversion).

Initially it is best not to challenge disordered thought and perception, although non-critical acceptance should never extend to confirming their validity. Any collusion, ironic or otherwise, will strengthen the patient's existing conviction, and detected insincerities will destroy any trust invested in the caring team.

Once a relationship has been established, it is more appropriate to help the patient explore the reality of his experience and discreetly offer alternative perspectives.

Some patients are less willing to ventilate their concerns, which must be deduced through visible preoccupation, agitation, or disturbed response. Rather than directly intrude, the nurse may be best advised to adopt a less direct manner, remaining quietly available without encroaching on the patient's personal space nor sacrificing alertness.

A calm, unhurried manner of approaching the patient should be adopted, prior reassurance given

Nursing Care Plan 9.1 Care plan for a patient with schizophrenia		
Problem	**Nursing actions**	**Rationale**
MAINTAINING A SAFE ENVIRONMENT		
1. **Imagined environmental threats**	❒ Allow patient opportunities for self-expression	Ventilation of fears is beneficial Facilitates development of therapeutic responses Allows critical exploration of patient's reality
2. **Episodes of agitation or aggression**	❒ Conservative measures ❒ Discreet observation ❒ Active measures (offer medication, engage patient in activity)	Perceived as non-threatening Monitors patient's behaviour May dissipate tension
COMMUNICATING		
3. **Mistrust of others**	❒ Clear, truthful communication	Establish and maintain a trusting relationship
4. **Inappropriate speech**	❒ Reinforce normal conversation	Replacement of odd with normal communication
5. **Lack of social skills**	❒ Demonstrate and provide opportunities for patient to practise these	Patient will acquire enhanced social attributes
6. **Social withdrawal**	❒ Consistent encouragement to gradually increase participation	Generate self-reinforcing momentum
EATING AND DRINKING		
7. **Refusal to eat, through belief food poisoned/ medicated**	❒ Allow patient to select meal from trolley Encourage patient to buy and prepare own provisions Ask relative to bring in what patient desires Nurse offers to taste patient's food (morsel only!) Provide bland food, enabling patient to season it himself	Minimize overt possibility to patient of malign contamination
PERSONAL CLEANSING AND DRESSING		
8. **Indifference to appearance**	❒ Provide incentives for improvement (praise, financial reward) ❒ Enable patient to select and purchase own toiletries and clothes ❒ Ensure warmth and privacy for personal hygiene ❒ Provide an inspiring role-model for patient	Instil motivation Encourages patient participation Encourages bathing and changing Patient liable to take indirect lead from nurse
WORKING AND PLAYING		
9. **Lack of social contact in community**	❒ Arrange outings Encourage visitors, correspondence, telephone calls and overnight home stays	Familiarizes patient with enjoyable social settings. Fosters outside contacts
10. **Employment difficulties**	❒ Liaise with statutory agencies (Disablement Resettlement Officer, Employment Rehabilitation Centre)	Facilitate occupational assessment and rehabilitation
11. **Lack of self-sufficiency after discharge**	❒ Place patient and relatives in touch with Mental Health Charitable Association	Provision of community-based advice and support promotes independence

of honest intent, and any unnecessary interactions avoided if the patient is temporarily perturbed.

Antipsychotic medication may prevent uncontainable tension developing, and should be offered with assurance of its anticipated benefits. In addition, physical exercise such as an accompanied walk in the hospital grounds or pummelling a punch-bag are useful safety-valves.

Schizophrenic patients may be impelled to self-injury by their distressing experiences. Unfortunately, it is seldom as straightforward to anticipate such behaviour in such clients as with depressed patients, which places the nurse's observational and intuitive powers at a premium.

Communicating

Social withdrawal is particularly characteristic of schizophrenic behaviour. This generally results either from a paranoid mistrust of others (discussed above), or because social interaction is felt to be inherently unrewarding. Lack of social fulfilment can in turn result from the negative impression made on others by persistent attempts to convey delusional or otherwise bizarre notions in a manner guaranteed to generate fear or ridicule. By selectively showing interest in and praising only appropriate speech, it is possible for the nurse to progressively engineer a normalization of the patient's conversation. Additionally, the patient is likely to adopt basic social skills (such as gestures, facial expressions and small talk) portrayed by nurses who demonstrate warmth and respect, particularly if they are given a secure forum in which to practise these new attainments. Initially, this may be in one-to-one encounters with a trusted nurse; later, once confidence expands, small patient groups provide a convenient supportive setting.

Progress is all too easily undermined by over-stressful exposure or minor social reverses. Communication with the patient should be caring, unambiguous and honest. Never appear to make the patient promises which it is impossible to be sure of keeping. Even confidentiality of information is not inviolable – significant material needs to be shared with professional colleagues, while a serious criminal confession might require still further dissemination!

Eating and drinking

Nutritional activities may be undermined in various ways, ranging from bizarre fads to apparent indifference, although perhaps paranoid food refusal is the most common obstacle.

Patients rarely persist far beyond normal limits of hunger and thirst, but the nurse can utilize a number of strategies to encourage the patient to eat a balanced diet.

Personal cleansing and dressing

Apathy often produces problems in this realm. To a large extent, appearances can be improved by diligent supervision and encouragement, although in the longer term the patient must be able to fulfil this basic need for himself.

Initially this transfer of responsibility may require incentive schemes in concert with the ward routine, in the hope that ultimately the intrinsic rewards of good self-presentation will sustain this behaviour after discharge.

Working and playing

Lack of motivation and capacity for enjoyment (anhedonia) can make these fundamental human activities immensely problematical. The resultant ability to tolerate a drab, idle existence makes schizophrenics especially vulnerable to institutionalization. Consequently it is vital for them to establish and maintain outside social contacts, and to find some source of remunerative occupation. Of particular help in these areas are several voluntary organizations, such as the National Association for Mental Health (MIND, or SAMH in Scotland) and the National Schizophrenia Fellowship, who organize local support groups and advisory services as well as fostering accommodation and employment projects for the mentally ill.

ORGANIC DISORDERS

INTRODUCTION

In contrast to functional disorders such as schizophrenia, organic conditions result from a clear physical cause or degenerative process. According to their characteristic course, such conditions are described as acute (sudden in onset and usually reversible) or chronic (slow, insidious onset followed by generally irreversible deterioration).

Five features are common to all organic disorders:

1. Disorientation in time and place (true CONFUSION). The patient is unaware of the hour, and may venture outside in nightclothes, miss appointments, etc. Gradually, the day of the week, date, month and ultimately the year cannot be recalled. When in hospital, the patient may believe he is still at home and so be bewildered by the presence of so many strangers.

2. Short-term memory loss. This refers to the inability to retain new information beyond about 15 seconds. As a result the patient may become upset at being 'kept in the dark' or not receiving due warning of events, particularly when nurses or relatives assure him to the contrary!

3. Impaired level of consciousness. The patient will be less aware of his surroundings, particularly when lighting is poor and he himself is tired. Consequently, problems are accentuated at night; nurses whispering to each other and moving the patient's belongings in the dark prior to providing care are liable to be perceived as burglars. Sensory information is less likely to register without clear repetition.

4. Personality change. All the above may contribute to arousing anxiety in the patient, creating either a fearful or hostile response. In addition, dementia is often accompanied by apathy previously uncharacteristic of the individual.

5. Intellectual dysfunction. Inevitably, inherently disordered perceptual and thought processes will erode the patient's ability to make sense of and respond to his environment. Personal awareness of this may understandably induce depression, although some patients deteriorate into euphoric oblivion.

ACUTE ORGANIC STATES

Delirium, the acute confusion caused by physical disturbances of the body's equilibrium, is commonest in early childhood and old age.

The following represent common types of cause:

1. febrile (e.g. juvenile infectious diseases, chest and urinary tract infections in the elderly)
2. nutritional (including dehydration, electrolyte imbalance and vitamin deficiencies)
3. cerebral (traumatic such as concussion, or following hypoxia or general anaesthesia)
4. environmental (sensory deprivation, e.g. isolation, poor lighting, and absence of sounds; unexpected changes of setting)
5. poisoning (e.g. constipation causing retention of waste products; drug side-effects including those of sedatives and alcohol).

Alcohol dependency and withdrawal

Relevant epidemiology and aetiology

Ethyl alcohol or ethanol, the favourite (legal) social lubricant of the western world, is basically a depressant drug (its 'stimulating' qualities are due to suppression of behavioral inhibitions) with significant toxic effects on most systems of the body.

Current British health recommendations suggest a maximum intake of 21 units for men and 14 for women, spaced throughout a week (a single pub measure of spirits or wine contains 1 unit, as does *half* a pint of standard beers). Recent research suggests that one in seven Britons regularly exceeds this, while one in four was ignorant of these guidelines.

Drinking over 36 units per week for men and 22 for women is thought likely to cause physical damage, although the timescale involved may be as long as 20 years for men. Women are vulnerable to damage within perhaps one-quarter of that period owing to certain physiological differences, which makes the apparent recent rise in female intake especially worrying. Also the recent rise in alcohol intake among young people in general is worrying; 18–25 year olds comprise the only European age group not currently enjoying increased life expectancy, due to alcohol and illegal drug-related mortality.

The potential physical ill-effects of alcohol are summarized in Figure 9.3.

Not surprisingly, as the liver metabolizes at least 95% of consumed alcohol, it is most prone to harm, involving gradual replacement of its substance by fatty and fibrous tissue (cirrhosis). This makes it harder for blood to leave the hepatic portal system (see Ch. 15), resulting in its diversion to collateral veins surrounding the oesophagus and rectum, which distend to form oesophageal varices (friable and prone to serious haemorrhage) and haemorrhoids respectively.

Other common alimentary problems include peptic ulceration and pancreatitis (possibly causing diabetes mellitus) caused by inflammation of the gut lining, producing in turn anorexia, malabsorption and anaemia.

Upper gut and lung carcinomas are thought to be related to the coincidence between heavy smoking and drinking; additionally, serious lung infections are common.

Fertility in both sexes is impaired by prolonged alcohol abuse; males commonly suffer diminished potency and increasing outward feminization, with profound effects on self-image, while pregnant women in addition risk provoking fetal damage (reviewed by Murray-Lyon 1989).

Alcohol wreaks particular havoc with nervous tissue, not least because the liver depletes the body's reserves of thiamine (vitamin B_1 is essential for nervous functioning) in metabolizing ethanol.

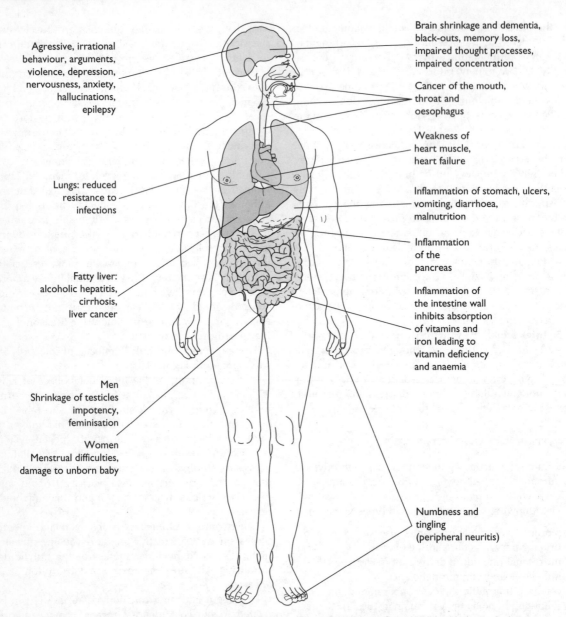

Agressive, irrational behaviour, arguments, violence, depression, nervousness, anxiety, hallucinations, epilepsy

Brain shrinkage and dementia, black-outs, memory loss, impaired thought processes, impaired concentration

Cancer of the mouth, throat and oesophagus

Weakness of heart muscle, heart failure

Lungs: reduced resistance to infections

Inflammation of stomach, ulcers, vomiting, diarrhoea, malnutrition

Inflammation of the pancreas

Fatty liver: alcoholic hepatitis, cirrhosis, liver cancer

Inflammation of the intestine wall inhibits absorption of vitamins and iron leading to vitamin deficiency and anaemia

Men
Shrinkage of testicles impotency, feminisation

Women
Menstrual difficulties, damage to unborn baby

Numbness and tingling (peripheral neuritis)

Fig. 9.3 Physical effects of prolonged alcohol abuse. (Reproduced from Cole 1990 by kind permission of Nursing Times where this diagram first appeared in an article on April 18th, 1990)

Effects range from painful or numb extremities (alcoholic neuritis) to irreparable cerebral atrophy, accompanied by poor co-ordination, epileptic seizures, abnormalities of mood and behaviour and the onset of dementia (Korsakov's psychosis).

Alcohol is firmly established as an intrinsic part of the British life-style. Under 5% of the adult population are total abstainers, while surveys suggest that by 15 years of age, 98% of young people have tried alco-

holic drinks (Hartz et al 1990). Average consumption per individual has more than doubled since World War II, partly attributable to a rise in disposable income accompanying a parallel fall in the relative price of alcohol. By 1991, the Scottish Council of Alcoholism noted that the £3.5 million spent by Scots per day on alcohol exceeded the amount they spent on clothes or heating their homes.

The cost of this indulgence is chastening; between a

third and a fifth of the admissions to **medical wards** are generally agreed to be alcohol related, while officially it accounted for 12 deaths per 100 000 of the mainland UK population in 1978 (more than double the 1965 rate).

Moreover, this latter statistic is thought to omit the contributory role of alcohol to many fatal accidents, including around a quarter of road accident deaths (and half of those involving drivers between 20 and 24 years) and drownings. As well as influencing around half the perpetrators (and victims) of murder and rape, alcohol was involved in 70% of the violent incidents which occurred in the casualty department of Edinburgh's Royal Infirmary in a 6-month period studied in 1984.

In addition, such intoxication has been associated with burglary, wife battery, child abuse and persistent work absenteeism – statistics alone are unable to fully gauge the social and economic harm caused by problem drinking.

Correlations have been detected between alcohol abuse and a range of factors, as shown in Table 9.4.

Common symptomatology

Prolonged intake of excessive amounts of alcohol induces both psychological and physical dependence. The former signifies that the person feels unable to function normally or even cope at all without alcohol, while the latter is established when physical

Table 9.4 Factors associated with alcohol problems	
Factor	Possible explanations
Geography Europe: highest in France, followed by Spain and Germany Scotland's alcohol-related deaths are double England's	Major wine-producers. Childhood introduction; associated with family and meal-time settings Economic hardship; restricted leisure facilities; communities isolated (highest in Highlands and Western Isles)
Social/cultural/ethnic Unusual in Mormons and Muslims Relatively high among American negroes and Irish compared with Jews there Common in Hebrides and Ireland	Religious taboo Social intolerance of drunkenness among latter Juxtaposition of teetotalism and inebriation creates ambivalence
Economic Incidence now low in Scandinavia (especially Norway) Prevalent in Social Classes I and V	Tax disincentives renders alcohol three times UK equivalent price Wealth may invite overindulgence; impoverished may seek oblivion (but alcoholism itself fosters penury)
Occupational Over-represented among: managers, publicans, seamen, salesmen, writers and journalists, for example	Such work may involve stress, tedium, peer-pressure, absence from home, lack of supervision and/or cheaply available alcohol (but may attract potential problem drinkers)
Gender and marital status Three males to every female alcoholic (but gap narrowing) Commoner in single/separated/divorced/widowed	Social attitudes; occupational patterns Loneliness; ? cause or effect
Familial A third of children of alcoholics develop same problem as adults Offspring also more likely to marry an alcoholic	? Genetic predisposition or learning from parental model
Personality Various personality 'types' and 'disorders' (see Ch. 10) implicated Aspirations toward masculinity (males) and sophistication (females)	Depression, anxiety, inadequacy and oral fixation relieved by intoxication Reflects appeal of advertising campaigns (but media bans don't seem to significantly reduce consumption)

signs and symptoms ensue in the absence of the drug.

The process of alcohol withdrawal may take three degrees of intensity. The mild form is often characterized by irritability, poor concentration and anxiety, often rooted in fear of experiencing delirium tremens (DTs). The alert nurse may pick up cues about a new patient 'feeling like a drink' during routine admission. Intense craving for alcohol is typically felt for episodes lasting about 60 minutes.

This may progress to a moderate stage where the patient becomes obviously restless, fearful, tremulous and perspires freely. Pyrexia and bounding tachycardia are often evident, while the patient may complain of muscle cramps and severe flu-like symptoms.

About 5% of patients experience severe withdrawal, with accentuation of moderate stage features plus those of DTs. This confusional state can involve severe tremor and inco-ordination of the whole body, along with vivid disturbances of visual perception. These can take the form of terrifying (often flying) animals, although amusing miniature figures may be seen (Lilliputians). The renowned pink elephants are largely mythical. Some patients are tormented by a sensation of crawling flesh (formication), while paranoid ideas concerning sexual betrayal by their partner may be reinforced by auditory hallucinations (the Othello or Jealous Spouse syndrome). The resulting distortion of reality can make the patient unpredictable, uncooperative and aggressive. Epileptic convulsions occur in about 10% of withdrawing patients.

Range of investigations

1. Blood tests. No laboratory tests at present permit certain diagnosis of alcohol dependence. However, the following provide useful indicators of problem drinking:

- Blood alcohol concentration above 80 mg/100 ml (the legal driving limit) in the morning, without any signs of inebriation (suggesting the development of **tolerance**).
- Raised levels of gamma-glutamyl transpeptidase (a serum enzyme) are found in 80% of problem drinkers, while increased mean corpuscular volume (MCV) occurs in 60% of cases.

Anaemia is characteristic of prolonged heavy drinking for two main reasons: malnutrition due to poor dietary intake and absorption, and blood loss from alimentary haemorrhage and reduced haemostasis. Consequently precautionary estimations of haemo-

globin content and prothrombin (clotting) time are made.

Owing to dietary neglect and the dehydrating effect of alcohol, it is important to ascertain that urea and electrolyte levels remain within safe limits. Similarly, as hepatic damage is the commonest complication, assays are performed to determine liver function.

2. Respiratory. Because of the increased susceptibility to lung disease, chest X-rays and analysis of sputum specimens are routine investigations.

3. Cardiovascular. An electrocardiograph is performed to detect any serious cardiac abnormalities caused by prolonged metabolic imbalance. Hypertension and heart failure are not common.

4. Neurological tests. Brain function can be systematically assessed employing psychological measures of memory, intellect and attitudes. Suspected brain damage may indicate the need for a CT scan (see Ch. 5) to demonstrate any cerebral atrophy and ventricular enlargement.

Therapeutic management

Ideally, withdrawal should be planned following discussion between the patient, carers and health professionals. This may take place at home, particularly if the family are supportive, supervised by the GP and community psychiatric nurse. More frequently, and invariably if complications occur, a general hospital setting is dictated. Not uncommonly, an inpatient unexpectedly displays withdrawal symptoms, usually after admission with a severe infection or following trauma, up to 72 hours following his last drink.

Conservative treatment generally suffices, with high-potency injections of vitamins B_1, B_2 and C (Parentrovite) being succeeded by oral supplements after 6 days, to prevent progressive deficiency complications. For the first 7 days, tranquillizing medication such as chlormethiazole (Heminevrin) or chlordiazepoxide (Librium) is administered to calm the patient, assist sleep, reduce craving by physically replacing alcohol, and prevent epileptic fits.

Sedation is gradually discontinued thereafter to forestall the development of secondary dependence.

Diligent attention is paid to dehydration (possibly requiring intravenous infusion) and nutritional status, and vital signs should be monitored closely (perhaps involving a cardiac monitor), as severe withdrawal carries a significant mortality risk (perhaps as high as 20%). Adequate rest is essential, until the acute phase is completed after 5–7 days.

Subsequently, the patient is invariably referred for psychotherapy, either to groups based at local psychi-

Nursing Care Plan 9.2	Care plan for a patient suffering from alcoholism	
Problem	**Nursing strategy**	**Rationale**
MAINTAINING A SAFE ENVIRONMENT		
1. **Tremor and poor grip**	❏ Provide 'hand warm' liquids in feeding beaker with large handles (or feed patient)	Prevent scalds
2. **Ataxia, restlessness, impaired vision**	❏ Constant observation; remove obstacles; provide assistance, adequate lighting, reassurance, sedation as prescribed	Minimize risk of falls
3. **Visual hallucinations and illusions**	❏ Ensure adequate, even lighting at all times; avoid shadows; provide rational explanations without antagonizing patient	Reduce possibility of misinterpretation
4. **Tachycardia, hypertension, dyspnoea, pyrexia**	❏ Monitor patient's pulse, blood pressure, respirations and temperature as patient's condition warrants	Early detection and reporting of significant changes in condition
COMMUNICATING		
5. **Poor concentration**	❏ Clear, simple, relevant instructions and responses	Facilitate attentional focus
6. **Disorientation from 'here and now' reality**	❏ Reorientate patient as appropriate; offer 'true' perspectives diplomatically	Assist patient to regain orientation
7. **Overambitious future aims**	❏ Help patient towards critical appraisal of self and goals; involve relatives where feasible	Direction of effort towards practicable targets; avoid disillusioning failure for all concerned
8. **Patient may reject responsibility for conduct, maintaining superficial facade**	❏ Be inwardly sceptical; show interest only in genuine therapeutic effort/discussion; refer to self-help group	Avoid reinforcing futile attitude and behaviour; fellow sufferers have to be honest with each other
EATING AND DRINKING		
9. **Alcoholic dehydration**	❏ Encourage high oral intake (fruit juice, squash, water). Manage intravenous infusion if required	Rehydrate; restore vitamin C and electrolyte balance. Quench patient's marked thirst
10. **Nutritional neglect**	❏ High protein diet	Rebuild wasted muscles. Preserves thiamine (used in carbohydrate metabolism)
	❏ Vitamin supplementation	Reverse effects of deficiency
	❏ Regular weight checks	Monitor progress
PERSONAL CLEANSING AND DRESSING		
11. **Personal neglect**	❏ Thorough inspection, cleansing and provision of clean clothing following admission (treat infestation as necessary)	Prevent further infection; boost patient's morale
12. **Pyrexia, excessive perspiration**	❏ Regular bed-baths, sponging down, deodorants, fanning	Maximize patient comfort and hygiene; reduce pyrexia
13. **Itch, formication**	❏ Keep skin clean and dry. Provide fresh, cool bed clothes and linen. Apply soothing lotions (e.g. calamine) as directed	Minimize discomfort

Nursing Care Plan 9.2 (*cont'd*)		
Problem	Nursing strategy	Rationale
WORKING AND PLAYING		
14. **Craving for alcohol during withdrawal period; brooding on past failure**	❑ Devise activities for patient (simple tasks of personal utility, existing hobbies, group activities e.g. run by occupational therapist)	Provide worthwhile distraction
	❑ Reassure craving is transient; listen sympathetically without fostering self-pity	Instil positive, future-oriented attitude
15. **Reliance on alcohol-related social settings and relationships**	❑ Assist patient to formulate alternative social outlets; enlist support of family, friends and voluntary organizations	Facilitate avoidance of undesirable associations and fill resulting social void
16. **Occupational unsuitability** a. Unemployment (actual or threatened)	❑ Negotiate with latest employer to consider trial employment following treatment. Liaise with social worker, occupational retraining and resettlement agencies	Establish or maintain remunerative occupation; self-esteem; avoid debt
b. Work environment encourages drinking	❑ Discuss means of resisting temptation or need to change work environment/occupation	Prevent relapse

atric facilities (e.g. day hospital) or those run by specialist voluntary organizations, of which Alcoholics Anonymous is the most ubiquitous. By entering discussions with fellow sufferers, the patient should find shared experience and encouragement within a sympathetic forum of mutual problem solving.

As well as involvement in group therapy, health professionals work with such patients on an individual basis to explore motivation (e.g. drawing up a list of the pros and cons of stopping), analyse potential difficulties (e.g. using drinking diaries to assess precipitants) and formulate realistic goals (e.g. degrees of abstinence rather than teetotalism). Psychological strategies are based on the belief that personal difficulties form the basis of problem drinking, and must be identified, confronted and resolved to enable a cure to occur – i.e. recognizing that alcoholism comes in people rather in bottles.

Some centres use aversion therapy to discourage relapse, for example drugs such as disulfiram (Antabuse) which when mixed with alcohol produce highly unpleasant side-effects. Such treatments have the disadvantages of not directly utilizing the patient's own motivation and of placing therapists in a punitive role, making their long-term effectiveness rather dubious.

Nursing strategies

These can be conveniently outlined using the Activities of Living scheme and are summarized in Nursing Care Plan 9.2.

1. Maintaining a safe environment. Common hazards here include scalding and falls due to poor motor control, and assault on other patients and staff due to disordered thought and perceptions. Consequently, during severe withdrawal the patient should be managed in a single room with minimal hazards, under constant nursing supervision.

2. Communication. Problems in this sphere are likely to revolve initially around the inattentiveness and general confusion accompanying withdrawal.

After recovery, patients often need help to focus honestly and realistically on the problems preceding admission.

3. Eating and drinking. Malnutrition and problem drinking are ultimately inseparable, often with lethal consequences. Early efforts to overcome this may be hampered by the severe nausea which often accompanies withdrawal. Initially, fluids are tolerated better, as precipitous resumption of a solid diet may induce or exacerbate diarrhoea.

4. Personal cleansing and dressing; controlling body temperature. Patients often present in an unkempt state, while the weakness, confusion and profuse sweating typical during acute withdrawal require active nursing interventions.

5. Working and playing. Time hangs heavily on withdrawing patients, inactivity giving scope to unhealthy preoccupations. In addition, reformed drinkers are faced with the probable need to totally restructure their social life. Manifold occupational problems generally follow alcohol abuse; either poor performance or attendance may precipitate dismissal, or the work environment may encourage drinking.

CHRONIC ORGANIC STATES

Gradual irreversible degeneration of healthy adult brain tissue, resulting in the loss of mental function known as dementia, occurs in several distinct conditions.

Traditionally, these have been classified, on the basis of age of onset, into presenile and senile conditions, with the arbitrary division set at 65 years (Table 9.5).

Alzheimer-type dementia (AD)

This condition is worth detailed consideration because of its current high profile, due not least to its high (and worryingly increasing) prevalence.

Physiology and anatomy

Microscopically, post-mortem studies demonstrate death of neurones throughout the cortex and their replacement by non-functional glial cells. Neurofibrils become tangled, and plaques (deposits) of useless protein develop, particularly in the hippocampus (an area associated with emotion and memory).

Gross inspection reveals widening of sulci and some ventricular enlargement, again implying relative degeneration of functional brain tissue.

Levels of acetylcholine, the neurotransmitter primarily implicated in mediating memory processes, appear markedly diminished in the brains of Alzheimer sufferers.

Epidemiology and aetiology

First described in 1907 (by the German psychiatrist Alois Alzheimer), AD is known to afflict at least 5–7% of the over-65 population, and up to one-fifth of those over 85 years.

Table 9.5 Features of various forms of dementia

	Incidence	Age of onset	Cause	Specific characteristics	Prognosis
PRESENILE DEMENTIAS					
Huntington's chorea	Around 6 per 100 000 population	Usually 20s–40s	Single autosomal dominant gene	Dysfunction of **basal ganglia** creates severe motor incoordination and overactivity	Death within 13–16 years
Pick's disease	Rare	During 50s	Possibly genetic (commonly runs in families and affects females)	Frontal lobes degenerate **disinhibited behaviour** and **inappropriate affect** ensue	Death within 2–10 years
Creutzfeld–Jakob disease (spongiform encephalopathy or SE)	Very rare	Non-specific	Probably viral (transmitted by contaminated neurosurgical instruments)	Cavities appear in brain and spinal cord, producing early **ataxia**. Human equivalent of **BSE** (mad cow's disease)	Rapidly fatal (1–2 years)
Alzheimer's disease	0.1% those under 65	Above 40 years	Uncertain (discussed below)	Rapid advance of dementia	Typically fatal within 7–10 years
SENILE DEMENTIAS					
Alzheimer type	High (5% those over 65)	Usually 70–90	Uncertain (discussed below)	Typical 'dementia' in relentless deterioration of intellect and personality	Death within 2–10 years
Multiple-infarct type	Relatively common (about 1–5% of those over 60 years)	60–80 years	Cerebral arteriosclerosis (progressive microscopic infarct development, equivalent to series of small thrombotic 'strokes')	Deterioration typically occurs in discrete 'steps' with intervening stability; insight and 'reactive' depression often present	Slightly longer course than AD; half may die of concurrent **cardiovascular disease**

Women roughly outnumber male AD sufferers by two to one, although this may simply reflect their greater life-expectancy.

Nearly three-quarters of all dementia cases are due to AD, estimated at about 1 million people in Britain alone. This figure is certain to increase with our ageing population. It is hardly surprising then that AD has been called the silent epidemic – silent largely due to the relative lack of attention it has hitherto generated, compared for example with heart disease and rare childhood conditions.

In the under-65 population, AD is relatively rare, with about one in 1000 developing the presenile form.

It may be useful to state that AD does **not** seem to be caused by old age itself, hardened arteries (as formerly held by expert opinion), over- or under-use of the intellect, stress or a sexually transmissible agent (although the terminal stage of AIDS may involve dementia).

Recently, suspicion has focused on aluminium, as high levels of aluminium have been detected in Alzheimer plaques and tangles. This has been brought to the national consciousness by the complaints of amnesia and other neurological symptoms among the populace of Camelford in Cornwall following the accidental contamination of the public water supply there with aluminium sulphate in 1988 (Sadler 1991).

Nevertheless, even normal regional variations in water aluminium are dwarfed by its high, almost universal presence in food, and it may be that AD itself merely makes the brain more prone to absorb and concentrate this commonest of metals.

Hereditary factors have been increasingly implicated in the genesis of AD. Although first-degree relatives of senile sufferers only seem at marginally increased risk, the early-onset form of AD does show a marked familial tendency. There is also considerable evidence that individuals with Down's syndrome as a result of trisomy 21 (an extra chromosome added to the normal pair is one of the causes of this condition) invariably develop AD if they live beyond their late 40s (Barr 1990). As a result, much research has centred around identifying a pathological AD gene on these chromosomes, in the hope of developing effective remedies.

As with multiple sclerosis, slow viruses have been proposed as aetiologically significant, but without much empirical substantiation.

Common symptomatology

The classic description of the typical course and fea-tures of AD was given by Irene Burnside (Burnside 1979), who identified three stages.

The initial stage is characterized by **memory loss** which interferes with the ability to cope with everyday tasks such as self-care and housework. Awareness of failing abilities often results in social withdrawal and depressed mood. Not inappropriately, AD has been called 'the thief of memory', stealing people's minds, which is especially significant as 'our memories are, in a sense, who we are' (Williams 1990).

The second stage is characterized by **confusion**, involving severe loss of cognitive functions such as language and sensory discrimination. Behavioural problems such as restless wandering, insomnia and repetitive questioning place great demands on carers, while the sufferer may exhibit severe anxiety or anger in the midst of her bewilderment.

The final stage of **terminal or profound dementia** consists of a progressive accentuation of the preceding phases, involving loss of perceptual recognition (of people as well as objects), immobility (with its attendant risks) and verbal unresponsiveness (patients may become mute). Ultimately, the patient may become totally dependent on carers for most activities of living, such as maintaining a safe environment (e.g. preventing falls, pressure sores, outside exposure), washing and dressing, elimination (double incontinence is common) and eating and drinking (patients may fail to recognize food and even actively resist feeding). The range of possible functional deterioration is well demonstrated in dementia behaviour scales such as that reproduced in Box 9.1 (McCracken & Fitzwater 1989).

Severe wasting occurs latterly, not entirely due to food refusal and dysphagia (Bucht & Sandman 1990).

Cachexia seems to render sufferers prone to fulminating bronchopneumonia, which most commonly occurs 7–8 years after the onset of this horrifying disease.

Range of investigations

It is important to distinguish AD from other at present reversible conditions with similar features, such as acute confusional states and depressive illness. The nurse has a major role to play in this, for example in monitoring the presence of any infection, the effects of medication and the apparent mood of the patient.

A variety of psychometric tests (e.g. orientation, memory and language skills) generally prove diagnostically useful, as may CT scan in delineating anatomical changes in the brain.

Box 9.1 Dementia behaviour scale

LANGUAGE-CONVERSATION
0 Is conversational
1 Repeats things, searches for synonyms, is reticent in conversation
2 Shows circumlocution, tells white lies, has mild vocabulary limitation, is easily led in conversation, uses automatisms
3 Loses thread of thought, has noticeable vocabulary loss
4 Is less aware of mistakes, has poor syntax and sequence, shows perseveration and neologisms
5 Parrots words, is incoherent and uncomprehending, has severe vocabulary limitation
6 Is mute and unresponsive

SOCIAL INTERACTION
0 Assists and/or takes initiative
1 Is an active participant and follower
2 Is a bland participant, is no longer empathic, shows loss of tact
3 Is observer only, misidentifies close relatives, is sometimes belligerent, defensive and/or suspicious
4 Is 'out of step', has poor recognition of persons, mistakes own reflection, is sometimes menacing
5 Wanders, shows frequent catastrophic reaction (is defiant, suspicious, and combative)
6 Is completely blank

ATTENTION-AWARENESS
0 Is bright and responsive
1 Requires guidance, can't recall date
2 Has shortened attention span, can't recall day, is easily distracted

3 Attention wanders, tires easily, has very few pleasures
4 Is distracted by illusions, picks at imaginary lint, misidentifies objects
5 Attention can be engaged only sporadically and briefly
6 Is oblivious to all surroundings

SPATIAL ORIENTATION
0 Is oriented well
1 Is oriented to immediate locus only (can't get home)
2 Is hesitant and loses things
3 Shows disorientation to place, hides things, is a 'pack rat'
4 Has body disorientation, can't seat self on chair, has bodily illusions, is oblivious to posture
5 Hallucinates
6 Is totally lost

MOTOR CO-ORDINATION
0 Is fully co-ordinated
1 Is underactive, but responds to commands
2 Shows poor co-ordination, moves slowly, stumbles
3 Occasionally requires manipulation and assistance
4 Has involuntary movements, is not self-mobile, neglects one side, requires manipulation and assistance
5 Is spastic, keeps chin on chest, requires wheelchair for safety, needs maximum physical assistance
6 Is unable to ambulate and has contracted limbs

BOWEL AND BLADDER
0 Cares for self
1 Asks to go, but needs cues to locate toilet
2 Is remindable, has occasional poor hygiene, forgets to flush

3 Needs regular supervision, requires assistance, is wet occasionally
4 Has occasional faecal incontinence
5 Shows unpredictable continence, is controlled by enema, needs occasional diapers
6 Is fully incontinent, needs full-time diapers and catheter

EATING AND NUTRITION
0 Cares for self, has steady weight, can cook
1 Needs prompting to eat, has history of weight loss, burns pots
2 Needs food cut up, wanders from table, can't cook
3 Uses utensils improperly, uses fingers, has slight weight gain
4 Is voraciously interested in sweets, steals food, shows marked weight gain *or* marked weight loss
5 Must be fed, will eat non-food items
6 Dysphagic, must be tube fed

DRESSING AND GROOMING
0 Is well groomed, shows appropriate self-care
1 Won't change clothing, is poorly groomed
2 Wears dirty, unkempt, inappropriate dress, ignores food on face
3 Misuses clothing, misidentifies clothes, wears others' clothes, needs clothes set out
4 Dresses only with help and instruction, is oblivious to grooming
5 Requires full assistance
6 Must be dressed, wears hospital gown

TOTAL SCORE: _____

Adapted with permission from Haycox J A 1984 A simple reliable clinical behavioral scale for assessing demented patients. Journal of Clinical Psychiatry 45: 23–24, figure 1, © 1984, Physicians Postgraduate Press

---

Recently it has become possible to demonstrate the characteristic protein plaques in skin and blood vessels, for example in the nasal mucosa of some patients, raising hopes of earlier positive diagnosis.

Therapeutic management

Unfortunately therapeutic developments have not matched such diagnostic advances. No cure exists, nor any significant form of active treatment.

Various drugs have been developed in an attempt to overcome the ascertained reduction of acetylcholine (ACh) activity in AD. These include THA, a drug inhibiting ACh breakdown, muscarine-like drugs which mimic the effects of ACh and nerve growth factor (NGF) which may hopefully promote the survival of ACh-producing neurones. However, it seems doubtful if any tangible benefits will result in human patients before the end of the present decade. Work continues to identify the specific genes which may mediate the physiological changes of AD, with a view to engineering their replacement.

Three distinct forms of interactive therapy have been developed by which nurses can adopt a therapeutic role in their daily management of confused patients.

1. Reality orientation (RO). This strategy aims to restore and maintain patients' contact with here and now reality, and takes two distinct forms.

The first of these is continuous, 24-hour, **informal RO**, wherein nurses present relevant details about time, location, impending activities and names to patients on each encounter, correcting misapprehensions as necessary. Such information is reinforced by environmental cues such as magnetic boards, large clocks and labels on ward areas (Bertram 1989).

Such constant reminders are usually backed up by formal or classroom RO, which takes the form of daily sessions where groups of patients of equivalent ability meet for around half an hour in a familiar, comfortable setting free of distraction. Activities, directed by a nurse or occupational therapist, include news media surveys, quizzes and identification of seasonal material, following mutual introduction of participants (perhaps by selection of name badges).

Consistently implemented, studies suggest RO may enhance individuals' orientation, and improve patients' ability to find their way about independently. Notable improvements undoubtedly boost nursing morale, although lapses in therapy and the inevitable progression of dementia will reverse gains (with varying swiftness).

More ambitious claims that RO increases patient independence in basic living skills are largely unsubstantiated, and this treatment has been criticized from both a practical and emotional standpoint (Morton & Bleathman 1988). If the patients won't be emerging from a centrally heated unit, and if every day carries an identical routine, should they be concerned about the weather or the stage of the week? Is it kind to confront amiably confused elderly people with the reality that their parents are long dead and the family home sold off or demolished?

2. Validation therapy. As a response to the concerns above, this alternative approach regards confusion as in part a form of withdrawal from an unpleasant, threatening present to past times when life was safe and rewarding. Rather than contradict confused speech and behaviour, validation therapy involves interpreting the meaning and feelings which the patient is unsuccessfully attempting to convey. Thus, for example, seemingly aimless overactivity might suggest the patient's need for useful occupation, while hoarding tissues may reflect a past career as a cashier (Goudie & Stokes 1989). Such interactions, maintained on the ground of the patient's choosing, may facilitate appropriate nursing interventions with minimal risk of distress, and are probably part of the intuitive repertory of all those experienced in nursing elderly people.

3. Reminiscence therapy. In 1963, Butler wrote of life-review in the elderly as a 'normal, naturally occurring, universal mental process, characterized by looking back over life lived, and recalling either pleasurable memories or unresolved conflicts, which can be surveyed and integrated'.

Reminiscence therapy consists of harnessing this natural process of reflection to provide an enjoyable, psychologically beneficial activity for small groups of matched patients, who often revel in discussing their undiminished long-term memories of shared experiences. The regular nurse therapist may stimulate reminiscence using a variety of materials, such as old photographs, catalogues, programmes, music-hall songs, sayings, coins and even the tools of former trades. During the meeting, the therapist should encourage and praise contributions, link themes and redirect topics as appropriate, so as to avoid isolation or painful topics affecting individual members.

None of these three forms of therapy are mutually exclusive; all have the advantage of offering potentially stimulating activities for patients, while expanding the nurse's role as a conscious therapist beyond that of custodian and provider of physical necessities.

Nursing strategies

For a detailed survey of the management of basic patient dependency created by AD, the reader is referred to Ironbar & Hooper (1989, topic 13) and Lyttle (1986, Chapter 34).

A recent initiative in the specialist care of Alzheimer patients in the USA is the introduction of closed units described by McCracken & Fitzwater (1989). Patients rated on behaviour competence scales (e.g. Box 9.1) are grouped according to their level of functioning, with more able patients remaining in standard unlocked conditions, while the more dependent residents are nursed in small enclosed areas, often adjacent to the main ward facility. Rather than incarcerating patients, the intention is to apply intensive rehabilitative techniques and, where necessary, physical care in fundamental activities, using a stable nursing team whose members become reassuringly familiar to patients and aware of their individual needs (e.g. those patients liable to fall or choke). In addition, it is felt that the *reduced* stimulation ensured by an environment free of demanding occupational therapies, overactive fellow patients and inviting exits is more beneficial to the psychological and functional well-being of profoundly demented patients.

The majority of AD sufferers are looked after at home by relatives, imposing huge emotional, physical and even financial stresses on carers (Williams (1990) gives a graphic personal account). Consequently, increasing demands have been made for improved respite facilities such as holiday admissions and day-hospital or day-centre attendance.

Voluntary organizations, for example Age Concern and the Alzheimer's Disease Society (see Lees 1989), have directed much of this campaign; their results include the Local Authority Homeshare Day-Care scheme in Ipswich. This pays members of the public to look after one or more patients in the formers' own homes for a few hours, akin to operating miniature domestic day-centres, allowing the carers some much needed personal space and time. In addition, those charities provide advisory services and organize local carer support groups throughout the country, concerning which all relatives should be informed. They also fund research and public education about a condition which is apparently still widely viewed (like other mental illnesses) as an unnatural, undesirable affliction against which sufferers and their families should persevere under a blanket of shameful secrecy.

Anorexia nervosa

Introduction and common symptomatology

This disorder is considered briefly in this chapter. Although the condition does not easily fit into any particular classification, as it has its own unique features, it carries some overtones of neurotic behaviour and inadequate personality as well as inherent accompanying oddities of thought and perception.

Thoughts related features include an overconcern with nutritional topics amounting to an obsession, a phobia of excess weight and a compulsive refusal to eat (bulimia nervosa is a related, less severe condition characterized by loss of control over eating). Distorted perception in anorexic patients seems confined to an exaggeration of body size and possibly of food portions (Yellowlees et al 1988).

Typical behaviour includes restriction of carbo-hydrate intake (sometimes replaced by excessive intake of very low calorie foods), occasional binges followed by self-induced vomiting and diarrhoea, and intensive exercising (to burn energy), often carried out surreptitiously with outward denial of any problem.

Serious weight loss is accompanied by somatic complications, including amenorrhoea, hypothermia, oedema (due to protein loss), hypotension and bradycardia. Cardiovascular collapse as a result of chronic electrolyte imbalance may cause premature death in up to 15% of sufferers, while pancytopenia renders survivors vulnerable to infections, particularly in the respiratory tract.

Epidemiology

The Eating Disorders Association reports that about one in 500 women between the ages of 15 and 25 are treated for anorexia nervosa, totalling around 6000 patients in Britain per year. Males can be affected, but only comprise between 2% and 10% of the total. The overwhelming majority of patients are young single women from affluent backgrounds, who nearly always develop the illness within 5 years of their first menstrual period.

Aetiology

As the incidence of anorexia has been increasing in recent years, and it remains largely restricted to females, connections have been suggested with the mass media promotion of slimness as the prerequisite of feminine fashion, success and desirability.

In view of the typical lack of sexual experience by the time of the patient's initial episodes of illness, it has also been proposed that girls may unconsciously retreat from adolescent sexual anxieties by suppressing secondary sexual characteristics through intense fasting. Many patients describe their thin figures as 'attractive, successful, safe and controlled', and equate fat or even shapely figures with ugliness, failure and frightening loss of self-control.

Much attention has also been paid to the family of anorexic clients, with varied reports of parental discord, maternal psychiatric illness (including eating disorders), prominence of food in family communication (meal-times often becoming battlegrounds for latent conflicts) and high expectations placed upon the patient. Parents often comment on the 'model childhood behaviour of anorexics', so perhaps rejection of lovingly prepared food represents an indirect expression of unacceptable rebellious impulses. Interestingly, the first illness often coincides with important school exams, a time of particular stress for those carrying intense parental aspirations.

Range of investigations

It is important to exclude conditions which also produce severe weight loss and possibly other features common to anorexia nervosa. These include:

- thyroid overactivity
- diabetes mellitus
- malabsorption states (e.g. Crohn's and coeliac disease)
- cancer (especially of the alimentary tract)
- disorders of the pituitary gland (source of gonadotrophins) and hypothalamus (which controls the pituitary and mediates appetite).

Therapeutic management

Generally treatment follows admission to a specialist unit, involving the patient's consent to a pre-arranged, non-negotiable contract (or compulsory detention if the patient's physical survival is in imminent peril). Intensive refeeding is commenced directed by a dietitian, initially with supplemented liquid feeds, (in extremis administered by nasogastric tube), progressing to increasingly solid meals containing up to 17 000 kJ per day, compared with the 9000 kJ daily intake recommended for the average adult female by the Government's Department of Health. Appetite stimulants such as chlorpromazine may be administered.

Management is based on a strict behaviour therapy regime, with the patient initially confined to bed (conserving energy) and having to earn rewards, such as use of bathroom facilities, reading materials, television and visits, through co-operation.

In recent years, criticism has been increasingly directed at such paternalistic methods, on the grounds that they are psychologically demeaning, fail to harness the patient's own motivation and are likely to generate rebellion (and so relapse) following discharge. Adherents would counter that this technique is demonstrably effective in reversing potentially fatal physical deterioration and precludes the very real possibility of covert sabotage by patients (e.g. by hiding or vomiting food when free of supervision).

Such arguments are expanded by Laywood (1989) and Gartside (1989).

What seems clear is that for physical recovery to

be maintained, psychological treatments and support are an essential supplement (or alternative). These include occupational and recreational therapy to diminish preoccupations, relaxation techniques and long-term psychotherapy.

The psychotherapy element includes individual and group discussion to embrace themes of adult sexuality, media pressures and attitudes to eating. Involvement of family members is seen as vital to overcome misunderstandings and tensions, and may be required for several years (so-called family therapy).

Following discharge, patient contact should be maintained through the community psychiatric nurse, day hospital and general practitioner, and both client and family made aware of the support available through such voluntary agencies as Anorexic Aid and Anorexics Anonymous.

Nursing strategies

Many nurses are well placed to develop caring empathetic relationships with anorexic clients, as they share many common characteristics (age, gender, conscientious personality, interests and life experience, to name a few). This makes them ideally placed to offer sympathetic listening, explanation and reassurance to patients who often contend with feelings of anxiety, guilt and poor self-esteem. Indeed, within a 'cruel to be kind' refeeding regimen, it may be all too easy for a nurse to internalize the patient's hostility and undermine consistency of management by unilaterally relaxing supervision. Such misgivings are better to be openly expressed and discussed honestly with approachable colleagues than left to fester unresolved.

A firm but relaxed manner is required when encouraging eating; this approach is acquired with practice and often learned by observing colleagues. Patient progress needs to be tactfully acknowledged.

Mention made of increasing freedom and privileges (such as outside contacts) may be more discreetly encouraging than telling the patient how much 'better' she's looking (which she may interpret as 'fatter' and further evidence of her tactical defeat). Every effort should be made to get to know the client's family and put them at ease, not least because of their integral importance to successful rehabilitation.

ETHICAL ISSUES

Individuals deemed to be experiencing abnormal

thoughts or perceptions are likely in our society to have their freedom of action and movement curtailed. For example, on the recommendation of one or more psychiatrists, under the Mental Health Act (1983, England; 1984 Scotland) they may be detained in hospital against their will if by reason of mental illness they are considered 'a danger to themselves or others'. Moreover, subject to periodic review, they may also be compelled to accept medication to remove or control such symptoms. While this argument may appear ostensibly reasonable, it begs two questions. First that some individual's ideas and experiences are less valid than those of others, and constitute ill or mad behaviour. This has been challenged by several eloquent authorities (e.g. Laing and Szasz), and psychiatry as a potential agent of social control is open to ideological abuse (e.g. the silencing of political dissidence). Secondly, that health professionals are able to judge what is in everyone's best interests. Although few would deny the need for protection of members of the public, this requires to be subjectively assessed in each case (and is therefore open to errors of caution or, sometimes, of highly publicized liberality), while removing personal responsibility from the patient ('as a danger to himself') infringes individual autonomy, however well intentioned (some might regard mountaineers and racing drivers as suitable cases for treatment!). Conversely, the ability of anyone suffering a serious mental illness to offer valid acquiescence (whether therapeutic, legal or sexual) must be open to question, even when professional opinion concurs with them!

Once the decision to admit and treat has been made, therapeutic management itself is not without controversy.

Again the principle of autonomy may be compromised. Should elderly confused patients be sedated or safely confined in geriatric chairs (often criticized as chemical and mechanical straight-jacketing), or left to roam unhindered, risking injury from falls and through aggravation of fellow patients? Are the issues here of *degree* of restraint (again a matter of subjective judgement) or of carer convenience?

Many authorities now believe that patients have a right to exercise a degree of risk in pursuit of free activity, and most psychiatric units have an open-door policy, which in fostering patient relaxation increases the stress on nursing staff responsible for preventing patients absconding.

Behaviour modification therapies have been discussed throughout this chapter, and are founded on the technique of operant conditioning developed in animal psychology experiments, a technique of encouraging desired behaviour by the selective rewarding of responses. The gut reaction of many health professionals (as well as laymen) is that such therapies, including token economy incentive schemes for self-care, or refeeding regimens in anorexia units, are inherently dehumanizing and erode our valued principle of 'respect for others'. Modern treatments go still further in employing what amounts to punishment for patients who fail to co-operate, in the forcible nasogastric feeding of anorexic (and some terminally demented) patients, the withholding of everyday privileges from the former, and the use of aversive drugs and electric shocks to treat problem drinking. Are these instances of 'the end justifying the means', and would health professionals be failing in their duty to care if they did not intervene out of respect for individual autonomy? Indeed, the voluntary nature of patient participation is often dubious in these instances, owing to the use of written contracts as a prerequisite of admission (Box 9.2), and the pressures frequently applied in various forms by relatives, friends and employers.

Even the much lauded recent moves to free patients from damaging institutional settings and restore them to their communities has proved a mixed blessing. Warner (1985) argues that cost savings have far outweighed humanitarian considerations as a political motivator generating this process, a suspicion re-

---

Box 9.2 Sample consent form required prior to admission for alcohol withdrawal

1. On admission you and all your baggage will be searched
2. Once on the ward, you will be expected to participate fully in the ward programme, including ward groups and occupational therapy sessions
3. Once on the ward, you will not be allowed off it during the 'withdrawal' period, other than to go to occupational therapy with other patients
4. You may be visited by only 'next of kin' during your initial assessment
5. Spot checks of your clothing and belongings may be made at any time
6. You will remain in nightclothes throughout the 'withdrawal' period
7. If you are found to be in possession of alcohol or have been drinking alcohol on the ward – immediate discharge will follow.

Signature .... Date ....

inforced by the persistent reports of underfunding of community support and accommodation facilities.

In saving patients from the evils of institutional neurosis, is our caring system merely propelling vulnerable individuals towards an existence of neglected hardship and exploitation, and precipitating their inevitable and rapid return through the revolving doors of streamlined modern psychiatric clinics? These represent a few of the ethical issues which psychiatric services must address in the coming years.

Suggested assignments

Discussion topics
1. Is there such a thing as 'mental illness', or is it an establishment 'label' for valid, non-conformist views and behaviour?
2. Are modern health professionals justified in infringing patients' rights of liberty and freedom of action?
3. What social measures might effectively reduce the incidence of problem drinking and anorexia nervosa?
4. With finite resources, how can the needs of psychiatric patients best be met in hospital and community settings?
5. Why, as we approach the twenty-first century, is there still a 'stigma' attached to mental illness?

REFERENCES AND FURTHER READING

Barr O 1990 Down's syndrome and Alzheimer's disease – what is the link? Professional Nurse June: 465–468

Barton R 1959 Institutional neurosis. Wiley, London

Bertram M 1989 The use of landmarks. Journal of Gerontological Nursing 15(2): 6–8

Bird J, Harrison G 1987 Examination notes in psychiatry, 2nd edn. Wright, Bristol

Bucht G, Sandman P O 1990 Nutritional aspects of dementia, especially Alzheimer's Disease. Age and Ageing 19: S32–36

Burnside I M 1979 Alzheimer's disease; an overview. Journal of Gerontological Nursing 17: 190–200

Butler R N 1963 The life review: an interpretation of reminiscence in the aged. Psychiatry 26: 65–76

Cole D 1990 Identifying the alcohol misuser. Nursing Times 18 April: 58–60

Gartside G 1989 The ultimate rebellion. Nursing Times 85(18): p 50

Gottesman I, Shields J 1982 Schizophrenia; the epigenetic puzzle. Cambridge University Press, Cambridge

Goudie F, Stokes G 1989 Understanding confusion. Nursing Times 85(39): 35–37

Gross R 1987 Psychology; the science of mind and behaviour. Edward Arnold, London, chs 28, 29

Hartz C, Plant M, Watts M 1990 Alcohol and health: a handbook for nurses, midwives and health visitors, 2nd edn. The Medical Council on Alcoholism, London

Ironbar N O, Hooper A 1989 Self-instruction in mental health nursing. Baillière-Tindall, London, topics 10, 13, 14 and 15

Laing R D 1967 The politics of experience and the bird of paradise. Penguin, Harmondsworth

Laywood A 1989 Anorexia nervosa: a view from the inside. Nursing Times 85(18): 48–50

Lees A 1989 Alzheimer's Disease Society: what it does and how it can help. Care of the Elderly 1: 146–147

Lyttle J 1986 Mental disorder: its care and treatment. Baillière-Tindall, London, chapters 20, 21, 24, 25, 28, 33, 34

McKracken A L, Fitzwater E 1989 The right environment for Alzheimer's. Geriatric Nursing November/December 293–294

Morton I, Bleathman C 1988 Does it matter whether it's Tuesday or Friday? Nursing Times 84(6): 25–27

Murray-Lyon I 1989 Alcohol and pregnancy. Maternal and Child Health June: 165–169

Paton A ed 1988 ABC of alcohol, 2nd edn. British Medical Journal, London

Rosenhan D L 1973 On being sane in insane places. In Gross R 1990 Key studies in psychology. Hodder and Stoughton, London, ch 29

Sadler C 1991 Poison from the tap. Nursing Times 87(9): 16–17

Szasz T 1972 The myth of mental illness. Paladin, London

Warner R 1987 Recovery from schizophrenia: psychiatry and political economy. Routledge and Kegan Paul, London

Williams C K 1990 Recovery from Alzheimer's disease: a caretaker's story. Topics in Geriatric Rehabilitation 5(3): 1–9

Yellowlees P M, Roe M, Walker M, Ben-Tovim D 1988 Abnormal perception of food size in anorexia nervosa. British Medical Journal 196: 1689–1690

10

Care implications of disorders of personality

Robert G. Mitchell

This chapter looks at the controversial subject of personality disorder. By definition, personality disorder is not an illness and it is not always clear if individuals thus afflicted require treatment. Some most certainly will not, but will live useful lives in the community, albeit perhaps with a reputation of being eccentric or somewhat difficult. Still others will have offended against society and may require to be cared for in a secure institution. This could be either a hospital or prison. In most cases, changes will occur only slowly, if at all, and it is useful to view an individual's personality as being relatively fixed in the short term.

Various theories of normal personality development will be explained before the disordered personality is considered. While the role of the 'expert' in treatment is not universally acknowledged, the role of nurses, doctors and society in general in caring for a number of individuals with different types of personality disorders will be addressed. Whenever possible the reader will be referred to appropriate material in other chapters of this book.

PERSONALITY

The concept of personality disorder is perhaps difficult to grasp and this may well be due to the fact that 'personality' itself is hard to define. Sometimes, it is prefixed with 'a' and wrongly used to describe individuals who open supermarkets, who are good at playing football or who appear regularly in the media: this is unhelpful. With only a little more sophistication, individuals may be referred to as **having** a nasty, nice or noxious personality, and this may be nearer the mark.

Uniqueness of personality

More accurately, personality refers to the relatively

constant and enduring aspects of a person which helps distinguish him or her as a unique individual. This uniqueness is central to the concept of personality which is a combination of many facets together making up a person who is like no other. Personalities are as different as fingerprints (Lyttle 1986).

Unique though every personality may be, it is possible to describe personalities and compare them with each other. This is because the total personality can be said to be made up of an indeterminate number of traits or characteristics, themselves recognizable, but in a combination that is entirely their own. Thus an individual may consistently display a number of merry or morose characteristics which would be seen by others as being part of their unique self. They might be described as having a friendly or depressive personality respectively.

Given the fact that no personalties are the same and recognizing the many imperfections that abound in everyone, it is hardly surprising that the act of identifying only certain personalities as being somehow disordered is controversial. This is the enigma of personality disorder.

Whereas certain individuals will exhibit psychiatric symptoms in such a manner and combination that will clearly identify them as being sick (see Chs 8 and 9), others, while displaying little in the way of definite symptomatology, still manage to conduct their lives in such a chaotic manner as to differentiate them substantially from their fellow beings (Mitchell 1986). When these maladaptive strivings become well established or characteristic and infringe on a large chunk of their life-style, they are said to have a personality disorder.

Since individuals ascribed as having a personality disorder do not display any symptoms of sickness, it is not at all clear if doctors and nurses are necessarily the best people to help them. In some cases they may come into conflict with the law and it can be argued that a prison sentence may be the most appropriate form of disposal. This debate is an ongoing and well rehearsed one and is often described as the mad or bad argument.

In order to more fully understand the concept of personality disorder, it is necessary to consider normal personality development.

PERSONALITY DEVELOPMENT

In introducing the concept of normal personality development, it is important to realize that much of our current thinking is based not on scientific facts, but rather on hypothetical theories first espoused by early, influential workers in this field. Foremost amongst these is Sigmund Freud.

Sigmund Freud (1856–1939)

Although originally a neurologist, Freud carried out exhaustive studies on large numbers of individuals, observing them closely and recording meticulously, all he thought he saw. His ideas were controversial, but represented a giant step forward in the understanding of human personality.

Freud claimed that the mind consisted of three territories or depths of functioning which he called the conscious, the preconscious and the unconscious mind. The conscious describes that part of the mind that relates to the here and now. It refers to everything that is in the immediate awareness, and therefore, only operates when the individual is awake. By necessity, the amount of material in the conscious at any one time is small since it would be impossible to wander around with one's head crammed full of large amounts of information of varying degrees of importance. Fortunately, therefore, the second level, the preconscious, accommodates material which is partially remembered and which can usually be recalled if required. It is here that inconsequential facts about schooldays, ageing pop groups and theories of nursing are stored; and it is from here that information about these and thousands of other topics can hopefully be recalled on demand.

The deepest territory is the unconscious. Here is stored the sum of all the memories, feelings and emotions experienced from birth. Although material stored here is completely 'forgotton' and cannot readily be brought to the surface, it continues to influence everything that is experienced. Memories which may be too upsetting to be handled may be relegated or 'repressed' to the unconscious where they are conveniently 'out of mind'. It is strongly argued by many theorists, however, that the contents of the unconscious reveal the clues to most psychological malfunctioning. Hints of what may be happening in the unconscious may sometimes be revealed in dreams, by slips of the tongue or apparently uncharacteristic behaviour (the so-called Freudian Slip), or as a result of psychotherapy. An acknowledgement of the existence of the unconscious is crucial to the understanding of Freud, as is the acceptance of the idea of repression.

Freud suggested that human personality development follows a specific, sequential pattern of various

Table 10.1 Freud's developmental stages		
Approximate age	Stage	Description
Birth–15 months	Oral	Pleasure principal, need for instant gratification. Everything goes into mouth
15 months–3 years	Anal	Reality principal, begins to delay gratification. Toilet training, 'battles of wills'
3–6 years	Phallic	Awareness of anatomical differences between the sexes, identification with same-sex parent. Oedipal and Electra complexes
6–13 years	Latency	Preference for playmates of same sex. Period of comparative calm
13–20 years	Adolescence	Period of extensive physiological and psychological growth on the road to maturity

stages as it progresses towards maturity (Table 10.1). Once one stage has been successfully negotiated the individual will advance towards the next.

At birth, he argues, the human infant presents with a set of basic, if keenly felt, biological needs. As parents everywhere can testify, the baby (for the sake of simplicity, a male child) cannot postpone gratification of any of these needs and will yell ferociously for nourishment or unconcernedly empty bowel or bladder at any time of day or night. At this stage in his development the infant is the centre of its own universe and conducts his life in accordance with the pleasure principle.

The importance of the mouth during these early weeks and months is apparent. It is impossible to know what emotions a distraught infant is feeling, but it can readily be seen how he will relax as soon as he is put to the breast or bottle. Important as the taking of nourishment is, it is not the sole purpose of the mouth. Thumb sucking, or the use of the commercial comforter – the dummy – is widespread; yet, if all that was desired was food, these comforters would be rapidly discarded on the realization that it was not forthcoming. That they are not, suggests that these oral activities are a source of pleasure, comfort or security in their own right. As he gets a little older, the infant quickly sets about exploring his environment; by sticking it in his mouth! With enviable dexterity he will locate and subsequently suck his toes, while rattles, teddy bears and his cot sides will all be given the same treatment during this period of intense discovery.

Because of the importance of the mouth during this time, the period from birth to around 15 months is termed the oral phase of development.

Gradually the child will develop the capacity to postpone his immediate desires. He will come to realize that mother is not around all the time and that he must wait for his meals. As toilet training begins, (according to Freud) he will discover that indiscriminate soiling will no longer be tolerated and eventually he will come to terms with the need to use a potty or toilet at an appropriate time. He is now beginning to function according to the reality principle.

At this stage the infant will be intensely aware of and increasingly interested in his excretory functions. The feelings of embarrassment or disgust attributed by many adults to the act of defaecation are conspicuously absent. The toddler will show off his faeces with the unqualified pride appropriate to this, the first thing he has produced unaided!

Because of the importance of excretion and the excretory organs during this phase, the period from approximately 15 months to 3 or 4 years is termed the anal phase of development.

From about the age of 3 or 4 the child will become vaguely aware of the anatomical differences between the sexes. Father, who may have been a somewhat shadowy figure in the early months or years, will loom ever larger and become increasingly important. By this time the chief area of interest and pleasure has switched to the genitalia, and this period is called the phallic stage of development. (Phallus is another name for penis, the male sex organ.)

At this stage, Freud claims, the small boy feels in competition with his father for the affection of his mother and may wish to take his place. This presents the youngster with a predicament: he may love his father and will also be impressed by his size; he is a formidable rival. Something similar is also happening with the small girl who may openly compete with her mother for her father's attention, but like the small boy may be anxious that her feelings might result in punishment.

This identification with the parent of the same sex may be seen as a good thing, since properly resolved, and assuming that the same-sex parent is an adequate role model, the youngster may be helped towards an eventual successful adjustment to adulthood. However, this crucial period of development, the so-called Oedipal stage, can be a very difficult time, and an unresolved Oedipal complex can be a recipe for future mental ill health. (Oedipus was a prince in Greek mythology, who separated from his parents at an early age, unknowingly slew his father in battle and married his mother.) Freud had an interesting, if eccentric, habit of using mythology to illustrate many of his theories and the female equivalent to the Oedipal complex is the **Electra complex**.

The few short years from birth until about 6 years of age as discussed above are hectic as far as personality development is concerned. They are followed, however, by a period of relative calm known as the years of latency. This takes the individual up to the turbulent years of adolescence which are usually traumatic, and which for some may even herald a psychiatric breakdown.

Before leaving Freud, it is important to consider his concepts of the id, the ego and the super-ego, essential to the understanding of personality disorder. These are notional, functional, parts of the mind which cannot be demonstrated, dissected or drawn.

The most basic level of function, concerned with the primitive, biological needs and governed by the pleasure principle is present from birth and is called the id. It is totally self-centred and the focus of all primary desire. It demands instant and total satisfaction and takes no account of reality.

With the development of the ego a more mature pattern of behaviour is seen. The infant learns to postpone id urges. It comes to realize that mother cannot always be around and futhermore, if she is summoned too often, her approach will be less tender and the experience will be spoiled. Behaviour now takes into account the demands of real life and the cravings of the id will frequently be thwarted. This stage of development is governed by the reality principle.

Even at this stage, although the individual may be able to guess at the possible outcomes of any piece of behaviour, an inner sense of rightness or wrongness will be totally absent. This arrives only with the development of the super-ego which corresponds roughly to the lay term conscience and produces internal checks on behaviour, which if ignored, cause the individual to experience feelings of guilt.

The super-ego does not develop until around the age of 6 or 7 years and varies greatly in its degree of strictness. Roughly, the individual adopts similar standards to those of his parents or significant others, so that a child brought up in a family where stealing is condoned will not feel guilty when he does likewise, whereas someone else may experience mountains of guilt over a misdemeanour that to others might seem trivial.

In the mature adult the id, the ego and the super-ego will learn to coexist, however uneasily, with most of the action taking place in the unconscious. The individual may not therefore, except in extreme circumstances, be aware of the desires of the id, the commonsense of the ego or the censorship of the super-ego, although if either is too dominant he may be storing up future mental ill health. Awareness of the foregoing theory is crucial to be understanding of the development of personality disorder.

Erik H. Erikson (1902–1994)

Erikson, like Freud, was a psychoanalyst, and he agreed with Freud that the developing individual must pass through a predetermined number of stages as he or she progresses through to adulthood and old age. Erikson, however, emphasized the importance of the social side of development. He proposed a series of eight psychosocial stages (Table 10.2), each of which is characterized by special developmental problems or crises to be confronted. Without mastering the first crisis it would not be possible to go on to successfully adapt to a more mature stage. The important aspect of Erikson's theory is the idea that each stage introduces the individual to a wider range of human contacts so that as each stage is mastered a well-adjusted social being results.

A sensory stage lasts from birth to approximately 18 months and the crisis to be overcome is that of developing trust. At this stage the infant's social network is based largely on the mother or mother substitute.

During the second stage, which lasts from about 18 months until 3 years, the social network expands to include both parents and others in the intimate circle. This is the muscular or toddler period during which autonomy begins to develop as the infant acquires self-control and self-confidence.

The third stage, between 3 and 5 years, is the locomotor stage and the critical task is to develop initiative and assertiveness. At this stage the child's social circle will include the basic family unit, but Erikson, like Freud, believes that the child desires to exclusively possess the parent of the opposite sex. If this situation is not adequately handled, a feeling of guilt

Table 10.2 Erikson's developmental stages

Approximate age	Stage	Description
Birth–18 months	Sensory	Social network based on mother. Need to develop trust
18 months–3 years	Muscular/toddler	Social network expands. Begins to develop autonomy
3–5 years	Locomotor	Social circle based on family unit. Desire to exclusively **own** parent of opposite sex. Development of initiative and assertiveness
5–12 years	Latency	Based on school life and classmates. Self-esteem should develop at expense of feelings of inferiority
12–20 years	Adolescence	Increased importance of peer group. Movement away from parents. Need to establish **identity**

Note: Erikson went on to discuss the further stages of young adulthood, middle age and old age and thus emphasizes the life-long characteristics of personality development.

may remain which could lead to complications in adulthood.

There next follows the latency stage by which time the child will be at school and the extent of his social interactions will have mushroomed. The critical task here is said to be to develop an orientation towards industry as against inferiority. Successfully managed, the child should leave this stage with relatively secure feelings of self-esteem, whereas if problems arise they may be left with feelings of inferiority and a tendency towards rebelliousness. Latency lasts from about the age of 6 years until puberty is reached.

The next stage is adolesence, said by Erikson to last from 12 to 20. The peer group assumes increased importance at this time, as the individual, moving somewhere between child and adult, begins to break away from his parents and assume independence. The critical task here is to establish a sense of identity with which to enter adulthood.

Erikson and Freud

It is easy to notice a similarity between the Eriksonian stages mentioned so far and the Freudian ones described earlier in the chapter. Erikson, however, goes on to discuss three other stages, early adulthood, middle adulthood and the ageing years and in so doing underlines the notion that personality development is life long.

Jean Piaget (1896–1980)

Piaget, a Swiss psychologist, also saw development as a series of sequential hurdles which had to be overcome one by one. He identified a series of four different stages (Table 10.3). Piaget's theories relate to the cognitive development of the individual, that is his ability to aquire rules that are used for thinking and solving problems and for dealing with and

Table 10.3 Piaget's developmental stages

Approximate age	Stage	Description
Birth–2 years	Sensorimotor	Differentiates him- or herself from environment. Realizes that objects exist even when out of sight
2–7 years	Preoperational	Rapid language development. Begins to use numbers and symbols in his/her mind
7–11 years	Concrete operational	Becomes capable of logical thought. Understands and calculates weights and volumes
11–15 years	Formal operational	Thinks in entirely abstract way. Capable of scientific reasoning

understanding his world. He believed that an individual's basic goal was to learn to master both his internal and external environment.

The first of Piaget's stages is the sensorimotor period which extends from birth to age 2. In this stage he progresses from the reflexive state of the newborn to a point where he can manipulate various objects and differentiate himself from his environment. He begins to realize that an object or person still exists, even though it is out of sight.

The second or preoperational period (from 2 to 7 years) is initially marked by rapid language development. He will begin to use the concepts of language and symbols to solve simple motor problems internally, that is, in his mind.

There follows the concrete operational period (7–11) in which the child is able to produce logical solutions to concrete problems and will develop the ability to understand and calculate weights and volumes.

The years from 11 to 15 are called the formal operational period, during which the ability to think in an entirely abstract way is aquired. Mature thought processes that enable the individual to think scientifically are developed. It is suggested that not everyone reaches the level of formal operations.

All the foregoing specialists believed in a sequential explanation of human development. Before leaving the subject, it is useful to consider the different approach of Bowlby.

John Bowlby (1907–1990)

John Bowlby, a British psychiatrist, is probably best known for coining the term maternal deprivation as a result of his work in the 1940s and 1950s (Bowlby 1951). He declared that it was essential for good mental health that the infant and young child experience a warm, intimate and continuous relationship with his mother (or a permanent substitute) in which both experience satisfaction and enjoyment. More colourfully, he claimed that 'mother love in infancy and childhood is as important for mental health as are vitamins and proteins for physical health' and that 'the prolonged deprivation of the young child of maternal care may have grave and far-reaching effects on his character and so on the whole of his future life'. When such deprivation exists (as for instance when mother or mother substitute and child are separated), specific characteristics may develop in the infant and weight loss and developmental delays may be the result. Perhaps significantly, some studies (e.g. Rutter

1972) suggest that boys may react more catastrophically than girls to early separations.

Developmental stages and mental health

The idea of an individual passing through a variety of stages on a quest towards maturity is attractive. The essence of such a progression is that it is natural, shared to some extent by all. Nevertheless, many of the specific mental health problems described in Chapters 8 and 9 tend to be associated with one or a small number of age groups.

PERSONALITY DISORDER IN PERSPECTIVE

Contrary to the conditions described in the previous two chapters, personality disorder is not an illness, but rather a combination of well-ingrained traits, which include poor social adaption, erratic interpersonal relationships and an inability or unwillingness to conform.

Relevant epidemiology and aetiology

Because of the controversial nature of the term personality disorder definitions are many, synonyms abound and consensus is rare. A marked, if confusing feature seems to be the fact that no distinguishable feature of psychiatric illness exists but that the disorder lies in the social or moral field.

In what can rapidly become a quagmire of subdivisions it is useful to differentiate between the primary personality disorder, whereupon the individual appears to experience no anxiety, and it is society who appears to suffer, (the psychopath) and secondary personality disorder which is characterised by maladaptive traits or tendencies which permeate all interactions and social situations. This combination of traits and tendencies, in themselves perfectly normal, may cause persistent disruption to self or others and may, for example, result in the individual being described as having a paranoid or depressive personality.

PRIMARY PERSONALITY DISORDER

An early definition of the disorder is that of Pinel (1801) who coined the term 'manie sans delire' to describe a state in which there was no alteration of intellectual functions but a marked disorder of affective (mood) functions including impulsive violence. In the nineteenth and early twentieth centuries, the term moral insanity and moral defective became popular to describe an individual with 'a morbid perversion of the natural feeling, affections, inclination, temper, habits, moral dispositions and natural impulses without psychotic features'.

These terms were largely superceded by that of psychopathy. One of the foremost experts in psychopathy was Sir David Henderson (1939) in Edinburgh, who used the term 'psychopathic state' to describe those individuals above subnormal intelligence who exhibit persistent antisocial behaviour and whose failure to conform is not 'mere willfulness or badness which can be threatened or thrashed out, but constitutes a true illness'. McCord & McCord (1956) described the psychopathic syndrome as that of 'a dangerously maladjusted personality who is asocial and driven by primitive desires and an exaggerated craving for excitement. He is highly impulsive, his actions are unplanned and guided by his whims. Guiltlessness and lovelessness conspicuously mark the psychopath as different from other men.'

The Mental Health Act, 1983, (England and Wales), revised the definition of the psychopath as follows: 'persistent disorders of mind (whether or not including significant impairment of intelligence) which result in abnormally aggressive or seriously irresponsible conduct on the part of the patient'. Mitchell (1986) spoke of the 'enigma' of the psychopath, 'charming, but heartless; superficially attractive, but cold; sane but capable of acts which can only be described as madness'.

Cleckley (1976) made an important contribution to the understanding of the condition by describing 16 characteristic features of the psychopath (Box 10.1) including superficial charm and good intelligence, unreliability, inadequately motivated antisocial behaviour, poor judgement and failure to learn by experience. He added that the psychopath's subjective experience 'is so bleached of deep emotion that he is invincibly ignorant of what life means to others'.

The term sociopath, first coined in America, is often preferred to psychopath since it highlights the social nature of the deviance and may help modify in the lay public the 'mad axeman' image of the psychopath often quite wrongly promoted in the popular media. Other synonyms include disruptive personality disorder, antisocial personality disorder as used by Cleckley and others, or less helpfully, aggressive personality disorder.

For the sake of consistency, the author will use the term psychopath throughout this chapter.

Box 10.1 Sixteen features of the antisocial personality disorder (Cleckley 1976)

1. Superficial charm; good or apparently good intelligence
2. Absence of delusions and other signs of irrational thinking
3. Absence of neurotic symptoms
4. Unreliability
5. Untruthfulness and insincerity
6. Lack of remorse and shame
7. Inadequately motivated antisocial behaviour
8. Poor judgement; failure to learn by experience
9. Pathological egocentricity; incapacity for love
10. General poverty in major affective reactions
11. Specific loss of insight
12. Unresponsiveness in general interpersonal relations
13. Fantastic and uninhibited behaviour with drink and sometimes without
14. Suicide often threatened but rarely carried out
15. Sex life impersonal, trivial, poorly integrated
16. Failure to follow any life plan

Types of psychopath

Although it has sometimes been argued that up to 14 different types of psychopath exist it is more common to cite two or three. Henderson (1969) describes the aggressive; the inadequate, or passive; and, more controversially, the creative, psychopath.

The aggressive psychopath

Here, the main feature is an impulsive resort to violence whether directed against others (the end result in extreme cases being homicide) or self (where suicide could be the end result). The individual's life is likely to be punctuated by a series of violent episodes ultimately resulting in hospitalization or a period of imprisonment. Punishment seems to have no effect on the aggressive psychopath and a feeling of guilt or a show of concern for the victim will be entirely absent.

The story of Michael, an aggressive psychopath, as told by Mitchell (1986), is illustrative of the condition. (See Case History 10.1).

Michael is typical of the aggressive psychopath who causes such a headache to society. Many go to prison; a course of action which quite legitimately helps protect the public. Less nobly, it also exerts a measure of revenge while doing nothing to rehabilitate the prisoner.

The passive or inadequate psychopath

These may be charming and plausible people, whose

Case History 10.1

Michael was the second son of a policeman. Like his brother, he was bright at school, but unlike him he showed no interest in going to university or embarking on a career. At 14, much to the embarrassment of his father, he was convicted of setting fire to a parked vehicle while fooling around with a gang of older youths.

Two years later he was given 7 years' detention for grievious bodily harm on a sub-post-mistress during a raid.

Despite an obvious attractiveness and likeability, Michael's nefarious career continued.

He is now serving a life sentence for the murder of a youth over a trivial argument. When questioned about the incident, he shrugs his shoulders and laughs. He has no regrets.

Michael's mother is dead. His father blames him for his lack of promotion in the police force, while his brother, a practising lawyer, has washed his hands of him.

Case History 10.2

Janice (Mitchell 1986), now in her early thirties, had a troubled childhood as the unwanted, illegitimate daughter of an alcoholic mother. A succession of hard drinking and unsympathetic men shared her mother's life, but usually had nothing but contempt for Janice. Her early years were spent being dragged around public houses, being left unattended at home, or worse, being ill-treated by the adults around her.

Quickly she learned self-reliance, and by the time she was 7 she was a regular truant and accomplished thief. She frequently ran off in search of her father, who in her fantasy world was kindly and rich, but who in reality, was unknown. She was demonstrably beyond her mother's control.

As Janice's need for care and attention became increasingly obvious, she was admitted to a short-term children's home. This heralded the start of her long association with institutions which has to date included spells in a variety of psychiatric hospitals and prisons.

At 15, she ran off with a 33-year-old alcoholic. Travelling in stolen cars, they committed a total of 27 offences in six different counties before being apprehended for obtaining free board and lodgings in a well-appointed seaside hotel.

Apart from a 2-year spell of comparative stability during which her own daughter was born, her life has been a continuing spiral of institutions, frauds and unfortunate sexual liasons. She shows little signs of changing. Janice is a good example of an inadequate psychopath.

---

lifestyle, although perhaps less dramatic than that of the aggressive psychopath, is nevertheless deeply ingrained and unlikely to be modified. Pathological lying (pseudologia phantastica) may be a feature and this may lead to swindling or thieving (see Case History 10.2).

The creative psychopath

The very existence of this group is open to question. An association between genius and madness has long been assumed by some individuals and many well-known historical figures seem to have been endowed with a certain quirkiness of personality. Although such a label may explain the excesses of various Hollywood stars or touring rock bands, it should be used with caution.

Incidence of primary personality disorder

It is not possible with any degree of confidence to predict the amount of personality-disordered individuals that exist in the community. The perfect personality almost certainly does not exist, and since there is no foolproof diagnostic indicator of psychopathy, individuals tend only to become statistics once they have offended against or deviated substantially from the norms of their society.

The author's tendency to use the pronoun 'he' while discussing psychopathy is not accidental. Psychopaths appear much more commonly to be male although the female psychopaths seem to have established for themselves a place in the folklore of many psychiatric hospitals. It is often argued that although fewer in number, female psychopaths may be particularly difficult to manage.

It has been noted that psychopathy is not spread evenly throughout the streets and glades of the civilized world. Although no location or social background is immune there is a definite tendency for numbers to be higher in the down-town ghettos of Social Class V. Early studies (Bowlby 1951, Goldfarb 1955) revealed a tendency for broken homes, illegitimacy, parental disharmony and early separation from mother to feature largely in the life history of psychopaths. Conversely, however, it is also comparatively easy to cite the names of notorious psychopaths from the arena of criminology who appear to have experienced none of those 'disadvantages', and Bowlby (1958) was later to announce that it was wrong to claim that early deprivation commonly lead to psychopathic or affectionless characters.

Psychopaths, may be 'discovered' following a para-suicide incident. It has been argued that individuals with severe personality disorders may account for between a third and a half of all suicide victims (Morgan 1979). Some may surface on seeking admission to hospital for some apparently unrelated disorder such as depression, or may initially present with a problem of addiction. Still others may only be encountered following a court appearance, and if hospital admission is at the behest of the authorities, some difficulty in complying with treatment can be anticipated.

Another group, of indeterminate size and impossible to quantify, is the so called successful psychopaths (Holmes 1991). If a generalized lack of guilt and a propensity to manipulate are deemed as psychopathic, then it is plain to see that we must look further afield than hospitals and prisons to find our prime samples. A cynic may examine the personal characteristics of successful entrepreneurs, leaders of industry and politicians and discover a remarkable cluster of many of Cleckley's 16 points.

Aetiology

Psychodynamic

Freud's explanation of personality development provides a compelling explanation of the cause of psychopathy. This theory would point to the psychopath's failure to develop a super-ego as being crucial. If this censoring mechanism is absent, then the lack of guilt so characteristic of the psychopath will result. Since the super-ego develops around the age of 6 or 7, events happening around or before that time may be crucial. Since the child is said to develop the standards of his parents or significant others the availability of a same-sex role model may be important, and this may be more likely to be missing in the case of the young boy. Boyle (1977) describes a childhood in which his father was dead and stealing seemed to be accepted as a way of life for many adults (although not his mother). In his remarkable autobiography, utterances of guilt are conspicuously absent.

This theory fits nicely with Bowlby's concept of maternal deprivation, which suggested that early separation from mother could lead to an affectionless personality which stood a good chance of developing psychopathy in later years. Although he later modified his views to include consideration of the quality of the relationship before and after separation, this does not diminish the importance of the early years.

There are two other important psychodynamic concepts. That of fixation, where an individual fails to develop beyond a certain psychological stage, and regression, where they slip back to an earlier stage, possibly when under stress.

The nature/nurture debate

Whether or not the reader finds the above explanation attractive, it is as yet impossible to be too dogmatic about the cause of psychopathy. Arguments commonly rage as to whether things like hereditary or environmental factors may be most important; a discussion that is commonly known as the nature/nurture debate.

Hereditary

Anyone working closely with the community will be aware of the existence of so-called problem families. Frequently, the problems may be partly attributable to personality-disordered members who may span more than one generation. Mitchell (1983), however, points out that the fact that a son and his father may both be diagnosed as psychopathic is insufficient to prove a definite hereditary link. An equally likely explanation would be that the behaviour was copied, or learned from the father, or because of frequent absences, the son may have been denied a suitably consistent role model.

Genetics

Lyttle (1986) argues that some important aspects of personality have a genetic component but this has not been consistently demonstrated. The discovery of an extra Y chromosome in a number of delinquent males led to a brief assumption that a sex chromosome abnormality, the so-called XYY male, was responsible for their antisocial behaviour. Further studies have failed to show a consistent link between this abnormality and a predisposition to crime except in males with a mental handicap and the significance of the earlier findings is unclear.

Neurological

A sizeable school of thought believes that psychopathy can be attributed to factors of a physical nature, which are identifiable, or which would be identifiable if instruments or techniques of sufficient scientific intricacy could be perfected. Antisocial, aggressive and uninhibited behaviour has commonly been identified in some individuals who are brain damaged, and psychopaths have been shown to have a higher number of abnormal EEG readings than a non-psychopathic control group. In addition, malfunctioning of the brain due to injury (especially to the hypothalmus), encephalitis, epilepsy, birth trauma and intrauterine damage would all at times seem to be implicated. However, the existence of a large number of psychopaths whose condition seems to flourish in the absence of any physical abnormality leads us naturally to the consideration of the environmental approach.

Environmental

Of all the different theories this has perhaps the most evidence to back it up. Despite many exceptions there is a definite tendency for psychopaths to come from a deprived social background. Illegitimacy, divorce and alcoholism are common factors, while tales of childhood beatings may be told.

Authorities who house a number of these families in poor areas of low amenity in large cities are guilty of creating a self-perpetuating cycle of deprivation. If this includes a high number of single-parent families with fathers who may be in prison or out of the picture altogether, the absence of the suitable same-sex role model may be crucial.

However, consideration must be given to the significant number of psychopaths who quite clearly do not fit into this category. Some come from professional or middle class backgrounds (like Michael) and do not suffer from material deprivation. Supporters of the environmental argument would claim, however, that these individuals might be emotionally deprived and, like their counterparts further down the social scale, still therefore suffering from a type of rejection in childhood.

The effects of psychopathy

The individual

The individual may believe that he is not being affected by this condition. Anxiety in primary personality disorder is absent and he may be able to boast a large number of sexual conquests and lead an exciting lifestyle. Kneisl & Wilson (1988), however, point out that these individuals are frequently in trouble with the law, have a poor work record and few close friends. Although they may appear to enjoy and to have chosen their way of life, it will be apparent to others that they are following a self-destructive path.

Significant others

Wives, husbands, parents and children of psychopaths are likely to be long suffering in the extreme. Sexual adventures are common and coupled with a difficulty in forming longstanding and stable relationships, this bodes badly for a happy marriage. Financial committments such as alimony or child maintainance are likely to be ignored and lying is commonplace. His significant others, like everyone else, are there to be manipulated and then abandoned when they have served their purpose.

Society

Society pays a huge price at the hands of the psychopath. Those who come to the attention of the authorities seem to require expensive and long-term disposal. Whether in prison or hospital, the financial demands on the state are likely to be large, the prospect of cure remote.

Society, too, must pick up the financial tabs when families are left unsupported; if their treatment at the hands of the psychopath makes them ill, more government money will be spent. Victims, whether family or strangers, may require counselling, treatment or compensation and the families of victims will require support in the meantime. All this expense to society comes on top of the regular unemployment giros which form a major part of the psychopath's income.

By far the greatest expense to society, however, but equally the most difficult to quantify, is the cost of broken hearts, broken promises and wasted potential.

Differential diagnoses

In this, the condition that isn't an illness, there are no differential diagnoses in the traditional sense. Psychopaths however may come to the notice of the nurse in one of several guises. It is generally the fate of the psychopath to be unwelcome in hospital. He who is not ill cannot get better, and he who cannot get better makes doctors and nurses uncomfortable. In the great debate about where the psychopath should go, hospital staff often say prison, while prison officers advocate a spell in hospital.

Consequently, psychopaths are often admitted for some other condition whereupon their psychopathy eventually emerges. They may be admitted with a real or apparent depressive illness; although apparently unperturbed by their lifestyle, it is reasonable to assume that it may eventually take its toll on their affect.

Similarly, they may arrive via the accident and emergency department following a parasuicide. Morgan (1979) estimated that between a third and a half of all incidents of suicide or parasuicide are carried out by individuals who have a severe personality disorder. Commonly, the initial diagnosis may be one of alcohol abuse, and this may be something of a chicken and egg situation. It is hard to say if the drinking is a direct result of the personality disorder or whether the two things are quite separate. Conditions which also seem to attract a large proportion of personality-disordered sufferers are other substance abuses and sexual deviances (see below).

Some psychopaths may deliberately feign illness to ensure admission when they may otherwise be refused, while in other cases, the true nature of the personality disorder may only reveal itself after the acuteness of the precipitating symptoms disappear. It is not helpful for staff to debate whether or not the admission is genuine, since such deliberations can only be subjective and must never be allowed to form the basis of a care plan.

For a condition that is so often overlooked, it is perhaps ironic that large numbers of individuals are falsely diagnosed as having a personality disorder. This is frequently the fate of those whose symptoms may be difficult for the practitioner to label with certainty.

Conditions associated with primary personality disorders

Before leaving primary personality disorders, it is useful to consider certain other conditions in which it is often a feature. Sufferers from the following conditions are not all psychopaths but the behaviours they manifest and the problems they experience and pose are sufficiently similar to warrant inclusion here.

The alcohol abuser

Alcohol is perhaps the most commonly used drug in the country. Almost universally used to aid relaxation, to celebrate life's minor successes and as a symbol of hospitality, alcohol nevertheless, for a sizeable number of individuals, represents a problem with which they just cannot cope.

There is no such thing as the typical alcoholic and it is particularly unhelpful to associate alcohol abuse purely with the 'skid row' drunk. Recent, unfortunate trends suggest that younger people and women are more frequently becoming involved in what for many

years had been a problem largely of the menfolk. Increased spending patterns and the changing role of women are probably important influences in this change.

Many people will obtain help for their alcohol problems from their general practitioner or through a large number of voluntary or self-help organizations, but some will require hospitalization. Many may be admitted to a general hospital for conditions caused or exacerbated by their abuse of alcohol.

The management of the alcoholic can ideally be described in three stages:

1. They must be withdrawn from alcohol (dried out) and physically patched up.
2. While remaining abstinent, they should be helped to explore the reasons for their addiction and to try to restructure a daily routine which is not dominated by a need to acquire the next drink.
3. They should be offered long-term support for the tough times which will undoubtedly lie ahead.

Other substance abuse

It is fashionable but nevertheless accurate to state that substance abuse has reached epidemic proportions in some parts of the western world. What is much less clear is the role of the psychiatric services in the management of those concerned.

Individuals abusing the so-called 'hard' drugs run the risk of addiction, physical and life threatening effects of needle sharing and almost definite involvement with the criminal underworld. Polydrug users who may use a mixture of whatever is available run additional risks of death from accidental overdoses or from any one of a number of common adulterants.

The abuser of other less dramatic substances (in many cases prescribed medication) should not be overlooked and the nurse is quite likely to be asked to care for someone being weaned from such an addiction.

Users are unlikely to present for treatment of their own free will and requests for help may follow an involvement with police. In such cases, nursing care is difficult to plan but will be covered below.

Sexual deviancy

This term has almost an old-fashioned ring to it nowadays, as the wide diversity of sexual activity indulged in by some people is slowly realized. In general, the trend seems to be towards regarding anything practised between consenting adults in private as acceptable. However, some people's sexual inclinations and orientation are such that they will invariably find themselves in sharp conflict with society and the law.

Paedophiles who desire sexual relationships with children are universally abhorred (but must be accepted and cared for by the nurse) while exhibitionists (men who feel compelled to show their penis to women, but who normally refrain from any closer contact) are pursued by the whole might of the law.

Unlike the primary personality-disordered individual, sexual offenders usually retain the capacity to experience guilt and consequently have to live with their own shame as well as the disapproval of society and the law courts. Treatment, which may include behaviour therapy (see Ch. 8), is of limited value, probably in part due to the offender's ambivalent motivation.

SECONDARY PERSONALITY DISORDERS

Many individuals who clearly do not show signs and symptoms associated with primary personality disorder as described above, nevertheless display a consistent combination of personality traits and characteristics which will tend to colour all their everyday experiences. Although all these traits may be present to some extent in everyone, it is their persistence and ability to cloud the individual's life-style that makes them maladaptive in some cases.

Anankastic personality disorder

This disorder is characterized by a slavish adherence to strict routine. The personality is marked with a rigidity and tendency towards excessive conscientiousness. Self-doubt is common and the individual may be ill at ease with their sexuality. Considerable stubborness may be displayed if their ritualistic approach to life seems threatened.

Cyclothymic personality disorder

Here, it is the person's mood or affect, (see Ch. 8) which is affected. Individuals will experience mood swings which are greater and more frequent than those which can be explained as being a result of the vagaries of normal living. Without missing work or seeking medical attention they may constantly be full of the joys or down in the dumps. For some the mood swing will tend to be in one direction only and the person will fairly consistently be either low or elated.

Hysterical personality disorder

The existence of this personality disorder is sometimes questioned, since traditionally it seems to have been a label used by men to describe women of whom they may not have approved. The features include an overall histrionic (that is theatrical) approach to all interactions. Behaviour may appear flirtatious, but feelings are said to be shallow and the individual may shy away from long-term physical or emotional intimacy.

Paranoid personality disorder

This disorder is characterized by suspicion. Innocent events at work or in the home may be misinterpreted as having special significance and offence can easily be taken where none was meant. It is common for people with this disorder to pursue lengthy court battles in their quest for 'justice'. Other features of this personality are a feeling of self importance and a tendency towards excessive jealousy.

Schizoid personality disorder

The main feature of this disorder is social isolation and aloofness. Individuals may prefer their own company and fantasies to the bustle of social interactions which is everyday life for most people. Shyness may have been a feature from early childhood and will have become more pronounced in adolesence. The adult will have a preference for solitary pursuits and a tendency to withdraw from social situations.

The observant reader will by now have noticed that some similarity exists between certain personality disorders described above, and some of the conditions described in earlier chapters. To some extent the difference is one of degree but the essential feature of the personality types described above is that they are so much part and parcel of the individual as to be virtually normal for him or her. The illnesses have temporarily crossed that boundary and are, by definition, not normal. It is reasonable to assume (but by no means definite) that if, for instance, someone with a cyclothymic or schizoid personality were to develop an acute psychiatric illness it would be an affective disorder and schizophrenia respectively.

RANGE OF INVESTIGATIONS

By its very nature personality disorder does not lend itself to a battery of diagnostic tests. However, in view of the largely pessimistic prognosis associated with the condition, the thrust of the investigations is directed towards the search for another, more treatable diagnosis. An EEG may be ordered if neurological problems are suspected, and a wide range of psychometric tests may be prescribed. Careful history taking, however, remains the best method of establishing a diagnosis.

THERAPEUTIC MANAGEMENT

This is an extremely grey area. One school of thought says that since psychopaths tend not to benefit from any form of therapy or punishment, medical treatment in hospitals has only a very limited role. Similarly, outpatient care would require a degree of co-operation and commitment which is unlikely to be forthcoming. Prisons, which provide incarceration and punishment as an alternative, traditionally fare little better in the quest for a long-term cure or change in behaviour patterns.

It would be very easy, therefore, to adopt an extremely pessimistic view, and it seems likely that this perfectly understandable, but unhelpful attitude has often been responsible for 'the self-fullfilling prophecy' which itself engenders even more pessimism. Equally, it would be foolish to expect miracle cures, particularly in the short term.

Any attempt at symptom reduction or personality change must therefore be seen as a long-term objective which may well involve the so-called 'one step back, two steps forward' maxim. Approaches, traditional and not so traditional, are considered below.

Pharmacological treatment

Traditionally this has been avoided. Unreliability in self-medicating, a tendency to sell or misuse prescribed drugs and a potential for habituation does not suggest that such an approach will be helpful. One group of drugs which are almost definitely better avoided is the benzodiazepines, although conceivably they could relieve some attendant anxiety, they are also capable of releasing aggression in predisposed individuals. Benzodiazepines also pose something of a dependency risk which may be a particular problem with some of this population.

Tyrer (1991) reports that several studies have shown that problems associated with severe personality disorder, such as impulsiveness, irresponsibility and aggression, may respond to antipsychotic drugs in low doses including depot injections such as fluphenazine decanoate. He also reports the use of other drugs such as amitriptyline, lithium carbonate and the anticonvulsive drug carbamazepine.

Too much credence should not be given to these studies as yet since at present pharmacological treatment is largely confined to the short-term use of medication to counteract associated conditions such as depression or alcohol dependency or withdrawal.

Individual psychotherapy

This expensive form of treatment which involves regular and prolonged interaction between the individual and his therapist is not recommended. This type of person demands instant results, and traditionally tolerates frustration very badly. When miracle cures fail to materialize the therapist is blamed and the treatment is usually abandoned. Vaillant (1975), who has a slightly more optimistic view than most, points out that this escaping behaviour is typical of the psychopath who will not, if given an alternative, face up to the reality of his situation. He espouses a common viewpoint that treatment can only hope to be successful if carried out within a secure environment from which physical escape is impossible.

The therapeutic community

This approach, which smacks of the liberal era of the 1960s, is based on the worth of the individual and the potential for everyone and everything in the environment to work either for or against a person's welfare. Thus other patients and ward cleaners are considered to be as potentially therapeutic as doctors and nurses, and all should have an equal right to be heard. Decisions are arrived at by the group as a whole and disagreements and conflicts must be talked through rather than ignored. This approach seems to offer some hope for the psychopath.

Given that a physically secure unit is usually required to ensure compliance with therapy and often the law, the atmosphere within the four walls can be rigidly disciplined or comparatively relaxed. Units specializing in the treatment of psychopaths using a therapeutic community type of approach are well established, with an early example being at Herstedvester in Copenhagen as long ago as 1933. In England the Henderson Hospital in Belmont, Surrey is probably the best known example of a therapeutic community geared towards the treatment of the psychopath, while Barlinnie Prison in Glasgow was the venue for an exciting experiment in 1973. Here the Special Unit was set up, introducing the concept of the therapeutic community to some of Scotland's most violent criminals, who because of their records had until that time been locked up in harsh and repressive circumstances. Despite the reactions of the more traditional prison officers and some sections of the media, the results were promising with the incidence of prison violence and serious assaults on prison staff being greatly reduced. It seems, however, that the regimen would fall considerably short of that in the maximum security ward of the Utah State Hospital where 'the inmates hold the keys both to the outside and to the seclusion rooms'! (Vaillant 1975).

The success of the therapeutic approach is only comparative and may be exaggerated due to shortcomings of all the alternatives. Its success may lie in the fact that staff deliberately avoid the authoritarian role symbolic of society and that psychopaths may be prepared to accept home truths from their peer group that would be totally rejected if they came from staff.

The passing of time

If all else fails the psychopath may eventually grow out of his chaotic lifestyle! Although the reasons are unclear, it is often said that there are no psychopaths over the age of 40 and while scientific evidence may not be forthcoming, it is a commonly reported observation that the once antisocial teenager may develop into the law-abiding middle aged man or woman.

NURSING STRATEGIES

Bearing in mind the fact that there is no definite agreement that hospitalization with its accompanying doctors and nurses is of any real value, readers should not be surprised to learn that there is no place for a dogmatic nursing approach. In what is traditionally regarded as a very difficult task for any nurse, important requirements are consistency, a sense of humour and infinite patience.

The main nursing approaches will be considered under three headings: nursing management of the manipulative patient, nursing management of the aggressive patient and nursing management of a parasuicidal gesture. In the sections below the nurse is portrayed as female, the patient as male for simplicity, no sexism is intended.

Nursing management of the manipulative patient

Psychiatric nurses, however experienced, will if they are being honest recall a time when they were manipulated by a patient. They may have lent him money, allowed him a special privilege or succumbed momentarily to his flattery. This may make them per-

---

Box 10.2 Management of the manipulative patient

1. Be consistent
2. Show unconditional positive regard
3. Confront inappropriate behaviour without anger
4. Do not coax, bargain or rationalize
5. Reinforce desirable behaviours, withdraw reinforcers when behaviour unacceptable
6. Role model 'acceptable' behaviour
7. Be aware of peer group pressure
8. Avoid 'special' relationships
9. Be sensitive to effect on ward team: air intrateam annoyances and grievances
10. Explore effects on other patients

---

manently on guard and may detract from their usual positive approach. In order to be fair to both patient and nurse, therefore, the following principles (as summarized in Box 10.2) should be followed.

1. The need for consistency

This golden rule overrides all others. The manipulative patient will have lived a lifetime of exploiting inconsistencies to his own advantage. Limit setting is a priority. In fairness to all it is important that the ground rules are spelt out and the penalties for any misdemeanours are unambiguously stated. Staff who deviate from the care plan or stray from the team approach are guilty of reinforcing the idea that rules don't matter and that authority is there to be flouted.

2. Unconditional positive regard

This principle coined by Carl Rogers is in the view of the author the most important tool in any communicator's repertoire. Manipulative patients may well try to test the genuineness of this approach by extreme forms of behaviour calculated to infuriate or disgust the nurse and thus leave her protestations of acceptance open to the accusation of being phoney. Unconditional positive regard does not mean the blind acceptance of any behaviour however malevolent, which could only be described as a sure fire recipe for disaster. On the contrary, it requires the careful separation of behaviours, which may or may not be entirely unacceptable and the individual himself who must always be seen as worthy of respect.

3. Confront inappropriate behaviours without anger

This becomes easier in a spirit of unconditional positive regard. Because of perhaps a mixture of intimidation and charm, the manipulative patient may frequently avoid the uncomfortable need to face up to the consequences of his behaviour in an adult fashion. When confrontation does take place it may frequently be in the torrid atmosphere of accusation and recrimination. Such scenes may actually fuel the thrill-seeking behaviour of these individuals, or alternatively can be readily dismissed as the ravings of an out-of-touch authority.

A quiet, unemotional statement of the facts accompanied by a request that the incident and its precedents be explored in a rational manner is more likely to be acceptable to all parties.

4. Do not coax, bargain or rationalize

Again the presence of an unambiguous care plan with strict limit setting is absolutely essential. Given any encouragement the manipulative patient may gladly spend hours arguing, negotiating or point scoring in an attempt to wrestle minor concessions from various staff members. Any deviation from the care plan by members of staff can then be interpreted as weakness and is liable to be exploited by the patient. In particular, such concessions are likely to be used to 'wrong foot' other staff members and encourage squabbling within the team.

5. Reinforce desirable behaviour: withdraw reinforcers when behaviour is unacceptable

In childhood, the reinforcement of our desirable behaviour and the lack of reinforcement of that considered to be undesirable, plays a major part in determining the type of individual that develops. It is to be hoped that a similar approach can modify the behaviour of the manipulative adult.

When manipulative behaviour is met by an angry tirade or a miscreant becomes the centre of attraction, his behaviour is being reinforced, and consequently is more likely to be repeated. It is often observed that the manipulative patient seems to thrive on attention and similarly, that it is undesirable behaviour that seems to be rewarded in this way.

Instead, the opposite approach should be encouraged, the childish outburst, if harmless, should be ignored, while any interest, however fleeting, shown to the welfare of others should be acknowledged with a positive remark.

6. Role model 'acceptable' behaviour

A similar boon in the process towards the maturation of the 'normal' individual is the ready presence of a suitable role model. In many instances this may be the parents. The nurse, often unwittingly, serves as a potent role model to those in her charge. As a constant reminder that success does not necessarily demand the exploitation of others, the mature nurse must act as an example of a more satisfying and less chaotic lifestyle.

7. Be aware of the power of peer group pressure

The importance of the peer group has already been mentioned. In this client group where the desires and opinions of those in authority may be considered worthy only of contempt, peer group pressure often offers the best likelihood of change. The growth of self-help groups and the comparative popularity of group therapy and a therapeutic community approach in the care of the manipulative patient acknowledges the importance put on the opinion of the fellow sufferer and underlines the lack of respect for more traditional experts.

8. Avoid special relationships

It feels good to be special. Unfortunately it is also a somewhat heady experience which may affect the straight thinking of even the most case-hardened individual.

Members of staff made to feel special by a manipulative patient may find themselves becoming increasingly wrapped up in their daily living. They may discover themselves becoming critical of the efforts of their colleagues and may start to believe that they are the only one capable of understanding this person's unique situation. These are danger signs.

It is a common experience that more than one member of staff is singled out for the flattery that makes them special and this can be particularly disruptive. Each time the patient succeeds in upsetting the team spirit it is fair to assume that such cleverness gives him a kick and acts as a damaging reinforcer which will encourage further manipulative behaviour.

9. Be sensitive to effects on the ward team

The nursing of a manipulative patient is punctuated with a series of intrateam conflicts. In fact it is often the slow realization that tensions between various team members have become dangerously high that alerts staff to the presence of such a person on the ward. It is frequently reported that these patients like to play one staff member off against the other and this can easily be done by exploiting any inconsistencies in approach, however minor.

Such disruptions can best be faced with calm confrontation involving all concerned and an increased attention to communication skills.

10. Explore effects on other patients

The nurse has a responsibility to all her patients. As important as the care of the manipulative patient is, it is also vital to realize that other more vulnerable patients may be easy prey to their irrascible charms. Less worldly wise or more acutely ill patients may be wide open to financial or sexual exploitation by an individual who is equally capable of charming his way into their bankbook or their bed. An important feature of the treatment contract must be the unambiguous statement that all debts to fellow patients must be repaid, while staff should refrain from lending money. Sadly, a broken heart is much less easily put right.

Nursing management of the aggressive patient

Aggression and violence is a small but anxiety-provoking feature in the life of most nurses. Incidents of direct violence are mercifully still rare. Nurses who spend their off duty in such activities as attending discos, football matches or pubs, or indeed, in walking down the street at night are almost definitely in greater danger than when they are at work. Most violent episodes probably take place in the domestic situation behind closed doors. Nevertheless, it is important that if the nurse is confronted with violence, she will know how to cope. It is not helpful to associate violence and aggression with one branch of nursing, (e.g. mental health) or with particular diagnoses (personality disorder or paranoid schizophrenia), when in reality, such instances occur in a variety of hospital and community settings and are usually perpetrated by individuals who are mentally healthy.

Although aggression is not always unhealthy and the expressing of anger may well serve as a useful safety valve, overt violence creates the possibility of injury and is disruptive to the therapeutic objective of the setting.

In the ideal scenario, the nurse will anticipate a likely flashpoint, minimize the risk of physical or psychological damage to the aggressor, witnesses and nursing staff, and in analysing the episode use it in such a way as to make a repetition less likely.

In order to meet these demanding objectives, the following principles (summarized in Box 10.3) should be followed.

Box 10.3   Management of the aggressive patient

1. Accept that verbal aggression is normal and can be healthy
2. Develop strategies to anticipate and minimize aggressive incidents
3. Remain, or try to remain calm, confident and objective
4. Do not be a hero; avoid one-to-one confrontations
5. Summon assistance if necessary: be aware of local alarm systems
6. Restraint, if used should be the minimal amount necessary to effect the required result
7. Strive to preserve the self-esteem of the patient throughout
8. Following the incident arrange for patient and, if necessary, staff to be examined for any injury
9. Arrange on the spot de-briefing to help avoid recurrences
10. Record fully, using the appropriate documentation

---

1. Accept that verbal aggression is normal and can be healthy

Since verbal aggression may, on occasion, be the precursor of physical violence it is understandable that some nurses might view it as something that should be avoided at all costs. It may be equally tempting to label the person voicing his anger as being aggressive, and particularly if he is an inpatient in a psychiatric hospital, attributing it to some character defect or symptom of his illness.

These assumptions are dangerously wrong. The controlled expression of anger can have the healthy effect of reducing tension and allowing the individual to let off steam without losing face. The suppression of this anger, however, can lead to the expression of frustration taking on a physical characteristic and the occurrence of an avoidable violent episode.

An individual who has learned that he can give verbal vent to his feelings, however angry, may well be an individual who does not need to resort to physical violence.

2. Develop strategies to anticipate and minimize aggressive incidents

Despite how it may appear, physical violence seldom occurs out of the blue. A nurse who knows her patient and who is familiar with what has gone before may well be able to head off potentially violent situations. Typically, violence may occur as a result of the individual feeling vulnerable and being unable to express himself in more socially acceptable ways.

A patient who is fobbed off when making a simple request or who is kept waiting for a cigarette or his medication is much more likely to erupt than is someone who is treated with the courtesy that he deserves. Environmental factors, like overcrowding, a poor patient/staff ratio or an unstructured day which leaves everyone with too much time on their hands can also be instrumental in causing increased violence.

Sometimes, but perhaps less often than is commonly supposed, the person's mental or physical health may be directly implicated in his resort to violence. The epileptic patient may be aggressive either before or after a seizure, the intellectually or physically handicapped person may become angry if urged beyond his capacity, while a patient who is experiencing pain may have a lowered tolerance threshold. The person who is experiencing delusions or hallucinations or who is disorientated through a confusional state may react violently to their perceived predicament.

The nurse who knows the patients as individuals and who approaches them with genuineness and empathy will be able to defuse many situations. If the nurse can anticipate which patient is likely to become disturbed, it may be possible to coax them away from the group to another part of the ward or to a quieter room where there are less potential stressors.

3. Remain, or try to remain calm, confident and objective

Aggression is frequently as frightening to the perpetrator as it is to the person to whom it is directed. A subjective feeling that they are somehow out of control can lead to escalating violence which could conceivably have been avoided.

The calm approach of the nurse can at least give the impression that she is in control and can be reassuring to the patient faced with his own frightening potential for mayhem. The nurse who is confident in her own ability and in the back-up system available in an emergency can best exude this confident air. Objectivity is essential, both during an incident when assessing the likely danger and also after it has died down. There is no place for the exaggerated telling of stories which although perhaps showing the nurse in a good light will also build a reputation for certain patients with the resulting risks of a self-fulfilling prophecy.

4. Do not be a hero: avoid one-to-one confrontation

In the event of physical violence, the one-to-one confrontation should be avoided at all costs. Such confrontations invariably personalize the issue, and can make it difficult for either party to capitulate without an apparent loss of face.

An aggressor faced with only one 'opponent' may realistically decide that he can emerge the victor if only he becomes a little more violent, and the situation can escalate. It is almost impossible for any one individual to be sufficiently on top of a situation to physically bring it to a safe conclusion. Instead, a struggle is likely to ensue in which the safety of neither party can be guaranteed.

5. Summon assistance if necessary: be aware of local alarm systems

Given that one-to-one confrontations are to be avoided, it is logical that an early response must be to summon help. This will be easier to achieve if someone in the vicinity knows the whereabouts of each member of staff. If the possibility of violence can reasonably be anticipated it is particularly important to ensure that the nurse is never isolated without the means of attracting immediate attention.

A variety of different local alarm systems are in common usage and staff in any unit should be introduced to them as a matter of priority. All staff have a duty to respond rapidly to any distress signal if at all possible, and equally, they have the right to expect a similarly unequivocal response from their colleagues should the need occur.

6. Restraint, if used, should be the minimal amount necessary to effect the required result

Sometimes the arrival on the scene of a calm, professional team in adequate numbers, is in itself sufficient to defuse a situation. This is the desired result and should not be seen as a waste of time of the individuals concerned.

The number of staff used may well depend on the amount available to respond to the call, and when urgent action is required, it will be limited to those in the immediate vicinity.

The amount of force used should be the minimum required to safely control the situation, and should be applied in a manner calculated to reduce rather than inflame further aggression.

Barnes (1992) suggests that if physical restraint becomes unavoidable, the nurse in charge should designate each nurse to gain control of a particular limb, with one nurse being responsible for controlling the patient's head and thus trying to ensure that the airway is protected. Clothing should be held in preferance to limbs, but when limbs are used they should be held near a major joint to reduce leverage and thus minimize the likelihood of serious injury. Pressure should not be applied to the abdomen, chest, throat or neck.

7. Strive to preserve the self-esteem of the patient throughout

Direct physical confrontations are invariably un-dignified and can be potentially degrading for all concerned. Unnecessary force or an injudicious or unprofessional remark uttered at a time of heightened emotion can permanently damage a therapeutic relationship long after any physical threat has evaporated.

However hard to implement, the need for un-conditional positive regard is never more important, and the message must be that however unacceptable the behaviour, the person himself remains worthy of value.

8. Following the incident arrange for the patient and if necessary, the staff to be examined for any injury

This needs little explanation but is nevertheless vital. The duty to care for patients never diminishes and they have the undeniable right to early medical at-tention. The possibility of legislation should not be overlooked and in such occasions, whoever the complainant, a medical report will be vital evidence.

9. Arrange on the spot de-briefing to help avoid recurrences

It is important that all concerned learn from the incident with the aim of reducing the likelihood of it happening again. Staff and patients (if agreeable) should openly examine events leading up to the outburst and should ask themselves whether it could have been anticipated.

Individuals should be helped to express their feel-ings openly and uncritically and to seek explanation and reassurance. Any constructive verbalization is acceptable but bickering or point scoring is not. If feelings are still running high it is best to postpone the meeting until everyone is more relaxed rather than risk another, avoidable flare-up. It is a fact that poor communication can itself be a potent factor leading to frustration and aggression and it makes sense to introduce a regular forum where irritants, minor or major, can be discussed.

10. Record fully, using the appropriate documentation

The nurse has a legal duty to record important hap-penings relating to her patient and must do so fully. It is important that such incidents are reported objec-tively and that incidents are not presented in such a way that the patient seemed more violent or the nurse more heroic. Any record of violence must form part of an overall patient profile which must be kept in perspective. The recording of three violent outbursts in a month is significant but must not be allowed to negate the fact that for 28 days the patient's frustration was controlled.

Nursing management of the parasuicidal gesture

Parasuicide is a deliberate attempt at self-harm which does not have a fatal outcome. This term is more satis-factory than its still common alternative, **attempted suicide**, since it does not speculate on whether or not the act was a genuine attempt to die.

Much of the care required by someone who has made a parasuicidal gesture will be that of the person deemed a high suicide risk and readers are reminded of the section on the suicidal patient (see Ch. 8).

People who indulge in parasuicide frequently do so more than once and each accident and emergency unit will have a quota of regulars who will be well known to staff and who may be viewed with a mixture of pity and intolerance.

Farmer & Hirsch (1980) describe three patterns of repetition with regard to parasuicide.

1. Chronic repeater. These individuals resort to parasuicide as a habitual method of coping with life's stresses. Approximately 30% of parasuicidal admis-sions to hospital may come into this category and the likelihood of a successful suicide some time in the future is high.

2. Clustering. Two or more episodes may occur within a short space of time as a result of prolonged or severe stress. There may then follow a long period of time without any further attempts.

3. One-off. A single parasuicide episode occurring at a time of severe crisis. Repetition in this group, must, by definition, be unlikely.

In order to meet the demands posed by parasuicide, the following principles (summarized in Box 10.4) should be followed.

1. Initiate or participate in first aid as required

Staff cannot afford to ponder too long on the

Box 10.4   Management of the parasuicidal gesture

1. Initiate or participate in first aid as required
2. Recognize that the person may genuinely want to die
3. Assess depth of suicide risk
4. Maintain a safe environment
5. Look out for trigger incidents
6. Avoid value judgements
7. Avoid overidentification
8. Discourage exaggerated use of sick role
9. Address loss of self-esteem
10. Set realistic short-term goals

---

genuiness of any parasuicidal gesture, nor can they be allowed to show that they resent the fact that their workload has been increased by what they may see as an avoidable occurrence. The expectation of staff is clearcut. Whether they are called on to carry out a stomach lavage, assist with suturing or provide nursing care on a longer term basis, they must do so without moralising or being tempted to take short cuts. Sadly this does not necessarily happen and so called 'self harmers' are frequently cited as among the least popular categories of patient.

2. Recognize that the person may genuinely want to die

It is a dangerous mistake to think that people who make a parasuicidal gesture are merely attention seekers with no serious intent to kill themselves. Indeed the opposite is just the case, and individuals who have involved themselves in deliberate acts of self-harm within the previous year are about 100 times more likely to commit suicide than is the population at large.

3. Assess the depth of suicide risk

Chapter 8 describes how suicide can be minimized and the observations that must be made on any individual classed as suicidal. Self-harmers must come into this category and their suicidal intent must be carefully assessed. The decision that any individual does not pose a suicide risk is one that is best taken by the team on the basis of careful observation. It can never be taken lightly.

4. Maintain a safe environment

The reader is again referred to Chapter 8. The risk of self-harm can be greatly minimized if a series of

commonsense precautions are implemented. Whether the injuries thus avoided are fatal or merely superficial is immaterial; the maintainance of a safe environment is paramount.

5. Look out for trigger incidents

People who self-harm once are well known to be likely to do so again. Since all acts of self-harm could be said to constitute a crisis for those concerned, any lessons which can be learned and used to minimize the likelihood of a repetition are to be welcomed.

Bancroft et al (1977) found that in the week prior to a parasuicide act it is common for the individual to have quarrelled with a significant other and it seems that such an event superimposed on chronic problems may spark a crisis in predisposed individuals. In a hospital ward, nursing staff may notice that such problems may occur for example, after an individual's plans have been thwarted, following a highly charged visit, or when the presence of a sympathetic audience may give maximum effect.

6. Avoid value judgements

Any attempt to moralize or debate the genuiness of an individual's distress is unforgivable. Staff may at times be aware of the histrionic nature of some parasuicidal gestures or may be struck by the apparent lack of serious injuries resulting from repeated gestures. Cynicism may be understandable at such times but is never helpful. Some individuals may not be aware of, for example, the amount of tablets required to initiate death, or the position of the major blood vessels and so may harbour intent far greater than their injuries may suggest. The reader is reminded again of the merits of unconditional positive regard.

7. Avoid overidentification

The typical parasuicidal person is said to be young and female. This is also a reasonable description of the typical nurse. A feature of these people can be their complicated life-styles and personal relationships which may cry out for the understanding of the sympathetic nurse. In striving to meet the undoubted needs of her patient the nurse may find herself becoming ever more drawn into an overexclusive relationship. While never losing sight of the need to offer unconditional positive regard, she must take care to ensure that all patients in her care are looked after according to their needs.

8. Discourage exaggerated use of the sick role

The patient, as has been seen, may require prompt first aid or medical treatment and will require to have his psychological distress acknowledged. Beyond that, it may not be helpfull to over-medicalize the situation. An inherent problem is the fact that to recognize the individual as genuinely ill may well be to provide the positive reinforcement that will lead directly to a repeat. A far better alternative is to encourage the patient to carefully explore the reasons for his behaviour and the likely effect it will have on others.

9. Address loss of self-esteem

Individuals who choose to disfigure their own bodies and risk permanent disablement or death are likely to have a very low opinion of themselves. This could well be reinforced by the unsympathetic attitudes of those around them who may on occasions be tempted to voice their frustrations. As on so many occasions the message must be, 'the behaviour is not acceptable, but the person is worthy of value'.

10. Set realistic short-term goals

Perhaps only one-third of parasuicides can be classed as suffering from a recognizable psychiatric illness (Newton-Smith & Hirsch 1979). Medical intervention, with the exception of first aid interventions, is therefore contraindicated.

In many cases the significant causative factor may be a plethora of social problems. In such cases, crisis counselling, the offering of a short-term listening ear, may be reasonably successful. This avoids treating the individual as a patient but helps them prioritize their problems and talk through various solutions. When obvious, real live problems are identified, such as impending eviction or an absence of child minding facilities, it may be possible to help the individual address and compare realistic, practical solutions.

Nursing strategies: the limitations

The foregoing paragraphs are noticably short on guarantees. Whether the problem is one of manipulative behaviour, aggression or self-harm, a common thread runs through its presentation. Each case is made more difficult by its unpredictability: the calm patient may suddenly lash out; the trusted companion may steal from his peers or a dramatic episode of self-injury may appear out of the blue.

Repetition may be a problem and despite the most valiant efforts of nursing staff it is never possible to decree that it will never happen again. Another enigma is the apparent lack of genuineness which may be exhibited and the difficulty in empathy that this may engender.

In the midst of such therapeutic negativism it is easy to understand how the problems addressed above are amongst the most difficult faced by the mental health nurse and why many of them question the validity of their taking part in any treatment programme.

ETHICS

This chapter should have highlighted the enigma that is personality disorder. Nowhere is this more evident than when it comes to deciding what should be done when an individual so designated presents as being in need of attention.

'Mad or bad?'

Traditionally the stark choice is between prison or hospital (often special hospitals) and the reason for the decision is not always clear.

Perhaps imprisonment is a more easily understood solution. If the individual offends it may seem both logical and just to visit him with the full might of the law. This disposal is probably justified in that it prevents the individual re-offending in the short term, while less nobly it extracts a measure of revenge for society. However, this treatment is notoriously inept at rehabilitating the offender, and entirely fails to address the 'mad or bad' question.

Hospital poses its own problems, however. A major feature of personality disorder is the apparent lack of psychiatric symptoms and the justification for treating it as an illness is not clear cut. When sections of the appropriate Mental Health Act are evoked to confine such an individual compulsarily to hospital even more questions are raised.

The indefinite sentence

Sentence to imprisonment, for whatever the heinousness of the offence, brings with it the prospect of eventual discharge. A release date will be known and may be brought forward if the behaviour of the inmate justifies it. No such date exists for the individual confined to hospital, and although this means that hospitalization could be short lived, it carries for others the threat of lengthy detention without even the safeguard of a trial.

Uncertainity of prognosis

The purpose of a hospital is to cure or ameliorate a condition, that of a prison to contain. A prerequisite of hospitalization therefore should be the susceptibility to treatment. Sadly this remains a grey area and one not overendowed with hope. The morality of confining a person in hospital for treatment which has not been shown to be particularly successful is suspect, as is the counter approach of operating hospital black-lists, banning certain individuals from being readmitted to hospital because of their lack of conforming during an earlier admission.

Best use of scarce resources

Increasingly, health service administrators and clinicians are forced to consider the cost of the service that they provide. Undoubtedly choices have often to be made between various options, and questions such as 'how many hip replacements are equal to a heart transplant?', although regrettable, have got to be asked.

Such questions are extremely relevant in the case of the individual with a personality disorder. The prognosis is uncertain and any treatment expensive. In such circumstances the special unit approach, high in physical amenity and client/staff ratio, may be prohibitive and mere containment might seem an attractive alternative.

Effect on other patients

The patient with personality disorder may exhibit antisocial behaviour which could include theft or violence towards either staff or fellow patients. Their cavalier approach to life may be frightening to other more timid patients whose treatment plans may then be in jeopardy. Again it must be considered whether the vague hope of amelioration of the personality disorder should take precedence over the more likely cure of other disorders.

PERSONALITY DISORDER: A CONCLUSION

Perhaps the best way to understand personality disorder is to know a little about personality development. After considering some theories of personality development this chapter went on to look at personality disorder in its various guises. Some nursing problems were explored and the prognosis discussed.

In caring for individuals described as being personality disordered, the nurse must guard against naivety and avoid being overoptimistic. She must never, however, lose sight of the capacity of the human being for change or of the need to recognize the worth of every individual in her care.

LEGAL IMPLICATIONS IN MENTAL HEALTH NURSING

Although it has been shown that individuals described as having a personality disorder may frequently get caught up in the legal process, this section applies to mental health in its widest context. It relies mainly on the Mental Health Act 1983 (England and Wales), and The Mental Health (Scotland) Act, 1984 for its contents and any reader with a specific legal query is advised to consult the act applicable to their appropriate country.

The law is often depicted by a set of scales, and this is particularly apt as far as mental health is concerned. Once it is acknowledged that some individuals may require to be admitted (however briefly) to hospital against their will, it must also be accepted that the might of the law must be equally available to protect their rights while they are thus incarcerated.

Various sections of the Act allow for individuals to be compulsorily admitted to hospital against their will. They must be shown to be a danger to themselves or others, or be refusing informal admission, and presupposes that their condition will be susceptible to treatment.

Admissions in the case of an emergency can be ordered by one doctor and will be for a short period only. This can be extended to intermediate or longer periods when circumstances decree, but further medical opinion will be sought, the courts will be called upon to adjudicate and patients will have the right of representation and to appeal in the event of the decision going against them.

In most cases patients legally detained in hospital will be discharged on the decision of their consultant often after a trial period at home on pass. In some cases, however, there may be a restriction on their right of discharge because of the heinous nature of an offence they may have committed or because of the danger they are thought to represent. In some cases, only the appropriate Secretary of State can order an individual's discharge.

Nurse's holding power

The current Acts introduced for the first time sections which allow certain trained nurses the power to legally detain in hospital an informally admitted patient determined to discharge himself. This holding power lasts for 6 hours in England and Wales and 2 hours in Scotland and can only be used when in the professional opinion of the nurse, the patient is suffering from mental disorder to such a degree that to leave would pose a great danger to himself or others. Crucially, the nurse can only take such action when the doctor (whose duty the ordering of such detention would normally be) is unavailable. The nurse must carefully note the time that she has evoked this procedure since it lapses at the end of the given time or on the arrival of the doctor, whichever happens first.

Consent to treatment

The broad principle has always been that informed consent should be sought from patients before any treatment is carried out. Patients should sign the familiar form and the doctor should countersign that he has explained the procedure. This course of events has its parallel in general hospitals and as a rule works smoothly. However, there will always be some patients who (possibly because of the very condition requiring treatment) will refuse the course of action deemed essential by the doctor.

For all but the most straightforward case (for instance, basic nursing care) the patient will have the right to have the doctor review his plans and if the problem remains, the right of the independent view of a specially approved psychiatrist from another geographical area. This independent psychiatrist must seek the opinions of a nurse and other non doctor who is familiar with the patient before he makes his decision. Only then will the decision be binding and treatment given.

In some very rare and irreversible treatments, both the written consent of the patient and a second independent medical opinion is required before approval can be given.

Protecting the rights of patients

Legislation also exists to protect the rights of patients in a number of other situations. They must be protected from sexual exploitation and from assault or theft (staff may be the victims of false accusations in these areas and must also be protected by the Acts). Individuals incapacitated by illness, age or handicap must have their financial affairs safeguarded and various sections of the Acts allow for family, friends or legal representatives to be made responsible for this in certain circumstances.

Conclusion

Because of the all-encompassing nature of the Mental Health Acts, it is hardly surprising that they are wordy and difficult for the ordinary person to understand. They strive to protect the patients' rights but at the same time, must protect the public from dangerous patients. They guard against unnecessary detention of a patient in hospital, but paradoxically make it possible for the nurse in certain circumstances to prevent him leaving. They must offer protection to patients from uncaring or sadistic members of staff, but at the same time must protect the very much larger numbers of caring staff from possible false accusations.

The earlier advice that the reader should consult the Acts in their entirety for clarification of any specific points is repeated with some feeling.

Suggested assignments

Discussion points
1. Divorce rates are said to be increasing in the western world. Bearing in mind the central role of the family in many theories of personality development, what effect may this have for society?
2. 'Just because a father and son have both been diagnosed as having a psychopathic personality this is insufficient to prove a definite hereditary cause' (Mitchell 1983). Discuss.
3. Convicted killers may be freed from prison within 10 years. Patients in a special hospital can remain there indefinitely. Is this fair?
4. Informed consent to treatment is a basic right. It should never be bypassed. Discuss.

REFERENCES AND FURTHER READING

Bancroft J, Skrimshire A, Casson J, Harvard-Watts O, Reynolds F 1977 People who deliberately poison or injure themselves: their problems and their contact with helping agencies. Psychological Medicine 7: 289–303

Barnes C A 1992 In: Brooking J, Ritter S, Thomas B (eds) A textbook of psychiatric and mental health nursing: Personality disorders. Chapter 34, pp 425–435 Churchill Livingstone, Edinburgh

Bowlby J 1951 Maternal care and mental health. WHO Geneva

Bowlby J 1958 A note on mother-child separation as a mental health hazard. British Journal of Medical Psychology 31: 247

Boyle J 1977 A sense of freedom. Pan Books, London

Cleckley H 1976 The mask of sanity. CV Mosby, St Louis

Costello T W, Costello J T 1992 Abnormal psychology, 2nd edn. Harper Collins, New York

Farmer R, Hirsch S 1980 The suicide syndrome. Croom Helm, London

Goldfarb W 1955 In: Hoch P H, Zubin J (eds) Psychopathology of Childhood. H. New York

Gross R D 1992 Psychology: the science of mind and body, 2nd edn. Hodder & Stoughton, London

Henderson D 1939 Psychopathic states. Norton, New York

Holmes C A 1991 Psychopathic disorder: a category mistake? Journal of Medical Ethics 17: 77–85

Kneisl C R, Wilson H S 1988 Psychiatric nursing, 3rd edn. Addison-Wesley Publishing, California

Lyttle J 1986 Mental disorder: its care and treatment. Baillière Tindall, Eastbourne

McCord W, McCord J 1956 Psychopathy and delinquency. Grune and Stratton, New York

Mental Health Act 1983 (England & Wales). HMSO, London

Mental Health (Scotland) Act, 1984. HMSO, London

Mitchell R G 1983 Psychopathic disorders. Nursing Times 80(11): 49–51

Mitchell R G 1986 Essential psychiatric nursing. Churchill Livingstone, Edinburgh

Morgan H G 1979 Death wishes? The understanding and management of deliberate self harm. John Wiley, Chichester

Newson-Smith J G B, Hirsch S R 1979 Psychiatric symptoms in self poisoning patients. Psychological Medicine 9: 493–500

Parry R 1983 Basic psychotherapy, 2nd edn. Churchill Livingstone, Edinburgh

Pinel P 1801 Traite Medico Philosophique sur l'allienation Mentale ou la Name. Richard Caille et Ravier, Paris

Rutter M 1972 Maternal deprivation. Penguin Books, Baltimore

Tyrer P 1991 Personality disorder in perspective. British Journal of Psychiatry 159: 463–471

Vaillant G E 1975 Sociopathy as a human process: a view point. Archives of General Psychiatry 32. 178: 178–183

Weber A 1991 Introduction to psychology. Harper Collins, New York

CHAPTER CONTENTS

11

Care implications of disorders of the locomotor system

Christine Donnelly

In health a person must be able to stand upright, sit, walk, run, jump and perform the many complex movements necessary in everyday life. To do this it is vital that the bones, joints, voluntary muscles, sensory and motor nerves are all in perfect working order and working together. Abnormalities within any of these systems can lead to a reduction in efficiency of the locomotor system.

Orthopaedic conditions, their prevention, treatment and nursing, is a specialty in its own right and there are many excellent textbooks on the subject from which a detailed knowledge of such disorders can be gained. The purpose of this chapter is to provide a basic foundation about the working of the locomotor system which can be related to the nursing care given to people suffering from orthopaedic conditions commonly encountered in general hospitals.

ANATOMY AND PHYSIOLOGY

Movement must be co-ordinated if it is to be efficient. In order to achieve this, bones, joints, muscles and nerves must function as a team. To aid understanding of how this team works it is necessary to study the structure and function of each of the above. (The nervous system is dealt with in detail in Ch. 5.)

BONE STRUCTURE AND FUNCTION

Bones are living tissue which come in various shapes and sizes but they have many common features:

Blood supply   Nutrient arteries supply bone tissue with oxygen, essential nutrients, vitamins and hormones, while veins remove waste products of metabolism from bone.

Periosteum   This is a tough, white membrane which covers the bone except where joints occur. It has two layers; an outer fibrous layer for protection and the attachment of muscles, and an inner osteogenic layer which mostly consists of osteoblasts (bone-forming cells) and oeteoclasts (bone-destroying cells). It also has a rich blood, lymphatic and nerve supply.

Compact bone Found just underneath the periosteum, compact bone forms a hard, dense bone which is necessary for strength and support. Although there are many spaces in compact bone, they are invisible to the naked eye. Compact bone is thickest in the shaft (diaphysis) of long bones and thinnest in flat bones. Calcium salts are responsible for giving bone its hardness.

Cancellous bone Found in varying amounts underneath compact bone, cancellous bone is less dense than compact bone and the spaces are obvious to the naked eye. Cancellous bone (spongy bone) is described as looking rather like a honeycomb. (Interestingly, the lines of bone follow the lines of greatest stress through the bone, adding support to the structure.) It is found in the epiphyses of long bones and forms the bulk of short bones and flat bones.

Red marrow Haemopoiesis (formation of blood cells) occurs within red marrow which is typically found in the spaces of cancellous bone.

Articulating cartilage Wherever two bones form a joint, the surface of each bone is covered in a hard, shiny cartilage. This smooth surface acts as a cushion and absorbs stress during movement. It is continuous with the periosteum.

Medullary cavity Peculiar to long bones, the medullary cavity contains yellow marrow. Yellow marrow consists of fat cells and a very few blood cells.

See Figure 11.1 for a diagrammatic representation of a typical long bone

Functions of bone

The functions of bone can be gleaned from its structure:

1. **Support**: strong bones provide support for the whole body.
2. **Protection**: vital organs, e.g. the brain, heart and lungs are protected within bony cavities.
3. **Movement**: bones provide attachment for muscles; joints allow movements to take place.
4. **Storage**: fat and mineral salts are stored by bone.
5. **Haemopoiesis**: new blood cells are formed within the red marrow.

JOINT STRUCTURE AND FUNCTION

A joint is any place in the body where two or more

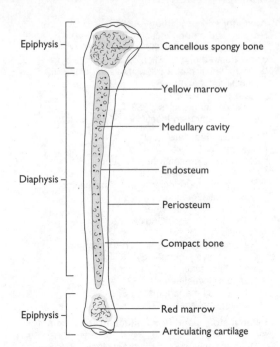

Fig. 11.1 Diagram of a typical long bone

bones touch (or articulate). Some joints are fixed, such as joints between bones of the adult skull, and no movement is possible. Some joints are slightly movable; here the union between the bones is formed by cartilage. A third type of joint which is of major importance in locomotion is the freely movable joint.

Characteristics of a freely movable joint

The articulating surfaces are smooth and complementary to each other – as in the shoulder, hip and knee joints on the skeleton. The bones which form the joint are separated by a fluid-filled cavity called a joint cavity. This cavity is formed by thickened ligaments called capsular ligaments which surround the joint and unite the articulating bones. The capsular ligaments give stability to the joint while still permitting movement to take place. Synovial membrane lines the joint capsule and secretes a viscous fluid (rather like the consistency of egg white) called synovial fluid. Synovial fluid helps to reduce friction between the bone ends during movement, it nourishes the articulating cartilage and it contains phagocytes which remove debris and microbes from the joint. Freely movable joints are surrounded by extracapsular ligaments which provide stability and prevent subluxation and dislocation. Intracapsular ligaments modify the shape of the articulating surface and thereby allow two different bone shapes to fit snuggly

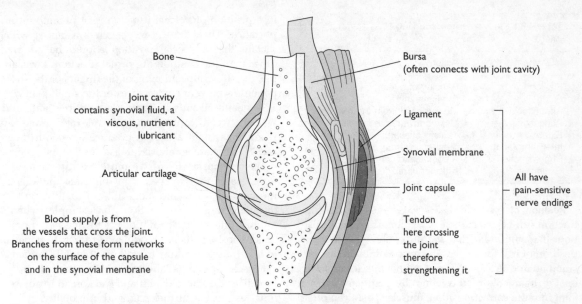

Fig. 11.2 Diagram of a synovial joint. (Reproduced from Gunn C 1984, Bones and Joints, Churchill Livingstone p. 10)

together. The shape of the articulating surfaces and the presence or absence of ligaments, determines the movements which can occur at different joints.

See Figure 11.2 for a diagrammatic representation of a synovial joint.

Functions of joints

There are two main functions of joints:

1. To hold all the bones together.
2. To allow movement in a skeleton made of rigid bone.

MUSCLE ACTION

Within the body there are three types of muscle: smooth, cardiac and skeletal (smooth and cardiac are mentioned in Chs 12 and 15). Skeletal muscle is so called because it is attached to bones and is involved in moving the skeleton. Although the structure of each type of muscle differs they have several similarities:

1. **Excitability**. This is the ability of muscle tissue to receive and respond to a stimulus, such as a neuro-transmitter substance, which generates an electrical current (action potential) that travels along the muscle cell.

2. **Contractility**. This is the ability of muscle tissue to contract, or shorten, in response to a stimulus.

3. **Extensibility**. This is the ability of muscle tissue to be stretched, or extended, beyond its relaxed length.

4. **Elasticity**. This is the ability of muscle tissue to regain its original shape following extension or contraction.

Functions of muscles

There are four important functions of muscles:

1. movement
2. maintenance of body posture
3. joint stability
4. generation of heat.

Movement

A muscle or group of muscles which produce movement must be attached to a fixed point on either side of a joint. When a muscle contracts the opposing muscle relaxes and movement is produced. The effect of this action is to decrease the angle of the joint and bring two distant points closer together, for example, flexion.

Table 11.1   Movements occurring at synovial joints

Movement	Action
Flexion	Bending of a joint
Extension	Straightening a joint
Abduction	Moving away from the midline
Adduction	Moving towards the midline
External rotation	Turning outwards
Internal rotation	Turning inwards
Circumduction	A combination of all the above
Gliding	Articular cartilages sliding

Position of rest (Fig. 11.3) Excessive muscle contraction can be caused solely by abnormal joint position. It is important that the nurse should know the position of rest for each of the major joints. In this position no undue tension is put on the muscles or strain on the ligaments of the joints. By gently moving a joint into the correct position, muscle spasm can often be relieved or minimized. This is of particular importance when moving and handling patients who have suffered paralysis of a limb. Ensuring that the patient is left with the limb adequately supported and in a position of normal function is of paramount importance. There are, however, circumstances which dictate that a special position should be adopted, other than the position of normal function, for example, the straight positioning of the fingers of the stroke patient to prevent contractures of the small joints.

In health all muscle fibres are held in a state midway between contraction and relaxation and are ready for instant action to produce a smooth movement. This state is referred to as muscle tone.

Muscle spasm Excessive muscle contraction is referred to as muscle spasm. In this state the affected muscles are rigid and stone like in quality. Sudden dramatic muscle contraction, for example, when a mother lifts a very heavy object to free her trapped child, can be sufficiently violent to fracture bones or to tear muscle tendons from their bony attachments.

Muscle spasm is always acutely painful. It immobilizes the affected joint and can spread to adjacent muscles causing further pain and immobility.

Simple measures to relieve muscle spasm Muscle spasm caused by inflammatory or other painful lesions can often be relieved by the application of local heat which aims to increase the circulation to the

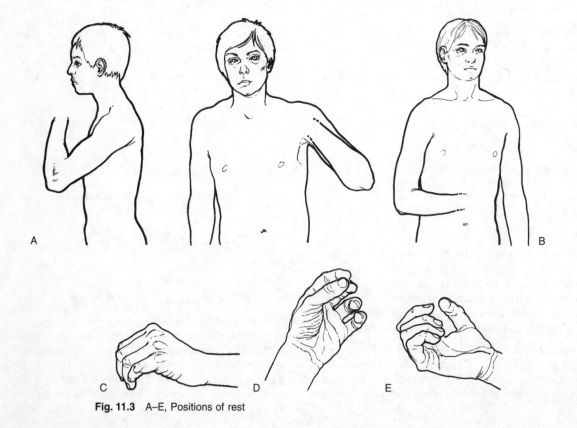

Fig. 11.3 A–E, Positions of rest

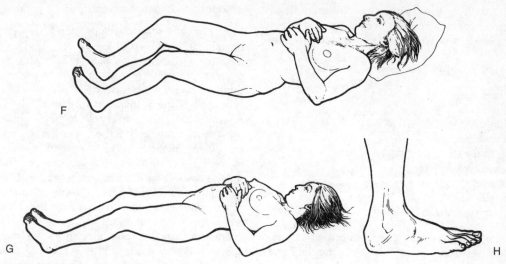

Fig. 11.3 F–H, Positions of rest

affected muscle, thus raising the temperature locally. The nurse should realize that safety precautions must be taken in order to prevent burning accidents occurring. Methods of applying local heat are:

1. Covered electric heat pad.
2. Hot baths/hydrotherapy – total immersion or immersion of the affected part only.
3. Wax baths – only the affected part is immersed.
4. Poultices – preparations such as kaolin contain a counter-irritant.
5. Massage – which should only be carried out by an **experienced practitioner.**
6. Ultrasonic massage; very high frequency sound waves penetrate tissue to the required depth and increase blood flow to the affected part.
7. Hydropacks – packs are preheated in a boiler then wrapped in blankets and placed over the affected joint which is covered with the patient's own towel.

8. Infrared therapy – rays from a special lamp provide superficial heat.

Posture and body movements

In order to maintain the upright position with minimum effort, it is vital that weight transmission and balance are efficient. If the head, thorax and pelvis are thought of as loads which have to be carried by the legs, it is obvious that if the weights are piled in a straight column and balanced on straight legs, the amount of muscular effort needed to maintain this position will be minimal. The load is further stabilized when the feet are apart, as this gives a broader base for weight transmission.

The same is true of sitting positions. The slouching position is more tiring as it causes strain and muscle tension (Fig. 11.4).

Posture during normal activity   It is vital that nurses

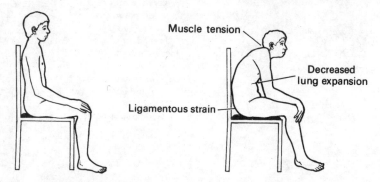

Muscle tension

Decreased lung expansion

Ligamentous strain

Fig. 11.4   Posture when sitting

maintain good postural habits since, by minimizing the amount of muscular effort needed for work, they can complete a task with less fatigue and also joint strain.

The major points of good posture are:

- head held high
- chin tucked in
- shoulders level
- lower abdomen flat
- curves of the spine maintained without exaggeration
- pelvis level
- knees relaxed
- feet pointing straight ahead.

Good body posture and alignment must be maintained during activity as well as when standing and sitting.

Moving patients is achieved by a series of dynamic movements. Not only has a load to be moved, but it has to be moved to a different relative position. Good postural habits and efficient movement techniques all aim to ensure that whether standing still or moving, the nurse maintains balance and equilibrium. Smoothness of action and easy transmission of weight are important if movement and handling of patients is to be carried out safely for both the patient and the nurse.

Efficient handling and moving

Most human beings develop a top-heavy pattern of movement, as shown in Figure 11.5(A). This type of movement threatens balance and creates excessive postural protective reflexes in order to prevent an individual from falling forwards. An excessive amount of muscle tissue is involved in maintaining balance, leaving little muscle available to help with the lift. Most of this muscle is in the upper limbs, making the movement inefficient. The sustained tension in the lower limbs creates physiological changes within the muscle tissue, which leads, over a period of time, to a cumulative effect resulting in tissue adaptation. The tissue becomes less able to cope with stress and strain and is more liable to injury.

Efficient handling and moving: a neuromuscular approach (Vasey & Crozier 1982) is one that achieves its objective with a minimum of muscle effort. It must include a conditioning programme that helps to neutralise the effects of cumulative strain and tissue adaptation. Conditioning prepares the body for movement and helps the individual to regain flexibility of their muscles and joints.

In efficient movement the emphasis is on balance. The base action enables the individual to move in such a way as to promote balance and reduce the degree of postural stiffening associated with top-heavy movement (Fig. 11.5(B)). This is known as recoil and it

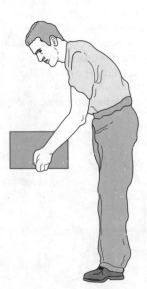

The basis of all harmful movement is:

Top heavy bending
Initial bending of head and upper trunk

Stiffens legs and back so feet do not adjust for movement

Hands have to reach out excessively

Elbows jut out from body

Excessive finger end pressure

A

Fig. 11.5(A)

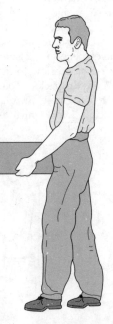

The basis of all good movement is:

Base action
Initial relaxation of both knees

Legs and back relax for movement

Feet adjust to allow follow-through with load

Elbows tend to remain into body

Good palmar hold

requires practice to become proficient at this type of movement.

Principles of efficient handling and moving
See Fig. 11.5.

1. **Relax the knees**: this begins to lower the centre of gravity of the body and helps to reduce unnecessary stiffening or tension building up in the muscles.

2. **Move the feet**: finding a comfortable position for the feet is very important. Having a comfortably wide stance and pointing a foot in the direction in which you wish to move helps to maintain balance and reduces muscle tension.

3. **Let the back relax**: when the back relaxes naturally, the centre of gravity is further reduced and allows the extensor muscles to be slightly over-stretched. This facilitates elastic recoil and achieves a position of optimum balance.

4. **Take an indirect hold**: objects should be supported from below using the palms of the hands. The arms should over-reach slightly before coming to rest on the object. This action stretches the muscles and therefore they will work more efficiently. The hold should be taken as low down the object as possible.

5. **Relax the knees again**: this relieves tension and slightly stretches the muscles.

6. **Lead up with the head**: the head leads the cervical, thoracic and lumbar curves into their safest position.

Throughout any moving and handling sequence it is necessary to re-adjust the **feet** and **hold** as neces-

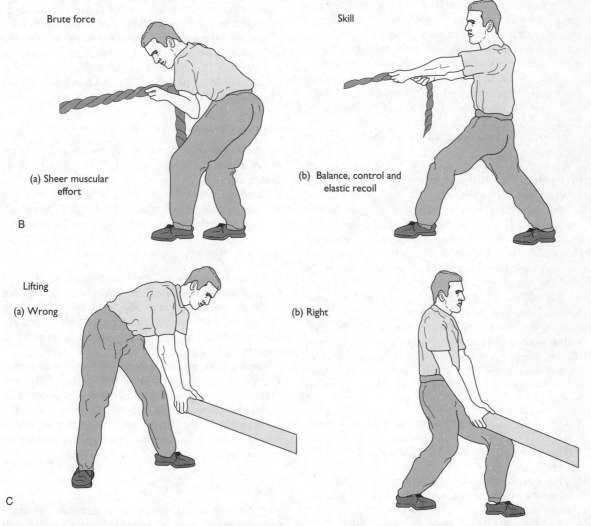

Fig. 11.5   A–C Diagrams to illustrate correct and incorrect methods of lifting and moving. (Adapted from Walsh 1988.)

sary so as to maximize the efficiency of the move. In particular it is important for nurses to 'get in close' to their patients and keep their arms as near to their bodies as possible. It is also worth bearing in mind that shifting a patient's position does not have to be completed in one movement. It is often better to make several small efficient movements which leave the nurses and patients feeling relaxed and comfortable than making one huge effort which leaves the nurses breathless and the patient embarrassed at the amount of effort needed to move him!

The commands to follow for efficient movement are 'knees and head' rather than the customary '1, 2, 3, go!' This serves to remind the operators that relaxing the knees and leading with the head results in smooth and efficient movement.

It is important to remember that the vital components in moving objects or patients are assessment and planning. If the immediate environment has not been adequately prepared then the potential for injury to the nurse and/or the patient is increased.

Before proceeding to move a patient, how the move will be accomplished should be assessed, taking into account the patient's condition. If necessary, furniture and equipment should be moved to create sufficient space and lifting aids should be used where appropriate.

When the assessment is completed it is important to communicate to the patient and colleagues how the move will be accomplished.

Back injuries are very common in areas where manual handling of loads is required and the cost to employers, in lost working days alone, is massive. Nurses in particular are prone to back injuries and this can have far-reaching effects on their careers. In 1992 the European Community published legislation on the safe handling and moving of loads and new laws came into force on 1 January 1993. Where reasonably practicable, mechanical aids should be used in the execution of moving heavy objects. In those circumstances where mechanical aids cannot be used, careful assessment of the situation must be made before any movement is carried out. The assessment involves:

- **The task**, e.g. bed to chair, chair to commode, sitting up in bed, assisted walking.
- **The load**, e.g. how heavy? Is the patient co-operative?
- **The environment**, e.g. condition of the floors, available space, temperature of the room, ventilation, humidity.
- **Characteristics of the handler**, e.g. height, weight, experience.

The Manual Handling Operations Regulations (Health & Safety Executive 1992) require individuals to report any instances where the assessment procedure has been inadequately carried out, placing them at risk of injury.

HAZARDS OF ENFORCED INACTIVITY

Problems associated with inactivity and bed rest are many and varied and it is appropriate at this point to summarize the major problems which the observant nurse can prevent or minimize.

Muscle atrophy

Muscle becomes smaller and its circulation diminishes, resulting in decreased endurance and rapid fatigue. This can occur over a few days and leads to increased inactivity which can take weeks to reverse.

Nursing intervention Active exercises by the patient should be encouraged at least once hourly. In a paralysed or unconscious patient, passive movements should be performed by the nurse and/or the physiotherapist.

Joint contractures

Tendons, capsular ligaments or the muscles themselves shorten, causing joint stiffness and possible deformity.

Nursing intervention Correct positioning of limbs and active exercises should be encouraged. Where appropriate, passive movements should be performed.

Drop foot deformity

If the foot is not adequately supported, tendons of the calf muscles tend to shorten while the muscles of the anterior portion of the leg tend to lengthen. Depending on the severity of the problem, the patient may not be able to put his heel to the ground when attempting to stand.

Nursing intervention Ensure the foot is maintained in a position of function at all times (Fig. 11.3H) and sheets are loose enough to allow active exercises to be performed. Ensure that any strapping around the leg is not too tight. Carry out passive movements, if necessary. In some circumstances special appliances may be used to maintain a good position.

Hypostatic pneumonia

Any position which results in a reduction of chest expansion can lead to hypostatic pneumonia (see Ch. 13).

Nursing intervention Ensure that the patient's posture allows optimum ventilation, within the limits of his/her condition. Encourage deep breathing and coughing exercises.

Pressure necrosis

This results from prolonged pressure on vulnerable areas of tissue. This is fully discussed in Chapter 6.

Nursing intervention Relieve pressure as often as the patient's condition demands by changing the patient's position and the use of appropriate aids.

Disuse osteoporosis

Inactivity and lack of weight bearing results in loss of calcium from the skeletal system. Bones become more liable to fracture.

Nursing intervention Nurses are unable to prevent osteoporosis, but can minimize the risks by encouraging active exercises and positioning limbs carefully. In some cases it may be appropriate to raise the head of the bed for several hours per day. This simulates weight-bearing stress.

Renal calculi

Calcium lost from the skeletal system is excreted by the kidneys. This increased calcium excretion may lead to the formation of kidney stones. Formation of stones is fully discussed in Chapter 17.

Nursing intervention Encourage an increased fluid intake and active exercises.

Difficulty with micturition

Lying supine and lack of privacy make it difficult for patients to relax the perineal and sphincter muscles.

Nursing intervention An empathetic manner and the use of slipper bedpans can help to overcome this problem.

Constipation

Neither lying supine nor sitting with the knees extended will promote the normal reflexes necessary for defaecation.

Nursing intervention Help the patient to achieve as normal a position as possible. An increased fibre intake may help, particularly with the elderly patient.

Thrombosis

This results from stasis of blood in the lower limbs, and is fully discussed in Chapter 12.

Nursing intervention Encourage active exercises hourly. Anti-embolus stockings can be worn in bed.

Postural hypotension

Postural hypotension (see Ch. 12) results from sudden pooling of blood in the abdominal viscera and legs following confinement to bed for long periods and is very common in patients with paralysis following spinal cord injury. On assuming the upright position the patient may experience vertigo. Fainting may occur.

Nursing intervention Application of support stockings while on bed rest helps to minimize the effects of blood pooling in the legs. Sitting the patient up for short periods prior to ambulation is also beneficial in preventing postural hypotension.

Disorders of the locomotor system can be classified as traumatic, inflammatory, degenerative, metabolic, congenital and neoplastic. The remainder of this chapter will cover the most common condition occurring in each category.

TRAUMATIC DISORDERS

FRACTURES

A fracture is an interruption in the continuity of bone. It is most commonly caused by injury but can also occur due to a pathological defect in the bone. All age groups are susceptible to fractures as a result of accidents, for example, falls, sports injuries, car accidents, accidents in the workplace, but some age groups are more susceptible to certain types of fractures. The elderly, in particular elderly women, are prone to falling and sustaining fractures to the neck of the femur, whereas sports players often sustain fractures of the lower leg due to the abnormal rotational forces applied to the bones.

Whether it is the small bones in the hand which are affected or the femur in the upper leg, fractures cause a great deal of pain for patients and result in periods of disability. For some individuals, a fractured bone may signal the end of a promising career; for example, musicians may lose the function in their fingers, sports players may damage their legs so badly that they never regain their former athletic ability. For others it may mean a few weeks of inconvenience; not being able to drive a car because their arm is in plaster. For some, such as the elderly, it may lead to

Nursing Care Plan 11.1   Care of an elderly patient with a fractured right neck of femur

Problem	Goal	Nursing action	Rationale
1. Difficulty with communication due to anxiety or confusion on admission	To relieve anxiety and orientate patient to time and place	❒ Introduction to staff and ward and explain actions in simple terms. Identify any anxieties the patient may have regarding home circumstances or hospital admission	If the patient understands what is happening to him/her, he/she will be more able to comply with treatment. Relieving anxiety will also help to promote a trusting relationship.
2. Pain/deformity	To overcome muscle spasm, relieve pain and immobilize affected limb, and prevent deformity To reduce pain and encourage active exercise post-operatively	❒ Carefully check the limb to rule out signs of skin damage, oedema, circulatory impairment, apply balanced skin traction to the affected limb with appropriate weights as directed by the surgeon (normally 2–4 lb). Leg may be supported on a pillow. Offer analgesia as prescribed. Foot of the bed may be slightly elevated	Traction is applied to overcome muscle spasm. This should help to relieve pain. Skin traction should not be applied to previously damaged or susceptible skin. Balanced traction requires the foot of the bed to be elevated but in some patients this may be contraindicated. Relieving pain also helps to reduce blood pressure and increases patient compliance
3. Possible complications of skin traction	Prevent	❒ Neurovascular checks carried out at regular intervals. Skin extensions should be re-applied 4 hourly or more frequently if necessary	Skin extensions may have been incorrectly applied. Loss of circulation, sensation or movement in the extremities must be identified quickly to prevent further damage to the limb, e.g. ischaemia
4. Loss of mobility prior to and following surgery	To restore function of the limb, achieve mobility To prevent complications of bed rest	❒ On admission identify previous mobility status, e.g. was the patient walking independently, or did she require the use of aids ❒ Pressure area care, active exercises, deep breathing and coughing exercises should be carried out at regular intervals	A knowledge of the patient's previous mobility status allows realistic goals to be set for the patient postoperatively Complications of bed rest can arise very quickly in elderly people, which could affect their mobility and lengthen their stay in hospital
5. Potential elimination problems due to bed rest, traction and pain	To prevent urinary retention or constipation	❒ Bedpans should be offered at regular intervals ❒ The affected leg should be supported on a pillow. Slipper bedpans may be more comfortable for the patient to use ❒ Protect the bed linen in case of accidents	Promote urinary continence at all times Promote patient comfort Very distressing for the patient if the bed linen has to be changed often
6. Fasting for theatre	To prevent dehydration occurring while the patient is fasting for theatre. Correct fluid/ electrolyte imbalance prior to surgery. To maintain or improve nutritional status	❒ Intravenous therapy should be administered as prescribed. Observe patient for signs of dehydration, e.g. dry mouth, skin, confusion. Also observe for signs of fluid overload	Safe administration of intravenous fluids Prevent problems during anaesthesia due to electrolyte imbalance Prevent postoperative urinary complications A good nutritional status promotes wound healing

Nursing Care Plan 11.1 (*cont'd*)			
Problem	**Goal**	**Nursing action**	**Rationale**
7. Surgery	To prevent/minimize complications	❑ Adequate physical preparation of the patient for theatre. Explanations offered about postoperative care	Reduce/prevent postoperative complications
8. Unconsciousness	Maintain airway and a safe environment	❑ Nurse the patient in the recovery position on her unaffected side. Oxygen and suction equipment should be nearby	Maintain airway without increasing pain
9. Inability to maintain position of affected limb postoperatively	To prevent deformity, to maintain function and prevent contractures developing postoperatively	❑ Nurse the patient with pillows between her legs while in bed. She may be nursed on her back or unaffected side	Abduction of the hips should be maintained Since the muscles have been divided at operation the limb must be supported until function is restored. If the joint has been replaced this also helps to prevent dislocation of the prosthesis
10. Pain	To reduce and encourage active exercise	❑ Offer analgesia as prescribed	If the patient is pain free, she will be more able to mobilize
11. Effects of anaesthesia and surgery	Early detection of postoperative complications	❑ Recordings of temperature, pulse, blood pressure, respirations, neurovascular checks, wound and drain checks are made at regular intervals. Urinary output is recorded and deep breathing and coughing exercises are encouraged	Early detection of complications allows appropriate nursing/medical intervention to be made as soon as possible. Drains can be removed when their output is minimal
12. Loss of mobility	To restore or improve mobility	❑ As soon as able, the patient should be sat up in bed and encouraged to carry out active exercises. Mobilization usually begins on the first postoperative day. Patient should be assessed for appropriate walking aids. Shoes or good fitting slippers should be worn ❑ Patient should be helped out of bed maintaining abduction of the hips ❑ A high chair should be used when sitting. Both feet should touch the floor and be pointing forward. Do not allow the patient to twist, swivel or flex at the hip to pick up things ❑ Gradually increase amount of mobility and re-assess for walking aids	Patient should be mobilized as early as possible to reduce complications of bed rest. Also helps to overcome fear when the patient realizes her leg will bear his/her weight. Weight bearing promotes bone healing. Good fitting shoes reduce the possibility of accidents and also give support Maintaining the normal position of function reduces the possibility of loss of mobility Correct positioning in the chair aids recovery and prevents contracture from developing As patient's confidence increases and as muscle power returns, he/she will be able to walk further, becoming more independent and relying less on aids

Nursing Care Plan 11.1 (cont'd)

Problem	Goal	Nursing action	Rationale
13. Difficulty with elimination	Prevent constipation, promote urinary continence and increase independence	❐ Well-balanced diet encouraged as soon as patient is able to eat	Reduces/minimizes the need for laxatives
		❐ Encourage mobility. Ensure that the patient understands the need to use a raised toilet seat	Promotes peristalsis. Understanding promotes compliance. Must prevent overflexion at the hip joint
		❐ Maintain safety in the toilet area, e.g. use of hand rails	Promotes independence
14. Difficulty with dressing	Promote independence	❐ Encourage patient to dress herself. Occupational therapy assessment may be necessary to identify need for dressing aids	Patient will feel better when dressed. Aids will help the patient to gain independence and prevent complications of twisting and bending
15. Discharge home	To prepare the patient physically and psychologically for discharge To promote independence and safety in the home environment	❐ If necessary a home visit should be arranged in order to assess the patient in their own environment	The home environment needs to be safe for a patient with limited mobility
		❐ Referrals to other agencies, e.g. social work, district nurse, should be made well in advance of discharge date ❐ Discuss any anxieties with the patient and her relatives. Ensure the patient understands the range of movements she can make to avoid complications. Offer information and advice about drug therapy and outpatient appointments	Arrangements need to be made in advance if raised toilet seats or hand rails or other aids are needed in the home. Any anxieties need to be aired prior to discharge to make the transfer as easy as possible for all concerned. Patient must be able to identify signs and symptoms of possible complications and who to contact if they arise

a loss of mobility which in turn leads to a loss of independence and probable admission to a long-term care of the elderly unit. (See Nursing Case Plan 11.1).

The majority of accidents are preventable and a great deal of emphasis is placed on accident prevention in all age groups by community health services, voluntary agencies, occupational health workers, schools, the police force and the media. Fractures are easily acquired, but not so easily resolved.

Very few people die as a direct result of sustaining a fracture. Those who do, generally have some other pathology such as the puncture of a major organ, multiple injuries, fat embolism (see 'Complications of fractures' below) or in the case of elderly patients, chest infection. People who suffer from fractures are generally not 'sick'. They are usually physically quite fit and are suffering from a mechanical breakdown rather than a physiological one.

Signs and symptoms of a fracture

1. **Pain** may be localized to the site of injury and throbbing in character. It is made worse by any attempt at movement.

2. **Loss of function** because of the instability of the bone and the pain.

3. **Swelling** caused by haematoma formation and local oedema.

4. **Deformity** resulting from the abnormal position of the bony ends.

5. **Shortening of the limb** as a result of the overriding of the bony ends and muscle spasm. This does not occur in impacted fractures (Fig. 11.6).

6. **Abnormal mobility** will occur in an unstable fracture, e.g. movement may be seen between the knee and ankle in a tibial fracture.

7. **Crepitus** is the grating sound which can be

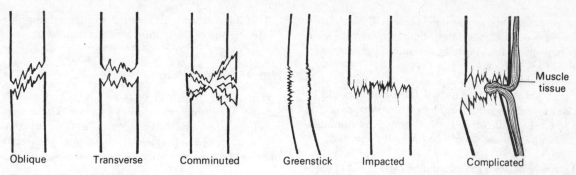

Oblique   Transverse   Comminuted   Greenstick   Impacted   Complicated — Muscle tissue

Fig. 11.6 Classification of fractures

heard when the two bony ends rub together. This should never be intentionally produced as it is extremely painful to the patient.

Classification of fractures

A simple (or closed) fracture is one in which the bone is broken but the skin remains intact. There may be some local injury to soft tissue.

A compound (or open) fracture is one in which the bone is broken and there is an open wound on the skin, allowing communication between the bone and the air.

Fractures are further classified into different types (Fig. 11.6).

A stable fracture is one in which either the bone ends are undisplaced and do not require to be re-aligned or, following realignment, they maintain their position easily. An incomplete fracture falls into this category. A complete fracture may be stable or unstable. An unstable fracture is one in which the bone ends are displaced and are easily displaced following realignment. Fracture stability is tested while the patient is under general anaesthetic – the surgeon attempts to displace the fracture once he has achieved a good realignment of the bone ends.

Table 11.2 shows complications that can arise from fractures.

Significance of nursing role in establishing differential diagnosis

Any person who has suffered a fracture requires to have observations carried out to assess the extent of damage to nerves, blood vessels and muscles.

Observations of circulation, sensation and movement (neurovascular checks)

Circulation If the blood supply to the extremities

Table 11.2	Complications of fractures
Immediate: occurring within the first few hours	Haemorrhage Damage to nerves and blood vessels Damage to internal organs Damage to surrounding soft tissue
Early: occurring within the first few days	Wound infection Fat embolism Chest infections
Late	Malunion of fracture Delayed union of fracture Non-union of fracture Avascular necrosis

has been interrupted as a result of a fracture, the tissue can become ischaemic in a very short space of time, resulting in permanent damage if appropriate treatment is not given. It is *essential* to note the colour and warmth of the affected fingers or toes and to check for pulses. There should be a quick return of blood to the area following release of digital pressure (blanching test). Limbs should be warm and a good colour but it is vital that a comparison is made with the unaffected limb as it may be 'normal' for an individual to have cold or mottled coloured feet, particularly in the elderly. It is also important to clean the toes or fingers and remove nail varnish so that their colour can be clearly seen. In individuals with heavily pigmented skin it is better to carry out the blanching effect on the toe or finger nails rather than the surrounding skin.

Sensation If nerves have been damaged the patient may suffer alterations to sensation and movement. Since different nerves supply different fingers or toes, it is important to check each one individually. It is not enough to pinch the great toe or one finger and conclude the sensation is good. Patients may complain of numbness and tingling, increasing pain on movement or a burning sensation, particularly if pressure is being applied to a nerve.

Movement The full range of movements available at each joint should be tested. The patient should be asked to fully extend and flex each toe or finger and to touch each finger with the thumb. Any diminishment in movement should be promptly reported.

The above observations should be carried out at regular intervals and any deterioration quickly reported. Accurate reporting of these observations can help the orthopaedic surgeon to identify the specific structures affected and initiate appropriate surgical intervention.

Patient history

During the admission procedure it is necessary for the nurse to record:

1. Previous conditions associated with the locomotor system.
2. An accurate account of the recent accident, if possible.
3. Level of function of the limb(s) prior to the accident.
4. Patient's occupation/life-style.

This information will be used to plan appropriate treatment and rehabilitation for each patient.

Range of investigations

Fractures are confirmed by X-ray examination. This can be a painful procedure for patients and they require support and encouragement in order to comply with the radiographer's instructions. Analgesia may be administered prior to X-ray examination.

Therapeutic management

Summary of bone healing (Fig. 11.7)

(A detailed description can be found in Dandy 1989).

1. For the first 2 weeks, bone healing forms the same pattern as the healing of any wound. The wound site is filled with blood and the broken ends of the bone become necrotic.
2. The blood clot is invaded by macrophages and osteoclasts which effectively clean the area and new blood vessels grow to provide an adequate blood supply.
3. Between 2 and 6 weeks after injury, new bone tissue develops and forms a firm mass, or callus, around the fracture. Osteoblasts are active in this phase.

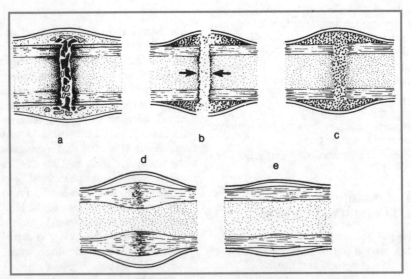

Fig. 11.7 Healing of bones. **A**, First 2 weeks, blood clot and macrophages form around the fracture. **B**, 2–6 weeks, sharp edges are removed by osteoclasts and callus forms within the haematoma and the medullary cavity. **C**, 6–12 weeks bone forms within the callus and bridges the gap between the fragments. **D**, 6–12 months, the cortical gap is bridged with bone. **E**, 1–2 years, remodelling occurs and normal anatomical architecture returns. (Reproduced with permission from Dandy 1989, p. 46)

4. Between 6 and 12 weeks, ossification occurs and the bone begins to regain some of its mechanical strength.

5. Between 6 and 12 months, depending on the site of the fracture, the gap between the fractured bone ends closes.

6. Between 1 and 2 years, remodelling by osteoclasts takes place to restore the bone's original shape.

There are three basic principles to be observed in the treatment of fractures:

1. Reduction or realignment of the fracture. The surgeon, by means of traction and gentle manipulation, counteracts the muscle pull and restores normal alignment to the bone.

2. Maintenance of the realignment by immobilization until healing (bony union) occurs.

3. Restoration of full physical function.

Methods of immobilizing a fracture

Some form of fixation or splintage is required to hold the bone ends in alignment until healing occurs. This may be achieved by:

1. External splinting such as a plaster cast. Usually used with closed fractures which are stable.

2. Internal fixation involving surgery, during which wires, nails, or screws are used to hold the fracture securely. This is indicated when the fracture cannot be controlled in other ways, the bone is broken in two or more places or the blood supply to the bones must be protected.

3. Traction (the application of a pulling force). Indicated by the patient's physical condition, type of fracture and surgeon's preference.

4. External fixation which involves the insertion of pins through the bones above and below the fracture and being held in place by a clamp. Usually used in severe open fractures where there is a large amount of tissue loss.

Emergency treatment of fractures

Following a fracture of a limb, a person is liable to suffer from shock, in particular hypovolaemic shock and shock resulting from the pain. The signs, symptoms and care of patients suffering from hypovolaemic shock are discussed in Chapter 12.

Resuscitation of the patient takes priority, ensuring that a clear airway is established. In people who have sustained small fractures, the degree of shock will be minimal compared to those individuals who suffer major or multiple fractures, therefore a quick assessment of the patient's general condition is needed to establish the degree of resuscitation required. The injured limb(s) must be handled with care in order to prevent disturbing clot formation and to reduce pain.

Obvious bleeding should be stopped by applying pressure over the bleeding point. In some cases this will not suffice and a tourniquet will be required. It is imperative that the **time of application** of the tourniquet is noted and that the tourniquet is **released** as soon as bleeding has been controlled or at least once every hour to prevent gangrene of the limb. If it is possible to raise the limb above the level of the heart this will assist in reducing bleeding and improve perfusion of the vital organs. Open wounds should then be covered with a clean dressing.

Pain can be relieved to some extent by temporary splinting. In an emergency situation the body and limbs can be used to provide splintage; for example, splint one leg against the other or splint an arm to the torso. A rolled-up newspaper provides excellent splintage for fractures of limbs or the neck. The homemade splint can be gently secured to the limb using ties or bandages.

It is unwise for untrained first-aiders to reduce fractures at the scene of the accident. It is more important that a safe environment is provided for the injured person. Injured people should not be moved any more than necessary and victims trapped in cars should be left there until emergency services arrive. Make sure it is safe to approach crashed vehicles and then switch off car engines to reduce the possibility of explosions. Check the victim's airway and pulses, offer reassurance and then stop oncoming traffic before further accidents happen. Keeping a regular check on the airway, pulse rate and carrying out neurovascular checks will help the emergency services in making diagnoses on their arrival at the accident scene. Once the emergency services have been contacted, keeping the victim warm and as calm as possible is the next priority.

Nursing strategies

Care of a patient in plaster

The diagnosis, reduction and immobilization of fractures is the province of the orthopaedic surgeon. If external splintage of the fracture is the chosen method of immobilization, the surgeon will be closely involved with its application. Diagnosis, reduction and immobilization all take place within a matter of a few hours or, at most, a day or two. The period of immobilization necessary for healing to occur extends for many weeks (6–8 weeks for an upper limb, 3 months and longer for a major weight-bearing bone). It is this period of healing which is the prime concern of the nurse.

Plaster of Paris is still widely used for making casts. It is comparatively soft and easily moulded around the affected limb. It is porous, so the limb can 'breathe' and it is easily removed. This is important in trauma because often a plaster will become loose after the initial swelling has subsided and it has to be replaced. Its disadvantage is that it can take 2–3 days to dry. There are many other materials available on the market today, including resins and fibreglass. They are much quicker drying and some are water-proof. Whichever material is used, the care of a patient wearing a plaster is similar.

Maintaining a safe environment Plaster of Paris is applied to a limb over padding which protects bony prominences. It is applied wet so that it can be moulded to the contours of the limb and into the best shape to maintain good reduction of the fracture. As the plaster dries, an exothermic reaction takes place and the plaster feels warm to the patient. It also feels very heavy. Preparation of the bed area is essential. A firm mattress and a bed cradle are important. Waterproof pillows covered with a towel are needed to support the wet cast. Blankets will be needed to keep the patient warm as the plaster begins to cool.

When the patient arrives in the ward a quick assessment should be made of his general condition. The plaster will immobilize the joints on either side of the fracture and any movement of the patient should be carefully planned to prevent damaging the plaster until the plaster is set. It is important to use the palms of the hands when handling a plaster and not the fingers as any indentations on the plaster could cause pressure on the underlying skin. The plaster should be supported along its length and the affected limb elevated. It is important that the plaster does not crack, as this will reduce its strength and allow movement to occur.

When the patient has been made comfortable in bed, colour, sensation and movement checks should be carried out at frequent, regular intervals. It may well be necessary to wash the skin around the plaster, as this not only improves the patient's comfort, but also allows more accurate recordings to be made. These recordings will continue until the plaster is dry and then the patient can be taught to check them himself so that he is confident in caring for the plaster on discharge and will be able to recognize any early signs of complications. Instructions on this

are usually given to the patient on discharge from hospital (Box 11.2).

It is important that the plaster is allowed to dry naturally. Artificial heat should not be used. To this end the plastered limb is often left uncovered or a bed cradle is used to allow a circulation of air around the plaster. The patient may require to be turned 1–2 hourly to allow different aspects of the plaster to dry evenly. If the towel under the plaster becomes wet it should be changed so as not to hinder the drying process. It is during this stage that the patient may complain of feeling cold because the plaster begins to become very cold and damp. While caring for the patient it is important that the nurse uses all his senses. The limb and plaster must be continually observed for signs of swelling, irritation, leakage from wounds and cracks. The nurse must use his sense of smell to detect any early signs of infections and he must listen to any complaints of discomfort or increasing pain that the patient makes. The nurse's sense of touch can help locate hot areas on a plaster which are covering a sore. Prompt and accurate re-porting of changes in a patient's condition will save him from unnecessary discomfort and the possible loss of a limb. As the patient feels better and the nurse is confident that his condition is stable, he should be encouraged, by explanation and reassur-ance, to take over the responsibility of caring for his own plaster.

The five problem signs to look out for in a plaster cast are shown in Box 11.1.

Mobility When a patient first fractures a limb, he is often afraid to move any part of the limb in case it hurts. It is most important that active exercises commence as soon as possible to minimize muscle wasting and joint stiffness. The patient should be given gentle encouragement and explanations of why movement is important. Active exercises should be carried out at regular, frequent intervals; for example, static quadriceps exercises are begun as early as possi-ble following the immobilization of a leg in plaster. This is achieved by straight-leg raising exercises and is important in enabling the patient to support the weight of the plaster cast when he is mobilizing. Patients wearing full leg casts are not allowed to use

---

Box 11.1 Cardinal symptoms of a tight plaster
• Pain
• Pallor
• Pulselessness
• Paraesthesia
• Paralysis

crutches until they can straight-leg raise, with the heel leaving the bed surface.

As the patient's condition improves, mobility will be encouraged. If the plaster encases the foot it is possible for the patient to wear a sandal with velcro fastenings. This can be easily removed before the patient goes to bed and is more hygienic than having a rocker attached to the plaster. When the patient is resting, the affected limb should be elevated to prevent oedema in the extremities. This also applies when plasters have been applied to the upper limbs.

Careful assessment of the patient and accurate identification of potential problems will help the nurse and physiotherapist to decide which type of walking aid is appropriate for each patient. There are many mobility aids available and generally speaking, as rehabilitation progresses and the patient gains independence, the use of mobility aids reduces from cumbersome, high zimmer frames or crutches, to tripods or walking sticks. It is important that patients are taught the correct use of walking aids and that they are seen to be using them safely prior to discharge. If necessary, they should be taught to climb stairs safely before going home.

Breathing Careful assessment of respiratory function is necessary to detect early signs and symptoms of fat embolism which can occlude the lumen of blood vessels. There are two theories on the occurrence of fat embolism: it may arise from fat globules which leave the bone marrow at the time of the fracture or, alternatively, as a result of trauma, chemical changes may occur within the blood and fat is produced which then circulates in the blood stream and finally lodges in the capillaries of the pulmonary circulation (see Ch. 13) leading to hypoxia and tissue death. Whatever the cause, symptoms develop within 24–48 hours following trauma. The nurse should assess the patient's mental state for mood changes or confusion which result from hypoxia in the brain. Often this is the first indication of developing fat embolism and if it is promptly reported, arterial blood gas analysis can be carried out and a low Po_2 content (see Ch. 13) would confirm the diagnosis. Later symptoms include drowsiness, worsening dyspnoea, respiratory distress, tachycardia and the development of a petechial rash (small pin-head-size red spots) over the upper chest, axillae and conjunctiva. The earlier a diagnosis is made, the better the prognosis. Treatment is largely with oxygen therapy and assisted ventilation if necessary. Should fat embolism develop, it is important that the nurse stays near the patient to offer quiet reassurance and encouragement. This situation is very distressing for the relatives who will require time, patience, explanations and support. Care of the patient during X-ray examination will be required and also during the transfer to a high dependency unit. It is unusual for fat embolism to occur more than 72 hours following injury.

Elimination This can cause embarrassment to patients wearing full-length leg plasters or plasters which include the hip joints and terminate at waist level. Plasters are carefully trimmed and bound to allow the patient to use a bedpan or urinal and to leave access for perineal and anal toilet. To prevent soiling or wetting the plaster, however, the nurse must develop some skill in the positioning of sanitary utensils. If the situation is adequately assessed before the utensil is positioned it can help to prevent accidents and reduce embarrassment.

1. If the hip joint is enclosed within the plaster it is better to use a slipper bedpan and to roll the patient onto it.
2. Place an absorbent pad at the cast edge as an additional safeguard but remove it with the bedpan.
3. Use pillows to support the patient's back and limbs whilst using the bedpan, particularly if the patient is wearing a long-leg plaster.
4. Taking time to position the bedpan properly pays dividends.

Immobility predisposes to constipation and urinary problems so tactful observation of elimination is important, particularly in the elderly. If the nurse anticipates problems she should encourage an increased fluid intake and a high fibre diet. Privacy and tact are also required. As mobility improves the nurse should see a reduction in elimination problems. If the plaster becomes heavily soiled the nurse should report it immediately and steps taken to protect the underlying skin. As the patient progresses he should be taught how to support his lower limbs while using the toilet to prevent damaging the plaster. It is useful to advise relatives to keep a foot stool in the toilet at home which can be used to support a plastered leg, and the use of raised toilet seats and handles are beneficial, particularly for elderly people. Occupational therapists or district nurses would be able to advise on the availability of the above aids for home use, and this should be arranged prior to the patient's discharge from hospital.

Work and play Because patients with fractures are rarely ill after recovering from the immediate trauma, they require a great deal of diversional therapy. Time can weigh heavily on their hands so it is useful to discuss with them ways of filling the hours. As previously stated, fractures can seriously affect an indi-

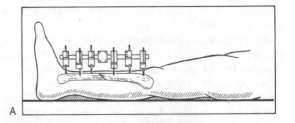

vidual's career and this should be borne in mind when dealing with a depressed patient. The nurse should aim to build up a trusting relationship with the patient in order to create the appropriate environment to allow these problems to be aired. Relatives may be included in discussions if the patient so wishes. Rehabilitation following a fracture can be a long and painful process and the nurse must be supportive, encouraging and realistic in her approach to the development of each patient's rehabilitation programme. Often the nurse has to take on the role of a referral agency by liaising with physiotherapists and social workers, to provide as comprehensive a rehabilitation programme as possible to facilitate the patient's return to maximum well-being.

When the patient is ready for discharge he, or his relatives, should be fully conversant with the care of the limb in plaster. The advice shown in Box 11.2 should be given.

Care of a patient following external fixation of fractures

Some forms of traction involve positioning a pin through a bone to ensure good alignment and provide immobilization of the fractures. In external fixation, several pins are inserted into the bones and are held together on the outside by a clamp (Fig. 11.8).

Maintaining a safe environment Once the external fixator is in position the fracture site is immobilized and the nurse is able to carry out wound care as required. Prevention of infection which could cause osteomyelitis is of paramount importance. Key-hole dressings are usually applied around each pin-site to keep them clean and dry. There has been much debate about dressing pin-sites but they do prevent patients picking scabs which form around the pins. Strict aseptic technique should be used during dressings. External fixators can be used to treat a wide range

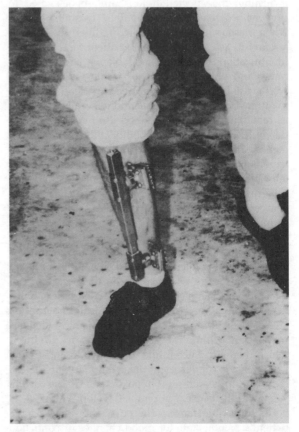

B

Fig. 11.8   External fixator. **A**, External fixation of the tibia. **B**, An external fixator in position. (Reproduced with permission from Dandy 1989, p. 126)

of fractures in long bones, from finger fractures to leg fractures. They can be worn for several months but, unlike traction, the patient has greater mobility, thereby reducing the complications of bed rest.

Caring for a patient following internal fixation of a fracture

Orthopaedic surgery has advanced rapidly over the last few years and many fractures can now be safely immobilized by internal fixation. Surgery is not always carried out immediately and is often delayed until local oedema settles and the numbers of osteoblasts present at the fracture site have increased. Dandy (1989) provides detailed information regarding the choice of method of fixation and the specific care required. The following is merely an overview of important aspects of nursing care. For the detailed nursing care of a patient following internal fixation of a hip fracture see Nursing Care Plan 11.1.

Maintaining a safe environment Prevention of infection takes high priority with orthopaedic surgery. Should any organisms enter the wound there is the possibility that they could invade the bone tissue, causing osteomyelitis (infection in bone). This is a very serious complication causing severe pain and discomfort to the patient, and in some instances can result in life-long, crippling deformity or disablement. If this occurs, the treatment is rigorous with antibiotics, strict bed rest and is prolonged. In order to prevent infection, the following points should be noted:

1. Preoperative skin preparation should be careful and meticulous.
2. Surgical techniques in the operating theatre should be scrupulous.
3. Care and attention must be paid to dressings to keep them clean and intact.
4. Aseptic wound dressing techniques must be used.
5. Patients with clean wounds should be kept away from any whose wounds have become infected.

Wound and neurovascular assessments should be carried out at frequent intervals and any dressings should be left undisturbed for as long as possible.

Mobility In order to prevent problems with mobility, the nurse should be aware of how to maintain limbs in positions of normal function using pillows as necessary. The nurse should encourage the patient to carry out active exercises as soon as possible following recovery from anaesthetic. Patients should be mobilized at the earliest opportunity, reducing the amount of time spent on bed rest with its inherent complications.

Caring for a patient in traction

Traction is applied to a limb for the following reasons:

1. To restore and maintain the alignment of fractures.
2. To overcome muscle spasm and reduce pain.
3. To correct deformities due to muscle contractures.

4. To rest painful joints and maintain their position of function.

Principles of traction When a force is applied to a limb to pull it in one direction, there must be an equal force pulling in the opposite direction. This opposing force is referred to as counter-traction and is necessary if effective traction (tension) is to be maintained. There are several methods used to achieve traction.

Skin traction Traction is applied to the skin and thus indirectly to the skeletal system. Various tapes or bandages can be used to provide adhesion and because they extend beyond the length of the limb, they are referred to as skin extensions. When these skin extensions are attached to a weight or splint, they allow a pull to be exerted on the skin and skeletal system. This pull must be in the correct direction to achieve maximum effect.

Fixed traction In fixed traction the limb is generally supported in a splint and the skin extensions are tied to the distal end of the splint. The ring at the proximal end of the splint rests against a fixed point such as

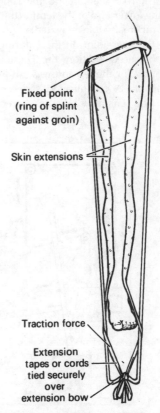

Fixed point
(ring of splint
against groin)

Skin extensions

Traction force

Extension
tapes or cords
tied securely
over
extension bow

Fig. 11.9 Fixed traction. (Note: the ring fits snugly into the groin, but the point of pressure (not shown) is the ischial tuberosity)

the axilla or, if a Thomas splint is used, the ischial tuberosity (Fig. 11.9). When a Thomas splint is used, slings support the leg in the splint and pads are positioned to maintain the optimum position of the knee. As this splint is heavy, it is usual to arrange a system of pulleys and weights to counter-balance the weight of the splinted leg. In this case, the weights act as a device to aid the patient's mobility in bed and are **not** involved in the maintenance of traction.

Balanced traction A state of traction is achieved by using metal weights as the traction force and the patient's body weight as the counter-traction (Fig. 11.10). The degree to which the bed is elevated and the amount of weight applied will depend upon the weight of the patient, but both must be sufficient to maintain a balanced pull. The patient must not slide up or be pulled down the bed by excessive weight in either direction. The greater the weight applied, the higher the bed has to be elevated.

Balanced traction can be achieved using skin traction (see p. 369) or skeletal traction. In skeletal traction a pin is inserted through the bone. The most common sites for insertion of the pin are the rounded prominences of the lower end of the femur (the condyles) or the tibial tuberosity (an elevated region of bone found below the knee joint on the anterior aspect of the tibia). In balanced traction, the Thomas splint is used as a support for the leg and it is not involved in achieving traction. A complicated series of weights and pulleys will ensure that the correct amount of traction is achieved and that the line of pull on the bone/joint is in the correct direction to achieve satisfactory healing.

Maintaining a safe environment Neurovascular checks should be carried out at frequent intervals when the traction is first applied and at regular intervals until it is removed. If balanced traction is being used (weights and pulleys), then the cords attached to the weights must be able to run smoothly over the pulleys. The weights should hang freely and be moved as little as possible since vibrations can travel up the cord and through the limb creating minute movement at the fracture site, prolonging bone healing and causing pain.

If fixed traction has been applied then the skin underneath the ring of the splint needs to be checked regularly. Generally speaking, the ring fits snugly over the skin and if there is any swelling present, pressure sores can develop. To avoid this the nurse must keep the area clean and dry by 2-hourly attention and teach the patient to ease the tissue gently under the ring to a different position every hour or each time he feels discomfort, whichever is the more frequent.

Most patients are allowed to sit up in bed for short periods. By alternating sitting and lying positions, pressure on the skin is redistributed and the function of the hip joint is maintained. It is important that the body remains in alignment to achieve traction. If a patient is lying to one side or slouched over while

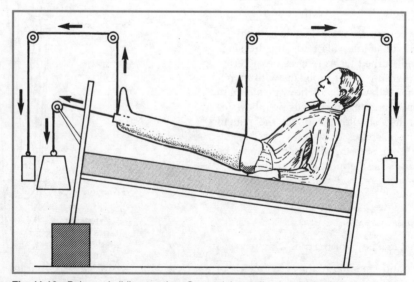

Fig. 11.10 Balanced sliding traction. One weight applies longitudinal traction and others are applied to the upper and lower ends of the limb so that it 'floats' in a gravity-free field. (Reproduced with permission from Dandy 1989, p. 121)

in a sitting position, the 'pull' will not be in a straight line and traction will not be achieved.

Active exercise to all joints must be encouraged and appropriate nursing care to prevent complications of bed rest (see p. 358) must be initiated. It is possible to have patients, young and elderly, in traction for 3–4 months without complications arising. (For care of pin sites, see p. 368.)

Controlling body temperature Ensuring the warmth and comfort of the patient on traction also requires some thought. The bed linen must often be arranged in a different manner to allow the traction cords to run freely or to accommodate a splint. This results in a series of very uncomfortable draughts for the patient. Use of warm socks and small extra blankets will help to prevent this discomfort. The patient may also feel exposed and vulnerable in the 'divided-bed' that is necessary to accommodate traction. As normal briefs cannot be worn because of the traction equipment, modesty pants which tie at the side should be provided for the patient's peace of mind.

Eating and drinking The nurse should take into account the patient's lack of mobility and position when serving food. The diet should be appetizing, with a high fibre content and 2–3 litres of fluid offered each day. Since some patients will require to eat in the supine position, food should be cut into manageable-sized bites and appropriate cutlery offered. For some people, a spoon may be preferable to a fork. Bendable drinking straws or plastic feeder-type mugs should be used to avoid unnecessary spillage.

Elimination Similar to caring for a patient with a plaster, a slipper bedpan is often more comfortable. The limb in traction should be well supported with pillows and with bed-fast patients it is especially important to ensure they are offered hand-washing facilities following elimination.

Work and play If the patient is trying to read while lying supine, prism spectacles can be used to make it less fatiguing.

AMPUTATION

Relevant epidemiology and aetiology

Loss of part, or all, of a limb can cause severe problems for a patient. Whether it is a finger tip or a leg, the impact of the surgery can be equally devastating for the patient concerned. Amputation is often carried out by surgeons to remove diseased limbs but for some individuals, accidents are the cause of the amputation. Indications for amputations are given in Box 11.3.

Amputations are not carried out without a great deal of consultation and counselling. For the majority of patients amputations bring tremendous relief from years of severe pain and markedly reduced mobility. For others it can mean a loss of independence, loss of self-esteem and loss of employment.

Common symptomatology

Mobility For those patients who are being considered for amputation because of disease process, lack of mobility, pain levels and presence or absence of ischaemia and infection help to make the decision. These patients will have been reviewed in peripheral vascular disease clinics or orthopaedic clinics and will have undergone many investigations and treatments before the decision to amputate is made.

Diabetes This is fully discussed in Chapter 16 and the patient's diabetes must be reasonably controlled, prior to surgery.

Atherosclerosis This condition is fully discussed in Chapter 12.

Patient implications

Weight loss and cessation of smoking prior to surgery are very important to promote wound healing postoperatively and achieve a successful rehabilitation. Such patients may need a great deal of support and encouragement if they are to change habits of a life-time.

Range of investigations

For details of investigations in atherosclerosis and diabetes, refer to relevant chapters.

Box 11.3 Indications for amputation	
Vascular disease	Diabetes or atherosclerosis can reduce the blood supply to a limb causing ischaemia and ultimately gangrene
Pain	Severe pain caused by ischaemia may only be relieved by amputation
Trauma	Limbs may be damaged beyond repair, severely crushed, or amputated in an accident
Frost bite or burns	Circulation to the limb is reduced causing ischaemia.
Tumours	Malignant tumours may metastasize
Infection	Osteomyelitis or gas gangrene which become uncontrolled necessitate amputation
Congenital deformities	

Therapeutic management

The level of amputation is dependent upon the severity of the disease process. In order to achieve successful recovery, the tissue must be healthy where the amputation is made.

In traumatic amputations it is important to protect the viable tissue, control bleeding and reduce the possibility of infection. If part, or all, of a limb is traumatically amputated, that part should be kept moist and cold and should accompany the victim to hospital. With the advances in microsurgery it is possible to save severed limbs, if the surgery can be carried out promptly and the amputated limb is in good condition.

Nursing strategies

The rehabilitation of a patient following amputation involves all members of the multidisciplinary team, consisting of nurses, physiotherapists, prosthetic consultants and social workers.

The aims in caring for an amputee are listed in Box 11.4.

Breathing Deep breathing and coughing exercises should be encouraged to prevent respiratory infection, particularly if the patient has been a heavy smoker.

Mobility Successful fitting of a prosthesis is dependent upon achieving a good stump shape and joint function. To achieve this the nurse must assess the stump regularly. In the initial postoperative phase the stump is bandaged and neurovascular and wound checks should be carried out without removing the bandage. The stump bandage should be kept on for at least 48 hours postoperatively, and should then be re-applied daily. Inexperienced nurses should not re-apply bandages as incorrect application can result in delayed healing and skin damage.

To maintain a good stump shape the foot of the bed should be elevated to help relieve oedema. Pillows should not be placed under the stump as this can lead to contractures of the hip joint in flexion. Correct bandaging methods should be employed and a stump shrinker bandage can be applied 10 days postoperatively. Exercise and ambulation should begin as soon as possible. When dressings are taken down, the incision line can be gently moved in order to prevent the formation of adhesions. Gradually, the stump should be handled more in order to desensitize it prior to limb fitting. Massage and transcutaneous electrical nerve stimulation (TENS) can also be used by experienced practitioners.

To prevent joint contractures, placing the limb in a position of function is necessary. Lying prone for a period each day is advocated to encourage extension of the hip joint and sitting for prolonged periods should be discouraged. When the patient is in a wheelchair, stump boards can be placed under the cushion and the stump can rest on it in the extended position. Active exercises and passive stretching should be encouraged.

Balance and ambulation with a prosthesis are taught by the physiotherapist.

Health education All amputees and their relatives need support to adapt to the altered body image. Nurses are involved in teaching patients the continuing care of the stump and the other limb. Exercise regimens must be emphasized. Explanations of 'phantom pains' are needed since some patients can still experience pain or itching in the amputated limb. Analgesia, or scratching the itch can help to relieve this distressing condition. Generally speaking, these pains disappear over time.

INFLAMMATORY CONDITIONS AFFECTING THE LOCOMOTOR SYSTEM

The most common inflammatory condition to affect the locomotor system is a chronic condition which affects synovial joints: rheumatoid arthritis (RA). Rheumatology is the term used to describe the study of diseases affecting connective tissue and rheumatoid arthritis is only one of many conditions which fall into this category. For this reason, it is not unusual to be caring for a patient who has a multiple pathology, for example, anaemia, ulcerative colitis, conjunctivitis, psoriasis, to name but a few. However, within this section the emphasis will be placed on caring for a patient suffering from rheumatoid arthritis.

Relevant epidemiology and aetiology

RA is a chronic condition affecting synovial joints.

Box 11.4   Aims in caring for an amputee
1. To help prepare the patient both physically and psychologically for the amputation
2. To adequately prepare the patient for prosthetic fitting
3. To re-educate the patient to mobilize with a prosthesis
4. To encourage the patient's return to maximum independence
5. To promote a positive approach to health care in the individual

The disease pattern is one of acute exacerbations followed by periods of remission and can result in severe disability for the sufferer. Women are more commonly affected than men (one in 200 women, one in 600 men) and the onset is often during the second to fifth decades, although it is not unusual for a diagnosis to be made during the mid-teens. Young children can also be affected (Still's disease). The prevalence of this disease is 1% with little world-wide variation, but the severity of the disease is worse in Europe. Out of 100 sufferers, 65% will continue having joint pain, 30% will recover within a few years and 5% will develop severe disease with extensive disability.

A great deal of research continues to attempt to identify a cause of RA although as yet no specific cause has been identified. It appears that many different factors may be responsible:

1. **Genetic make-up**. Although RA does not appear to be directly inherited, genetically controlled chemicals found on the surfaces of cells increase the likelihood of developing RA. Also, evidence is arising to suggest that individuals who are lacking a galactose sugar on the glycoprotein molecule are more susceptible to developing RA. This condition is referred to as Gal-zero.

2. **Infection**. From time to time different organisms have been isolated from joints affected by RA, but as yet none of the research has produced consistent results which would prove that viral or bacterial organisms cause this condition.

3. **Altered immunity.** It is possible that foreign proteins enter joints and in doing so stimulate lymphocytes and plasma to infiltrate the lining of the joint in order to combat the infection. This, however, begins to affect the joint itself as the plasma cells can produce an antibody called rheumatoid factor which combines with the patient's globulin. When this combination occurs within a joint an inflammatory process begins which is deleterious to the joint structure.

Common symptomatology

In most cases, rheumatoid arthritis has a gradual onset occurring over many months or even years.

Mobility

Generally the individuals complain of morning stiffness, particularly in the small, proximal joints of the hands or feet. The joints become uncomfortable and they may swell. Numbness and tingling in the hands are common complaints. Usually just one or two joints give rise to problems in the early stages, but occasionally, many joints can be affected. Patients will often say that they have difficulty in 'getting-going' in the morning or complain of not being able to hold a pencil very well first thing at work. However, it is not so much the stiffness that takes patients to their GPs as the feelings of tiredness, irritability, general malaise and depression. These symptoms commonly arise during the winter months and it is careful assessment by the GP which elicits a tentative diagnosis.

Rest and sleep

Pain is the most debilitating and constant symptom in RA sufferers. It arises initially from the effects of inflammation of the synovial membrane and the swelling which also results from the increased production of synovial fluid. The pain may be so severe as to keep the patient awake at night and often it is worse in the morning on getting out of bed. Exercising a joint too much will make the pain worse while resting the joints too much increases stiffness. Lack of sleep combined with anaemia, which is common among RA sufferers, can seriously affect an individual's life-style.

Patient implications

There are many factors which will adversely affect the prognosis for RA sufferers:

- insidious onset
- age – older patients generally do worse than younger patients
- early symmetrical arthritis, e.g. same joint in both hands affected
- late presentation at the clinic
- presence of rheumatoid factor
- female sex.

Being diagnosed as having rheumatoid arthritis is a traumatic experience for many sufferers. Having said that, once a diagnosis is made, appropriate treatment can begin and suffering can be alleviated to a great extent in some cases. For others, it will signal the beginning of a long relationship with the nearest rheumatology clinic and the possibility of many months in hospital and a rapidly changing life-style. The nurse plays an important role in listening to the patient and their loved ones and identifying the hidden fears and misconceptions they may have.

This requires a great deal of time, patience and understanding, coupled with factual knowledge about the disease process and the prospects for individual patients. The nurse must inspire in the person confidence and belief that even if a cure is not possible, the treatment will lead to an improvement in his condition.

Range of investigations

1. **X-ray examination** of symmetrical joints to identify joint changes.
2. **Arthrography** – this involves the injection of contrast medium into the joint which is then gently inflated with carbon dioxide. The patient should be warned to expect squelchy noises from the affected joint for up to a week following this procedure.
3. **Synovial fluid examination** – an increase in lymphocytes and protein content would be expected in RA.
4. **Synovial membrane biopsy** – examination of the synovium would show inflammatory changes.
5. **Arthroscopy** – Visual examination of the joint carried out usually under general anaesthetic using a fibreoptic instrument. Care of a patient following anaesthesia is required. Many patients can have this performed as a day case.
6. **Sheep Cell Agglutination Test (SCAT)** – this blood test is used to identify the presence of rheumatoid factor and can be carried out by the general practitioner.
7. **Blood tests** – e.g. haemoglobin, erythrocyte sedimentation rate, white cell count.

None of the above tests should be used in isolation when diagnosing RA. Results from a range of these tests are considered together and as a picture begins to develop, the physician is able to make a diagnosis. Taking an accurate patient history, observing the joints for swelling, inflammation and deformity, X-ray examination and blood tests will help to monitor the progress of the disease. Generally speaking, invasive procedures are the last investigations to be carried out because of the risk of infection to the patient. Because diagnosis can take a long time, the patient and his family must be well supported either in the community or in hospital.

Therapeutic management

The management of rheumatoid arthritis can be approached in two ways: conservative (medical) and surgical. Conservative treatment is always carried out first and surgical treatment can be considered at leisure. The principles of treatment for RA sufferers are:

1. to reduce pain
2. to reduce joint destruction
3. to avoid joint deformities
4. to help the patient to overcome/adjust to disability.

Pain reduction

Striking a happy balance between rest and exercise can go a long way towards achieving this objective. If a joint is overexercised, inflammation will increase and pain will result. However, if too much rest is taken the joints will become stiff (Fig. 11.11).

Drug therapy is also used to help relieve pain. The drugs are divided into two main categories – first-line drugs and second-line drugs. First-line drugs include:

- analgesics, e.g. coproxamol, paracetamol
- non-steroidal anti-inflammatory drugs, e.g. mefanamic acid, ibuprofen.

Either one or other or a combination of the two may be helpful in alleviating pain but they may not be enough to control the progress of the disease.

Second-line drugs include:

- antimalarials, e.g. chloroquine
- immunosuppressants, e.g. azathioprine
- antirheumatoids, e.g. Myocrisin (gold)
- corticosteroids, e.g. prednisolone
- corticotrophins, e.g. Synacthen.

These drugs will help to slow down the progress of the disease and are used in conjunction with first-line drugs. Their main disadvantage is the side-effects, particularly as some of these drugs need to be taken over a long period of time before improvements are seen. The nurse must be familiar with the effects and side-effects of drug therapies to ensure that appropriate nursing observations are carried out to enable early identification of complications.

Reduction in joint destruction and avoidance of deformity

Splints are used to help maintain joints in position of function during rest periods. These splints can take many forms but very often plaster of Paris splints are made because they can be moulded easily around the painful joints (Fig. 11.12). These splints can be removed at regular intervals to allow exercise to be carried out. In an acute exacerbation the amount of exercise carried out is closely monitored, usually by

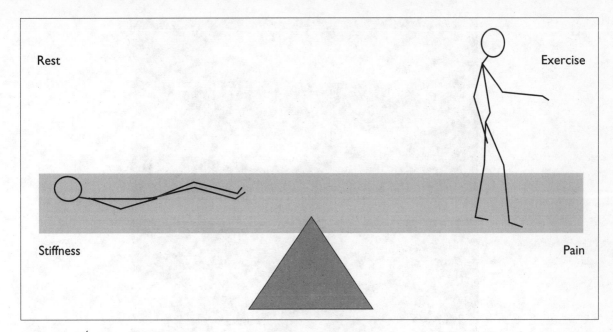

Fig. 11.11 The effects of rest and exercise on an individual suffering from rheumatoid arthritis

a physiotherapist. As pain and swelling reduce, the amount of exercise undertaken can be increased. Splints are often worn at night to rest joints in positions of optimum function and can be used to counteract soft tissue contractures. Should medical treatment become less effective, resulting in poor pain control and deteriorating function, surgery is indicated.

Box 11.5 indicates the types of surgery that can be offered to reduce pain and deformity.

Specialist textbooks should be used to gain detailed information about the above types of surgery. Before surgery is contemplated there must be close liaison between members of the multidisciplinary team, physicians, surgeons and the patient. Surgery to the large joints is usually carried out first, to reduce stress on smaller joints. Medical treatment with drugs continues during the following surgery but the regimen may change following surgery.

For some individuals the fear of living with a chronic, disabling disease is very distressing and they look for other alternative remedies to help cure their condition.

Diet

Many sufferers try exclusion diets. It is thought that sensitivity to particular food types may cause RA. In an exclusion diet only certain foods are taken for 4–6 weeks (Box 11.6). If the condition seems to improve, other foods can be added one at a time to the diet. In trials, most patient's condition improves during the diet but this might only be as a result of the weight loss. Research still continues in this area.

Green-lipped mussel treatment   Extract of this New Zealand mussel is taken daily either in tablet, granule or capsular form. There are no dangerous side-effects and this extract has been shown to relieve sufferers of any age.

Herbal remedies   The philosophy of herbal remedies is that the whole body can be restored back to health. Specialist advice should be sought before trying them out.

Homeopathy   As above, the whole body is treated by homeopathic remedies. Medicines are given in extreme dilutions in order to enhance their curative properties. Again, specialist advice should be sought.

For some patients it may be appropriate to use a combination of orthodox and complementary remedies. It is important that the nurse is able to support the patients if they choose to try complementary medicines and liaise with medical staff on the patient's behalf if necessary.

Nursing strategies

Rest and sleep

RA sufferers become fatigued very easily, especially

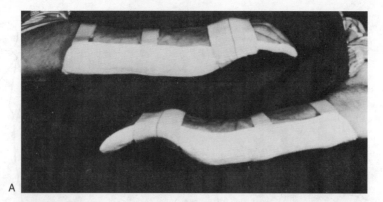

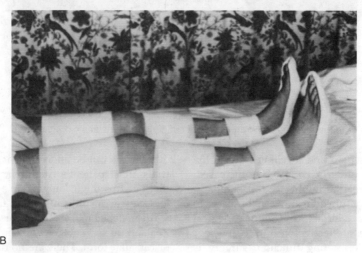

Fig. 11.12 Splints used to support painful joints. (Courtesy of Dr T. M. Chalmers, Consultant Rheumatologist, Northern General Hospital, Edinburgh)

Box 11.5 The types of surgery which can be offered to reduce pain and deformity

Soft tissue surgery
Decompression of nerves
Decompression of tendons
Division of tendons (tenotomy)
Synovectomy

Bone surgery
Osteotomy (division of bone)

Joint surgery
Arthrodesis (fusion of a joint)
Arthroplasty (removal/replacement of a joint)

Box 11.6 Exclusion diet

- Oily fish
- Chicken
- Carrots
- Bananas
- Rice
- Green beans
- Spring water (only)

---

during an acute flare-up of the disease. Rest and sleep help to:

- relieve pain
- prevent injury to the joint

- overcome muscle spasm
- aid healing within the joint and
- prevent tiredness and exhaustion.

If patients are wearing splints the skin must be examined carefully for signs of redness and irritation and neurovascular checks should be carried out regularly (as described in p. 363). The bed should have a firm mattress, a back rest and sufficient pillows to keep the patient upright. Limbs should not be supported by pillows but should be maintained in positions of function. Bed linen should be light-weight and a bedcradle used if necessary. Careful movement of the patient is required to prevent jarring of the joints and tearing of the skin, which can become paper thin as a result of the disease process and drug therapy. In an acute phase, nursing care to prevent hazards of immobility should be employed.

Mobility

Active exercises should be encouraged. Each joint must be put through its full range of movements on a daily basis. Most RA sufferers develop their own exercise regimen and should be encouraged to continue with this while in hospital. Mobility aids, raised toilet seats and high seats increase a patient's independence as their condition improves.

Hygiene

In an acute phase the patient will be totally dependent on the nurse for care. Skin checks and pressure care must be carried out regularly. If the patient has subcutaneous nodules, which form around the elbows and other bony prominences, they must be inspected to prevent skin breakdown and infection. There are many aids available to help relieve pressure and protect the skin. Once the acute phase has passed, patients may have a bath or shower. Many patients prefer a shower since they are more accessible. Water should not be too hot as it adds to the patient's fatigue. Many patients find a sponge easier to wring out than a face cloth. Patients should be unhurried to compensate for joint stiffness.

Occupational therapists are able to help patients gain independence in washing and dressing techniques and can give invaluable advice on aids that are available to make life easier for RA sufferers.

Maintaining a safe environment

As RA is an inflammatory disease, temperature, pulse and respiration rate are recorded at least twice daily and joint inflammation/stiffness accurately recorded. Any alterations in recordings should be promptly reported. The nurse must be able to report on the effectiveness of the prescribed drugs or any side-effects which occur. Urinalysis is important. Albuminuria may be present if there is renal involvement. Certain drugs may also produce proteinuria, and glycosuria may develop in patients receiving high doses

of steroids. Patients receiving treatment with chloroquine should have full eye screening, at least annually, since this drug can cause retinal damage.

Communication

These patients become fully conversant with their condition and treatment very quickly. As a result, it is important that all members of the multidisciplinary team convey the same information to the patient, otherwise trust will be lost and the patient–nurse relationship will break down. It is important to listen to these patients carefully when they are identifying their needs as they know what suits them and their family. Many of them will already have made major changes to their life-style and this should be acknowledged by the multidisciplinary team. Relatives and loved ones should be included in planning care since they will have to help implement that care at home. It is important not to set unrealistic goals for the sufferer, as there comes a point when the disability has to be accepted and the appropriate care and support have to be given. It is depressing enough having a chronic disability without feeling a failure into the bargain.

Rehabilitation

This begins from the moment a GP suspects a diagnosis of RA. The rehabilitation programme involves the whole multidisciplinary team which includes the patient and relatives. Physiotherapists and nurses need to work closely together to help the patient maintain independence and mobility. While in hospital the patient may spend large periods of the day in the physiotherapy department and the nurses must facilitate progress in the ward by ensuring that the rest and exercise programme is adhered to. These patients can become fiercely independent and it can be difficult for an inexperienced nurse to adopt a 'hands-off' approach. This independence is important if the patient is to cope at home successfully and return to work. Occupational therapists can teach new skills to patients to help them to adapt to independent living and social workers can help provide the much-needed community support and arrange for modifications to be made to the patient's home.

The Arthritis and Rheumatism Council provides an excellent information and support service for sufferers and their loved ones. Their money-raising activities allow research to continue into seeking the cause and a cure for RA.

Surgical intervention

The care of a patient with RA undergoing surgery is similar to that of a patient with fractures:

Special precautions include:

- Preoperative neck X-ray to exclude RA and prevent fractures occurring during anaesthesia.
- Careful limb positioning postoperatively and close observation of wounds.
- Wounds which are leaking or showing signs of infection should not be exercised.

DEGENERATIVE DISORDERS

The most common degenerative condition affecting the locomotor system is osteoarthrosis. Should a secondary inflammation occur within the joint the more commonly used term osteoarthritis describes the condition.

OSTEOARTHROSIS

Relevant epidemiology and aetiology

Osteoarthrosis (OA) is a condition which commonly affects the large weight-bearing joints such as the hips, knees and spine. It affects both males and females equally aged below 55 years, but over this age a higher percentage of women are affected.

Osteoarthrosis is characterized by the deterioration of the central articular cartilage and the underlying bone. In order to compensate for the loss of surface area, osteophytes (abnormal lateral outgrowth of bone) grow. This serves to increase the weight-bearing surface area. Complications of osteophyte growth include damage to other joint structures and surrounding soft tissue. Osteoarthrosis can occur following previous injury or damage to a joint, in which case it is called secondary osteoarthrosis. If there is no previous history of disease it is called primary osteoarthrosis. Unlike rheumatoid arthritis, this condition is not associated with general systemic illness.

OA sufferers generally find that pain and limitation of movement cause reduced mobility as they get older and in many cases, surgical intervention in the form of arthroplasty, markedly improves quality of life. OA is not a natural consequence of ageing but may be associated with obesity, sporting activity, congenital joint deformities and previous surgery.

Common symptomatology

The pain associated with OA is usually worse during movement and eases with rest. Secondary synovitis can cause stiffness following periods of rest.

Mobility

Limitation of movement occurs as a result of the alteration in shape of the joint surface, protective muscle spasm and the conscious efforts of the individual to reduce/avoid pain. If synovitis occurs, the joint can become swollen because of the excessive amounts of synovial fluid produced.

Range of investigations

Diagnosis is confirmed by X-ray examination which shows a narrowing/loss of joint space, destruction of the articular cartilage, osteophyte formation and possible joint deformity.

Therapeutic management

There are two options available: conservative and operative treatments.

Conservative treatment

When OA is diagnosed in its early stages, it is possible, through health education, to modify the course of the disease. Advice which should be given to sufferers includes:

1. Explanation of the disease process and prognosis.
2. Nutritional advice to help with weight reduction.
3. Modifying lifestyle to reduce joint destruction, e.g. reducing sporting activities, reducing physical stresses at work, and to find a balance between rest and exercise.
4. Using aids to improve mobility, e.g. high chairs, walking sticks.
5. Drug therapy, e.g. analgesics and/or NSAIDs (see p. 374).

Operative treatment

See the surgical care of patients with RA (see p. 378).

There are a wide variety of prosthesis available for joint replacement surgery and often the decision regarding choice of the prosthesis depends on the individual characteristics of the patient and the surgeon's own preference. On average, the life-span of a major weight-bearing prosthesis, for example, a hip or knee joint, is 10 years. This will vary depending on individual patient's demands of the joint. The age at which a patient undergoes surgery is therefore an important consideration for the surgeon. Often patients require to have their prosthesis replaced.

Nursing strategies

Care is similar to that for patients with RA. Health education and explanations of the disease can help to prevent further joint deformity occurring. The majority of OA sufferers will be treated in the community and will be admitted to hospital for surgical procedures such as total hip replacement or knee replacement.

Box 11.7 shows advice that should be given to patients following a total hip replacement.

Box 11.7   Advice to patients following a total hip replacement

1. Do NOT bend at the hips too much. This may cause dislocation of the prosthesis
2. Do NOT cross your legs. In bed, keep two pillows between your legs to maintain a good position and prevent dislocation. (Adduction must be avoided)
3. Do NOT pivot on the affected hip. Walk in small circles if you wish to turn around
4. WEAR good fitting, supportive shoes
5. GET OUT OF BED from the affected side if possible. (This will help to prevent adduction of the hip)
6. USE a raised toilet seat and a high chair. This helps to reduce mobility problems
7. USE walking aids appropriate to your needs

METABOLIC DISORDERS

Relevant epidemiology and aetiology

Bone is a living tissue and it has the ability to replace itself during life. Different bones will replace bone material at different rates and several factors are involved in bone growth and replacement. Should something go wrong with the mechanisms involved in bone growth and replacement, abnormalities can occur within the bone which can seriously weaken it. These conditions are classified as metabolic disorders and include rickets, osteomalacia and osteoporosis.

The factors necessary for bone growth and replacement are:

- good blood supply
- growth hormone
- sex hormones
- parathormone
- calcitonin
- calcium
- vitamins C and D.

Factors contributing to bone growth are also illustrated in Figure 11.13.

Rickets

Rickets is a condition which affects the young and it results mainly from an inadequate intake or synthesis of vitamin D. As a result, there is decreased mineralization of osteoid tissue and the bones become soft and curved, leading to a bowing of the lower extremities. Mobility is severely affected. This condition is most often encountered in underdeveloped countries where health provision for children is poor and the diet is lacking in calcium, phosphorus and vitamin D. The disease progress can be halted by administration of these three factors on a daily basis. Genetic predisposition, kidney defects and malabsorption syndromes can also cause a condition known as resistant rickets. Large doses of vitamin D are required to treat this condition.

Osteomalacia

Osteomalacia, or sick bones, is an adult form of rickets. It occurs in bones after fusion of the epiphyseal plates has taken place and is the result of mineral deficiency and lack of vitamin D. Poor diet, disturbances in calcium or vitamin D absorption and loss of serum phosphorus from the kidneys can be held accountable for the development of this condition. X-ray examination shows a typical lack of mineral salts in normal osteoid tissue, similar to rickets, and serum calcium and phosphate levels are low, with a raised alkaline phosphatase. Symptoms include bone pain and general malaise resulting from malnourishment. Pathological fractures can . occur. Treatment involves administration of vitamin D and the correction of dietary insufficiencies.

Osteoporosis

This is the most common of the metabolic disorders which affect bone and is commonly seen in postmenopausal women. It is a long-term condition affecting bone for which there is no known cure. Osteoporotic bones become thinner, less strong and

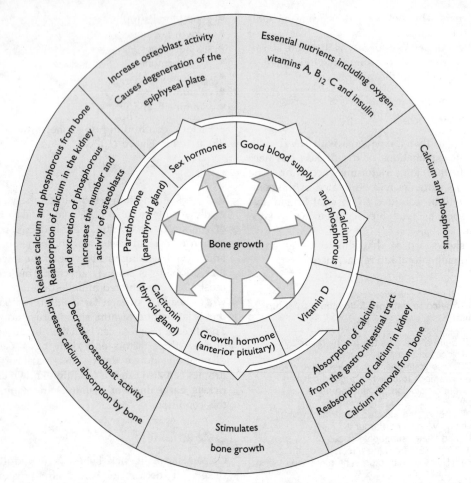

Fig. 11.13 Factors affecting bone growth

are liable to fracture. One in four females are affected as compared to one in 40 males. There is an increased risk after the menopause when oestrogen levels fall but it may also develop as a result of inactivity, poor diet or endocrine dysfunction. It is seen in astronauts after prolonged periods of weightlessness.

Common symptomatology

Mobility Often back pain is the presenting symptom in osteoporosis. It may have a sudden or gradual onset and mobility can be badly affected. The individual usually complains of odd aches and pains in the lower back and hip regions in particular. In many cases, it is only when an individual falls and fractures a bone that osteoporosis is diagnosed.

Patient implications Many individuals never suffer

as a result of osteoporosis, but for some it can mean years of agonizing back pain and reduced mobility leading to possible isolation and loneliness in the elderly. Independence is lost and quality of life is markedly reduced.

Range of investigations X-ray examination is used to diagnose osteoporosis. During this procedure the nurse should be aware of the need to adequately support fractured limbs (see p. 365) and be able to advise the patient on how to move efficiently and maintain a good posture if she is suffering from severe back pain.

Therapeutic management

There are three principal methods of treatment of osteoporosis, although none are very successful.

1. exercise
2. diet
3. hormone replacement therapy.

Exercise can help prevent disuse osteoporosis (see 'Hazards of enforced inactivity' p. 358) and the elderly should be encouraged to walk about and take regular exercise. Many health clubs encourage older people to make use of their facilities and day centres will include dancing and movement to music in their list of activities.

A diet rich in calcium and vitamin D can help to prevent osteoporosis and many elderly people are given calcium and vitamin D supplements on a daily basis. It is being suggested that women in particular should increase their calcium intake long before the menopause in order to prevent osteoporosis, that is before 35 years of age.

The most controversial therapy available is that of hormone replacement therapy (HRT) which puts back hormones that have been lost, namely oestrogen and progesterone. Oestrogens increase osteoblast activity and when they are absent this activity is reduced. As a result, osteoclast activity becomes greater than osteoblast activity which causes a thinning of bones. Replacing oestrogens either as pills, skin patches or vaginally, reduces osteoporosis as well as relieving other symptoms associated with the menopause (see Ch. 17).

Nursing strategies

Since successful treatment of osteoporosis is unlikely in the majority of cases, the nurse must take on the role of health educator in order to allow individuals to take responsibility for improving their physical well-being and reducing the risk of developing osteoporosis. A sound knowledge of the affects of diet and exercise on the locomotor system is essential and the nurse should make the most of every opportunity available to offer factual information to people about the prevention of osteoporosis. It is also important for nurses to keep themselves up to date with current debates and research about controversial issues, such as HRT. Only then can the nurse offer factual, im-partial information to his/her clients or patients to enable them to decide whether or not they wish to accept a particular therapy.

Ethical issues

There is much debate about the long-term safety of patients receiving HRT. Treatment generally lasts from 1 to 5 years but it can go on for much longer. Research suggests that if HRT is properly prescribed there should be no harmful side-effects, but concern is still expressed among some professionals that HRT causes an increase in the risk of developing breast cancer. Other common adverse effects of HRT include: fluid retention, premenstrual tension, breast tender-ness, changes in menstrual flow, gastrointestinal dis-turbances, intolerance to contact lenses, headaches and depression.

Since only one in four women develop osteoporosis and of that number only one in four will suffer a frac-ture, perhaps the cost-effectiveness of treating all postmenopausal women with HRT is debatable.

CONGENITAL DISORDERS

Abnormalities which are present before birth are termed congenital. With the advent of improved maternal health care, prenatal care and perinatal care, the incidence of congenital deformities has reduced dramatically, so much so that there are few children's orthopaedic wards now.

Congenital deformities may result from:

1. Genetic factors.
2. Environmental factors, e.g.
   a. rubella infection in the mother
   b. poor nutritional status of mother
   c. oxygen deficiency
   d. hormonal disturbances
   e. chemical poisons, such as quinine, thalidomide.

The types of deformities that can arise are absence of, maldevelopment of, or extra parts of a limb. Some common disorders are given in Box 11.8.

Some conditions are more easily treated than others but for many children it can result in long periods of hospitalization and separation from the parents and other siblings.

Box 11.8   Some common congenital disorders

- Dislocation of the hip
- Talipes equinovarus (club foot)
- Hammer toe
- Infantile scoliosis
- Amelia (absence of a limb)
- Torticollis (wry neck)
- Flat foot

Therapeutic management

Conservative and operative management are available for the treatment of congenital abnormalities. The treatment centres around the correction of the resultant deformity. In some instances, correcting soft tissue contractures using physiotherapy and splintage are all that is necessary. For other children, long periods of treatment with traction are required. Surgical intervention is used to correct bony deformities, remove excess digits or refashion new digits. Whichever form of treatment is used, the fact that children are growing needs to be taken into account. This factor can either be advantageous or disadvantageous to the surgeon.

Nursing strategies

The care of a child in plaster or in traction is the same as for adults (see pp. 365–371).

Psychological support

Parents of children who are born with a deformity can have a great deal of difficulty rationalizing what has happened and can be overwhelmed by feelings of guilt. Much of the nurse's work is involved in helping to support the parents during the phase of hospitalization. Health visitors, medical social workers and other members of the multidisciplinary team will already have been involved in the community. Giving clear, concise information to the parents allows them to become involved in their child's care and rehabilitation. The parents will be largely involved in the rehabilitation when the child is discharged, so they must be given the opportunity to ask questions, observe care and be involved in decision making before the child goes home. Building up a trusting relationship between parents, child and staff also makes separation easier. Not all parents can stay in hospital with their child because of other family or work commitments, and if parents know their child will be well cared for in their absence, they will be more able to cope with their other responsibilities. Where appropriate, other agencies should be involved in giving support, reassurance and practical advice to parents. It is worth remembering that the parents know their child best and nurses should listen to their advice on the child's general management. Once again the 'hands-off' approach is required.

Children will adapt quickly to being in hospital and many of these children will have repeated admissions over a number of years. Anxiety can be reduced if the child is admitted to the same ward and, where possible, is cared for by a familiar person.

NEOPLASTIC DISORDERS

Bone tumours may be classified as benign or malignant, primary or secondary.

Relevant epidemiology and aetiology

Primary bone tumours arise from any tissue associated with bone; for example, blood vessels, nerves, fibrous tissue, cartilage or bone. These tumours occur mostly in the metaphysis (see p. 352) of growing bone. Benign, primary tumours do not invade any other structure.

Malignant, primary tumours are most often seen in children and adolescents. They occur most commonly in the medulla of long bones and spread to affect other structures. These tumours can spread to the lungs, resulting in death usually within 5 years.

Malignant, secondary tumours arise in bone having originated in other structures; for example, breast, lung, thyroid, prostate, kidney. These are generally blood-borne and are referred to as metastases or metastatic bone disease. Prognosis is generally poor when metastases are diagnosed.

Common symptomatology

1. Pain, increasing in severity if malignant.
2. Pathological fractures in susceptible bones.
3. Swellings, often painful in malignant tumours.
4. Tenderness   ⎫ Common in
5. Anorexia and weight loss ⎬ malignant tumours.
6. Dry, unproductive cough ⎭

Mobility

This can be markedly reduced in sufferers. They may limit movement consciously to avoid pain.

Work and play

Because treatment can have drastic side-effects, many changes are necessary in the patient's life-style. Family life can be severely affected.

Range of investigations

1. Patient history and observation.
2. X-ray examination.
3. Blood tests – Low haemoglobin, raised ESR or hypercalcaemia.
4. Bone scan – this involves the injection of a radioactive element which collects in areas where there is an increased blood supply. These 'hot spots' indicate areas of bone tumour and are easily recognized on the bone scan.
5. Bone biopsy.

Throughout any of the above procedures, psychological support of the patient is necessary.

Therapeutic management

Options include surgery, radiotherapy or chemotherapy. Care of a patient undergoing treatment for cancer is discussed in Chapter 4 and applies equally to children, adults and the elderly.

Suggested assignments

Discussion points

1. Osteoarthrosis is a condition which is more prevalent in the overweight person. Should such people be offered expensive surgery to relieve joint pain without first demonstrating a commitment to losing weight?
2. Complementary treatment such as aromatherapy, reflexology, massage and manipulation are increasing in popularity as a first line of treatment for many orthopaedic conditions.

   Discuss the implications of this shift in preference for nurses who are working with patients in a more traditional setting.
   You may wish to consider the following points:
   - How can a nurse offer advice to a patient about the use of complementary treatments when she lacks knowledge in these areas?
   - Should provision be made to allow nurses to train in these specialist areas during their training?
   - How can nurses maintain their expertise if they are unable to practise these specialist skills on a regular basis?
3. EC Directives advocate the use of the ergonomic approach to handling and moving objects/patients. Does this have implications for nurses working with patients who are immobile or wearing heavy plasters?
4. How can the nursing profession ensure that the number of back injuries and resulting loss of working days is reduced and that safe handling and moving techniques are being employed by the workforce?

REFERENCES AND FURTHER READING

Dandy D J 1989 Essential orthopaedics and trauma. Churchill Livingstone, Edinburgh

Gunn C 1984 Bones and joints, a guide for students. Churchill Livingstone, Edinburgh

Health & Safety Executive 1992 Manual handling, guidance on regulations. HMSO, London

Marieb E N 1992 Human anatomy and physiology, 2nd edn. Benjamin Cummings, Wokingham

Miller M, Miller J H 1985 Orthopaedics and accidents illustrated. Hodder and Stoughton, London

Tortora G H, Anagnostakos N P 1990 Principles of anatomy and physiology, 2nd edn. Harper and Row, London

Vasey J, Crozier L 1982 A move in the right direction. Nursing Mirror 28 April pp 42–47

Vasey J, Crozier L 1982 Get into condition. Nursing Mirror 5 May pp 22–27

Vasey J, Crozier L 1982 At ease. Nursing Mirror 12 May pp 28–31

Vasey J, Crozier L 1982 Handle with care. Nursing Mirror 19 May pp 30–32

Vasey J, Crozier L 1982 Easy on the back. Nursing Mirror 26 May pp 36–41

Vasey J, Crozier L 1982 Safety first. Nursing Mirror 2 June pp 44–48

Walsh R 1988 Conflicting ideas of movement (human kinetics) Nursing Times 84(36): 51

12

Care implications of disorders of the cardiovascular system

Mary Bronte and Morag A. Gray

INTRODUCTION

Cardiovascular disorders cause the deaths of 40% of men aged 35–44 years and 50% of men aged 45–54 years. They are second only to cancer as a major cause of mortality in women. Coronary heart disease is the largest element of cardiovascular disease and is alone responsible for more than a quarter of the total deaths in the UK (Fig. 12.1). More than one in five men will have a heart attack before retirement.

Cardiovascular disease creates major human costs through bereavement and disability as well as major economic costs through lost working days as a result of sickness and premature deaths, and increasing demands on the NHS.

There are therefore major implications for both primary and secondary prevention, and the involvement of nurses in health education as well as teaching and rehabilitation is becoming increasingly important. As there continue to be major advances in medical research and clinical practice, and as understanding of the causes and treatment of cardiovascular disorders increases, the management of

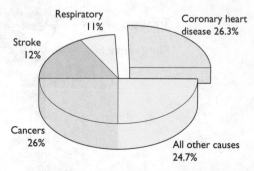

Fig. 12.1 Percentage mortality by cause in the UK. (Source: The Coronary Prevention Group 1992)

these patients is one of the most progressive areas in nursing today.

This produces new responsibilities and challenges for nurses, particularly those in special care units such as coronary care, who need to develop a high level of knowledge and skills related to both physical and technical care. However, effective and holistic management of the patient requires much more than this. The nurse needs to be competent in assessing the various needs of the patient and family and must be able to provide physical comfort, safety and psychosocial support (Thompson 1985).

The area of cardiovascular nursing is both vast and complex and the aim of this chapter is to emphasize the broad goals of nursing care. The reader is encouraged to refer to more specialized texts for further detail. The areas of cardiac and vascular disorders and their implications have been dealt with in separate sections.

ANATOMY AND PHYSIOLOGY

The main function of the cardiovascular system is to provide an adequate circulation of blood to the tissues to ensure the transport of oxygen and nutrients to body cells and carbon dioxide and metabolic waste products from cells. In order to maintain a stable internal environment, the cardiovascular system must be able to maintain an adequate flow to tissues under a variety of circumstances, including periods of stress such as exercise, illness and changes in emotional state.

The cardiovascular system is a closed circulatory system, comprising the heart and blood vessels, containing approximately 4.8 litres of blood in a 70 kg adult male.

The heart

The heart is enclosed in a fibrous sac, the pericardium, which provides a protective covering and attaches it to the large blood vessels, the diaphragm and to the sternal chest wall. There is a potential space between the heart and the pericardium called the pericardial cavity. This cavity contains pericardial fluid which alleviates friction as the heart beats (see Fig. 12.2).

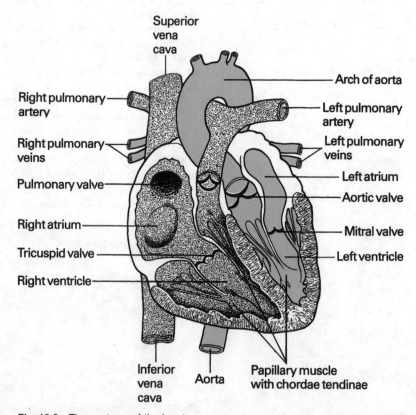

Fig. 12.2 The anatomy of the heart

The heart has three layers:

1. **Epicardium** – the outer visceral layer which forms part of the pericardium.

2. **Myocardium** – the middle layer, consisting of specialized muscle tissue, which is responsible for the heart's contraction, pumping blood into the arterial circulation.

3. **Endocardium** – an inner layer of endothelium which lines the chambers of the heart and covers the heart valves.

The heart is divided by a muscular septum into left and right sides which normally do not communicate with each other after birth. Each side is subdivided into upper and lower chambers, the atria and ventri-

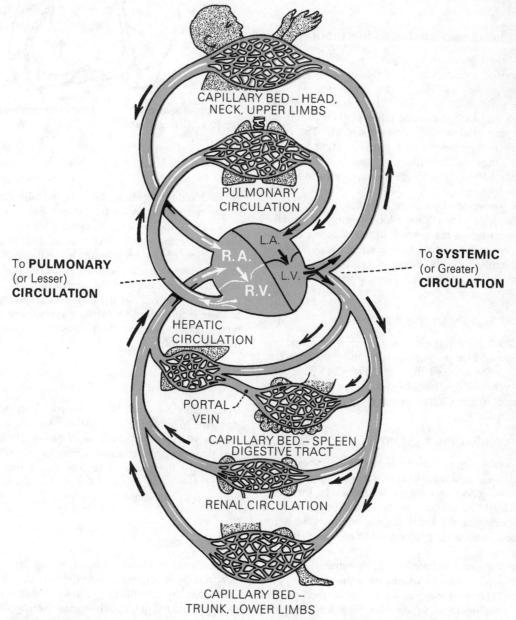

Fig. 12.3 Pulmonary and systemic circulations. (Reproduced with permission from McNaught & Callander 1983, p. 91)

cles. Each atria is separated from its respective ventricle by an atrioventricular valve (the tricuspid and mitral valves) which allows blood flow in one direction. The valves are attached to muscular projections of the ventricular wall (papillary muscles) by fibrous strands called the chordae tendinae. The semilunar valves (pulmonary and aorta) lie between the ventricles and the major arteries and prevent backflow of blood into the ventricles.

Pulmonary and systemic circulation

There are two distinct circulations within the cardiovascular system; the pulmonary and systemic circulations (Fig. 12.3).

The pulmonary circulation is where exchange of oxygen and carbon dioxide takes place between the blood and the alveolar air (see Ch. 13). The heart pumps deoxygenated blood from the right ventricle to the lungs via the pulmonary artery and receives oxygenated blood via the pulmonary veins to the left atrium.

The systemic circulation supplies all the body tissues. During contraction, blood is pumped from the left ventricle, via the aorta, into the systemic circulation, where the exchange of nutrients and products of metabolism occurs. Blood is returned to the right atrium via the inferior and superior vena cavae.

Blood supply to the heart

The heart muscle itself is supplied with blood via the right and left coronary arteries and their branches, which originate from the aorta (Fig. 12.4). The coronary veins return blood from the myocardium to the right atrium via the coronary sinus.

The conducting system

The conducting system is composed of specialized muscle cells which are concerned with the initiation and conduction of electrical impulses in the heart (Fig. 12.5). The purpose of the conducting system is to ensure that the heart muscle contracts in a co-ordinated and orderly manner, thus ensuring effective pumping.

The impulse is initiated in the sinoatrial (SA) node, hence the SA node is often called the cardiac pacemaker. The electrical impulses spread through the atria, causing them to contract. The impulse then enters the atrioventricular (AV) node, where it is

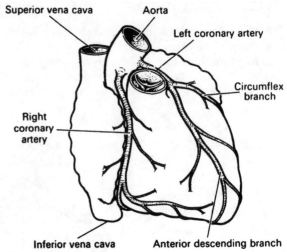

Fig. 12.4 Coronary arteries

delayed sightly to allow the atria to finish emptying before the ventricles contract. Once through the AV node, the impulse spreads rapidly through the remainder of the conducting system, bringing about contraction of the ventricles. This wave of electrical impulses spreading through the heart is termed depolarization and brings about contraction of the heart muscle. As the cells of the conducting system return to their resting electrical state, the resulting wave of repolarization brings about relaxation of the heart muscle.

Cardiac cycle

Contraction of the heart muscle generates the pressure to effectively pump the blood, while the cardiac valves direct the flow of blood. The contraction phase of the atria and ventricles is termed systole, whilst the phase of relaxation is term diastole. The cardiac cycle refers to the period of one systole followed by one diastole.

Cardiac output

The volume of blood pumped by the left ventricle per minute is termed the cardiac output. It can be calculated by multiplying stroke volume (volume of blood ejected with each contraction) by the heart rate (number of contractions per minute)

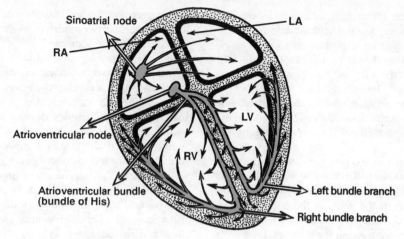

Fig. 12.5   Conducting pathways

Cardiac output = Stroke volume x Heart rate

Cardiac output may be modified by altering the heart rate, the stroke volume, or both.

A normal cardiac output is approximately 5 litres/minute and this can increase to as much as 25 litres/minute in a normal person performing strenuous exercise, or even further in a well-trained athlete. The heart is therefore normally able to increase its output to meet the demands of the body. Cardiac output is central to the functioning of the cardiovascular system as it determines the amount of blood available for transport of oxygen and nutrients to body tissues.

The blood vessels

Apart from the capillaries, all blood vessels (Fig. 12.6) are similar in structure, but the proportion of the components varies in relationship to their function:

- Tunica adventitia – outer layer of fibrous connective tissue, collagen and fibroblasts.
- Tunica media – middle layer of smooth muscle and elastic tissue.
- Tunica intima – inner layer of endothelium.

Arteries differ from veins by having a smaller lumen, more muscle and elastic fibres in the middle layer and thicker walls. Most veins have valves, which direct the blood towards the heart. The arteries distribute the cardiac output to the body tissues and help maintain an adequate blood pressure by offering resistance to blood flow. The arterioles, due to their

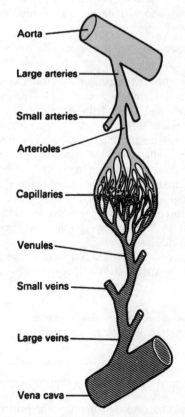

Fig. 12.6   Components of the vascular bed

smaller radius, offer the main resistance to blood flow (peripheral resistance) as they contract and relax.

The capillaries play an important part in cell respiration and nutrition by bringing blood into close contact with all body cells and are sometimes known as exchange vessels. The thin capillary wall allows the exchange of water, oxygen, carbon dioxide and low molecular weight substances between the blood in the capillaries and the interstitial fluid and subsequently the cells.

The veins return deoxygenated blood from the body tissues to the heart. They act as a store of blood and return it at the rate required to maintain cardiac output. The action in the veins of the legs is of particular importance during exercise. When the veins are compressed by contracting leg muscles, the valves ensure that blood flows in the direction of the heart.

Blood pressure

Blood pressure refers to the pressure exerted by the blood against the walls of the blood vessels. Blood pressure is a function of blood flow (equivalent to cardiac output) and vascular resistance (total peripheral resistance). Therefore:

$$\text{Blood pressure} = \text{Cardiac output} \times \text{Total peripheral resistance}$$

The pressure in the major arteries rises and falls as the heart contracts and relaxes. The maximum pressure exerted against the artery walls when the heart contracts is known as systolic pressure. The diastolic pressure is the force of blood exerted against the artery walls when the heart is relaxing. Blood pressure varies from person to person and even under varying circumstances, for individuals. Parameters such as age, sex and race influence blood pressure values. However, normal pressures are said to range from 100 to 150 mmHg systolic and from 60 to 90 mmHg diastolic.

For further detail on anatomy and physiology refer to Tortora & Anagnostakos (1990) and Ross & Wilson (1990).

DISORDERS OF THE HEART AND CIRCULATION

EPIDEMIOLOGY AND AETIOLOGY

Cardiovascular disorders are now the principle cause of death in developed countries. Much research has been carried out into the causes of these disorders and their prevention. So far, however, the causes of many of them, especially coronary (ischaemic) heart disease, are still not fully understood.

The heart may be affected directly by congenital defects and structural abnormalities such as atrial septal defect or vascular disorders, or by impaired blood supply to its structure, for example, from diseased coronary arteries causing angina and myocardial infarction. The heart may also be affected by infection both directly by a variety of bacterial and viral infectious and indirectly, as in rheumatic fever.

Changes in cardiac function are associated with many other disorders such as hypertension, thyrotoxicosis and anaemia and the cardiovascular changes of pregnancy and childbirth may place a strain on an already diseased heart. Whether the structure and function of the heart are affected directly or indirectly, in time the heart muscle itself may fail and heart failure results.

The main types of heart disease and the percentage mortality in the UK are shown in Figure 12.7. The six common symptoms of heart disease are discussed below prior to dealing with specific disorders.

Dyspnoea

Difficult or laboured breathing, although not peculiar to cardiac disorders, is the most common and often the earliest symptom. This symptom is most severe when the patient's lungs are congested and oedematous and the heart is in failure, and can cause great distress and anxiety. Unlike the anxious individual who has deep sighing respirations, the patient with cardiac dyspnoea breathes rapidly and shallowly. There are several types of dyspnoea, and with cardiac disorders, dyspnoea is usually progressive. It may however, be suddenly exacerbated.

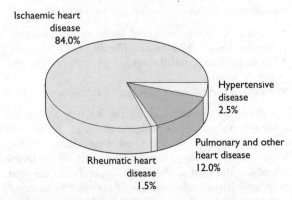

Fig. 12.7 Percentage of mortality for types of heart disease in the UK. (Source: CSO Annual Statistics 1990)

Dyspnoea on exertion

This is the most common form of cardiac dyspnoea and first appears when climbing hills or stairs, or when doing heavy housework. Various non-cardiac conditions such as poor physical health, old age and obesity can lead to dyspnoea on mild exertion. Gradually, less strenuous exercise will cause shortness of breath, for example walking slowly on level ground.

Dyspnoea at rest

Eventually dyspnoea is present even when the patient is resting and ultimately orthopnoea occurs, that is the need to sit upright in order to breathe more easily. When the individual lies flat, there is an increase in venous return to the heart, which in a patient developing left heart failure may increase venous congestion. This decreases lung compliance and vital capacity, which is further reduced by the elevation of the diaphragm when lying down. Assuming the upright position makes it easier to use the accessory muscles of the shoulders to help breathing.

Paroxysmal nocturnal dyspnoea (cardiac asthma)

In people with disorders which cause overwork of the left ventricle, for example, aortic stenosis or heart failure, an attack of dyspnoea may develop without an obvious precipitating cause. Attacks commonly occur at night during sleep. After a few hours of sleep the person may wake up suddenly, gasping for breath and feeling very frightened. He will quickly sit up on the edge of the bed and may go to an open window for fresh air to ease the distress. An unproductive cough and wheeze which resembles asthma can occur, hence the term cardiac asthma. The mechanism involved is probably the same as that of orthopnoea, but because the person is sleeping, he is unaware of the situation and therefore unable to correct it by sitting up.

Chest pain

Pain in the chest is a very common complaint occurring in disorders such as myocardial ischaemia and infarction, and pericarditis. There are however, many other causes of chest pain and therefore it is important to differentiate not only between the different types of cardiac pain, but between cardiac pain and pain caused by disorders of other structures within the chest such as pulmonary disorders, musculo-skeletal pain and gastrointestinal disorders. The two main causes of cardiac pain are myocardial ischaemia and pericarditis. A transient and reversible inadequacy of blood supply to the myocardium gives rise to the type of chest pain known as angina pectoris. Angina commonly occurs in response to exercise in people with coronary heart disease and was first described by Heberden in 1722 as a 'painful and disagreeable sensation in the breast, which seems as if it would extinguish life if it were to increase or continue; but the moment they stand still, all this uneasiness vanishes'. If the reduction in blood supply is sufficient to cause death (infarction) of an area of myocardium, the pain is usually more severe and prolonged and is not related to exercise. The typical characteristics of angina pectoris and the pain of myocardial infarction and pericarditis are described in Table 12.1.

It is important however to remember that pain is unique to each individual and therefore individual assessment of pain is vital (see Ch. 4). In addition, these classical characteristics may not always be clear cut, for example, the pain may or may not radiate or may be felt in the arm and not the chest. In other forms of angina, such as unstable angina, pain may occur at rest and therefore be confused with the pain of myocardial infarction.

Palpitation

Palpitation is an awareness of the heart beat. It may be experienced by healthy people as well as those with cardiac disorders. The sensation is described in several ways: as a racing of the heart, an awareness of irregular or missed beats, a thumping in the chest and as a throbbing in the neck. In healthy individuals, emotion, excitement or anxiety and stimulants such as nicotine and caffeine can be associated with a fast heart rate and extra beats, creating the sensation of palpitation. It is an important symptom in people with dysrhythmias. Someone with a tachycardia may be aware of the sudden onset of rapid, regular beating of the heart, whereas those with atrial fibrillation may be conscious of its irregularity.

Oedema

The mechanisms of oedema formation are described in Chapter 4. The location of oedema in congestive cardiac failure is determined by gravity and the patient's position and is known as dependent oedema. Oedema accumulates first in the lower parts of the body. When the patient is ambulant or when sitting, it

Table 12.1 Characteristics of chest pain

	Angina pectoris	Myocardial infarction	Pericarditis
Location	Retrosternal – can be located in the centre of the chest but is more often felt across the chest	Retrosternal	Retrosternal
Radiation	The pain may radiate to the arms, neck, jaw, back or abdomen. This is known as referred pain and is due to the shared nerve supply in the thoracic area	The pain may radiate to the arms, neck, jaw, back or abdomen	The pain may radiate to the neck, back or abdomen Rarely radiates to the arms
Severity	Mild to moderate discomfort, sometimes described as an ache rather than a pain. Individual's perception of pain differs	Severe pain	Mild to moderate pain
Nature	Tightness, pressure, constriction, burning, aching or heaviness. Often tightness is perceived as breathlessness. The person often clenches his fist over the chest in an attempt to describe the pain	Crushing, choking, strangling, oppressive pressure May have a feeling of impending doom	Sharp Pain is usually sharp but may be aching in nature
Duration	Brief, usually less than 20 minutes. The pain usually builds up gradually over seconds or minutes	Prolonged The pain is continuous and lasts longer than 30 minutes	Usually constant
Precipitating, aggravating factors	Exercise, emotions, extreme temperatures, heavy meals. Angina pectoris is brought on by an increase in myocardial oxygen demand	Usually no precipitating factors The pain may occur at rest or during sleep	Aggravated by inspiration, lying flat, coughing and swallowing
Relieving factors	Rest and/or glyceryl trinitrate (GTN). Rest reduces the heart's demand for oxygen	Unrelieved by rest and GTN Rest and GTN may decrease the intensity of the pain Opiates are usually required to relieve it	Sitting up and quiet, shallow breathing
Associated symptoms	Uncommon	Nausea, vomiting, dyspnoea, sweating and pallor Symptoms often appear shortly after the onset of pain They may or may not be present	Pericardial friction rub A dry scratchy sound may be heard on auscultation

collects initially in the feet and ankles and then in the legs. When in bed, oedema gathers in the sacral area and thighs. In right-sided heart failure oedema first shows in the dependent parts, whereas in acute left-sided heart failure fluid may accumulate in the lungs causing pulmonary oedema. The oedema increases with the progression of the heart failure.

Fluid may accumulate in the peritoneal cavity (ascites) and in very advanced failure total body oedema (anasarca) may develop. Cardiac oedema is said to 'pit' on pressure. This means that if an oedematous area is pressed by the finger, an indentation remains when the finger is removed.

Fatigue

People with cardiac disorders frequently complain of fatigue on mild exertion, which is relieved by rest. Fatigue in disorders affecting the heart is a sign that the heart is unable to pump out sufficient blood and oxygen and is unable to meet even a small increase in the metabolic demands of cells and tissues.

Syncope

Syncope or fainting is a transient loss of consciousness as a result of a sudden decrease in blood flow to the brain. Syncope can often occur in response to emotion, but physical factors such as pain, blood loss and debility after infection can contribute to its occurrence. Fainting of this kind usually develops when standing and is usually preceded by yawning, sweating, nausea and a 'sinking feeling' in the stomach. In those individuals with cardiac disorders, syncope occurs when cardiac output has fallen dramatically. This is common as a result of a very slow or fast heart rate or severe cardiac dysrhythmias. Sycnope on exertion is a characteristic feature of severe aortic stenosis.

A more important and dangerous form of syncope is the Stokes–Adam's attack, which is a brief episode of cardiac arrest due to either asystole or ventricular fibrillation.

DISTURBANCES OF BLOOD VOLUME

Adequate cardiac function and output is dependent on a sufficient volume of blood being returned to the right side of the heart (venous return) and therefore indirectly on the total blood volume. If venous return is too small, then cardiac output may fall, resulting in an inadequate circulation. In situations of increased venous return, for example, during exercise, the heart can normally increase its cardiac output. However, if the volume is too great and/or the heart is pumping inefficiently the heart will become overworked, resulting in circulatory overload. A decrease in circulating blood volume can result from dehydration (see Ch. 4), haemorrhage or circulatory failure (shock).

Haemorrhage can be caused by trauma to a blood vessel causing it to rupture, or by spontaneous rupture; for example, rupture of an aortic aneurysm or a vessel in the brain of a hypertensive person. Haemorrhage may also be the result of a deficiency in certain blood factors (see Ch. 4). Bleeding may be local or systemic.

The terms circulatory failure, low output state and shock are used to describe a clinical picture of overall tissue perfusion which is inadequate to meet the body's needs. This can occur in a number of disorders, such as haemorrhage, burns and other states involving a reduction in fluid volume (hypovolaemic

shock), as well as other disorders such as heart failure (cardiogenic shock), severe allergic reactions (anaphylactic shock) and severe sepsis (septic shock).

Fluid overload may occur as a result of excess water intake which is usually iatrogenic in nature (e.g. excessive or rapid intravenous infusion) or in patients with heart, kidney or neurological disorders. As a result, venous return may increase to the extent that the volume of blood in the ventricles becomes too great, reducing the force of contraction and causing the heart to dilate. The effectiveness of the heart is thereby reduced and cardiac output falls.

Common symptomatology

The effects of haemorrhage or fluid loss depend on the volume and rate of fluid lost, and the site of haemorrhage. The clinical features of acute haemorrhage are similar to those of circulatory failure or shock of any type, and include restlessness, dizziness, syncope, pallor, a rapid thready pulse and a low blood pressure. The patient's skin is usually cold and sweaty and the urinary output will be reduced. These signs and symptoms are due to a fall in cardiac output and a resultant diversion of blood away from less vital areas, for example, skin and kidneys to vital organs such as the brain and heart.

Patient implications

Almost every patient, regardless of diagnosis, is susceptible to fluid imbalance as illness, by its very nature, upsets the body's delicate homeostatic mechanisms. Certain patients are however particularly susceptible, for example those with cardiovascular and renal disorders or patients undergoing surgery. The implications vary with severity. For example, small local haemorrhages are not usually dangerous unless they occur within the pericardial space causing cardiac tamponade, or in the brain (see Ch. 5). Large systemic haemorrhages are however always dangerous as they may greatly reduce blood volume and cardiac output. The development of shock has severe implications, as if untreated it will result in death.

Nurse's role in establishing differential diagnosis

The nurse has an important role in identifying signs and symptoms at an early stage, thus ensuring early treatment. This is of particular importance for example in internal haemorrhage where in addition to the symptoms mentioned there may be pain in the area of bleeding due to swelling of tissues along with fever.

CONGENITAL ABNORMALITIES

A congenital abnormality of the heart is present in nearly one in every 100 babies born. If untreated, about half of the affected babies would die from their heart disorder or some associated anomaly during the first year of life. However, a person with a minimally malformed heart may go through life symptomless and completely unaware of the defect until the child or adult is much older and perhaps is being examined at school, for employment or insurance purposes. Little is known of the causes of congenital heart disease, although in some cases there is evidence of either a genetic abnormality or environmental factor affecting the mother during the early months of pregnancy. If a mother contracts rubella (German measles) during the first 3 months of pregnancy, her child may have a heart defect as a result of arrested or faulty fetal development. Other viral infections may occasionally be responsible, as may some drugs, including alcohol. Congenital defects may also be found in auto-somal chromosome abnormalities such as Down's syndrome.

The most common form of congenital heart disorder is a ventricular septal defect, with Fallot's tetralogy being the most common cause of cyanotic heart disorder in children surviving infancy. The different types of congenital heart disorders and their effects are summarized in Table 12.2, with some examples given in Figure 12.8.

Many congenital abnormalities can be corrected by surgery.

DISORDERS OF HEART VALVES

The function of heart valves is to ensure one-way flow of blood through the heart and therefore damage to valves can disrupt blood flow. Disorders of valves may cause their cusps to stick together, thus narrowing the opening (stenosis), which can damage the edge of the cusps, with the result that they are unable to close completely. This causes backflow (regurgitation) of blood through the valve. Such a valve is said to be incompetent or insufficient. Stenosis and incompetence can occur together but usually one or other exists independently.

Table 12.2 Types of congenital heart disorders

Types of disorders	Examples	Effects	Clinical features
Abnormal communications between the left (systemic) and right (pulmonary) circulations	Persistent ductus arteriosus Atrial septal defect Ventricular septal defect (Fig. 12.8)	Left to right shunt:- re-oxygenated blood from left to right side of heart and an increase in blood flow through lungs Severe pulmonary hypertension may result leading to a reversal of shunt i.e. venous blood from right to left side of heart	Eventually leads to breathlessness and fatigue and cardiac failure Dyspnoea Cyanosis Fatigue
Obstructive lesions	Coarctation (constriction) of the aorta Aortic stenosis Pulmonary stenosis May be combined with abnormal communications e.g. Tetralogy of Fallot	Cause a strain to the related ventricle May cause cardiac failure Severe pulmonary hypertension may result leading to a reversal of shunt i.e. venous blood from right to left side of heart	Dyspnoea Cyanosis Fatigue
Displacement or absent chambers, vessels or valves	Dextrocardia (heart in the right side of chest) Right-sided aorta Transposition of the great arteries	Limited importance Associated with high mortality Heart failure and death usual within first month	Cyanosis develops at/or shortly after birth Difficulty in finishing feeds Increased breathlessness and deep cyanosis

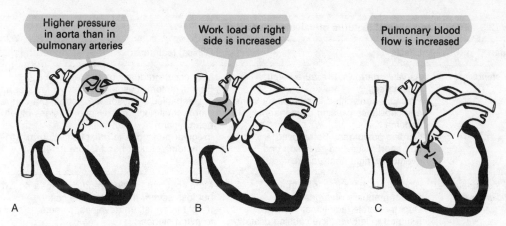

Fig. 12.8 Examples of congenital defects. (A) Persistent ductus arteriosus. (B) Atrial septal defect. (C) Ventricular septal defect

Valvular disorders are most commonly the result of infection or congenital abnormalities, but may also be due to trauma. The mitral valve is affected most frequently followed by the aortic valve.

Mitral valve disease

Disease of the mitral valve is frequently due to rheumatic endocarditis, resulting from acute rheumatic fever, and taking the form of mitral stenosis, although some degree of regurgitation may be present. Acute rheumatic fever is a febrile illness which follows infection with and an abnormal response to the Group A haemolytic streptococcus. Rheumatic endocarditis may smoulder on for many years producing chronic rheumatic heart disease and presenting sometimes in early adult life, but more often many years later. In many countries including the UK, rheumatic fever has been becoming progressively less frequent over the past 50 years. Mitral valve disease, particularly mitral incompetence, may also be due to ruptured or disordered chordae tendinae, papillary muscles or valve cusps, or to dilatation of the valve ring as a result of left ventricular enlargement. Mitral valve prolapse syndrome results in incompetence of the mitral valve as a result of a dysfunction of the valve cusps.

Aortic valve disease

Aortic valve disease may be rheumatic in origin and then usually associated with mitral valve disease or may be due to congenital or degenerative change. Most instances of aortic stenosis occur in middle or old age with no evidence of other valves being

involved. Many of these people tend to have only two cusps to the aotic valve and in later life, the valves tend to become calcified and stenosed.

Pulmonary and tricuspid valve disease

Tricuspid valve disease, which is relatively uncommon, is nearly always rheumatic in origin and usually occurs in combination with mitral and/or aortic valve disease. Pulmonary valve disease is extremely rare.

The effects and clinical features of valvular disorders are summarised in Table 12.3.

Patient implications

A patient may experience no symptoms of valvular disorders for many years, but when symptoms do occur they may, depending on their severity, greatly affect an individual's normal activities of living. Symptoms such as fatigue, dyspnoea on exertion and in some cases angina can have an increasingly debilitating effect. In later stages of the disease, dyspnoea may occur on minimal exertion and the symptoms of heart failure lead to increasing immobility, anxiety and restrictions in normal activities. Cardiac surgery may be required, either valvotomy or valve replacement.

ENDOCARDITIS

Endocarditis is an inflammation of the inner lining of the heart, affecting predominantly the heart valves, and represents less than 1% of all cardiac disorders. The main cause is infection, although it may be due to

Table 12.3 Effects and clinical features of valvular disorders

Disorder	Effects	Clinical features
Mitral stenosis	As valve narrows, pressure in left atrium rises Pressure transmitted to pulmonary veins and capillaries causing pulmonary oedema Cardiac output may be reduced Left heart failure may develop and eventually, right heart failure	May occur gradually or suddenly First symptom – usually excessive fatigue, may be accompanied by dyspnoea, cough, orthopnoea, paroxysmal nocturnal dyspnoea (signs of left heart failure) Irregular pulse due to atrial fibrillation (p. 401) Symptoms of right heart failure (p. 403)
Mitral incompetence/ insufficiency	Blood flows back into left atrium Atrium gradually enlarges During diastole, additional volume returned to left ventricle causing dilatation (hypertrophy) and left heart failure	Most common – fatigue and dyspnoea on exertion but less severe than mitral stenosis If right heart failure develops, symptoms similar to mitral stenosis
Aortic stenosis	Increased workload for left ventricle Ventricle hypertrophies (compensation) but eventually blood flow unable to meet demands of heart muscle for oxygen – myocardial ischaemia In severe stenosis: fall in cardiac output, left heart failure	May be asymptomatic for many years First symptom – usually fatigue followed by angina pectoris (p. 399), dyspnoea and syncope on exertion Late in disease – orthopnoea, paroxysmal nocturnal dyspnoea, pulmonary oedema
Aortic incompetence/ insufficiency	Backflow of blood to left ventricle during diastole Increased workload for left ventricle, leading to hypertrophy and left heart failure	Symptoms may not appear for many years First symptom – usually fast pulse (sinus tachycardia, p. 400) followed by dyspnoea on exertion and dyspnoea Late in disease – symptoms similar to aortic stenosis

non-infective causes such as rheumatic heart disease. Bacterial (infective) endocarditis may be acute, subacute or chronic. It is characterized by the formation of loosely adherent vegetations on the heart valves and by the spread of bacteria from the valves, via the blood to various tissues and organs.

DISORDERS OF THE PERICARDIUM

Pericarditis

Inflammation of the pericardium is most commonly a complication of myocardial infarction. Idiopathic pericarditis is also common, but is probably due to a viral infection or to an allergic or immune reaction. Other causes include connective tissue disorders, malignant disorders and trauma. Pericarditis may be acute or chronic (constrictive).

Common symptomatology

Acute pericarditis produces pain, which is similar in distribution to the pain of myocardial infarction –

retrosternal pain which may radiate to the neck, back or abdomen. However, unlike ischaemic heart pain, it is worsened by inspiration, movement and by lying flat (Table 12.1). Diagnosis may be confirmed by the presence of a pericardial friction rub, which is heard as a scratching or grating noise over the heart on auscultation. Dyspnoea and an elevated temperature may be present.

Chronic constrictive pericarditis is a chronic inflammatory disorder in which the pericardium thickens and compresses the heart. The symptoms are those of congestive heart failure (see p. 403).

Pericardial effusion

Pericarditis may be accompanied by a pericardial effusion which is a collection of fluid in the pericardial space. This fluid is often serous in nature, but may be purulent or blood stained (from trauma or malignant disease). Large effusions may be detected by percussion, although it is most frequently noticed on a chest X-ray. Treatment is not usually required unless there is tamponade.

Cardiac tamponade

An accumulation of pericardial fluid may cause compression of the heart impairing venous return and normal filling of the ventricles. As a result, cardiac output and blood pressure fall, the heart rate increases to compensate and the clinical signs of shock appear.

In addition, there is a rise in central venous pressure (see p. 407), the neck veins may appear distended on inspiration (Kussmaul's sign) and a diminished pulse pressure may be detected during inspiration (pulsus paradoxus). The most common cause of cardiac tamponade is haemorrhage within the pericardial cavity due to cardiac rupture, perforation during cardiac catheterization (see p. 406) or aortic aneurysm dissection (see p. 432). Tamponade due to pericardial effusions as a result of infection tends to occur more slowly.

Patient implications

The implications of pericarditis for an individual depend on the cause and treatment depends on the severity of the symptoms, with pain relief being a priority. However, the development of cardiac tamponade can lead to sudden death and requires emergency intervention which involves aspiration of the fluid under local anaesthesia.

Nurse's role in establishing differential diagnosis

The nurse has a vital role to play in the early identification of the signs and symptoms of developing cardiac tamponade. A falling arterial blood pressure should always be reported. In cardiac tamponade the diastolic pressure tends to remain stable while the systolic pressure falls. Prompt recognition and reporting of vital signs can prevent the possibility of sudden death.

DISORDERS OF THE MYOCARDIUM

The heart muscle is involved in most types of cardiac disorders, most commonly in association with coronary heart disease (see p. 498). The terms myocarditis and cardiomyopathy however are used in association with relatively uncommon types of myocardial disorders which are not attributable to coronary heart disease, congenital and valvular disorders or hypertension. The myocardium may be affected by diverse factors such as tumours, toxins, chemicals, physical trauma (electric shock and radiation), immunological responses, autoimmune diseases and nutritional disorders. Many are of unknown origin.

Myocarditis

The term myocarditis is used to describe inflammatory disorders of the myocardium due to infections and toxins. It is commonly associated with pericarditis and varies in severity.

Common symptomatology

Some patients may only develop a rapid heart rate and non specific electrocardiograph (ECG) changes, while others may develop symptoms of heart failure and abnormal heart rhythms. There is a risk of acute circulatory failure and sudden death.

Cardiomyopathies

The cardiomyopathies are a group of chronic disorders of the heart muscle, the most common type being congestive or dilated cardiomyopathy. The ventricle dilates and enlarges and the muscle thickness diminishes, leading to a reduced force of contraction. In hypertrophic cardiomyopathy there is extensive hypertrophy and increase in muscle mass and blood flow may be obstructed.

Common symptomatology

Cardiomyopathy results in an impairment of the pumping ability of the left ventricle leading to left and eventually right heart failure. Most patients therefore present with the symptoms of heart failure (see p. 403).

Patient implications

There is no specific treatment for myocarditis and with rest and alleviation of symptoms, many people recover completely, while others may be left with permanent damage causing a form of cardiomyopathy. Minor forms of cardiomyopathy are common and the person may remain well for many years. The main concern, however, is sudden death which is often preceded by abnormal heart rhythms. When the patient becomes unresponsive to the treatment of heart failure, heart transplant will become the only hope for survival.

DISORDERS OF THE CORONARY ARTERIES

The primary disorder affecting the coronary arteries is atherosclerosis, a gradual pathological process which results in changes in the lining (intima) of arterial blood vessels (see p. 424).

Almost everyone by the age of 40 has a small amount of narrowing of the coronary arteries, although this usually goes unnoticed. Significant narrowing of arteries however, causes a reduction or sometimes total obstruction to blood flow resulting in coronary heart disease (ischaemic heart disease) as well as peripheral arterial disease (see p. 426).

CORONARY HEART DISEASE

Coronary heart disease is a major threat to the health of middle-aged and elderly people in the western world. In the UK, more than 170 000 people die from coronary heart disease each year, 25% of whom are below 65 years of age. An estimated 200 million working days are lost each year due to this disease and it is a major cause of morbidity and mortality in the elderly. In 1991 approximately 17 000 coronary bypass operations and 261 heart transplants were carried out in the UK and over 320 000 people consult their doctor about angina each year (British Heart Foundation 1994). There are therefore major economic as well as human costs for the country. Scotland has one of the highest mortality rates from coronary heart disease in the world.

The exact mechanism responsible for the development of atheroma in the coronary arteries is not known. However, various studies have provided important information on life-styles and risk factors and although there is no single cause, three major risk factors have been identified: cigarette smoking, high blood cholesterol and hypertension. Many other factors are also involved, some which are avoidable and some which are not (Box 12.1). For further information refer to Julian & Marley (1991) and Williams (1992).

The symptoms of coronary heart disease depend on the degree of obstruction of the artery and range from ischaemic chest pain due to moderate obstruction, to death in some instances of complete obstruction. If the narrowing occurs over a number of years, small communications may develop between arteries (collateral vessels), which help to supply blood to the heart muscle beyond the narrowed artery, and may help protect the myocardium from ischaemia, particularly at rest.

Box 12.1   Risk factors for coronary heart disease (CHD)

MAJOR RISK FACTORS
Raised blood cholesterol:
Strong relationship between a serum cholesterol > 5.7 mmol and CHD
The low density component of cholesterol (LDL) is most responsible
The high density component (HDL) carries a lower risk
Smoking
Smokers have a 2–3 times greater risk than non-smokers
Cigarettes are more dangerous than cigars or pipes
Giving up smoking reduces risk of death from CHD (passive smoking also increases the risk)
High blood pressure
There is a 2–3 times greater risk at systolic blood pressures over 150 mmHg and diastolic over 95 mmHg

OTHER RISK FACTORS
Age
Risk increases with age
Gender
Mortality rates higher for males
Incidence almost equal > age of 60
Family history
Strong familial tendency
Diabetes mellitus
Increased risk. Reason uncertain
Obesity
Increased risk at > 20% over ideal body weight
Physical inactivity
Physical activity protects against development of CHD
Stress and personality
Role of stress uncertain. Certain types of behaviour patterns may increase risk
Socioeconomic and geographical factors
Marked international differences in incidences of CHD throughout UK (highest in Scotland, N. Ireland and North England) More common in Social Classes IV and V
Other factors
Relationship between oral contraceptives, heavy drinking, a high uric acid level and CHD

Myocardial ischaemia

Ischaemia is the condition of oxygen deprivation, accompanied by inadequate removal of metabolites, consequent to reduced perfusion.   (Braunwald 1988).

The heart utilizes nearly all of its available oxygen supply even with normal levels of activity and therefore, when the heart requires additional oxygen for increased activity, coronary blood flow must increase. If there is substantial deficit in the blood supply (due to narrowing of the coronary arteries) in proportion to the demands for oxygen and nutrients, myocardial ischaemia results. Ischaemia can therefore also be defined as an imbalance between oxygen supply and demand.

Angina pectoris

The majority of people with myocardial ischaemia develop the symptoms of angina pectoris. Angina is a discomfort or pain, usually in the chest, which is precipitated by increased in activities such as exertion, emotion and exposure to cold, when the demand for oxygen is increased. It is relieved when the oxygen demanded of the myocardium falls or by taking a glyceryl trinitrate tablet sublingually (see p. 409). A typical anginal attack lasts 3–5 minutes. Although atherosclerosis is by far the most common cause of myocardial ischaemia and anginal pain, other disorders such as spasm of the coronary arteries, severe anaemia and very fast heart rates may also be responsible. Conditions such as cardiomyopathies, hypertension and aortic stenosis increase the demand of the myocardium for oxygen and therefore may cause angina pectoris. Unstable angina is the term used to describe prolonged episodes of angina occurring at rest.

Myocardial infarction

When there is profound and sustained ischaemia to a part of the myocardium, the cells deprived of oxygen are unable to survive, and death (necrosis) of an area of heart muscle results. The overall process is termed acute myocardial infarction and is often referred to as a coronary occlusion or heart attack. It occurs usually when an artery is occluded by a thrombus forming on an atheromatous plaque (see p. 426). The location and size of the myocardial infarction depends upon the area of muscle supplied by the occluded artery and on the collateral blood supply.

The heart responds to a reduced blood supply in different ways, hence many people have an uneventful recovery while others develop more serious complications. Most myocardial infarctions affect the left ventricle and since this ventricle is the major pumping chamber responsible for ejecting adequate blood volume to maintain an adequate cardiac output, infarction can have severe consequences.

Common symptomatology

The patient usually presents with a history of chest pain, difficulty in breathing, nausea, vomiting, sweating and sudden weakness. The pain of acute myocardial infarction is usually more severe than anginal pain and is not relieved by rest or glyceryl trinitrate (Table 12.1). Not everyone however, presents with this typical picture. Some may have few symptoms, the position, type and severity of the pain may vary, while others develop more severe symptoms.

Abnormal electrical activity of the cells can produce abnormal heart rhythms (dysrhythmias): 'Within the first 30 minutes of the onset of chest pain, 80% of patients experience a disturbance of cardiac rhythm' (Dawkins 1987). Approximately 25% of people die within the first hour, usually due to ventricular fibrillation, many of whom experience no warning. Sixty per cent of sudden cardiac deaths occur outwith the hospital setting. Infarction of the left ventricle also results in a decreased force of contraction and may lead to acute left heart failure (see p. 402) or cardiogenic shock.

Cardiogenic shock

This is a serious complication and mortality is high. It results when the heart is unable to sustain the circulation and provide adequate oxygen to vital organs and tissues.

The individual is pale, extremities are cold and clammy, blood pressure is below 90 mmHg systolic and urinary output low. The person may also be confused.

Other complications of myocardial infarction such as pericarditis (see p. 439), rupture of the interventricular septum, myocardial wall or papillary muscles and ventricular aneurysms may also develop.

Myocardial infarction is diagnosed by the patients history, ECG changes and serum enzyme studies (see investigations p. 405–407).

Patient implications

The implications of myocardial ischaemia or infarction depend not only on the severity of the disorder and its symptoms but also on factors such as age, life-style, current state of health and dependence, etc. Not only do symptoms have an effect on normal activities of living, but there may well be major implications for alterations in life-style with modification of various risk factors.

The symptom of angina pectoris is a warning to the patient that his heart is not receiving enough oxygen and therefore it is important that he/she:

- knows what causes angina

- recognizes its onset
- treats the angina immediately
- alters some aspects of his life to reduce the workload of the heart.

The occurrence of acute myocardial infarction may have serious implications depending primarily on the amount of damage to heart muscle, the development of complications and the patient's age (mortality rises steadily with age).

Most deaths occur within the first few weeks, with the majority of these being caused by serious cardiac dysrhythmias before the patient reaches hospital. Excluding these early deaths, the overall mortality is 15–30% (Julian 1988). The experience of having a 'heart attack' can be very frightening, causing a sometimes abrupt interruption in the life of the patient and that of his/her family and friends.

Following discharged from hospital, patients who have previously been active and energetic can become very frightened, unnecessarily restricting their normal activities, and their family and friends may become overprotective. A planned rehabilitation programme is therefore important (see p. 424).

The diagnosis of coronary heart disease may have major implications for alterations in life-style, with the modification of actual or potential risk. The prevention of coronary heart disease is discussed on page 414.

Significance of nursing role in establishing differential diagnosis

The nurse has an important role to play in identifying patients who are at risk of developing coronary heart disease, enabling preventative measures to be instituted at an early stage. She should also have a knowledge of the signs and symptoms of angina and myocardial infarction so that they can be identified at an early stage and medical intervention requested. Pain assessment is of particular importance in differentiating between ischaemia and infarction as well as other cardiac and non-cardiac disorders. Accurate observation of the patient and recording of vital signs, and prompt reporting of alterations in the patient's condition can be extremely important in the early recognition of complications in the coronary patient.

DISORDERS OF CARDIAC RATE, RHYTHM AND CONDUCTION

Disorders in rate, rhythm and conduction (dysrhyth-mias) occur in both normal and diseased hearts. Dysrhythmias (also called arrhythmias) develop when the heart is unable to initiate and/or transmit electrical impulses in the normal manner. People with normal hearts may develop a dysrhythmia as a result of exercise, fever, emotion, fear, anaemia or hyperthyroidism. Dysrhythmias are also a common complication of coronary heart disease, in particular myocardial infarction, and of rheumatic heart disease, and many are caused by electrolyte imbalances and drug toxicities.

The normal heart rate ranges between 60 and 100 beats per minute, with higher rates being found in young children and lower rates in athletes. The impulse normally originates in the SA node, as its rate of discharge is faster than other myocardial cells. The normal heart rhythm is therefore referred to as sinus rhythm: sinus = originating in the SA node, rhythm = normal regular rhythm, at a rate of 60–100 per min. There are many different dysrhythmias and some potentially affect the circulation more than others. Two potentially lethal dysrhythmias causing cardiac arrest are ventricular fibrillation and cardiac standstill (asystole;) (see p. 412). Dysrhythmias may be classified in a number of ways, for example, fast rhythms or slow rhythms, atrial or ventricular rhythms. Table 12.4 gives examples of cardiac dysrhythmias and some of the more common ones are mentioned here. ECG monitoring of these rhythms is discussed on page 405.

Sinus tachycardia

The SA node is the pacemaker, the rhythm is regular, but the heart rate is greater than 100 beats per minute.

Sinus bradycardia

The impulse originates in the SA node, the rhythm is regular, but the heart rate is slower than 60 beats per minute.

Sinus arrhythmia

Impulses originate in the SA node but not with a completely regular rhythm. This irregularity is due to a variation of autonomic nervous system influence, resulting in alternating periods of slow and fast rates. It is usually related to the phases of respiration and is a relatively normal phenomenon, being common to young people.

Table 12.4 Examples of cardiac dysrhythmias

Site	Type of dysrhythmia	Explanation
ABNORMAL IMPULSE FORMATION AND ECTOPIC BEATS		
SA node	Sinus arrhythmia	Normal variation in sinus rhythm
	Sinus bradycardia	'Sinus rhythm' slower than 60 beats per minute
	Sinus tachycardia	'Sinus rhythm' faster than 100 beats per minute
Atria	Atrial ectopic beat	Premature atrial impulse followed by normal QRS complex
	Atrial tachycardia	Rapid discharge of abnormal pacemaker, within atria, rate 160–250 beats per minute
	Atrial flutter	Rapid, regular atrial activity giving rise to 'saw-tooth' waves. Every 2nd, 3rd or 4th impulse reaches ventricles
	Atrial fibrillation	Atrial activity appears as small, rapid, irregular waves (Fig. 12.15). Ventricular activity is completely irregular
Atrioventricular	Junctional ectopic beat	Premature junctional beat followed by normal QRS complex
	Junctional rhythm	Impulses arise in AV junctional area. Atria and ventricles may be stimulated simultaneously. Rate 40–60 per minute
	Junctional tachycardia	Fast, regular rhythm arising in the AV junctional area
	Ventricular ectopic beat	Premature ventricular impulse. QRS complex is wide and distorted
	Ventricular tachycardia*	Rate is 140–220 per minute. No visible P waves. QRS complexes wide and bizarre
	Ventricular fibrillation*	No visible P waves. Ventricular rhythm rapid and chaotic. Most serious dysrythmia – death results if not rapidly corrected
DISTURBANCES OF CARDIAC CONDUCTION		
SA node	SA block	SA node fails to initiate one or more impulses
AV node	1st degree AV block	PR interval prolonged. QRS complex normal
	2nd degree AV block	Only every 2nd, 3rd or 4th atrial impulse conducted to ventricles
	3rd degree AV block*	No relationship between atrial and ventricular rhythms
	(complete heart block)	Ventricular rhythm slow and regular
Ventricles	Asystole*	Ventricular standstill. No QRS complexes
		Potentially lethal dysrhythmia

Note: All dysrhythmias may lead to alterations in haemodynamics. Some can, however, produce critical haemodynamic alterations and are marked*.

Ectopic beats (premature beats)

When an ectopic focus, either in the atria, ventricles or AV junctional area, discharges prior to the SA node, a premature impulse takes place. Following this, there is a slight pause before the next normal sinus impulse arises.

Atrial fibrillation

In this common dysrhythmia, ectopic foci in the atria discharge electrical impulses in a very fast and irregular manner, and as a result the atrial muscles merely twitch or fibrillate. The AV node is unable to conduct all the impulses through to the ventricles and some pass through at irregular intervals. As a result, the ventricles contract in an irregular way and at a rate of usually 100–150 per minute.

Further information can be obtained from Hampton (1986) and Bennett (1989).

Common symptomatology

The effects of dysrhythmias vary considerably, depending on the type (Table 12.5) and on the clinical circumstances. Minor dysrhythmias do not usually affect the circulation and therefore may produce no symptoms, whereas major dysrhythmias tend to reduce the efficiency of the heart as a pump thereby affecting cardiac output. However, it is important to remember that even a sinus tachycardia increases the workload of the heart and therefore the demand for oxygen; hence, in association with for example myocardial infarction, it may produce more serious symptoms. Likewise, a sinus bradycardia may be slow enough to reduce cardiac output significantly. If the dysrhythmia has an adverse affect on the circulation, the person may complain of palpitations (in fast rhythms), dizziness, anginal pain or dyspnoea. Blood pressure may fall, sycope may occur and the pulse may reflect the heart rate by being fast, slow or irregular. Some dysrhythmias may produce cardiac arrest and collapse. Dysrhythmias are diagnosed by the patient's history, cardiovascular examination and ECG (see investigations on p. 405).

HEART FAILURE

Heart failure (cardiac or pump failure) is present when the ability of the heart as a pump is impaired and it is unable to meet the metabolic needs of the body. The heart will fail if there is damaged or poorly functioning muscle (e.g. myocardial infarction, cardiomyopathy), if the heart has to cope with an increased workload (e.g. systemic or pulmonary hypertension) or if there is abnormal blood flow within the heart (e.g. valvular disorders). 'High output failure' may occur where there is an increased metabolic demand which requires an above normal cardiac output (e.g. thyrotoxicosis).

Heart failure may be acute or chronic. Chronic heart failure is commonly referred to as congestive cardiac failure.

Congestive cardiac failure

Heart failure can be best understood by considering the heart as two pumping chambers; the left side being the pump for the systemic circulation and the right side the pump for the pulmonary circulation (see p. 387). One side may fail independently of the other but usually failure occurs almost together, one closely following the other.

Left-sided heart failure

When the left side of the heart fails, the left ventricle is unable to empty effectively and pressure within it rises. This is followed by increased pressure in the left atrium, pulmonary veins and pulmonary capillary bed. When the pressure becomes sufficiently high, fluid is forced out of the pulmonary capillaries and into lung tissues causing pulmonary oedema. The cardiac output will also fall, resulting in a decreased perfusion of body tissues and various compensatory mechanisms will occur. These include an increase in heart rate and dilatation and hypertrophy of the ventricle.

Right-sided heart failure

When the right ventricle fails and is unable to empty effectively, the subsequent rise in right ventricular and atrial pressures leads to back pressure into the vena cavae and the hepatic and systemic veins leading to oedema (see Ch. 4). A reduced amount of blood is pumped from the right ventricle and the resulting decrease in blood in the left side of the heart results in a fall in cardiac output.

Common symptomatology

The symptoms of congestive cardiac failure may be due to a low cardiac output, but are often the result of the body's compensatory mechanisms which serve to maintain the cardiac output. The symptoms of left- and right-sided heart failure are shown in Table 12.5.

Acute left ventricular failure (acute pulmonary oedema)

Acute left ventricular failure develops rapidly when the heart muscle suddenly loses its effectiveness as a pump, for example following acute myocardial infarction. Acute pulmonary oedema results from grossly inadequate cardiac function, due to a rapid rise in left ventricular volume and pulmonary venous pressure. Fluid exudes into the pulmonary alveoli, causing lung stiffness and impaired gaseous exchange. This leads to the following symptoms:

- breathlessness
- cold, clammy skin
- pallor
- fast (often irregular) pulse
- hypotension
- restlessness
- anxiety
- dry, unproductive cough and wheezing.

Patient implications

The patient with congestive cardiac failure may experience increasing activity intolerance and anxiety as a result of his symptoms. He may therefore require a great deal of support in adjusting to any necessary changes in life-style.

Table 12.5   Symptoms of heart failure: congestive cardiac failure

Symptom	Cause
LEFT-SIDED HEART FAILURE (SYMPTOMS RESULT FROM CONGESTION OF THE LUNGS AND REDUCED CARDIAC OUTPUT)	
Dyspnoea **Orthopnoea** **Paroxysmal nocturnal dyspnoea**	Fluid in alveoli
Cough	Large amounts of frothy blood-tinged sputum. May be unproductive
Altered renal function **Oedema** **Weight gain**	Decreased renal blood flow Increased sodium and water reabsorption
Anxiety **Restlessness** **Irritability**	Cerebral anoxia
Fatigue **Muscular weakness**	Low cardiac output Impaired oxygenation of tissues and removal of metabolic wastes
RIGHT-SIDED HEART FAILURE (SYMPTOMS RESULT FROM VENOUS CONGESTION OF THE VISCERA AND PERIPHERAL TISSUES)	
Dependent oedema **(usually pitting)** **Weight gain** **Distended neck veins**	Venous congestion Impaired sodium excretion
Coolness of extremities	Decreased peripheral blood flow due to venous congestion
Abdominal pain **Liver enlargement**	Hepatic congestion with venous blood
Anorexia **Nausea**	Venous engorgement and stasis within abdominal organs
Anxiety **Fear**	Symptoms and condition

Acute left ventricular failure is an emergency which requires urgent treatment.

Nursing role in establishing differential diagnosis

The nurse needs to carefully assess the patient with heart failure, observing for signs and symptoms of pulmonary and systemic fluid overload, recording and reporting findings promptly. Identifying alterations in the patient's breathing pattern or increasing oedema for example, helps to identify developing problems at an early stage enabling appropriate treatment to be given.

DISORDERS OF BLOOD PRESSURE

Hypertension

Blood pressure varies from person to person, and within one individual it varies throughout the day. It is however, considered that a resting blood pressure exceeding 150/90 mmHg indicates hypertension (raised blood pressure). Occasionally hypertension occurs in relation to toxaemia of pregnancy, endocrine disorders, cerebral disorders, etc., and is then called secondary hypertension. Hypertension in those under 40 years of age is usually secondary, unless there is a strong family history. In the majority of individuals no definite cause can be found and this type is called essential or primary hypertension, constituting 90% of all cases. There are many risk factors involved in the development of essential hypertension, including high alcohol and salt intake, and some drugs such as oral contraceptives and cortiosteriods. In normal individuals, a transient increase in blood pressure occurs with anxiety, cold and exercise. Pressure also rises with age. Obesity and emotional stress are contributory factors and there is definite evidence of an hereditary factor and strong familial tendency to hypertension.

Essential hypertension can be further subdivided into two groups, benign and malignant. Benign hypertension is characterized by a gradual onset and prolonged course. It is usually mild and may be symptomless. Malignant hypertension on the other hand has an abrupt onset and a short dramatic course. The diastolic pressure is usually very high, cardiac failure may develop and there may be involvement of the kidneys, brain, eyes and other organs. The increased workload of the heart leads to left ventricular hypertrophy and failure. The prognosis is poor and few survive more than a year without treatment.

Common symptomatology

These are extremely variable and there may be no symptoms for many years. Often the hypertension is only diagnosed as part of a routine medical examination. The severity of hypertension is not judged by the level of blood pressure alone as the course of the disease can vary in people with similar levels of blood pressure. At first the blood pressure is 'labile', that is it becomes abnormally high in response to emotion, anxiety and exercise. Eventually hypertension is found at rest and in the later stages the clinical features indicate cardiac, renal and cerebral involvement. Severe occipital headaches associated with nausea and vomiting, drowsiness, giddiness, anxiety and mental degeneration may occur as a result of cerebral impairment. Blood vessels in the brain may haemorrhage causing a cerebral vascular accident (see Ch. 5). Dyspnoea is usually the first symptom of left heart failure and eventually right heart failure may develop. As hypertrophied myocardium demands increased oxygen and blood supply, if atherosclerotic disease is present, it may be aggra-

vated or accelerated by hypertension and thus myocardial ischaemia or infarction may occur. Changes in the eyes, particularly the retina, are significant and directly proportional to the severity of the disease. There may be retinal haemorrhage and in severe hypertension, oedema of the optic disc (papilloedema) occurs.

Hypotension

A persistently low blood pressure is relatively rare and in fact chronic hypotension, with a systolic pressure in the range of 85–110 mmHg, is not pathological and may be associated with a longer life expectancy. Sudden development of hypotension, particularly in a patient who is recumbent, is usually associated with alterations in cardiac output and perfusion as a result of, for example, haemorrhage, shock, low blood volume, dysryhthmias or cardiac failure.

Postural hypotension may occur when there is loss of vasomotor tone leading to impairment of normal compensatory mechanisms which serve to overcome the initial gravitational effects associated with an upright position. This may occur during antihypertensive drug therapy, in disorders of the peripheral or central nervous systems, diseased or varicose veins causing pooling of blood in the lower extremities or after a long illness requiring prolonged bed rest, especially in elderly people. When the person stands up suddenly, there is a rapid fall in blood pressure due to impairment of peripheral vasoconstriction.

Common symptomatology

The principal clinical manifestation of hypotension is dizziness or syncope, which is a transient loss of consciousness due to temporary impairment of cerebral blood flow. When acute hypotension occurs as a result of, for example, dysrhythmias, haemorrhage, acute heart failure or shock, the clinical features of low cardiac output and associated compensatory mechanisms will be evident. These include tachycardia, cold and moist peripheries, decreased urinary output, restlessness and confusion.

Pulmonary hypertension

In pulmonary hypertension, the pressure in the pulmonary rather than the systemic arteries is elevated. This condition most commonly results from chronic lung disorders but may also be caused by thrombosis.

RANGE OF INVESTIGATIONS

The patient with a cardiac disorder may undergo various investigations in order to aid diagnosis and to monitor therapy given. These may range from simple procedures such as the taking of blood pressure to complex procedures such as cardiac catheterization. The nurse has a vital role to play in helping to maintain the dignity and well-being of each individual during procedures which are at times perhaps seen as routine but nevertheless very frightening for the patient.

History

Investigations of cardiovascular disorders should begin with a detailed history of the patient's past health, current illness and family history. Relevant information would include details of the onset of the disorder, signs and symptoms and their effect on normal activities, and the identification of risk factors. The nursing history (see p. 415) can contribute significantly together with the medical evidence to build a picture of the patient's problems.

Clinical examination

A physical examination will be carried out in order to collect objective information. This involves monitoring pulses and blood pressure as well as inspection of the patient's skin, extremities, neck veins, chest movement and body build. Palpation of the anterior chest wall will be carried out for pulsations and vibrations. Listening to heart sounds with the aid of a stethoscope (auscultation) is important in identifying abnormal heart sounds and murmurs.

The electrocardiogram

An electrocardiogram (ECG) is a graphic representation of the electrical activity in the heart. The electrical forces generated in the heart spread through the heart in multiple directions as waves of depolarization and repolarization (see p. 388). The ECG records these waves by means of electrodes attached to the limbs and specific points of the chest wall. The wave form recorded has been labelled the PQRS and T waves, with the P wave representing depolarization of the atria, the QRS complex depolarization of the ventricles and the T wave repolarization of the ventricles (Fig. 12.9).

These waves are made up of a series of positive and negative deflections – impulses which move towards

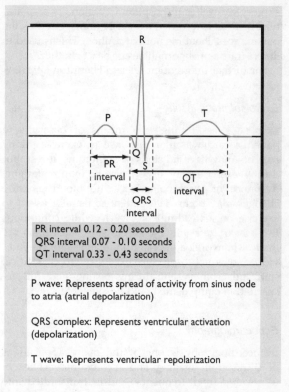

P wave: Represents spread of activity from sinus node to atria (atrial depolarization)

QRS complex: Represents ventricular activation (depolarization)

T wave: Represents ventricular repolarization

Fig. 12.9 The normal ECG complex

a recording electrode give rise to an upright (positive) deflection whilst those moving away from the same electrode display a downward (negative) one.

The standard ECG consist of recordings from 12 different leads which view the electrical activity from different angles, hence providing information about different sections of the heart. It is important to note that the ECG records only electrical activity and not contraction of the heart muscle, albeit the electrical activity spreading through the heart brings about contraction.

Continuous recording of the ECG can be carried out using a single lead to record the heart rhythm (see p. 417). The ECG is an important diagnostic aid in cardiac disorders. For example, it is used for the detection of dysrhythmias and diagnosis of myocardial infarction and ischaemia. It also helps to identity the specific area of heart muscle affected.

When the ECG is being recorded, the patient should be asked to remain as still as possible, to avoid distortion of the tracing by muscle activity. It is also important to ensure that all traces of the electrode gel are removed from the skin following the procedure. An ECG may be recorded at home or in the doctor's surgery as well as in hospital. Occasionally a special type of ECG is recorded over a 24-hour period as the patient goes about his normal routine. This is used to detect transient abnormalities of heart rhythm.

For further information refer to Hampton (1986).

Exercise stress testing

Exercise stress testing is a means of observing a patient's cardiovascular response to exercise. Many patients may have no signs or symptoms at rest, but during exercise may experience premature fatigue, dyspnoea or chest pain. ECG and blood pressure changes may occur. The patient is usually asked to exercise on a treadmill or bicycle while continuous ECG, heart rate and blood pressure recordings are made. The workload is carefully planned for the individual so as not to produce excessive stress. Medical staff must be present during testing and full resuscitation equipment should be available.

Echocardiography

Echocardiography is one of the many applications of ultrasound imaging and records the echoes of ultrasound (high frequency) pulses transmitted into the chest and reflected back by heart structures. When the ultrasound pulses meet a boundary between structures of different acoustic densities, for example heart valve tissue and blood, soundwaves are reflected back and these can be amplified and displayed on an oscilloscippe (monitor) or graphically.

Echocardiography is a useful method in assessing cardiac structure and function in a non-invasive manner. It is particularly useful in studying disorders of heart valves and for identification of pericardial effusion.

Chest X-ray

Enlargement of heart chambers, displacement of vessels and lung congestion in pulmonary oedema may be examined on chest X-ray (see Ch. 4).

Cardiac catheterization and angiography

Cardiac catheterization is a widely practised technique which involves the passing of a flexible catheter into one or more of the heart chambers. It is carried out to:

- record the pressures within the heart
- measure cardiac output

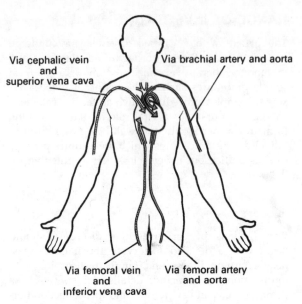

Fig. 12.10 Cardiac catheterization routes

- identify abnormalities of structure and function
- visualize the coronary blood vessels by angiography.

The right and left sides of the heart may be investigated independently or together.

Right heart catheterization A radio-opaque catheter is passed into a basilic or saphenous vein and advanced into the right atrium, through the tricuspid valve, into the right ventricle and then into the pulmonary artery (Fig. 12.10).

Left heart catheterization The catheter is introduced into the femoral or brachial artery and is passed back into the left ventricle via the aorta. This route is also used to examine the coronary arteries by angiography.

Angiography Contrast medium can be injected into the heart during cardiac catheterization and simultaneous high speed cine-radiography carried out, demonstrating the anatomy of the heart, any defects in myocardial contraction, abnormal blood flow through valves or septal defects or occlusion/narrowing of the coronary arteries.

Preparation Adequate explanations should be given and the patient should be aware of the need to lie on his back on a hard table in the catheterization laboratory during the procedure (approximately 90 minutes). He should also be warned to expect a sudden burning sensation when the dye is injected into the heart. The patient should be prepared in the normal way for a local anaesthetic.

The nurse has an important role to play in minimizing anxiety prior to and during the procedure by assessing the individual's needs and coping strategies, and giving appropriate support.

Aftercare   The nurse should assess and monitor the patient following the procedure and identify potential complications. The catheterization site should be observed for excessive bleeding, or formation of a haematoma especially following an arterial puncture. A pressure dressing is applied and the limb should be kept straight for 1–2 hours. If the femoral artery has been used, the patient is usually kept on bed rest for 6–8 hours to prevent occlusion. Frequent recordings of pulse, blood pressure and temperature should be carried out and the limb needs to be inspected regularly for adequate perfusion, indicated by the presence of a pulse, warmth and sensation. The patient should be assessed for pain and appropriate analgesia given as prescribed.

Nuclear imaging

Nuclear imaging can be used to provide additional information about ventricular size and contraction, and blood flow through coronary arteries. Although relatively costly, it has the advantage of being non-invasive, using special cameras, computers and radio-isotopes. The most common nuclear scans are the thalium scan, the pyrophosphate scan and nuclear ventriculography.

Blood tests

Various blood tests may be carried out in the diagnosis and assessment of cardiovascular disorders. For example, measurement of serum enzymes such as creatine phosphokinase (CPK) in myocardial infarction. These enzymes are released into the bloodstream when heart muscle is damaged.

Haemodynamic monitoring

A number of techniques are now available which enable cardiovascular haemodynamics to be assessed at the bedside and many require careful monitoring by nurses with advanced knowledge and skills.

Central venous pressure monitoring (Fig. 12.11)   The central venous pressure (CVP) reflects the pressure in the right side of the heart and is determined by the blood volume, vascular tone and cardiac function. The CVP catheter is inserted via the subclavian vein and lies in the superior vena cava or right atrium. The catheter is usually attached to an intravenous infusion, with a three-way tap connecting the infusion to a manometer which monitors the pressure. Insertion is usually carried out at the bedside and the patient is required to lie flat, usually with the head of the bed tipped slightly downwards. The nurse should ensure that the patient fully understands the procedure, offering support and reassurance. The nurse is usually responsible for the CVP recording and must ensure that recordings are accurate and also minimize any discomfort for the patient. For example, a patient with dyspnoea may find it uncomfortable to lie flat during recordings and therefore these should be carried out as swiftly as possible.

Pulmonary artery pressure monitoring   The valve of CVP measurement can be somewhat limited in many cardiac disorders as it reflects primarily right heart function which does not always parallel that of the left side. Measuring the pressure in the pulmonary artery with a special balloon-tipped catheter provides valuable information about left heart pressure and is

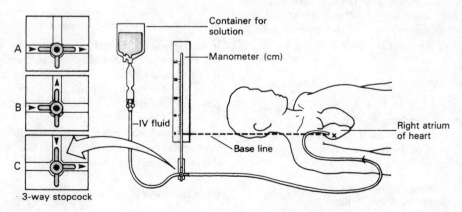

Fig. 12.11   Central venous pressure (CVP) monitoring. IVI, intravenous infusion

useful in patients with, for example, acute myocardial infarction and left ventricular failure. Cardiac output may also be measured. Catheters are usually inserted in specialized units, such as coronary care units, as management of the patient requires a high level of nursing skill and expertise.

THERAPEUTIC MANAGEMENT

The various disorders of the cardiovascular system have one thing in common – they all eventually lead to a decrease in cardiac reserve, that is the ability of the heart to meet the increased demands placed upon it. Specific therapeutic techniques and medications differ slightly for each major cardiovascular disorder. However, since the problems in all disorders tend to be similar, the important goals of therapeutic management can be applied to most dysfunctions of the cardiovascular system.

These are to:

1. Improve cardiac output and increase cardiac reserve.
2. Supply adequate oxygen, fluids and nutrients to all body tissues.
3. Correct dysrhythmias.
4. Control symptoms.
5. Minimize the undesirable effects of therapy.

Common drug therapy

Analgesics

Pain relief in the cardiac patient usually requires pharmacological intervention, although other methods may be of benefit. Opiates are used to relieve moderate to severe pain, the most commonly used being diamorphine and morphine. These agents help to relieve pain, reduce fear and anxiety and promote sleep, and may also help to decrease the risk of dysrhythmias. Diamorphine may also help to reduce the workload of the heart by vasodilatation.

Antiarrhythmic drugs

Antiarrhythmic drugs act by blocking the stimulus to the dysrhythmia, blocking the impulses or blocking the conduction of the impulse. Different drugs tend to act at specific sites of the conduction system.

For example:

- AV node – verapamil, digitalis, adenosine
- Ventricles – lignocaine, mexilitine
- Atria and ventricles – amiodarone, flecainide.

Anticoagulants

Anticoagulants may be used to prevent or treat thromboembolism which might occur in, for example, atrial fibrillation or myocardial infarction. They may also be used to prevent the recurrence or progression of thrombosis in coronary artery disease or prevent deep venous thrombosis or embolism in the patient with reduced mobility. Heparin and aspirin are the most common agents used.

Antihypertensive drugs

Antihypertensive drugs work by reducing peripheral vascular resistance or by decreasing cardiac output. Drugs include diuretics, beta-blockers, vasodilators and other agents such as methyldopa.

Beta-blockers

Beta-blockers are commonly used in the treatment of coronary heart disease, dysrythmias and hypertension. They reduce the workload of the myocardium and oxygen consumption by reducing the heart rate, strength of muscle contraction and systemic blood pressure. The patient's heart rate therefore needs to be carefully monitored and observations made to identify adverse effects such as heart failure, peripheral coldness, nightmares, insomnia and depression.

Calcium antagonists

These drugs interfere with the uptake of calcium by cells, causing a decrease in cardiac work, vasodilatation and a reduction in dysrhythmias. Drugs such as nifedipine and diltiazem are used in angina, whereas verapamil is useful in the treatment of supraventricular tachycardias.

Diuretics

In cardiovascular disorders, diuretics are used primarily in left ventricular failure and pulmonary oedema. By causing a diuresis of water and solutes, they reduce blood volume, venous return to the heart and pressure in the left ventricle. The resulting reduction in pressure in the pulmonary capillaries will help the patient to breathe more easily with the reduction in ventricular pressure decreasing cardiac workload and therefore its oxygen requirements.

Inotropic drugs

Positive inotropic drugs increase the strength of

contraction of heart muscle, thereby increasing cardiac output. These drugs are commonly used in the treatment of heart failure and cardiogenic shock and examples include dobutamine, dopamine and digitalis.

Vasodilators

Vasodilators are used in the treatment of angina, heart failure and hypertension. Nitrates, for example glyceryl trinitrate (GTN), have been the main treatment of angina for many years and can be administered by several routes, the most common being sublingually (see Ch. 4), other routes include oral sprays, ointment and skin patches.

Thrombolytic therapy

In the majority of cases, the occlusion of a coronary artery which causes myocardial infarction is caused by thrombosis. This thrombus can be dissolved by giving thrombolytic agents intravenously, allowing the ischaemic area of muscle to be reperfused and minimizing the amount of resulting muscle damage. Since necrosis of myocardium which is starved of blood is usually complete within 6 hours, it is crucial that the thrombolytic agent is given as soon as possible within this period of time. The thrombolytic agents currently available include streptokinase, recumbinant tissue type plasminogen activator (rtPA), anisoylated plasminogen-streptokinase activator complex (APSAC), urokinase and prourokinase. Following thrombolysis, anticoagulants are used to prevent reocclusion of the coronary artery. The patient may develop various problems as a result of this therapy; for example, bleeding, alterations in cardiac output, pain, anxiety, allergic reactions, dysrythmias and alterations in perfusion of tissues.

It is important that the nurse carefully explains the rationale for this therapy and its implications and observes for complications and reduction of pain and anxiety.

Percutaneous transluminal coronary angioplasty (PTCA)

Coronary angioplasty is a procedure by which stenosed (narrowed) coronary arteries are dilated, with the aim of restoring blood flow. This involves the passing of a thin double lumen balloon catheter into the coronary artery. The balloon is advanced so that it lies within the stenosis and then inflated for about 30–60 seconds. This is repeated several times until

there is evidence that the patency of the artery has improved. The best results from this procedure occur when there is disease of just one artery and in younger patients with a recent history of coronary heart disease.

Circulatory assist devices

Various mechanical devices are sometimes used which assist circulation and decrease cardiac work. For example, the intra-aortic balloon pump (IABP) can be used in patients with cardiogenic shock following myocardial infarction or cardiac surgery. This involves the insertion of a deflated, long, sausage-shaped balloon into the descending thoracic aorta, usually via the femoral artery. The balloon is inflated during cardiac diastole, before systole, aiding blood flow from the aorta to the coronary arteries, and deflated just before systole helping to 'suck' blood out of the left ventricle. Nursing care of a patient on an IABP requires a high level of expertise by specially trained nurses, who need to be able to deliver a high standard of care in a very technological environment.

Other forms of ventricular assist devices can be used to increase oxygen supply to the myocardium, reduce cardiac work, support the systemic circulation and allow for recovery of heart function.

Anti-shock trousers

The anti-shock trousers, commonly known as MAST (military anti-shock trousersuit), are used for the emergency management of patients with loss of blood volume, usually haemorrhage. The various chambers of the suit are inflated and the pressure exerted against the patient's legs and abdomen forces blood out of these areas, aiding return to the heart and improving perfusion of vital organs.

Cardiac pacemakers

Artificial pacemakers are often used to control the electrical activity within the heart. Pacemakers may be temporary or permanent, both consisting of a pulse generator which acts as a power source and a lead or insulated pacing wire with an electrode at its tip, which carries impulses to the heart.

Temporary pacemakers

Temporary pacemakers are used to maintain an adequate cardiac output in situations such as severe bradycardia, heart block and asystole. The generator or pacing box is external and portable, and the pacing wire is usually inserted via the subclavian vein and advanced into the tip of the right ventricle.

Permanent pacemakers

Permanent pacemakers are used in patients who have disorders of cardiac conduction which, following cardiac assessment, are considered to be long-term problems, with a high risk of recurrent symptoms. The permanent pacemaker is usually implanted under local anaesthesia in the cardiac catheterization laboratory. The pulse generator is inserted in subcutaneous tissue in the chest wall and the pacing wire inserted through a large neck vein into the heart. The pulse generators can be set to deliver a fixed rate or more commonly set 'on demand'. The demand form of pacing means that the artificial pacing beat can be inhibited when a normal cardiac impulse occurs, thus reducing the risk of competition between the two impulses. Nursing care of a patient with a cardiac pacemaker involves:

- Providing information regarding the procedure and its implications.
- Ensuring patient comfort and safety during and following insertion.
- Assessing pacemaker function.
- Preventing and dealing with complications, e.g. dysrhythmias, haemorrhage, haematoma and infection at pacemaker site.
- Teaching the patient about his condition and management.

CARDIAC SURGERY

There are two main types of cardiac surgery: open and closed. In closed heart surgery, the circulation continues to flow through the heart during the operation; for example, mitral valvotomy is used to relieve stensosis of the mitral valve. A dilator is inserted into the left atrium and positioned into the valve to stretch it, separating the cusps and thus relieving the obstruction.

Open heart surgery necessitates the emptying of the heart and lungs of blood (cardiopulmonary bypass) to enable the surgeon to operate. During cardiopulmonary bypass, venous blood is drained from the right atrium and vena cavae and passed through an oxygenator which removes carbon dioxide from the blood and adds oxygen. The blood is then passed through a heat exchanger and a filter, which removes air bubbles and other emboli, before being returned to the aorta or femoral artery. The patient's body

temperature is reduced to 28–32°C and cardiac arrest induced. This technique is commonly used for replacement of heart valves and for coronary artery bypass surgery. It may also be used for the correction of congenital heart defects and intracardiac repairs.

Valve replacement

Valvular heart disease is almost always treated surgically. The damaged valve may be repaired, or it may be removed and a prosthetic valve sutured in its place. Various types of mechanical and tissue valves are used.

Mechanical valves

There are three major groups of mechanical valves:

1. The ball-in-cage valve, e.g. Starr–Edwards.
2. The tilting disc valve, e.g. Bjork Shiley.
3. The bileaflet valve, e.g. St Jude.

Because of the risk of thrombus formation on these valves, the patient requires anticoagulant therapy, sometimes for life. A further problem with mechanical valves is turbulence of blood flow; the action of the valve destroys red blood cells causing anaemia.

Tissue valves

Tissue valves fall into three main groups:

1. The xenograft (pig) aortic valve, mounted on a stent, e.g. Carpentier Edwards.
2. The xenograft pericardium (bovine), fashioned into cusps and mounted on stents, e.g. Bioflow.
3. The homograft (human tissue) aortic valve.

Coronary artery bypass graft surgery

Coronary artery bypass graft (CABG) surgery is a technique in which an occluded or stenosed section of a coronary artery is bypassed using part of a vein or artery from somewhere else in the body, usually the long saphenous vein or the internal mammary artery. The aims of CABG are to improve the quality of life in patients whose activities are restricted due to coronary heart disease. By relief of angina pectoris and an improvement in cardiovascular function, many patients can return to their previous life patterns. Although cardiac surgery is not without its risks, in patients with good left ventricular function and no other systemic disorder, overall mortality is less than 3%.

Heart transplantation

Some patients with end-stage cardiac disorders undergo heart transplantation, when other therapies have been successful. The number of suitable donor hearts available for transplantation however is limited at present. Heart transplants are carried out in specialized centres. The ethics of transplantation are discussed in Chapter 17.

Nursing management

Patients undergoing cardiac surgery require skilled observation and a wide range of emotional, physical and technical care. In the immediate postoperative period, this care is given by a specially trained team of professionals in an intensive care unit.

Patients require careful and thoughtful preparation for surgery. It is important that the patient knows what will happen to him before and after surgery and what to expect during the recovery period. Initially, he needs to know what to expect on regaining consciousness from the anaesthetic in the intensive care environment. For example, he should expect to have an endotracheal tube in situ along with various chest drains, infusions and monitoring equipment. The patient's family also need to be prepared for the first time they see the patient following surgery.

Most cardiac units have specially prepared booklets giving information about different members of hospital staff, admission, intensive care and convalescent areas, the operation itself, drug regimes, rehabilitation, etc. Nurses need to be sensitive to the many fears which patients undergoing heart surgery experience; for example, fear of the unknown, fear of pain, fear of their own families future and fear of death itself.

Good recovery has been shown to be associated with low anxiety regarding pain, reduced stress levels and a positive response to preoperative preparation.

For further information refer to Behrendt & Austen (1985).

EMERGENCY INTERVENTION

Cardiac arrest

Cardiac arrest is the sudden failure of the heart to contract, with a subsequent cessation in circulation and breathing. The brain is the organ of the body most sensitive to lack of oxygen and circulation must be restored within 4–6 minutes to prevent irreversible brain damage. Cardiac arrest may be caused by primary factors such as acute myocardial infarction or secondary causes such as drugs, electrocution or electrolyte imbalance. The majority of cardiac arrests occur when the patient is not in hospital, although it is not an uncommon occurrence in the hospital, and nurses as well as other health care professionals need to learn how to carry out basic cardiopulmonary resuscitation (CPR) effectively. It is also desirable for the lay public to learn these skills.

The nurse must know:

1. how to recognize a cardiac arrest
2. how to summon appropriate help
3. how to initiate CPR
4. where to find necessary equipment.

Cardiac arrest is recognized by:

1. abrupt loss of consciousness
2. absent carotid pulse
3. absent respirations.

Cardiopulmonary resuscitation

There are two main phases of CPR – basic life support (BLS) and advanced life support (ALS). The aims of BLS are to restore an oxygenated blood supply to the brain until spontaneous cardiac output returns or until medical treatment (ALS) can be initiated.

Basic life support

The steps to be taken in BLS are given in Box 12.2.

Advanced life support (ALS)

ALS combines basic life support with the use of specialist techniques and equipment for maintaining circulation and respiration. This may include:

1. **Airway management** – use of airway adjuncts, including endotracheal intubation (see Ch. 13).
2. **Electrocardiographic monitoring** – monitoring should be established as soon as possible following cardiac arrest. Three dysryhthmias are commonly associated with cardiac arrest:
   a. Ventricular fibrillation is the most common. The ventricles contract in an unco-ordinated manner due to chaotic electrical activity within the heart. The ECG shows an irregular, bizarre pattern (Fig. 12.13).
   b. Asystole is characterized by total standstill of the ventricles. The ECG tracing shows a flat trace which must be differentiated from faulty connections of the leads or monitor.
   c. Electromechanical dissociation is characterized by a normal ECG trace but with collapse of the circulation.

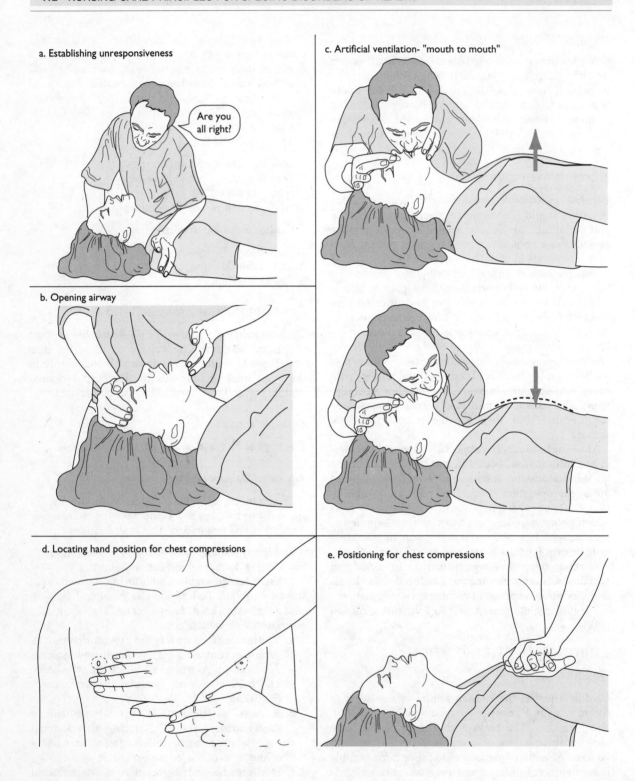

Fig. 12.12 Cardiopulmonary resuscitation (CPR)

Box 12.2   Basic life support

Assessment
- *DANGER*
  Ensure that there is no continuing danger to yourself or the patient.
- *RESPONSE*
  Establish if the patient is conscious by shaking him/her carefully and asking 'are you alright?' (Fig. 12.12 (a))

  Assessment then follows an **A B C** sequence
- **A** – *AIRWAY*
  Open the airway by tilting the head and lifting the chin using one hand on the forehead, pressing down to tilt the head and two fingertips of the other hand to lift the chin (Fig. 12.12 (b)).
- **B** – *BREATHING*
  Check if the patient is breathing by:
  Looking – for chest movement
  Listening – for breath sounds
  Feeling – for exhaled air (on your cheek)

LOOK, LISTEN AND FEEL FOR 5 SECONDS
- **C** – *CIRCULATION*
  Check the carotid pulse for at least 5 seconds

Action
- If there is no response but breathing and pulse are present:
  Treat any other life-threatening condition
  Place patient in the recovery position
  Summon help
- If there is no response and no breathing but a pulse is present:
  Give ten breaths of artificial ventilation (see below)
  Summon help (dial 999 if outwith hospital)
  Reassess before continuing with appropriate action
- If there is no response, no breathing and no pulse
  Summon help (dial 999 if outwith hospital)
  Start artificial ventilation and chest compressions (see below)
                        (Resuscitation Council (UK), 1993)

ARTIFICIAL VENTILATION. (Fig. 12.12 (c))
If the patient is not breathing artificial ventilation must be carried out. This is usually carried out by the 'mouth-to-mouth' method but nurses should also practise more complex techniques with the use of various airway adjuncts.

- Keep the patient's head tilted fully back and pinch the nose closed
- With the other hand, lift the patient's chin and allow the mouth to open
- Take a deep breath and making an airtight seal around the patient's mouth, give two slow breaths (approximately 2 seconds for full inflation)

- The rescuer's mouth should be removed between breaths to allow passive exhalation and he/she should ensure that the chest falls between inflations

An alternative method is 'mouth-to-nose' ventilation.

CHEST COMPRESSIONS
If there is no pulse cardiac compressions at approximately 80 per minute should be commenced.
  To carry out cardiac compressions:

- Ensure patient is on his back on a firm surface
- Locate the base of the sternum (Fig. 12.12 (d))
- Place the heel of one hand two finger breadths above this point – over the lower third of the sternum
- Place the heel of the other hand on top and interlock the fingers (the fingers should be clear of the chest) (Fig. 12.12 (e))
- Keep the arms straight and elbows locked and bring the shoulders up until they are directly over the patient's chest
- Depress and release the sternum 4–5 cm (in adults)

Artificial ventilation should be carried out with chest compressions at a ratio of two breaths to fifteen compressions (2:15). If there are two rescuers, one should carry out chest compressions while the other delivers a breath after each fifth compression, i.e. ratio of 1:5. There should be a slight pause to ensure that the delivered breath is sufficient to cause the patient's chest to rise.

VARIATIONS IN CHILDREN
Airway – in infants especially, the head should not be hyperextended otherwise kinking of the airway may occur.
Breathing – if breathing does not restart after opening the airway, give five breaths of artificial ventilation. In infants (up to 1 year) give artificial ventilation by covering the baby's mouth and nose with your mouth and blowing gently into the lungs until the chest rises. Ventilation should be at a rate of 20 per minute.
Circulation – in infants palpate the brachial pulse. If there is no pulse or it is less than 60 per minute, start chest compressions
Chest compressions – If chest compressions are required on a child, they should be given with proportionately less force than with an adult.
For infants:
  Compress the lower half of the sternum (below nipple line)
  Use only two fingertips at a rate of 100 per minute
  Use a ratio of 1:5 for both one and two rescuers
In children over 1 year:
  Give compressions with the heel of one hand at a rate of 100 per minute and a ratio of 1:5.
For further information see Resuscitation Council (UK) (1993).

Defibrillation   Ventricular fibrillation may be corrected by electrical defibrillation. The defibrillator delivers a preprogrammed electrical shock to the heart muscle in order to stop the chaotic electrical activity and allow normal heart rhythm to return. The defibrillator paddles are first covered with electrode jelly or conducting gel pads are placed on the skin to prevent burns. One paddle is placed on the chest,

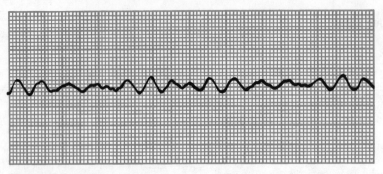

Fig. 12.13 Ventricular fibrillation

to the right of the upper sternum, with the other at the apex of the heart, so that the electrical current passes through the heart muscle. To avoid getting an electric shock, everyone should stand well clear of the patient and bed during defibrillation.

Drug therapy Intravenous access is essential for administration of drugs and fluid. Various drugs can be used to increase or decrease heart rate, stimulate heart contraction, suppress abnormal electrical activity and correct hypoxia and acidosis. Examples of drugs used include adrenaline, atropine, calcium chloride, lignocaine and sodium bicarbonate.

Further information can be obtained from Baskett (1993).

NURSING STRATEGIES

Health education

The nurse has an important role to play in the prevention of cardiac disorders, in particular coronary heart disease. Although there is insufficient evidence to prove that any specific measures will prevent coronary disease, the differences in incidences between countries and the changes which have taken place within countries suggest that modification of risk factors is important.

As suggested on page 400, this may involve minor modifications or major changes in an individual's life-style and the population as a whole. Health education is a process which aims to influence behaviour by producing the changes in knowledge, attitudes and skills necessary to maintain and improve health.

Prevention of coronary heart disease

The prevention of coronary heart disease is a major challenge for all health care professionals. Ideally, it should begin in childhood since atheroma has been shown to develop slowly over time. A high pro-

portion of people, for example, take up smoking as teenagers and many school children are physically inactive. Some of the risk factors may be reduced therefore by health promotion in schools and in the antenatal period, when mothers are receptive to information about health. Screening programmes are becoming increasingly popular in an attempt to identify risk factors at an early stage. Modifying behaviour is a difficult and long-term process. Nurses, however, need to be aware of current research evidence and be able to assist individuals in the interpretation of information and in modification of life-styles as appropriate. Health education is concerned with helping people make informed choices.

Modifying risk factors

While it is not possible to reduce some risk factors, for example family history, sex and race, others such as a high blood cholesterol, smoking and hypertension (see p. 398) may often be modified, hence minimizing the progression or development of coronary disease.

Diet Although there is still some controversy regarding the benefits of reducing cholesterol in the diet, it is generally recommended that the intake of saturated (animal) fats should be reduced to 11% of food energy and total fats to 35% (Department of Health 1991). Food should ideally be grilled rather than fried, fat trimmed from meat, and poultry rather than animal meat is recommended. Salt should be omitted in cooking and a high fibre diet incorporating more whole grains, vegetables and pulses may be beneficial in increasing the amount of indigenous cholesterol excreted. Individuals with hyperlipidaemia may require further dietary restrictions or drugs.

Alcohol Moderate amounts of alcohol are not harmful and may in fact reduce cardiac workload.

However, heavy drinking should be avoided as it increases blood pressure and may lead to weight gain and abnormalities of blood lipids. The recommended upper limit of alcohol intake for men is 20 units per week with restrictions of 15 units advised for women.

Weight The development of obesity predisposes to hypertension, increasing cardiac workload. An ideal body weight for height, age and sex is desired and those who have a weight problem should aim to reduce calorie intake and increase energy expenditure.

Smoking There is a strong correlation between cigarette smoking and coronary heart disease and although pipe and cigar smokers have a reduced risk, people should be advised to stop smoking. Smoking also exacerbates hypertension.

Hypertension Although there is some question as to whether reducing blood pressure in patients with existing coronary disease actually decreases mortality and morbidity, hypertension in these patients does increase the risk of developing coronary heart disease. Control of blood pressure may be brought about by partaking in regular exercise, balanced with adequate rest and sleep. Maintaining an ideal body weight is of benefit, as is the avoidance and management of stress.

Exercise Regular physical exercise is a vital element in the prevention of coronary heart disease. Physical activity in patients who have existing cardiac disorders however, needs to be carefully monitored and is an important element of any rehabilitation programme (see p. 424).

Stress Learning how to cope with stress is thought to significantly reduce blood pressure, serum cholesterol and the type A behaviour pattern. Type A behaviour pattern is defined by Friedman & Rosenman (1974) as:

a characteristic action–emotion complex which is exhibited by those individuals who are engaged in a relatively chronic struggle to obtain an unlimited number of poorly defined things from their environment in the shortest period of time and if necessary against the opposing efforts of other persons or things in the same environment.

There are many methods of stress management and relaxation available, for example listening to music, meditation, yoga, etc., and a suitable method for each individual should be found. The role of physical exercise is also important in reducing tension.

Further information may be obtained from Williams (1992).

Assessment

The nurse's initial contact with the patient with cardiac problems may be in the community, an outpatient department or on admission to hospital. Assessment involves observation, the taking of a nursing history and physical examination. This information is used to identify actual and potential problems.

Nursing history

When obtaining a nursing history from a patient with a cardiac disorder, the nurse needs to be aware of whether the patient is acutely ill or whether he has more chronic problems and his condition is stable. A patient who is acutely ill, for example following acute myocardial infarction or left ventricle failure, will require immediate medical and nursing intervention, and therefore an extensive interview at this point will not be a priority. At the same time as the nurse is monitoring the pulse and blood pressure, she may also gain important information regarding key symptoms such as pain, dysponea, palpitations, oedema, the patient's colour, level of consciousness, etc. When the patient's condition is more stable a more detailed history can be taken.

Various biographical and health data should be obtained, as well as information regarding activities (Box 12.3). The patient's pattern of living should be described. This will usually be based on a model of activities of living (see Ch. 3).

Physical assessment

Observing and talking to the patient will assist in the assessment of his physical and emotional state. However, a more detailed physical assessment will supply the nurse with more subjective information, confirm information obtained in the nursing history and provide suitable baseline data.

Pulse A pulse is the wave of expansion palpated in the artery wall when a superficial artery is compressed by the finger. As the ventricle contracts, the blood ejected distends the arteries, which contain elastic tissue in their walls. Common sites used for the examination of pulse are illustrated in Figure 12.14. The rate, rhythm and volume of the arterial pulse should be assessed.

Rate The pulse rate normally reflects the heart rate. In a resting adult the normal range is 60–100 beats per minute.

Rhythm The normal heart beat is regular, but sinus arrhythmia (see p. 400) is common in children and young adults and is considered normal. Ectopic beats (see p. 401) may appear as isolated irregularities in an otherwise regular pulse. These extra beats will be

---

Box 12.3   Nursing history

BIOGRAPHICAL AND HEALTH DATA
Brief description of patient
e.g. name, age etc.

Reason for admission

History of present illness
Details of onset of problem
Identification of risk factors
Signs and symptoms
Diet and physical activity

Previous history

Family history
Relevant information would include history of cardiac disorders, hypertension, diabetes, hyperlipidaemia

Psychological history e.g. interpersonal relationships, support systems
Helps to identify problems which may have a bearing on the patient's condition or affect the course of his illness or rehabilitation

PATIENT ACTIVITIES
Should include detailed information on:

Breathing
e.g. dyspnoea associated with exertion or at night, smoking, cough
Eating and drinking
e.g. normal dietary intake, alcohol intake, knowledge regarding dietary risk factors
Eliminating
e.g. normal patterns and use of diuretics or aperients
Personal cleansing and dressing
e.g. preference for bath or shower and frequency, condition of skin
Mobilizing, working and playing
e.g. normal mobility and any recent restrictions due to pain, dyspnoea, etc.
normal and altered work, leisure, sexual activities and rest periods, etc.
Sleeping
e.g. sleep patterns, hours per day, use of sedatives
Dying
e.g. patient's and family's fears and anxieties, spiritual needs, etc.

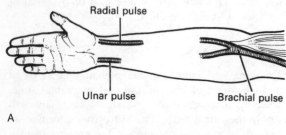

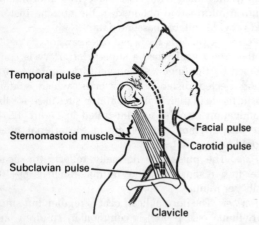

Fig. 12.14   Arterial pulses in: (A) upper limb; (B) head and neck

palpated as one which follows quickly upon the previous beat and is usually followed by a compensatory pause. In irregular heart rhythms, for example atrial fibrillation (see p. 401), the pulse will also be irregular. In addition, when the heart is contracting irregularly, not every contraction is strong enough to produce a palpable pulse and the pulse will be irregular in both rhythm and volume. This creates what is known as a pulse deficit where the heart rate is greater than the pulse rate. The deficit is estimated by the simultaneous recording by two people of heart rate by auscultation at the apex of the heart and of the pulse rate by measuring the radial pulse. Rates should be counted for not less than 2 minutes.

Volume   Pulse volume is reflected in the amount of movement felt by the palpating finger, caused by the pulse wave. Volume is related to cardiac output.

Blood pressure   Blood pressure (see p. 391) should be recorded when the patient is resting and relaxed. Blood pressure is usually assessed using a sphygmomanometer and by auscultation of the brachial artery. Sometimes postural hypotension (see p. 404) occurs and it may therefore be appropriate to measure the blood pressure in both the upright and supine positions.

Respiration   Dyspnoea is a common symptom in patients with cardiac disorders and may be observed both on exertion and at rest, especially when the patient lies flat. The rate, rhythm and depth of respiration should be assessed (see Ch. 13).

Temperature Increases in body temperature may be observed in some cardiac disorders which are related to infection; for example, bacterial endocarditis and rheumatic fever. A low-grade pyrexia may also occur following myocardial infarction, beginning within 24–48 hours and subsiding during the first week. This is thought to be a reaction to myocardial necrosis.

Weight Patients with cardiac disorders are sometimes weighed as often as daily, particularly if cardiac failure is present. Gradual weight gain might suggest the development of fluid retention whilst gradual weight loss can indicate the success of diuretic or other drug therapy.

Examination of head, limbs and abdomen In cardiac patients, the lips, earlobes, nose and hands should be examined for signs of cyanosis. The patient's skin should be observed for moistness and temperature as well as pallor. The feet, legs, abdomen, sacral area and hands should be observed for the presence of oedema.

Assessment of chest pain The nurse has a very important role to play in the assessment of chest pain. Pain in the chest may occur not only as a result of various cardiac disorders but also because of non-cardiac disorders (see p. 391). Assessment of the location, severity and nature of chest pain is therefore vital in establishing differential diagnosis (Table 12.1).

The nurse can assess pain by observing facial expressions and body posture, heart rate and blood pressure and by talking to the patient. The patient is the only person who can give an accurate, subjective description of the pain.

Open rather than closed questions should be asked where possible, as in the example given in Box 12.4.

Cardiac monitoring Assessment of the patient should be a continuous process. Frequent assessment of pulse, blood pressure, respirations and temperature should be carried out as appropriate, as well as the assessment of symptoms, and the effectiveness of nursing and medical intervention. Continuous monitoring of the patient is sometimes carried out using special equipment; for example, continuous blood pressure monitoring, central venous pressure monitoring (see p. 407). More commonly continuous monitoring of heart rate and rhythm is carried out.

Cardiac monitoring is a means of displaying the ECG (see p. 405) continuously on a small screen. This is especially valuable when disturbances of heart rhythm are present or suspected.

The value of cardiac monitoring is dependent on the presence of skilled nursing staff who are able to

Box 12.4	**Examples of methods of questioning patient in assessment of chest pain**
Location	Ask the patient to identify the location of the pain. Is it localized?
Radiation	Does the pain spread to any other parts? If so, where?
Severity	Ask the patient to describe the pain and its severity. Rating scales can be used (see Ch. 4). Compare with any previous pain, e.g. angina
Nature	Ask the patient to describe the type of pain, e.g. stabbing, burning, crushing, etc.
Duration	When did the pain start? How long did it last?
Precipitating/ aggravating factors	What brought the pain on? What were you doing at the time? Does anything make it worse, e.g. movement, deep breathing?
Relieving factors	What relieves the pain, if anything?
Associated symptoms	e.g. nausea, vomiting, sweating

recognize and interpret the significance of dysrhythmias. Some dysrhythmias (see p. 401) can endanger life and careful observation of changes on the monitor, and prompt treatment may prevent sudden deterioration. Examples of cardiac rhythms are shown in Figure 12.15.

Generally, cardiac monitors are found in intensive and coronary care units where an individual bedside monitor can be linked to oscilloscopes and alarm systems at a central nursing station. It is important to ensure that the patient and his family understand the purpose of cardiac monitoring, including the fact that the monitor does not affect the patient's heart.

Nursing intervention

Following assessment of the patient, and identification of problems, goals of care should be established and nursing intervention planned. It is important to set priorities for care. Priorities, for example, on admission to hospital, may include the alleviation of pain and anxiety and the relief of dyspnoea. As previously stated (see p. 408), cardiac disorders lead to a decrease in cardiac reserve and therefore initial intervention is aimed at decreasing the heart's requirement for oxygen (myocardial oxygen demand) alongside medical therapy which may increase the myocardial oxygen supply (e.g. the administration of

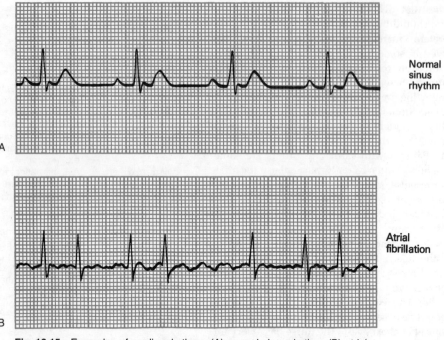

Normal
sinus
rhythm

A

Atrial
fibrillation

B

Fig. 12.15 Examples of cardiac rhythms: (A) normal sinus rhythm; (B) atrial fibrillation

oxygen therapy or thrombolysis). Myocardial oxygen demand can be reduced by the relief of pain and anxiety, promoting rest and by meeting the basic needs of the patient such as comfort, safety, elimination and giving adequate information.

The patient's immediate concern may be that of contacting family, or care of his pets, and he may be very frightened and fearful of dying. The nurse therefore needs to establish a close rapport with the patient and family in order to be effective in reducing fear and anxiety, helping to adjust to change and planning together for a successful recovery. The principles of nursing management are outlined below and examples of the care of patients with common cardiac disorders are included.

Control of symptoms

Chest pain Pain is a complex and personal experience and relief of pain is an important nursing responsibility. A careful and detailed assessment of pain is essential so that effective relief can be given as quickly as possible. People may respond differently to the same pain in different situations and anxiety seems to increase the severity of pain. For example,

chest pain may seem very severe when the patient is at home but may lessen on admission to hospital where he believes something can be done to relieve it. On the other hand, a patient who believes his chest pain is due to indigestion may feel the pain more severe if told he may have suffered a heart attack. Pain can have many adverse effects on the patient, including anxiety, sleeplessness and an increase in the workload of the heart. It is important, therefore, that pain relief is rapid and effective.

The pain experienced by cardiac patients is usually linked with an inadequate myocardial oxygen supply in relationship to demand and therefore measures should be taken to decrease the demand. These include minimizing patient activities, providing a relaxed atmosphere and maintaining a friendly and concerned approach.

The amount of analgesia required depends on the degree of pain, the size of the patient and the effects of any previous analgesia given. Although it is the doctor who prescribes the analgesia, the nurse usually administers it and evaluates its effectiveness.

Pain relief in a patient with an acute cardiac disorder such as myocardial infarction necessitates pharmacological intervention, usually with opiates.

The nurse must monitor the patient for hypotension, nausea and vomiting, dry mouth and a drop in respiratory rate. Oxygen therapy (see Ch. 13) is often used as a method of pain relief in the cardiac patient, aimed at increasing oxygen supply to the myocardium. Other pain-relieving strategies may also be employed by the nurse, including careful positioning of the patient, ensuring comfort and providing reassurance.

In the management of the patient with angina pectoris prevention of pain is an important element of care, as is education regarding nitrate administration (Nursing Care Plan 12.1).

Dyspnoea   Dyspnoea commonly occurs in patients with heart failure due to pulmonary venous congestion, and intervention is therefore aimed at reducing this congestion. For example, assuming the upright position not only directly aids breathing but reduces the venous return to the heart, thereby reducing pulmonary venous congestion. This effect is evident in orthopnoea and paroxysmal nocturnal dyspnoea (see p. 391). In the cardiac patient activities may require to be modified, as dyspnoea commonly occurs on exertion. Severe or acute dyspnoea is frightening for the patient and the nurse. The patient is often overwhelmed by feelings of panic, extreme anxiety and fears of suffocation and death, and therefore requires skilled care and support. Management of the dyspnoeic patient is discussed in Chapter 13.

Oedema   Various methods may be employed to reduce oedema, including dietary restriction of sodium, fluid restriction, rest and diuretic therapy. The recording of fluid balance is essential in monitoring fluid intake and the effect of therapy in producing a diuresis. Weighing the patient also helps to assess fluid gain and loss. The patient should be weighed on the same scales and at the same time each day (usually before breakfast) and wearing the same clothing. It is essential that rest is encouraged as periods of recumbency favours diuresis in patients with heart failure. The patient should be observed for signs of dehydration from rapid diuresis; for example, changes in blood pressure, urinary output and skin turgor.

The oedematous patient requires meticulous skin care as tissue is prone to develop pressure sores. Frequent changes of position and reduction of pressure on affected parts should be carried out.

Syncope   Syncope or fainting occurs as a result of a fall in cardiac output, which may be due to an abnormal heart rhythm and may be associated with other symptoms such as pallor, perspiration and the skin may feel cold to touch. At the onset of symptoms the patient should lie flat or sit down and lower his head between the knees. The nurse should check his blood pressure and pulse whilst summoning assistance. It is important to differentiate between syncope and cardiac arrest (see p. 421) by ascertaining the presence of breathing and pulse.

Meeting basic needs

Meeting the patient's basic needs, such as comfort, rest and sleep, is an essential component of nursing intervention and the patient may require assistance in meeting these needs. However, the balance between what the nurse does and what the patient does for himself is continually changing, keeping in mind that the goal of nursing practice is always to encourage and facilitate patient independence.

Communication   If nursing intervention is to be effective, communication between the nurse, patient, family and other personnel has to be effective (see Ch. 3). The cardiac patient often feels very stressed and anxious due to the nature of the disorder, since any disorder affecting the heart poses temporary or permanent threats, including altered self-image, changes in work, social and family circumstances, alterations in physical activity and even death. Cardiac patients may often experience very rapid changes in circumstances, such as being suddenly brought into a strange environment with a resulting loss of control over their own lives.

Effective communication can greatly influence the speed of recovery and patients' feelings of well-being and the nurse is the primary source of communication.

Comfort   Helping the patient to feel as comfortable as possible necessitates skilled nursing intervention. The alleviation of pain and discomfort is an essential primary component. Positioning of the patient is also of prime importance and requires effective communication and co-operation between nurse and patient. The presence of monitoring lines and equipment may make this difficult and the patient may be frightened to change his position due to fear of disturbing the equipment or developing pain. Giving appropriate information will help to ensure that unnecessary immobilization and discomfort do not occur. Minimizing unnecessary noise and control of light and temperature are also important, as are planned periods of rest.

Activity and rest   With many patients, bed rest is an important planned intervention aimed at reducing myocardial oxygen demand. Total bed rest, however, should be enforced for as short a time as possible due

Nursing Care Plan 12.1   Care plan for a patient with angina pectoris

Problem	Aim	Nursing action	Rationale
1. Anginal pain due to myocardial ischaemia	Prevention of pain	❐ Encourage patient to identify factors which cause his/her angina or make it last longer ❐ Advise patient to recognize his/her limitations and moderate activities accordingly. For example:	
		— Limit walking up several flights of stairs and steep hills — Avoid heavy exercise or mental stress just after eating — Avoid isometric exercise — Participate in activities which do not cause angina, dyspnoea and excessive fatigue — Balance activities with periods of rest	Greater risk is caused by placing sudden or unaccustomed demands on the heart Rest after meals allows for adequate blood flow to digestive tract Isometic exercises cause excessive increases in heart rate and blood pressure
		❐ Encourage patient to: — Avoid overeating and rest after meals	
		— Maintain proper body weight — Avoid excessive caffeine intake	Obesity increases cardiac workload
		— Stop smoking — Avoid extremes of temperature — Try to avoid stressful situations	Smoking increases the workload of the heart and decreases oxygen supply
		❐ Encourage patient to lead a normal life in all other respects, e.g. he can continue to have an active sex life	
	Relief of pain	❐ Advise patient to take nitroglycerin prophylactically ❐ Advise patient to carry nitroglycerin at all times ❐ When pain occurs, advise to:	Avoid pain known to occur with certain activities
		— Stop all activity and rest until pain subsides	Rest decreases myocardial oxygen demand
		— Take nitroglycerin tablet or spray every 3–5 minutes until pain relief obtained — If pain persists more than 15 minutes doctor should be called	Reduced myocardial oxygen consumption, decreasing myocardial ischaemia and relieving angina
		❐ Advise patient on correct storage and administration of nitroglycerin	Optimizes effectiveness of medication
2. Anxiety regarding angina and fear of heart attack	Reduction in anxiety levels	❐ Assess for presence of anxiety ❐ Stay with patient to provide support and minimize fear ❐ Provide appropriate explanations regarding the disorder, environment and intervention for patient and family	Anxiety may predispose to or worsen angina pain
3. Potential knowledge deficit regarding disorder and possible complications	Increase patient's and family's understanding	❐ Explain angina in terms the patient understands	

Nursing Care Plan 12.1 (*cont'd*)			
Problem	**Aim**	**Nursing action**	**Rationale**
3. (cont'd)		❐ Provide relevant written information	
	Prevent complications	❐ For example:	
		— How to stop smoking	Smoking is a major cause of coronary heart disease
		— Eating a healthy diet	
		— Adequate exercise	Regular exercise eventually improves coronary blood flow and enhances well-being
		— Alcohol intake	
		— Finding ways to relax	Alcohol in moderation may help to prevent angina whilst large amounts may cause hypertension and increase blood lipid levels

to the risk of complications. Early mobilization is important, especially in the elderly, and should be carefully planned for each individual. It is common nowadays to keep the patient in bed for a maximum of 24 hours following uncomplicated myocardial infarction (Nursing Care Plan 12.2). During the period of bed rest, active and passive exercises should be planned. These not only reduce the risk of complications but also help overcome boredom and give the patient a psychological boost. It is vital that the patient understands the reasons for enforced bed rest and is closely involved in the plans for mobilization. He may require assistance in performing daily activities, but should be allowed to remain as independent as possible. The nurse should contribute to the creation of a restful and relaxing environment.

Diet Adequate nutrition is essential in the promotion of recovery. If the patient is inactive and feeling unwell, he may not feel very hungry and it may be appropriate to offer small meals and nourishing fluids. Dietary salt may be restricted as may fluids, especially in the patient with cardiac failure. The patient and his family may require advice regarding altering dietary habits, and nurses can play an important role in nutrition education (see Ch. 4).

Hygiene Assistance with personal hygiene may be necessary if the patient's activities have been restricted because of the need to reduce energy expenditure or the presence of symptoms such as pain, dyspnoea or fatigue. The nurse needs to be sensitive to the possibility of the patient feeling embarrassed and should avoid fostering dependency. However the patient may feel very uncomfortable if he is sweating or has vomited for example, and may require mouth care, change of clothing or general assistance with hygiene.

It is relevant to note that the patient uses more energy when taking a shower than when bathing, and the patient's need to conserve energy requires to be assessed when planning washing and other appropriate interventions.

Minimizing stress and anxiety The patient requires to rest emotionally as well as physically. The development of a trusting and caring relationship with the patient is vital in reducing anxiety and stress. The breathless patient may be very anxious and restless and the patient experiencing chest pain may have a strong fear of death. In these circumstances, staying with the patient will help to reduce these anxieties and increase his sense of security. It is important that the nurse creates an atmosphere in which there is acceptance of fear and anxiety and where frequent and private opportunities to share concerns are available. The provision of carefully planned and relevant information can help reduce feelings of fear and isolation.

Sleep Various factors may result in alteration of normal sleep patterns. The symptoms of the disorder, the interventions and monitoring instituted, and an unfamiliar environment may be contributing factors. The nurse must assess the patients needs for sleep and take measures to promote adequate sleep for the patient. These measures may include the careful planning and timing of interventions, control of the environment and reduction of pain and anxiety as discussed in the previous sections.

Elimination Reduction in normal activity levels may predispose the patient to constipation, and straining must be avoided as it may encourage alterations in heart rate, particularly bradycardia; laxatives may therefore be required. The use of a commode rather than a bedpan may be easier for the patient as well as being more pleasant and comfortable. Careful attention needs to be paid to diet and in particular

Nursing Care Plan 12.2   Care plan for a patient with a myocardial infarction

Problem	Aim	Nursing action	Rationale
1. Chest pain and discomfort	Freedom from pain and discomfort Reduction in anxiety	❏ Assess pain and discomfort Give analgesia promptly as prescribed (usually opiates) Observe for adverse effects, e.g. hypotension, respiratory depression Provide a calm, relaxed atmosphere and give support and reassurance to reduce anxiety Administer oxygen as prescribed (usually be nasal cannulae) Minimize unnecessary activity Promote comfort by careful positioning of the patient	Reduces pain, anxiety and fear and promotes sleep Anxiety increases cardiac workload and pain May increase oxygen diffusion into ischaemic myocardium Nasal cannulae do not restrict communication, eating and drinking Activity increases cardiac workload and pain Good positioning can be of value in reducing pain and discomfort
2. Risk of further myocardial damage and complications	Limit infarct size	❏ Bed rest: normally maximum of 24 hours if free from complications Promote adequate rest by reducing noise, controlling temperature and humidity, adequate pain relief, comfort, sleep and relaxation Minimize unnecessary activity during first 24–48 hours, e.g. prevent straining during bowel movements (see problem 3) — Provide privacy for elimination — Provide assistance with personal hygiene as required — When mobile, encourage bathing rather than showering — Ensure call bell, locker, etc. are within easy reach Minimize stress and anxiety (see problem 5) Assist with administration of thrombolytic therapy and observe for complications, e.g. hypersensitivity and bleeding problems	Rest decreases the oxygen demand of the heart allowing the myocardium time, oxygen and nutrients to recover Oxygen consumptions higher during showering Thrombolytic agents promote revascularization of occluded coronary arteries and reperfusion of ischaemic heart muscle
3. Potential complications of bed rest and immobility	No complications of immobility	❏ Gradual, early mobilization as condition permits (see rehabilitation programme) Encourage active and passive leg exercises Encourage patient to carry out deep breathing exercises Ensure skin is kept clean and dry, and bedclothes free from wrinkles Ensure proper lifting of patient Ensure patient takes adequate fluids and uses laxatives as required to prevent constipation	Reduce the risk of complications of immobility Prevention of deep venous thrombosis (DVT) Prevention of pulmonary embolis Prevention of pressure sores Constipation may encourage straining which may predispose to cardiac dysrhythmias

Nursing Care Plan 12.2 (*cont'd*)			
Problem	**Aim**	**Nursing action**	**Rationale**
4. **Potential haemodynamic instability**	Haemodynamic stability	❏ Continuous monitoring of heart rate and rhythm If dysrhythmias occurs, report promptly and observe for signs of a fall in cardiac output Measure and record blood pressure, pulse, respirations and temperature 1–4 hourly as prescribed Observe for signs of dyspnoea, pulmonary oedema and cyanosis Observe peripheries for warmth and colour Record fluid intake and output and monitor balance	Early detection and treatment of dysrhythmias Early detection of abnormalities enables prompt intervention and may reduce the risk of complications, e.g. left ventricular failure, cardiogenic shock
5. **Fear and anxiety, worries about immediate and long-term future**	Reduction in fear and anxiety Development of a realistic outlook for the future	❏ Listen to patient's concerns in a calm, unhurried and empathetic manner Encourage the development of a relationship of mutual trust	The patient needs to feel able to ventilate his feelings and fears
		Orientate patient and family to environment Ensure close and constant contact between patient and nurse, e.g. call bell Facilitate open, flexible visiting and protect patient from feeling over-tired Explain all procedures	Increases feelings of security and decreases sense of isolation
		Choose a suitable time to discuss concerns with both patient and family	It is important that both the timing and environment are suitable
		Help patient to identify his own risk factors and encourage to consider what modifications may be necessary (see rehabilitation programme p. 425) Provide literature to read and discuss with patient at a later time	Patient education improves understanding and relieves stress
6. **Lack of knowledge regarding condition and treatment**	The patient and his family will understand what is happening and why	❏ Establish current level of knowledge Discuss condition fully with patient and family Provide clear and relevant explanations of all intervention	Adequate knowledge reduces stress and anxiety and enhances compliance with treatment and advice and ability to cope with the problems of illness
		Explain what a heart attack means in language the patient and family understand Provide appropriate written and audiovisual material	Assists in understanding and retention of information
7. **Loss of control**	Preservation of self-esteem and independence	❏ Encourage patient to perform usual activities as soon as possible Involve patient in decision-making about care Provide privacy for washing, family visits, etc.	Minimizes sense of loss and helplessness Increases feelings of self-worth and independence

the fluid and fibre content. If the patient is receiving diuretic therapy he needs to be aware of the increased amount and frequency of micturition and facilities need to be readily available and privacy maintained.

Support of the family

Disorders affecting the heart can frequently cause great anxiety for the family members as well as the patient. Often they feel isolated, helpless and frightened and may even experience feelings of guilt, thinking that somehow they may have contributed to the illness. The family requires information, reassurance and support. They need to be able to express their feelings and they also need to feel involved in caring for their relative. The family are also an important resource for the nurse as they may be able to provide valuable information regarding, for example, the patient's likes and dislikes. By meeting the family's needs the nurse, in turn, will be more able to give support to the patient so aiding recovery.

It is vital that the family are involved in the process of education and rehabilitation. Unnecessary problems can be prevented by including, in particular, the spouse in all aspects of decision making, including planning for discharge and preparation for management at home.

Rehabilitation

The goal of rehabilitation is to restore the patient to an optimum level of recovery and where possible prevent progression of the underlying disease. Its aims are to extend and improve the quality of life.

Cardiac rehabilitation programmes for patients following myocardial infarction and cardiac surgery are now commonly offered. The individual needs of the patient however, must be central to all programmes. Rehabilitation ideally should begin as soon as the acute episode occurs. The major components are that of early ambulation, education and support of the patient and family. The first step in this process is careful assessment of the patient's needs, desired health state, motivation, educational readiness, support mechanisms and physical and psychosocial state. Realistic goals can be set and individually tailored strategies planned. The programme should include both psychological and physical aspects of rehabilitation.

Patient education, teaching and counselling

The patient and his family require teaching and counselling to assist in their understanding of the illness and its management and to enable them to assume responsibility for their care.

Educational elements may include:

- information regarding hospital stay
- information about the nature of the disorder
- recognition of signs and symptoms
- names, dosages and side-effects of drugs
- knowledge of risk factors and their modification
- emergency treatment
- resumption of activities
- physical, psychosocial and financial problems
- sexual activity
- how to take a pulse.

The nurse is usually the most appropriate person to the teach the patient. Information needs to be given in a clear and structured manner and needs to be tailored to meet individual needs. Various physical, printed and audiovisual aids are available and form a useful part of the educational process.

Physical conditioning

A programme of physical activity should be carefully planned during the acute and rehabilitation phases and for long-term maintenance. Physical conditioning leads to improvements in cardiac risk factors such as blood cholesterol levels, blood pressure and body weight and improves cardiac efficiency. Physical activity should be graduated, starting with gentle passive exercises and subsequent activities should be individualized depending on the extent and severity of the disorder, the patient's previous level of activity and speed of recovery. An example of a rehabilitation programme is given in Nursing Care Plan 12.3.

For further information refer to Wenger & Hellerstein (1992).

VASCULAR DISORDERS

DISORDERS OF ARTERIES

Epidemiology and aetiology

Arteries are affected by arteriosclerosis and atherosclerosis and by thrombosis and embolism. Thrombosis, however, is seen less often in arteries than veins, as the arterial circulation is more rapid. Coronary artery thrombosis (myocardial infarction) (see p. 399) and cerebral artery thrombosis (see Ch. 5) are considered elsewhere. Arteriosclerosis literally means hardening of the arteries. It is characterized by thickening

---

Nursing Care Plan 12.3 Planning a cardiac rehabilitation programme. Goal: to restore the patient to an optimum level of recovery and limit the progression of coronary heart disease

Education	Activity
Aim: To increase the patient's understanding of his illness and its management To provide information which will help the patient to assume responsibility for his care and future health	**Aim:** To restore the patient fully to his normal activity. — Gradual, early mobilization
Assessment: — Pre-existing knowledge — Life-style and risk factors — Importance placed by patient on various activities — Readiness to learn	**Assessment:** Advice about specific activity should be individualized and taken into account: — The extent and severity of the disease — Patient's limitations — Patient's previous level of activity — Current condition and extent of recovery — Normal/usual circumstances

Education

Planning:
— Information should be structured for the individual and given in an easily understood and sympathetic manner
— Written, verbal and audiovisual information should be given
— Timing should be appropriate
— Counselling should also be provided

Information regarding hospital stay:
— Purpose of equipment, e.g. cardiac monitoring, intravenous infusions
— Procedures and routines
— Restrictions on activities, e.g. bed rest
— Visiting, telephones, etc.
— Staff

Information regarding disease:
— Structure and function of the heart
— Development of coronary heart disease
— Myocardial infarction: risk factors, warning signs

Plans for discharge:
— Resumption of activity, e.g. sexual, work, leisure, driving, etc.
— Exercise programme
— Diet
— Modification of risk factors, e.g. smoking
— Outpatient appointments and health checks
— Medications
— Involvement of spouse and family
— Signs and symptoms to be reported
— Resources available, e.g. associations, self-help groups, etc.

Activity

Planning:
Any exercise programme should be tailored to suit the individual and should be carefully monitored and evaluated. Early ambulation is recommended in the uncomplicated individual. The following is just an example:

Day 1	Bed rest, self-feeding, wash with assistance, passive limb movements Use of commode
Day 2	Sit out of bed for 20 minutes, twice per day Wash unassisted Active limb movements
Day 3	Sit out of bed for 1 hour, twice per day Walk to bathroom
Day 4–5	Walk up to 50 yards and short flight of stairs

Recovery process:
Psychological implications
Walking should be gradually and progressively increased in both time and distance e.g.

Week 2	Walk approximately 100 yards on flat Increase by 5–10 yards each day Do not become over-tired Use stairs 4–5 times daily
Week 3	Gradually increase walking to 250–300 yards, 2–3 times daily Increase activities, e.g. light gardening May use a bus and do light shopping Make sure you get as much sleep as possible
Week 4	Start to resume a normal way of life Increase daily walking and attempt a slight incline Do not do heavy work
Months 2–5	Gradually resume normal activities except heavy work Keep as active as possible

IF CHEST PAIN, EXCESSIVE BREATHLESSNESS, DIZZINESS OR TIREDNESS OCCUR – STOP!

---

of the walls of small arteries and arterioles. Since atheroma and arteriosclerosis often occur together, the term atherosclerosis is used to describe the resulting disorder.

Atheroma is deposited in the intima of arteries, eventually affecting the media. Atheroma is composed of cholesterol, macrophages and sometimes calcium, surrounded by fibrosis. It narrows, roughens and weakens the vessel wall. The narrowing of the arterial lumen leads to stenosis and a reduced blood supply to the tissues (ischaemia). Blood cells which would otherwise glide over a smooth intima, now have a greater tendency to stick to the roughened area to form thrombosis which further complicates matters by totally occluding the vessel. The weakness of the vessel predisposes to the development of aneurysms.

The initial development of atheroma is thought to begin in the first decade of life with fatty streaking. There is little progression during the second decade but in the third decade, if there are other predisposing factors, the formation of plaques of atheroma accelerates. It is not until the fourth and fifth decades of life that true atheroma and its effects are seen.

Atherosclerosis is a generalized disorder which not only affects the peripheral arteries but is usually present in other arteries, for example in the cerebral and coronary arteries. The predisposing factors in the development of atherosclerosis are the same as those associated with the development of coronary heart disease (Box 12.1).

It is important to recognize that there is a gradual narrowing of arteries by atheroma. This allows time for the formation of a collateral circulation which involves the formation of new blood vessels in an attempt to bypass the stenosis. Thus the body attempts to offset the effects of the atheroma.

In the UK the incidence of atherosclerosis is highest in South West Scotland and Northern Ireland, with the highest rates occurring amongst manual and unskilled workers and in those individuals who have relatives who developed the disorder before the age of 60 (Rose 1992).

Peripheral arterial disease

Disorders of the peripheral arteries invariably cause acute or chronic ischaemia.

Acute ischaemia

Acute ischaemia is caused by a sudden occlusion of a major artery which prevents the flow of blood to the area normally supplied by the affected artery. It is treated as a surgical emergency since muscle tissue can only survive without a blood supply for 6–8 hours. Thereafter amputation of the limb is necessary.

The two most common causes of acute ischaemia are embolism and thrombosis of an artery already affected by atherosclerosis.

Epidemiology and aetiology Ninety-five per cent of limb emboli originate from thrombi which have

developed in the heart as a result of atrial fibrillation, myocardial infarction, infective endocarditits or congestive cardiac failure. They become detached and are swept along in the arterial blood flow and stop when they reach a vessel too small for them to pass through, thus occluding it. Trauma to an artery is also an important cause of acute ischaemia. The number of iatrogenic injuries is increasing due to the many types of percutaneous catheters being used for diagnostic and therapeutic purposes (Mansfield & Wolfe 1992).

Common symptomatology The six 'Ps' summarize the clinical features of acute ischaemia (Campbell 1990):

1. **Pain** – this is usually extremely severe in nature and emanates from the ischaemic muscle.
2. **Pallor** – the affected limb is either white or mottled in colour.
3. **Paraesthesia** – objective sensory loss is an important sign of acute ischaemia, indicating the need for urgent treatment.
4. **Pulselessness** – the pulses distal to the occlusion will be absent.
5. **Paralysis** – the degree of paralysis of the limb varies.
6. **Perishing cold** – since the temperature of the skin is dependent on blood flow, an occlusion causes cooling of the limb.

Significance of nursing role in establishing the differential diagnosis It is imperative that nurses are aware of the signs and symptoms of acute ischaemia and are vigilant in their observations of patients who are at risk of developing it. Hence the need for circulation checks of patients whose limbs are encased in plaster or following cardiac catheterization or arteriography. Any abnormalities must be reported promptly so that action may be taken to save the patient's limb.

Range of investigations

1. **Clinical examination** – both limbs are compared and diagnosis made from the above signs and symptoms and the patient's clinical history.
2. **Doppler ultrasonography** is a non-invasive technique used to determine the extent of blood flow and obstructions in blood vessels. Conducting gel is applied over various pulse sites and a hand-held probe is positioned over an artery. High frequency sound waves are created which are used to elicit the Doppler effect. The sound waves are transmitted via the probe and conducting gel and as the sound waves 'hit' red blood cells they are reflected back to the

Doppler machine where the reading is displayed. The reflected sound depends on the velocity of red blood cells and is directly proportional to blood flow. Apart from explanation of the procedure to the patient, no special preparation or aftercare is necessary. In acute ischaemia it is performed to establish the presence or absence of blood flow and to differentiate between arterial and venous occlusions.

3. **Arteriography** – this is usually performed under local anaesthesia but children or very anxious adults may require general anaesthesia. It involves the injection of a radio-opaque contrast medium into the arterial tree most often via the femoral artery. A series of X-ray films are then taken in quick succession down the length of the limb, demonstrating filling of the leg vessels and narrowing, occlusions or other arterial abnormalities.

Preparation If the patient is to have a general anaesthetic, they should be prepared accordingly (see Ch. 4). More commonly, the patient is prepared for a femoral arteriography under local anaesthetic. The patient should be informed that the examination may be lengthy and that as the contrast medium is injected they may experience a feeling of heat and nausea. For the latter reason, the patient receives fluids only for 6 hours prior to the investigation. The groins may be shaved and bladder and rectum emptied (by suppositories if necessary) before the procedure. The latter is to allow a clear unobstructed view of the contrast medium within the vessels. A consent form should be signed and circulation and sensation checks should be performed on both legs to form a baseline for postprocedure observations. These checks involve observing and comparing both limbs for colour, warmth, the presence or absence of pedal and limb pulses and sensation.

Aftercare The aim of aftercare is to prevent and/or detect postprocedure complications of haemorrhage and occlusion. The puncture site is firmly padded to prevent haemorrhage. The patient should remain on bed rest for 24 hours; their blood pressure, pulse, groin puncture site, circulation and sensation should be checked on a regular basis as instructed. Circulation checks should always be compared with baseline observations. After-effects should involve no more than local groin stiffness or bruising. In acute ischaemia arteriography is performed to establish the extent of arterial injury.

Therapeutic management Surgery to restore the circulation to the limb is required. The type of surgery is dependent on the cause of the acute ischaemia.

If the ischaemia is caused by an embolus, an em-bolectomy is performed, whereas if it is a result of trauma, the injured artery will be repaired or replaced with a graft. In cases where acute ischaemia is due to a thrombosis occluding an atherosclerotic artery, a bypass vein graft is performed (see p. 429).

Following embolectomy, patients receive heparin and are discharged on warfarin which they must continue to take for 3 months. These anticoagulant drugs are prescribed to prevent thromboembolic com-pilations which cause about 50% of postoperative deaths following embolectomy. Twenty-five per cent of all patients undergoing embolectomy die in hospital and 16% of patients require amputation (McPherson & Wolfe 1992).

Nursing strategies

Preoperative care The patient undergoing embolec-tomy requires the minimum of preoperative care since surgery is an emergency. It should be remembered that the combination of pain and the haste in prepar-ing for surgery will be alarming for the patient and the reasons for carrying out emergency surgery must be calmly and carefully explained with reassurance to the patient and his family. A consent form requires to be signed, skin preparation is contra-indicated and the patient is fasted. If the patient has eaten recently a nasogastric tube may be inserted to empty the stomach and then the patient is prepared for theatre.

Postoperative care An account of the basic post-operative care required can be found in Chapter 4 (see Ch. 4). The specific care the patient requires following embolectomy is discussed in Nursing Care Plan 12.4.

Health education Patients discharged on warfarin require important advice and guidance. This is discussed in Table 12.6.

Chronic ischaemia

Epidemiology and aetiology Chronic arterial insuf-ficiency or peripheral vascular disease is principally caused by atherosclerosis (see p. 424) and usually occurs in the lower extremities. It is found pre-dominantly in men over the age of 50. It is stated by Rose (1992) that 40% of middle-aged men have evidence of ischaemia caused by atherosclerosis. 'Women's protection wanes gradually with age, and by "old age" the risks are similar for the two sexes. At any age the protection is wiped out by diabetes'. (Rose 1992, p. 1.)

Common symptomatology Early symptoms include cold extremities and the characteristic pain known

Nursing Care Plan 12.4   Specific postoperative care following femoral embolectomy

Problem	Aim	Nursing action	Rationale
		MAINTAINING A SAFE ENVIRONMENT	
1. Potential haemorrhage due to surgery and anticoagulant therapy	To detect early so that bleeding may be arrested promptly	❏ Record blood pressure and pulse as instructed	Haemorrhage would be detected by falling blood pressure and a rising pulse rate
		❏ Observe the patient's skin and report pale, cold and clammy skin	Indicates the presence of shock
		❏ Observe wound site and report signs of bleeding or haematoma formation	Indicative of haemorrhage occurring around operation site
		❏ Observe wound drainage bottles for patency and amount of drainage, report abnormalities	Patency of system prevents the formation of haematoma. Large amounts of drainage indicate bleeding from operation site
		❏ Observe patient for other signs of bleeding such as epistaxis, haematuria, bruising. Report promptly	May indicate over-anticoagulation of patient. Recognition and reporting allows for remedial action to be taken
2. Potential postoperative thromboembolism	To prevent these from occurring	❏ Perform circulation and sensation checks in both limbs as often as instructed	Circulation checks which involve the palpation of limb pulses, the observation of colour and temperature and asking the patient about sensation to his limbs allows prompt recognition of any further occlusions. By performing these observations in both limbs a comparison can be made with his non-affected limb. This enables detection of abnormalities.
		❏ A bed cradle should be used to lift weight of bed clothes off lower limbs	Allows patient to move his limbs more freely.

as intermittent claudication. The course of the disorder is usually progressive with the development in time of severe ischaemia and pain at rest. Eventually skin ulceration and gangrene may occur. For more details see Table 12.7.

Significance of nursing role in establishing differential diagnosis Since many middle-aged and elderly people are unaware of the presence of atherosclerosis until vessel narrowing causes symptoms due to ischaemia, the nurse plays an important role in requesting early medical advice for the patient should he/she identify the presence of cold limbs, absence of arterial pulses (Fig. 12.16) and intermittent claudication.

Range of investigations

1. **Clinical examination.**

2. **Doppler ultrasonography** (see p. 426).

3. **Arteriography**. This is performed to demonstrate the extent and severity of stenosis or occlusion. It is also necessary to determine whether reconstructive surgery is possible (see p. 427).

Therapeutic management The aims of management are to increase the blood supply to the affected limb in order to relieve the symptoms the patient will be experiencing and, if possible, halt the progression of the disorder.

In the absence of a specific cure, management of a patient with peripheral vascular disease includes control of risk factors, education of the patient in the care of their limbs (both discussed in the nursing strategies) and measures to improve the blood supply.

From the results of the investigations, the best course of surgical intervention will be determined

Table 12.6 Advice and guidance to patients receiving warfarin anticoagulant therapy	
Advice/guidance	Rationale
Follow prescription of dosage and timing of anticoagulant drug precisely	Ensures appropriate dosage is taken and blood level of drug remains within therapeutic range
Wear/carry identification indicating that they are receiving anticoagulant therapy	Allows for prompt recognition if they are involved in an accident so that reversal of the anticoagulant effects can be considered
Avoid taking vitamin supplements, aspirin, antibiotics, anti-inflammatory drugs or over the counter medicines without the consent of their GP	These medications can affect the way in which warfarin acts, resulting in either over or under coagulation
Do not stop taking warfarin unless directed to do so by the Doctor	Abrupt cessation of anticoagulant therapy can cause thrombi to form
Ensure that dentists, other doctors and chiropodists are informed that the patient is receiving anticoagulant therapy	It is important that this is known prior to any surgery, however minor, or any dental extraction
Keep all appointments with GP for blood tests	Regular blood tests allow for monitoring of the effectiveness of the warfarin therapy and recognition of over or under coagulation. If the latter occurs, the prescription can be altered accordingly
Be aware of the side-effects of warfarin and the importance of obtaining medical advice promptly, i.e. a. bleeding that will not stop b. appearance of bruises which increase in size c. passing red or brown urine d. passing red or brown bowel movements e. headache, faintness or dizziness f. stomach pains or vomiting blood	The presence of any of these signs must be taken seriously and investigated further

for patients on an individual basis. Several types of surgery are possible, and these will be discussed in order of the more minor to more major.

Sympathectomy involves the division of the sympathetic nerves supplying the peripheral blood vessels. Nowadays it is more common for patients to undergo phenol sympathectomy rather than a lumbar sympathectomy which involves an operation under a general anaesthetic. Phenol is injected, under X-ray control, into the appropriate level of the lumbar sympathetic chain to destroy the sympathetic ganglia which result in vasodilatation of the vessels supplying the legs. It is most useful in aiding the healing process in patients with leg ulcers.

Percutaneous transluminal angioplasty may be performed in patients with localised stenosis. This procedure is described on page 409.

When intermittent claudication has become severe and disabling, bypass grafting or endarterectomy

may be performed. Bypass grafting involves the bypassing of an obstructed section of an artery with either the patient's own long saphenous vein (reversed) or by using a synthetic grafting material such as Dacron. In endarterectomy, the thickened diseased inner layer of the artery is cored out. These techniques often prevent the need for amputation and allow many elderly people to retain their independence. However, despite success in retaining limb function it must be remembered that many of these patients will also suffer from other conditions related to their generalized atherosclerosis, such as cerebrovascular accident and myocardial infarction.

In patients whose disease has developed beyond responding to bypass grafting or endarterectomy, amputation of the affected limb is the only possible course of action.

Nursing strategies The nursing care involved when caring for patients with peripheral vascular

Table 12.7 Clinical features of peripheral vascular disease

Clinical feature	Rationale
Coldness of limbs	Insufficient blood supply to limbs
Pallor of limbs	Insufficient blood supply to limbs Blanching occurs when limb is elevated above heart
Reddy/blueness of skin of affected limb	As ischaemia progresses the remaining blood quickly loses its oxygen to the tissues causing the limb to become reddish/blue in colour
Absence of pedal pulses	When an artery is blocked it is unlikely that the pulses will be palpable below the block
Dry and scaly skin, muscle wasting and hair loss from affected limb and thickened ridged nails	These are all due to the decreased nutritional and oxygen supply to the tissues
Intermittent claudication	During exercise, metabolites are released. If there is ischaemia, the metabolites accumulate causing cramp-like pain. The pain disappears after a few minutes rest during which time the circulation to the muscle is restored and the metabolites removed
Rest pain	Eventually the blood supply is so precarious that the metabolites produced by muscles at rest cannot be removed resulting in rest pain being experienced by the patient. It can often prevent the patient from sleeping. A degree of relief can be gained by uncovering the foot and leg and hanging it out of bed
Gangrene	Finally the blood supply to the limb is so poor that even the viability of the skin cannot be maintained and gangrene intervenes

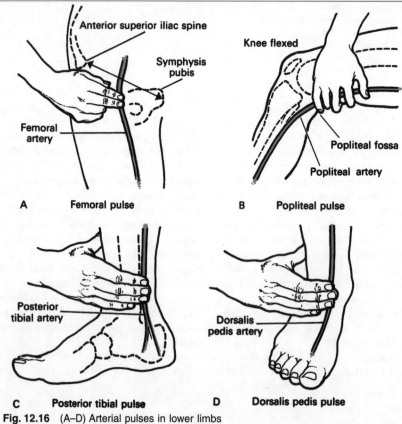

Fig. 12.16 (A–D) Arterial pulses in lower limbs

Nursing Care Plan 12.5 General principles in nursing patients with peripheral vascular disease

Problem	Aim	Nursing action	Rationale
		MAINTAINING A SAFE ENVIRONMENT	
1. Reduced blood supply to lower limbs	To improve circulation and prevent skin damage	❐ Elevate the head of the bed as instructed by medical staff	The use of gravity in this manner assists arterial flow
		❐ Explain to the patient that he should stop smoking	Smoking worsens his condition and prognosis
		❐ Avoid injury to legs:	These measures should ensure that the patient's skin remains intact. For the patient with peripheral vascular disease, even a small break in the skin can lead to tragedy. Ulceration and breaks are slow to heal and may cause the patient a great deal of pain and the eventual removal of the damaged part
		i. Great care should be taken when moving patient	
		ii. Ensure no one stands on patient's feet during transferring or mobilizing	
		iii. No attempt should be made to cut the patient's nails. A chiropodist should be employed	
		iv. Perform pressure care as often as indicated as necessary by their Norton or Waterlow score	
		v. Observe the patient's skin for its integrity each time pressure care is performed	Allows prompt reporting of abnormalities
		PERSONAL CLEANSING AND DRESSING	
		❐ Avoid extremes of hot and cold water. Tepid water should be used	Placing patient's lower extremities in hot or cold water will not only be painful for him but also serves to increase tissue necrosis
		❐ Pat skin gently to dry	Rubbing the skin dry may cause injury since the skin is usually thin and fragile
		❐ Avoid applying talcum powder to lower limbs	Talcum powder prevents the true skin colour being observed and causes further drying of the skin
		❐ Ensure environment in which personal cleansing is taking place is warm. Replace patient's garments as soon as possible	Patients with peripheral vascular disease lose their peripheral warmth quickly. They should therefore not be left exposed for any length of time
		MOBILIZING	
2. Reluctance to mobilize for fear of pain returning	To educate the patient so that he may mobilize within the limits of his disease	❐ Encourage the patient to mobilize but to rest if or when pain occurs	Exercise helps to promote blood flow and encourages the development of collateral circulation. Patients should not exercise through pain as this causes further tissue damage
		❐ Reinforce the exercises taught by physiotherapist:	These exercises contribute to the promotion of blood flow to the lower limbs
		i. Isometric leg exercises	
		ii. Active postural exercises – Buerger Allan exercises	
		❐ Administer analgesia as prescribed. Evaluate its effectiveness	Analgesics will help to reduce the pain felt by the patient. By evaluating the effectiveness of the drug given, an assessment can be made of the degree of pain control achieved by the drug. Medical staff can review prescription if inappropriate pain control is apparent

Nursing Care Plan 12.5 (*cont'd*)			
Problem	**Aim**	**Nursing action**	**Rationale**
		WHEN SITTING	
2. (cont'd)		❐ Always remove slippers	Slippers invariably have some sort of elastic device to keep them on. This can cause constriction around the feet and pressure at the back of the heels
		❐ Keep the patient's legs supported on a footstool Legs should never be elevated above heart level	Keeping the patient's legs supported in this manner aids venous return without compromising arterial flow
		❐ Discourage the patient from crossing his legs	Leg crossing inhibits arterial flow to extremities
		EATING AND DRINKING	
3. **Presence of disorder made worse by a high saturated fat diet and obesity**	To educate the patient in adopting a healthier diet	❐ Arrange for the patient to be seen by dietitian so that a reduction of dietary cholesterol intake and if appropriate a reducing diet may be discussed	Dietitian has specialist knowledge and will be able to negotiate with the patient the best diet for them as an individual encompassing as many of their favourite foods as possible It is important for compliance that the patient has an active role in the decision making
		❐ Nurse to reinforce advice and answer any questions raised by dietitian's visit	Helps to ensure patient's understanding of his diet
		❐ Encourage patient to drink fluids on a 1–2 hourly basis	This not only prevents urinary tract problems but prevents dehydration Dehydration increases blood viscosity which adversely affects the blood flow to the extremities

disease should follow general principles, regardless of the type of surgery performed. These general principles are discussed in detail in Nursing Care Plan 12.5. For information regarding the specialist care required following vascular surgery see Chapter 9 in Brunner & Suddarth (1992).

The primary health care team is vital for the continued and successful care at home of patients with peripheral vascular disease.

Careful assessment of the impact of the disease upon the person's ability to carry out his usual range of activities of living will be required.

As the disease progresses and exercise tolerance decreases, some patients may have to change to lighter, more sedentary work. For the housebound, the GP, community nurse and chiropodist may all give support and visits to a day centre can be valuable in providing the stimulation of change of environment, interest and friendship.

Health education Regardless of whether the patient is able to work or is housebound, they need to know about their disease so that they may limit the extent to which the disease may affect them. An example of the advice which should be given to patients can be found in Box 12.5.

Disorders of the aorta

The major disorder affecting the aorta is aneurysm. An aneurysm is a sac formed by dilatation of an artery at a point of weakness in the vessel wall. Aneurysms are very dangerous because they can rupture leading to haemorrhage and death.

Epidemiology and aetiology

The most common cause of aneurysm formation is atherosclerosis. Other causes include congenital defects of the arterial wall, trauma and infection.

There are various types of aneurysms (Fig. 12.17):

1. **True aneurysms** involves all three layers of the arterial wall. They can take the form of fusiform, saccular or dissecting.

Box 12.5 Discharge advice which should be given to patients with peripheral vascular disease

1. Impress upon the patient the dangers of smoking and particularly inhaling smoke. They should be aware of the reasons why smoking impairs their circulation as this is more likely to enhance compliance with advice to stop smoking
2. Patient should be advised to use mild soap and lanolin-based lotions to discourage dryness and cracking of the skin
3. Advise the patient against wearing constrictive garments such as girdles and garters
4. Advise the patient to avoid extremes of hot and cold to their extremities, i.e. hot water bottles, electric heat pads, hot or cold water
5. Patient should keep their feet warm in winter by wearing warm socks and sheepskin-lined boots
6. Impress upon the patient that adherence to any special diet they have been prescribed is vital
7. Advise the patient to attend the chiropodist regularly
8. Advise the patient never to go barefoot and to wear well-fitting shoes. Shoes should be checked for protruding nails and seams and linings for lumps. New shoes should be broken in gradually. Stockings, preferably seamless, must fit correctly
9. Advise the patients against crossing their legs whilst sitting or in bed
10. Patients should avoid crowded areas such as supermarkets where foot injuries are likely
11. Patients should examine their skin and feet regularly. Elderly patients can be advised to place a mirror on the floor in order to inspect the undersurface of their feet for lesions – can be difficult to accomplish otherwise
12. Impress upon the patient the importance of reporting any damage/injury however small to their GP immediately

2. **False aneurysm**: this describes complete rupture of the layers of the artery with blood being retained by the surrounding tissues.

Aneurysms may occur within different parts of the aorta. They occur more often in men than women with a ratio of five to one and the incidence is increasing within Great Britain.

Common symptomatology

The thoracic aorta is the most common site of dissecting aneurysms. Symptoms include the onset of sudden, severe and persistent pain arising from the chest or scapulae which is often described as ripping or tearing. The patient often displays signs of shock. Dyspnoea, cough or dysphagia may also be present.

Only approximately 40% of patients with abdominal aortic aneurysms have symptoms. These symptoms vary depending on the size of the aneurysm but include an abdominal pulsation, abdominal discomfort or pain, back pain and vascular insufficiency to legs. Signs of rupture/leakage include the sudden onset of severe pain, abdominal rigidity and guarding, cold pulseless legs and signs of hypovolaemic shock (see Ch. 4).

Range of investigations

The diagnosis of aneurysm and identification of its exact position and size can be confirmed by the following investigations:

1. ultrasound scanning (see p. 426)
2. arteriography (see p. 427)
3. computerized axial tomography (see Ch. 4).

Therapeutic management

Generally speaking, surgery is performed to remove the aneurysm and restore vascular continuity by using artificial graft material such as Dacron. Surgery of this nature is not without its risks and these should be explained to the patient.

Patients with ruptured aneurysms require major emergency surgery which carries a high mortality.

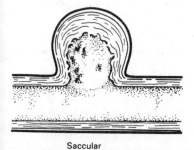

Saccular

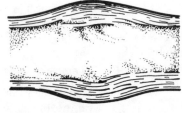

Fusiform

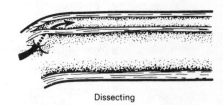

Dissecting

Fig. 12.17 Types of true aneurysms. (Reproduced with permission from Wilson 1990, figure 5.45)

Nursing strategies

The nursing care of patients requiring surgery for aneurysms is most specialized and outwith the scope of this text. For detailed information see Chapter 9 in Brunner & Suddarth (1992).

DISORDERS OF VEINS

Superficial phlebitis and thrombophlebitis

Epidemiology and aetiology

Superficial phlebitis or inflammation of the superficial veins is a common disorder caused by injury to vessels following surgery, childbirth or intravenous infusion therapy. As veins have thinner walls than arteries they are more prone to endothelial damage. The intima thickens and narrows and thrombus may form causing superficial thrombophlebitis – a condition often seen after prolonged infusion of intravenous fluids. Phlebitis of leg veins is often associated with varicosities.

Common symptomology

The affected area becomes swollen, red and tender. Such inflammation may be seen tracking along a length of affected vein.

Significance of nursing role in establishing differential diagnosis

Caring for patients with an intravenous infusion is discussed elsewhere (see Ch. 14). The nurse plays a vital part in alerting the medical staff to the presence of these disorders by observing for inflammation, abnormalities around infusion sites, and reporting complaints of pain or discomfort from patients.

Range of investigations

Diagnosis is made from clinical examinations.

Therapeutic management

Pain is relieved by analgesia and the application of local heat in the form of a kaolin poultice may be soothing. If an intravenous infusion is involved, the cannula is removed and the infusion recommenced at a different site.

Nursing strategies

The nurse's role here is to administer prescribed anal-

Box 12.6   Predisposing factors to varicose vein formation
1. Gender. Varicose veins occur more commonly in women
2. Occupations requiring prolonged standing such as nurses, shop assistants, hairdressers, dentists and soldiers on sentry duty
3. Hereditary weakness of vein walls
4. Pregnancy due to hormonal changes and the weight of the fetus compressing the main vessels in the pelvis
5. Age. Incidence increases with age due to the loss of tissue elasticity

gesia and evaluate its effectiveness and also to apply kaolin poultices.

Varicose veins

Epidemiology and aetiology

Varicose veins (varicosities) are the most common vein disorders being present in 12% of the British population. The long and short saphenous veins are affected most. Varicose veins occur when the valves become defective or incompetent, resulting in back pressure and stasis of blood which further dilates the veins. Venous congestion and oedema interfere with the oxygen and nutrient supply to the subcutaneous tissue causing fibrosis to occur and the possibility of complications such as varicose ulcers, thrombophlebitis and deep vein thrombosis.

Varicose veins occur more commonly in women with the ratio of five to one. The predisposing factors to their formation can be found in Box 12.6.

Common symptomatology

If only the superficial veins are varicosed the patient may be asymptomatic but complain of the unappealing sight of tortuous dilated veins.

Range of investigations

1. Clinical examination and history.
2. Doppler ultrasonography (see p. 426) may be used to detect degree of retrograde blood flow.

Therapeutic management

Management consists of either conservative or surgical treatment. Conservative management involves educating the patient in prevention of worsening their condition (Box 12.7) and the prescription of elastic

---

Box 12.7   Advice given to prevent recurrence of varicose veins

1. Avoid wearing tight garments such as corsets and garters
2. Avoid crossing legs at thigh, knee or ankle as this reduces venous circulation by 15%
3. Avoid sitting or standing for long periods
4. Walk upstairs rather than taking the lift
5. Walk at least 2–3 miles daily
6. Keep fit and keep weight within optimum limits. Swimming is a very useful form of exercise
7. Support stockings or tights can be useful

---

stockings which relieve symptoms, conceal unsightly veins and prevent further deterioration.

Surgery involves either the injection of a sclerosing fluid (sclerotherapy), ligation or stripping of the vein.

Nursing strategies

Sclerotherapy is often performed on a day case basis with the patient being advised to wear elastic stockings for 3–6 weeks and walk a minimum of 2–3 miles a day after treatment. The other operations involve a short hospital stay of 1–2 days. Preoperatively, the patient has his skin marked by the surgeon whilst he is in a standing position. The nurse should ensure these marks are not washed off inadvertently.

Postoperatively the patient returns to his bed which is elevated at the foot to aid venous return and has a bed cradle in place. Surgeons differ in their preference for the type of compression used postoperatively but whether bandages or graduated compression stockings are used, the nurse must ensure these are correctly applied and not proving to be uncomfortable. Analgesia is given as required and its effectiveness evaluated.

Observations of blood pressure and pulse are taken as often as ordered to identify the presence of any haemorrhage or lack of circulation to the toes which may occur if the compression stocking or bandages are applied too tightly. The patient is mobilized early since deep vein thrombosis is the main postoperative complication. For this reason, the patient may also be prescribed prophylactic low dose heparin. The nurse must advise the patient to perform exercises taught by the physiotherapist and that they should avoid standing for long periods. The patient should either be walking or sitting with their legs elevated to promote venous return. On discharge, they should be given advice to prevent the recurrence of varicose veins (Box 12.7).

Vein thrombosis

Epidemiology and aetiology

Thrombosis is the process of coagulation of circulating blood in the vessels. A thrombus is the solid substance formed from the blood constituents (a clot). A thrombus which becomes detached is termed an embolus.

Several factors are known to precipitate venous thrombosis.

1. **Injury to endothelial lining**. Intravenous infusion or injections, trauma, surgery and inflammation may damage the intima to which platelets then adhere.
2. **Increased blood coagulation.** Dehydration and polycythaemia both cause an increase in blood viscosity. The abrupt withdrawal of anticoagulant drugs, use of the oral contraceptive pill, myocardial infarction, childbirth and malignancy can all lead to increased coagulation of the blood.
3. **Slowing of venous circulation**. Venous stasis occurs when muscle action is reduced, as is experienced in prolonged bedrest, immobility and paralysis. Venous return may also be sluggish due to cardiac failure.

Thrombosis can occur in any vein of the leg but deep vein thrombosis commencing in the deep veins of the gastrocnemius muscle is by far the most common.

It is estimated that thrombi occur in some 25–35% of patients postoperatively and in 20–50% of patients post myocardial infarction or cerebrovascular accident.

Common symptomatology

Deep vein thrombosis produces limb oedema due to inhibition of venous drainage. The skin of the affected limb may be warm, red and the superficial veins engorged and prominent. The patient may have a low grade pyrexia. Some 50% of patients are asymptomatic. When the thrombus is only loosely adherent to the vessel wall, the first symptoms may be sudden collapse or the onset of clinical features of pulmonary embolus, the thrombus having detached from the vessel wall and travelled in the venous circulation to lodge in the pulmonary artery or one of its branches. It can be fatal.

Significance of nursing role in establishing differential diagnosis

The nurse should ask the patient, particularly if he

Nursing Care Plan 12.6 Specific nursing intervention in the prevention and treatment of deep vein thrombosis

Problem	Aim	Nursing action	Rationale
1. **Patient at risk of developing deep vein thrombosis**	Prevent deep vein thrombosis from occurring by ensuring good venous return	❒ Encourage early mobilization and discourage prolonged bed rest	One of the causes of deep vein thrombosis is venous stasis. Early mobilization prevents this
		❒ If bed rest is necessary, active and passive leg exercises should be carried out. The patient should dorsiflex and plantarflex his feet against resistance (active exercise) or the nurse should put the patient's ankle and knee joints through their full range of movements (passive exercise)	Active and passive leg exercises encourage use of the calf muscle pump, thereby aiding venous return to the heart and avoid stasis
		❒ Encourage patient to perform deep breathing exercises as taught by the physiotherapist	By deep breathing, there is an increase to the negative pressure within the thorax which helps to drain blood from the large veins into the right side of the heart
		❒ Handle and position lower limbs carefully, particularly during and after surgery. No pillows should be placed under the knee or calf	Avoids leg vein compression and injury to the vein – both predisposing factors to thrombus formation
		❒ Advise the patient not to cross their legs at the knee or sit in a chair which compresses the space behind the knee	Avoids leg vein compression and injury to vein – both predisposing factors to thrombus formation
		❒ Use elastic compression stockings as prescribed	Elastic compression stockings compress the superficial veins which results in an increased blood flow in deeper veins
		i. Ensure patient's calf is measured and appropriate size of stocking is used	If stocking is too tight it will cause ischaemia; if too loose it will serve no purpose
		ii. Apply stockings whilst patient is in bed, ensure there are no wrinkles and that the top of the stocking is not folded down on itself	Wrinkles may cause pressure sore development. If stocking top is folded down it can act as a tourniquet, producing stasis rather than preventing it
		iii. Remove stockings for a brief period twice daily	Allows for inspection of skin for any signs of irritation, sore formation or presence of calf tenderness
2. **Patient has a deep vein thrombosis**	To prevent pulmonary embolism or extension of thrombus	❒ Patient is nursed in bed – usually for 5–7 days	This length of time is required for the inflammation and associated symptoms to subside and for the thrombus to adhere firmly to the vessel wall
		❒ Elevate the foot of the bed as per instructions	Increase venous return
		❒ Use pressure-relieving aids such as sheepskin and perform pressure area care as often as the patient's Norton or Waterlow score suggests	Pressure sores may be prevented by these interventions
		❒ Use bed cradle	Keeps the weight of bed clothes off patient's leg. Allows for more freedom of movement
		❒ Prevent hazards of immobility such as chest and urine infections and constipation	See Chapter 4 for a detailed account of these nursing interventions

Nursing Care Plan 12.6 (*cont'd*)			
Problem	**Aim**	**Nursing action**	**Rationale**
2. (cont'd)		❏ Administer analgesics as prescribed and evaluate its effectiveness	Analgesics will help to reduce the pain felt by the patient. By evaluating the effectiveness of the drug given, an assessment can be made of the degree of pain control achieved by the drug. Medical staff can review prescription if inappropriate pain control is apparent
		❏ Apply compression stockings or bandages as requested by medical staff	Opinion differs about this aspect of treatment. Some doctors feel that they are necessary to increase the blood flow in the deep veins
		❏ Encourage patient to perform limb exercises in bed under the guidance of the physiotherapist	To prevent deep vein thrombosis developing in unaffected limb
		❏ Prevent dehydration by ensuring that the patient drinks something every hour	Dehydration increase blood viscosity which enhances further thrombus formation
3. Patient receiving anticoagulants	Recognize signs of over coagulation and report promptly	❏ Check infusion pump hourly for signs of kinks or leaks in tubing and that the correct dose is being administered. Report abnormalities promptly	Ensures that the patient receives the level of anticoagulation prescribed
		❏ Observe patient for signs of over coagulation: i. Test urine daily for haematuria ii. Test faeces for faecal occult blood iii. Observe for signs of bleeding gums, nose and bruising	Allows for prompt recognition of over coagulation. Medical staff can reverse the effects of heparin with protamine sulphate and warfarin with vitamin K
4. Patient now able to mobilize	To promote good venous return and advise the patient against actions which may cause further problems	❏ Instruct the patient that he may mobilize only with his elastic stockings on	Enhances venous return, preventing stasis
		❏ Advise and encourage the patient not to stand or remain sitting for long periods of time	Standing or sitting for long periods of time encourages venous stasis
		❏ Advise and encourage patient not to smoke	Smoking encourages platelet aggregation and potentially thrombus formation
		❏ Encourage patient to perform leg exercises hourly, during waking hours	Encourages venous return by using the calf muscle pump

is at increased risk of developing a deep vein thrombosis, if he has any calf pain or tenderness. If not contraindicated, the practice of placing each foot in a basin of water during bedbathing can often help in the recognition of a deep vein thrombosis. The calf rests on the rim of the basin and the slight pressure it exerts can sometimes elicit calf tenderness which may otherwise remain unnoticed.

During bathing, the nurse should also observe both legs noting and reporting any differences such as increased temperature or swelling.

Range of investigations

1. **Clinical examination**.

2. **Venography**. Peripheral venography involves the injection of a radio-opaque contrast medium and a series of X-rays taken as it enters and fills the venous system. Venography will detect the presence of thrombi.

3. **Doppler ultrasonography** (see p. 426) is sometimes used to establish the presence of occlusive thrombi in the femoral or iliac veins.

Therapeutic management

Prevention of deep vein thrombosis occurring in at-risk patients involves nursing interventions which have been discussed and the administration of subcutaneous low dose herapin and the application of antiembolism stockings in high risk patients.

The treatment of deep vein thrombosis involves the administration of the anticoagulant herapin intravenously. Heparin works by preventing the conversion of prothrombin to thrombin. Oral anticoagulation with warfarin is usually commenced 36–48 hours prior to discontinuation of heparin to allow uninterrupted therapeutic action, since warfarin takes about 24 hours to exert its effects. Warfarin therapy will be continued for 8–12 weeks. Patients with extensive thrombi may be treated with thrombolytic agents such as streptokinase (see p. 409 for more details).

Nursing strategies

The nurse's role in prevention and treatment of deep vein thrombosis can be seen in Nursing Care Plan 12.6.

Health education Since the patient will be discharged home on warfarin, he/she requires advice and guidance. This should take the form of explaining the purpose and need for warfarin. The advice and guidance which should be given is described in Table 12.6.

Suggested assignments

Discussion topics
1. Should all patients be resuscitated? Who should decide? What factors need to be taken into consideration?
2. Given the rising cost of treatment and limited resources, should all patients be considered for cardiovascular surgery/treatment, even if they refuse to reduce their own risk factors or alter their life-style? For example, should the individual who refuses to loose weight if obese or refuses to stop smoking be considered for cardiac surgery?
3. Does advertising affect you? What influence, if any, has publicity about risk factors and ways of preventing heart disease had upon your way of life?
4. Consider the anxieties a patient and his/her family might experience following an acute myocardial infarction. How can the hospital nurse and the community nurse help to relieve these anxieties?
5. Should all patients with acute myocardial infarction be admitted to the coronary care unit? In fact should all patients be admitted to hospital? Consider the advantages and disadvantages of home versus hospital care, and coronary care versus care on a 'general' ward.
6. How would you explain to a patient or relative the meaning of the terms 'angina', 'heart attack' and 'pacemaker'?

REFERENCES AND FURTHER READING

Basket P J F 1993 Resuscitation handbook, 2nd edn. Wolfe, London
Behrendt D, Austin G 1985 Patient care in cardiac surgery, 4th edn. Little, Brown and Co, Boston
Bennett D H 1989 Cardiac arrhythmias: practical notes on interpretation and treatment, 3rd edn. Wright, Bristol
British Heart Foundation/Coronary Prevention Group Statistics Database 1994 Coronary heart disease statistics, 1993 edn. British Heart Foundation, London
Brunner L S, Suddarth D S 1992 Textbook of adult nursing. Chapman & Hall, London
Braunwald E (ed) 1988 Heart disease: a textbook of cardiovascular medicine, 3rd edn. Saunders, Philadelphia
Campbell W B 1990 Acute limb ischaemia. Surgery 81: 1937–1941
Dawkins K D 1987 A manual of cardiology. Churchill Livingstone, Edinburgh
Department of Health 1991 Dietary reference valves for food energy and nutrients for the UK report of the Panel on Dietary Reference Values of the Committee on Medical Aspects of Food Policy. HMSO, London
Friedman M, Rosenman R H 1974 Type A behaviour and your heart. Knopf, New York

Hampton J R 1986 The ECG made easy, 3rd edn. Churchill Livingstone, Edinburgh
Julian D G 1988 Cardiology, 5th edn. Baillière Tindall, London
Julian D, Marley C 1991 Coronary heart disease: the facts. Oxford University Press, Oxford
Kaye W, Bircher G 1989 Cardiopulmonary resuscitation. Churchill Livingstone, Edinburgh
Mansfield A O, Wolfe J H N 1992 Trauma. In: Wolfe J H N (eds) ABC of vascular diseases. BMJ, London
McNaught A B, Callander R 1983 Nurses' illustrated physiology, 5th edn. Churchill Livingstone, Edinburgh
McPherson G A D, Wolfe J H N 1992 Acute ischaemia of the leg. In: Wolfe J H N (ed) ABC of vascular diseases. BMJ, London
Resuscitation Council (UK) 1993 Resuscitation for the citizen, 3rd edn. Resuscitation Council (UK) London
Rose G 1992 Epidemiology of artherosclerosis. In: Wolfe J H N (ed) ABC of vascular diseases. BMJ, London
Thompson D R 1985 Intensive care nursing: neglected areas Nursing Mirror 160(12): 38–42
Tortora G, Anagnostakos N 1990 Principles of anatomy and physiology, 6th edn. Harper Collins, New York

Wenger N K, Hellerstein H K (eds) 1992 Rehabilitation of the coronary patient. Wiley, New York

Williams K (ed) 1992 The community prevention of coronary disease. HMSO, London

Brown S S, Cowell G 1990 Treatment of varicose veins. Practice Nurse November 3(6): 356–358

Brunner L S, Suddarth D S (eds) 1992 Assessment and care of patients with vascular and peripheral circulatory disorders. In: Textbook of adult nursing. Chapman and Hall, London

Jowett N I, Thompson D R 1989 Comprehensive coronary care. Scutari Press, London

Keachie J 1992 Making sense of Doppler ultrasound. Nursing Times 8(10): 54–56

Kinney M R, Packa D R, Andreoli K G, Zipes D P 1991 Comprehensive cardiac care, 7th edn. Mosby Year Book, St Louis

Kirklin J W, Barrat-Boyes B C 1993 Cardiac surgery, 2nd edn. Churchill Livingstone, Edinburgh

Morison M 1991 A colour guide to the assessment and management of leg ulcers. Clinical Skills Series. Wolfe, London

Murie S 1990 Surgery for varicose veins. Update 15 December 1011–1016

Pritchard A P, David J A 1988 The Royal Marsden Hospital manual of clinical nursing procedures, 2nd edn. Harper and Row, New York

Stasser T (ed) 1987 Cardiovascular care in the elderly. WHO, Geneva

Thompson D R, Webster R A 1992 Caring for the coronary patient. Butterworth-Heinemann, Oxford

Thompson D R 1990 Counselling the coronary patient and partner. Scutari Press, London

Underhill S L, Woods S C, Sivarajan-Froelicher E S, Halpenny C J 1989 Cardiac nursing, 2nd edn. Lippincott, Philadelphia

Wilson K J W 1990 Ross & Wilson: 1990 Anatomy and physiology in health or disease, 7th edn. Churchill Livingstone, Edinburgh

13

Care implications of disorders of the respiratory system

Morag A. Gray

ANATOMY AND PHYSIOLOGY

The functions of the respiratory system are to distribute air to the alveoli via the bronchial tree and exchange gases between the alveolar sacs and the surrounding capillaries.

The lungs are situated within the thoracic cavity (Fig. 13.1). They are covered with a serous membrane called the pleura which is in two layers. The inner layer adheres to the lung and is called the visceral pleural and the outer layer lines the chest wall and is called the parietal pleura. The potential space between the two layers is called the pleural cavity and contains a small amount of serous fluid that prevents friction between the two layers during respiration. There is a negative pressure within the thorax, that is, the pressure is less than that of atmospheric pressure. During respiration the negative pressure increases; conversely it decreases during expiration. It is the negative pressure within the thorax which keeps the lungs expanded by exerting a pulling force.

Breathing is achieved by increasing and decreasing the size of the thoracic cavity. As a result of the intercostal muscles and the diaphragm contracting, enlargement of the cavity occurs and air is drawn into the lungs (inspiration). When the muscles relax, the elastic recoil of the lungs expels the air (expiration) (Fig. 13.2).

When inspired air reaches the alveoli it has already passed through what is known as the **dead space**, which is given the volume of 150 ml. The upper respiratory tract, the trachea, bronchi and bronchioles comprise the dead space. It is called the dead space because it is not involved in the diffusion of oxygen from the alveoli into the capillaries and carbon dioxide from the capillaries to the alveoli.

It should be noted that the diameter and patency of the bronchi and bronchioles can markedly affect the

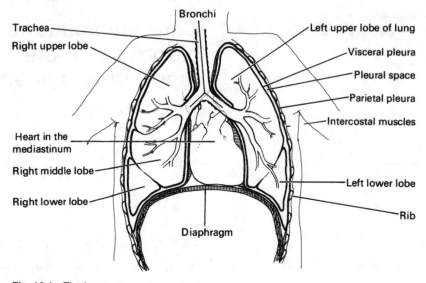

Fig. 13.1 The lungs

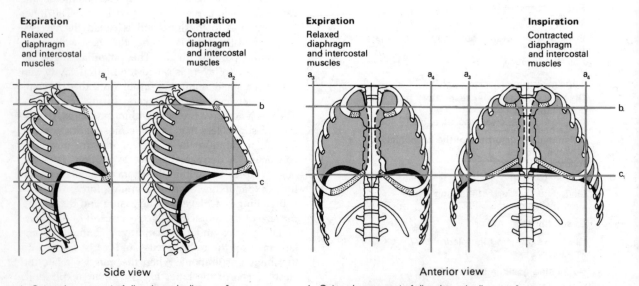

Expiration
Relaxed diaphragm and intercostal muscles

Inspiration
Contracted diaphragm and intercostal muscles

Expiration
Relaxed diaphragm and intercostal muscles

Inspiration
Contracted diaphragm and intercostal muscles

Side view

1. Outward movement of ribs shown by lines a_1 & a_2.
2. Upward movement of ribs & sternum shown by lines b & c.
3. Lowering of diaphragm shown by line c.

Anterior view

1. Outward movement of ribs shown by lines a_3 & a_4.
2. Upward movement of ribs shown by lines b_1 & c_1.
3. Lowering of diaphragm shown by line c_1.

Fig. 13.2 Diagram of changes in capacity of the thoracic cavity (and the lungs) during breathing. (Reproduced with permission from Wilson K J W 1990, figure 7.23)

oxygen and carbon dioxide levels in the blood. The diameter of the bronchioles can be altered by the autonomic nervous system. Parasympathetic stimulation causes bronchoconstriction whilst sympathetic stimulation causes bronchodilatation. In addition, the bronchi and bronchioles are lined with ciliated columnar epithelium which is covered by a mucous layer. The function of the mucus is to humidify inspired air and protect the epithelium protection from inhaled irritants and bacteria. The latter is achieved by the presence of antibacterial agents such as lysozyme within the mucus. The cilia facilitate the removal of inhaled particles by continuously moving the mucus upwards so that it may be coughed up. 'In health, the mucous layer in man moves at about 5–20 mm/min, but this can be reduced tenfold in patients with chronic bronchitis and emphysema' (Flenley 1990, p. 18).

The process of respiration is controlled by a group of nerve cells located in the medulla oblongata known as the respiratory centre (Fig. 13.3). It is influenced by the level of carbon dioxide (CO_2) and oxygen (O_2) in the blood. Specialized cells called chemoreceptors found in the aortic arch and carotid arteries detect the levels of CO_2 and O_2 in the blood. When high levels of CO_2 and low levels of O_2 are detected, the respiratory centre is stimulated causing an increased rate and depth of respiration in an attempt to 'wash out' or reduce the CO_2 level. Conversely, when low levels of CO_2 are detected, there is a reduction in the stimulus of the respiratory centre resulting in slow shallow respiration.

The maintenance of normal levels of O_2 and CO_2 in the blood depends on an adequate amount of oxygen in the inspired air and efficient respiratory and circulatory systems.

The effect of ageing on the respiratory system

As a result of the ageing process elderly people have a less efficient gaseous exchange and cough reflex. This is due to a decrease in lung elasticity, enlargement of alveoli, dilatation of bronchioles and a reduction in ciliary action.

Osteoporotic changes cause the thoracic cage to alter shape, inhibiting the elderly person from fully expanding their lungs.

EPIDEMIOLOGY AND AETIOLOGY

Disorders of the respiratory system account for the greatest number of days off work and are responsible for approximately one-fifth of all deaths in the UK (Davies 1990).

The high incidence of respiratory disorders in temperate climates, especially in the UK, is associated with cigarette smoking, air pollution and cold, damp, foggy weather. These unfavourable conditions greatly aggravate any infective or allergic inflammatory changes present in the respiratory tract. The gravity of the situation in many countries has led to a greater control of atmospheric pollution and of working conditions in occupations where dust, irritants and chemicals are a problem. Health education to reduce cigarette smoking has had some effect. According to Davies (1990) men are smoking less, women are smoking more and adolescent girls smoke more cigarettes than boys. When comparing incidence of smoking by occupation, it is noted that more professionals have stopped smoking than manual workers. A policy statement produced by the Scottish Office (1992) states that one of the priorities of health education in Scotland is to achieve a 30% reduction in the number of smokers in the 12–24 age group and a 25% reduction in the 25–65 age group in the period between 1986 and 2000.

More attention is also being focused on the dangers of passive smoking. It has been estimated that every year, passive smoking causes 1000 deaths in the UK (Roper et al 1990).

Passive smoking affects us all: 'An average room

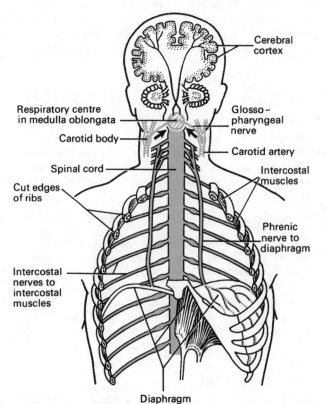

Fig. 13.3 Diagram of some of the nerves involved in the control of respiration. (Reproduced with permission from Wilson K J W 1990, figure 7.25)

Labels in figure:
Cerebral cortex
Respiratory centre in medulla oblongata
Glosso-pharyngeal nerve
Carotid body
Carotid artery
Spinal cord
Intercostal muscles
Cut edges of ribs
Phrenic nerve to diaphragm
Intercostal nerves to intercostal muscles
Diaphragm

has three times the CO (carbon monoxide) level when smoking has occurred, while in small confined spaces (cars, submarines, unventilated offices), concentrations can be raised thirty-fold' (Parrott 1991, p. 202). Non-smokers are at real risk of developing lung cancer from the effects of passive smoking. It is estimated that one-third of non-smokers who develop lung cancer do so because they live with people who smoke (Cull 1991). Women who continue to smoke during their pregnancy put their unborn children at risk. Children exposed to smoke are more likely to develop respiratory tract infections and it has also been implicated in the development of glue ear. These problems can lead to a deterioration in the child's development and absences from school. In some countries, the dangers of smoking are being taken seriously and legislation has been passed to prevent smoking in all public places.

Developing a respiratory disorder can have short- or long-term implications. In an acute disorder, the patient's life-style is usually only affected during the acute phase. However, in the more chronic conditions such as chronic bronchitis, the patient's activities of living can be greatly affected leading to a reduction in the quality of life.

Further consequences of having a chronic respiratory disease are job loss leading to loss of self-esteem, loss of work and social role (see Ch. 1), financial worries and a dependency on others.

COMMON SYMPTOMS OF DISORDERS OF THE RESPIRATORY TRACT

Cough

Coughing is a means of keeping the respiratory tract clear. The cough reflex is stimulated by an irritant touching the lining of the tract.

The respiratory centre is the controlling factor in this reflex action, which causes forced expiration of mucus (if present). A cough is said to be productive if sputum is expectorated and unproductive if it is not.

Sputum

It is not normal to produce sputum. Sputum is produced in response to irritation of the respiratory tract by agents such as smoke, dust and bacteria. It is composed of mucus, cell debris and micro-organisms.

Haemoptysis

This is the production of bright red frothy blood from the lung. It is usually associated with lung disease and vigorous coughing. The severity of the haemoptysis varies greatly, from a few blood-stained streaks in the sputum to a very large haemorrhage that may be fatal.

Chest pain

Pain associated with respiratory disorders may be:

1. Retrosternal pain which is made worse by coughing but not by deep breathing and most commonly caused by tracheitis.
2. Pleurisy which is the term used to describe inflammatory changes in the pleura. It is one of the symptoms of pneumonia, tuberculosis and malignant invasion of the pleura. There are two forms of pleurisy:
   a. dry pleurisy is characterized by a sharp, stabbing pain on deep breathing and coughing which restricts respiration;
   b. pleurisy with effusion is caused by changes in the pleura which prevent the normal secretion and reabsorption of pleural fluid; this causes fluid to accumulate in the pleural space and inhibits lung expansion, causing dyspnoea and necessitating pleural aspiration by thoracentesis (see p. 449).

Dyspnoea

Difficulty in breathing which produces obvious changes in the respiratory pattern is called dyspnoea. Breathing is laboured and requires considerable exertion. Patients with chronic respiratory disorders are often dyspnoeic even at rest.

Cyanosis

This is a blue discoloration of the skin or mucous membranes. It results from an abnormally high proportion of desaturated haemoglobin in the circulation. It is a sign of hypoxia. Hypoxia occurs when there is an inadequate level of oxygen to supply the body tissues and can be due to a shortage of oxygen in inspired air, cardiac disease or to lung disease preventing oxygen reaching the blood.

Finger clubbing

The cause of this is unknown but it manifests itself as a drumstick-like swelling at the end of the fingers. It is associated with chronic hypoxic conditions such as bronchiectasis and bronchial cancer.

SIGNIFICANCE OF NURSING ROLE IN ESTABLISHING DIFFERENTIAL DIAGNOSIS

The nurse plays a vital role in the observation and assessment of the patient's symptoms. Reporting her findings to the medical staff can contribute greatly to making a diagnosis.

Cough

The type of cough should be noted. A dry (unproductive) cough is characteristic of an upper respiratory tract viral infection. However a productive cough, particularly on waking, is suggestive of chronic bronchitis.

A cough which changes in nature over a period of time may indicate bronchogenic carcinoma.

Sputum

The nurse should note the amount, colour, odour and consistency of sputum. Sputum produced in response to irritants is clear, white and mucoid, when infected, sputum will be purulent (yellow or green) and on occasions it will contain blood. Smelly sputum is suggestive of a lung abscess or bronchiectasis. The consistency of sputum may be thin and watery or thick and tenacious (sticky).

Haemoptysis

It is important to establish whether the patient has in fact coughed up the blood or vomited blood. Blood from the lungs is bright red, frothy and mixed with sputum. Blood from the stomach is usually dark red or coffee ground and may be mixed with food. Testing the blood with litmus paper will help to establish whether acid is present or absent.

Chest pain

The patient's pain should be assessed for its location, severity, its characteristics, when it occurs, what makes it worse and what makes it better.

A pain assessment chart can be used to monitor the patient's pain over a given period of time to establish any recurring pattern. See Chapter 4 for an example of a pain assessment chart.

Dyspnoea

The patient's breathing should be closely observed. The respiratory rate should be counted whilst the patient is unaware that his breathing is being observed. It is difficult to maintain a normal pattern of breathing when one is conscious that every rise and fall of one's chest is being counted. For this reason it is normal practice to take the patient's pulse and then, continuing to hold the patient's wrist, count the respirations. A rapid rate of breathing is called tachypnoea whilst a slower than normal rate is termed bradypnoea.

Bradypnoea may occur as the result of depression of the respiratory centre by morphine. The depth of breathing may be shallow, indicating minimal chest expansion and gaseous exchange. Deep respirations demonstrate full lung expansion.

The rhythm of the breathing should be noted. A healthy person breathes with a regular rhythm. An irregular rhythm indicates disease. Cheyne–Stokes breathing is characterized by a cycle of very deep and rapid breathing, followed by bradypnoea and more shallow respirations which eventually cease (apnoea) and then gradually become deep and rapid again. When this type of breathing occurs the patient's condition is poor and it frequently occurs when a patient is dying.

The noise of the patient's breathing should be noted. Normal breathing is silent. A wheeze can indicate asthma or chronic bronchitis due to the changes in the diameter of the bronchioles. Noisy laboured breathing (stridor) can indicate airway obstruction.

Observation of chest movement should be made. Chest movements should be even on both sides. Uneven chest movement could indicate pneumothorax or atelectasis. Also by observing the chest, the nurse may note whether the patient is using his accessory muscles of respiration; the flaring of nostrils, the sternomastoid and abdominal muscles.

The position that the patient adopts whilst breathing should also be noted. Patients who cannot tolerate lying down because of breathlessness are said to be orthopnoeic.

Cyanosis

The nurse observes for the presence of cyanosis (see p. 444) by looking at the patient's lips, ear lobes, mucous membranes inside the mouth and nail beds.

COMMON INVESTIGATIONS OF THE RESPIRATORY TRACT

Clinical examination

The doctor will take a clinical history from the patient and assess his breathing by means of palpation, percussion and auscultation using a stethoscope. During the examination the patient's comfort and safety is the nurse's main concern. The patient requires an explanation of the procedure, reassurance, warmth and privacy. He will also need help and support whilst moving into suitable positions during the examination. Once the examination is complete, the patient should be settled comfortably and well supported by pillows. A sputum container, tissues and a glass of water should be within easy reach.

Sputum specimen

Sputum is obtained either to identify pathological organisms or the presence of malignant cells. Where a bacterial infection is suspected, a specimen of sputum is obtained for culture and sensitivity. An early morning sputum specimen is best as this is more likely to be copious in nature. The investigation of sputum is important as treatment is based on the results of microbiological or cytological examination (see Ch. 4).

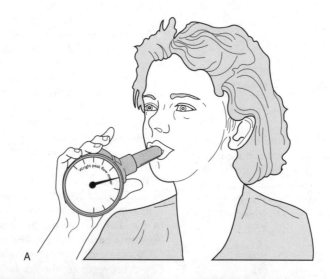

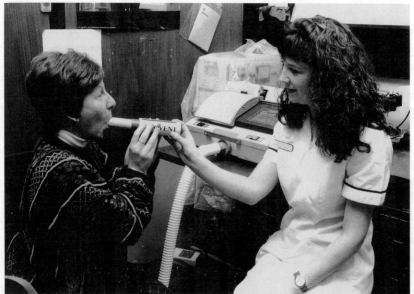

Fig. 13.4 (A) Wright's peak flow meter. (Reproduced with permission from Grenville-Mathers 1983, figure 1.21) (B) Peak flow meter

It may be necessary to support and assist the patient during expiration to ensure that an adequate specimen is obtained. A sterile specimen container should be used. Once obtained, the specimen should be correctly labelled and sent to the laboratory as soon as possible.

Chest X-ray

This is performed to detect abnormalities in the respiratory tract. Lung tissue is normally radiolucent and abnormalities appear as densities on the X-ray. Before any X-ray is taken, the patient requires a full explanation. The patient must be warmly clad whilst being taken to the X-ray department; he should be wearing his identification band and all previous X-rays should accompany the patient to allow comparison by the radiologist.

If the patient's condition is poor, a portable chest X-ray may be taken in the ward. The nurse, wearing a lead apron, may need to support the patient during the procedure. If this is not necessary, the nurse should leave the room or stand well away from the bedside to protect himself from the X-rays.

Blood gas analysis

By taking a specimen of arterial blood, the doctor is able to assess the efficiency of the patient's exchange of gases between the alveolar air and the capillaries.

The blood is taken from the brachial, radial or femoral artery.

The nurse, wearing gloves, may be required to apply pressure to the puncture site for a minimum of 3 minutes to prevent the formation of a haematoma. Once bleeding has been arrested, an Elastoplast or hypoallergenic dressing can be applied over the puncture site.

Pulmonary (lung) function tests

These are performed in patients with chronic respiratory disease. Pulmonary function tests involve the use of peak flow gauges and a spirometer (Figs 13.4, 13.5) to assess and measure the effectiveness of the patient's respiratory system to move air in and out of the lungs. The results can be used to determine the extent of the abnormality and/or to assess whether a patient is fit enough to have a general anaesthetic administered. The results can also be used to indicate how the patient is responding to treatment. Common terms associated with these measurements can be seen in Table 13.1.

Bronchoscopy

This allows the direct vision and examination of the larynx, trachea and bronchi. It permits the doctor to examine tissue, identify the extent of the disease and judge whether for example a tumour is amenable to

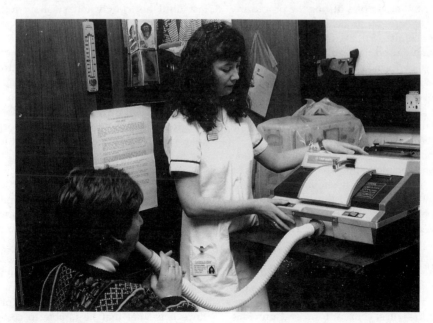

Fig. 13.5 Spirometer

Table 13.1   Common terms used in the measurement of lung function

Term	Definition	Normal average volumes (litre)
Vital capacity (VC)	The volume of air that can be expelled from the lungs by maximal expiration following maximal inspiration	3.5 (male) 2.3 (female)
Forced vital capacity (FVC)	As above but with a maximally forced expiration	4.0
Expiratory reserve volume (ERV)	The volume of air expelled by a maximal expiration following a normal inspiration	1.5
Inspiratory reserve volume (IRV)	The maximum volume of air which can be inhaled after a normal inspiration	2.0
Residual volume (RV)	The volume of air left in the lungs after a maximal expiration	1.5
Tidal volume (TV)	The volume of air moved during one respiratory cycle	0.5
Total lung capacity (TLC)	This is the sum of IRV, TV, ERV and RV	6.0
Forced expiratory volume (FEV)	The volume of air that can be expired forcefully at 1, 2 and 3 seconds after a maximal inspiration	3.0
Peak expiratory flow rate (PEFR)	Measured by rapid expiration into a peak flow meter (see Fig. 13.4)	Men 600 Women 400–500 Child (9)–175

surgery. The doctor can also take specimens of secretions and biopsy tissue samples during the procedure.

There are two type of bronchoscope, rigid and flexible fibreoptic (Fig. 13.6). with the latter being the more commonly used. Regardless of whether the bronchoscopy is performed under general or local anaesthesia, the patient must fast prior to this investigation to prevent regurgitation and inhalation of stomach contents.

The patient should sign a consent form once the procedure has been explained.

Since the thought of this type of investigation can cause considerable apprehension, not only because of the nature of the examination but also because of what may be found, the patient requires a great deal of support from the nurse.

The patient is prepared as for theatre. The patient is required to empty the bladder, then premedication is given as prescribed. A further identification band is applied, prostheses such as contact lenses and false teeth are removed and valuables are dealt with as per hospital policy. The patient is escorted to the diagnostic theatre with his notes, consent form and previous X-rays.

Following bronchoscopy, the patient continues to fast until his cough and swallow reflexes have returned. Mouth care should be performed to make the patient feel more comfortable. On return of the reflexes, sips of water may be given and the patient observed for any signs of pain or distress. The nurse should observe the patient and promptly report any signs of shock, dyspnoea, cyanosis and haemoptysis. Fluids and diet are introduced if no abnormalities are detected. The patient is warned to expect blood in his sputum and a sore throat for the next few days.

Pleural aspiration

The aspiration of pleural fluid for diagnostic or therapeutic purposes involves a procedure called thoracentesis. A needle biopsy of the pleura can be taken at the same time.

The procedure is usually performed in the ward using an aseptic technique. The patient is not required to fast before or after this investigation. It is important that the patient understands the explanation given since it is vital that he is able to co-operate during the aspiration.

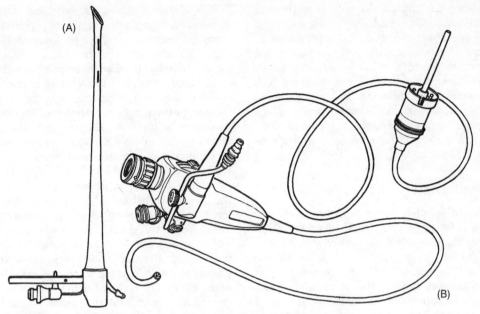

Fig. 13.6   (A) Rigid bronchoscope. (B) Flexible fibreoptic bronchoscope

The nurse should position herself by the patient's head so that he can give support and reassurance and also observe the patient's pulse, respirations, colour and signs of pain during the procedure.

To withdraw fluid from the pleural cavity, the patient must sit in the upright position, sitting either on the side of the bed or astride a chair with his feet supported and his arms and head resting on a bedtable or on the back of the chair. In this position, the shoulders and arms are raised, the rib cage elevated, the intercostal spaces increased, thus facilitating the introduction of the aspirating needle into the pleural space (Fig. 13.7). To prevent the aspirating needle puncturing the visceral pleura, the patient is asked to remain quite still and not to cough without warning and if possible not to cough at all.

At the end of the procedure, an occlusion dressing is applied over the puncture site and the amount of fluid aspirated is measured and recorded on the fluid balance chart. Specimens of pleural fluid are sent off in correctly labelled sterile containers for microbiological or cytological examination.

PRINCIPLES OF NURSING PATIENTS WITH RESPIRATORY DISORDERS

The nursing care of a patient with a respiratory disorder must be directed towards meeting his physical, psychological and social needs. One must

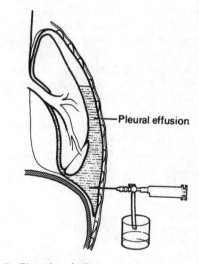

Fig. 13.7   Pleural aspiration

consider the symptoms the patient is experiencing and choose the most effective means of relieving the patient's discomfort. It must be remembered that the patient's needs and degree of dependence will relate directly to the severity of the illness.

In Nursing Care Plan 13.1 the nursing care of a breathless patient with a respiratory infection is discussed using the activities of living and the nursing process approach (see Ch. 3).

Whilst caring for the patient with a respiratory disorder, it is important to evaluate the care given and change the implementation of care as appropriate.

It would be hoped that with medical and nursing intervention, the patient's condition would improve over a few days. Once signs of improvement (e.g. reducing pyrexia, less dyspnoea and less purulent sputum) are apparent, the nursing care will be changed to encourage and allow the patient more independence and regain his autonomy in readiness for discharge home.

Patient education

It is important for the patient who has a chronic disorder to learn to live his life to the full within the limits of the disease. If the patient still smokes, he should be strongly persuaded to stop as even at this late stage there would be some improvement in respiratory function. Patients should be advised not to go out in cold damp weather unless necessary and will be advised to have an influenza vaccine every year in an attempt to prevent further exacerbations. In some patients whose condition is very severe, home oxygen therapy is prescribed. The patient has the necessary equipment installed at home and, with his family, is taught how to use it and the precautions that have to be taken. The GP will assess the patient's condition at home and arrange for the services of members of the primary health care team and/or voluntary services as required.

TYPES OF DISORDERS

DISORDERS OF THE LOWER RESPIRATORY TRACT

Bronchitis

Epidemiology and aetiology

Bronchitis is a general term used to describe an inflammatory condition of the bronchi. It may be acute or chronic.

Acute bronchitis may result as a complication of coryza (common cold), influenza or measles. Acute bronchitis affecting previously healthy individuals is normally viral in origin. However, patients, especially if they smoke, may develop a secondary bacterial infection.

Chronic bronchitis can be defined as a productive cough which persists for at least 3 months of the year for two successive years. It is a progressive degen-erative disease affecting the bronchial mucosa. It is caused by irritants associated with personal pollution of cigarette smoking and/or environmental air pollution. An acute exacerbation (often during the winter months) of the condition can be precipitated by a viral or bacterial infection of the respiratory tract.

The changes which occur during the course of the disease greatly reduce the number of cilia and destroy their normal function. The mucous glands enlarge, producing an increased amount of secretions which block bronchioles and impair alveolar ventilation. Loss of elasticity of lung tissue prevents adequate expiration and may cause the typical barrel chest of the chronic bronchitic. The respiratory centre is no longer stimulated by high levels of carbon dioxide but by the lower than normal level of oxygen. This is very important to remember when administering oxygen because to overoxygenate patients with chronic bronchitis results in a higher than normal level of O_2 in the blood. There would then be no stimulus to the respiratory centre and the patient would develop complete respiratory failure, requiring assisted ventilation with a positive pressure ventilator.

As a result of infection, fibrosis and stenosis of bronchioles occur. This can further lead to emphysema which describes the destruction of lung tissue with alveoli joining together making large irregular airsacs or cysts (bullae) which do not take part in gaseous exchange. Nearly all patients with chronic bronchitis have some emphysema and hence the terms are often used together. Eventually, right-sided heart failure (cor pulmonale) can occur. Chronic obstructive airways disease (COAD) is a term which is used to describe the condition in which patients have chronic bronchitis and emphysema. Some doctors would use the term to also include patients who exhibit signs of bronchial hyperreactivity (asthma).

Chronic bronchitis and emphysema occur in 17% of men and 8% of women in the UK in the 40–64 age group. Cigarette smoking is the major factor in its development as the disease is almost exclusively found in smokers and there is a definite link to the number of cigarettes smoked per day. Davies (1990) reports that those who smoke 30 cigarettes daily are twenty times more at risk of dying from chronic bronchitis and emphysema than non-smokers.

The socio-economic burden of chronic bronchitis and emphysema is considerable. Between 1976 and 1977 in the United Kingdom chronic bronchitis and emphysema were certified as causing 26 million lost working days for men and 2.6 million lost days for women, accounting for some 10% of all days of sickness absence from work, much the highest of any defined disease entity.

(Davies 1990, p. 656)

Those suffering from the disease have to come to terms with the fact that they have a chronic condition which will cause them significant illness and disability. Recent figures from the Scottish Office (1992) estimate chronic bronchitis and emphysema kills approximately 3000 Scots every year.

Common symptomatology

Cough In acute bronchitis there is an irritating dry unproductive cough which may become productive due to secondary infection. The patient with chronic bronchitis has a productive cough, especially in the morning.

Sputum Patients with chronic bronchitis will produce copious amounts of a clear white thick and tenacious sputum. However, when a secondary bacterial infection occurs, the sputum will increase in volume and become purulent.

Chest tightness and wheeze In bronchitis, retrosternal pain is present and the patient usually experiences chest tightness and wheezing. The patient with chronic bronchitis will undoubtedly suffer this especially on waking before the bronchial secretions have been expectorated. Their chest expansion will be poor and expiration slow and difficult, leading to an elevated level of carbon dioxide in the blood. Patients with chronic bronchitis characteristically breathe out through pursed lips because in this way they are able to exhale more air than would be possible if they allowed air to escape more quickly. To overcome the loss of elastic recoil of their lungs, patients will use their accessory muscles of respiration to aid expiration.

Dyspnoea As discussed on page 445, this can occur even when the patient is at rest.

Cyanosis This occurs as a result of hypoxia (see page 445).

Pyrexia and general malaise Patients with either acute or chronic bronchitis who develop a secondary bacterial infection will develop a pyrexia and general malaise.

Significance of nursing role in establishing differential diagnosis

This is discussed on page 445.

Range of investigations

- Clinical examination (for more detail see p. 445).
- Sputum specimen for culture and sensitivity (for more detail see p. 446).
- Chest X-ray (see Ch. 4).
- Pulmonary function tests to assess the chronicity of the condition (see p. 447).

Therapeutic management

Acute bronchitis Gradual improvement occurs in 4–8 days in the majority of cases. However, those patients who smoke or live in areas of high atmospheric pollution may have a prolonged illness. Antibiotics may be prescribed. Pain caused by the inflammation can be relieved by medicated steam inhalations. The nurse must ensure the patient's safety during this procedure since there is a potential danger of scalding if the Nelson's inhaler is not used properly. The irritating unproductive cough can be eased by the administration of a cough suppressant drug. Advice about rest and diet during the convalescent period may be required.

Chronic bronchitis During an acute exacerbation of the disease, bed rest is essential. Oxygen therapy will be necessary. It is vital that the correct mask is used as the respiratory centre in a chronic bronchitic patient is insensitive to carbon dioxide levels and a lack of oxygen becomes the stimulus to breathing. The administration of oxygen to such a patient is therefore very important. If the patient receives too much oxygen, respiration slows down and will eventually cease. Oxygen therapy via a Ventimask will be prescribed as this mask allows a regulated percentage of oxygen to supplement the atmospheric air. Arterial blood gas analysis results will guide the percentage of oxygen to be given and the duration required.

Antibiotic therapy will depend on the culture and sensitivity report on the sputum. Bronchodilator drugs such as salbutamol or terbutaline sulphate are given via a nebulizer (Box 13.1, Fig. 13.8). Chest physiotherapy and the use of drugs to reduce the viscosity of mucous help to prevent the accumulation of excess mucus which would obstruct the airway.

Nursing strategies

The nursing care of a patient with an acute exacerbation of chronic bronchitis is described in Nursing Care Plan 13.1.

Health education

Breathing The patient should be advised how to prevent further exacerbations. In the winter months especially the patient should avoid crowded areas in an attempt to avoid infections. They should go out as

---

Box 13.1   Nebulizer therapy

Definition:
The administration of a drug in solution which is converted into a fine mist of droplets by either oxygen or compressed air. The fine droplets can be inhaled directly into the bronchial tree.

How a nebulizer works:
'The production of droplets is achieved by passing compressed air (or oxygen) through a narrow hole. The jet of gas leaves the hole, creating an area of partial vacuum (the Bernouilli effect) into which the fluid is drawn from the reservoir and then broken up into droplets by the jet (this is the same mechanism that is used in an aerosol can). These droplets are filtered by a baffle structure within the nebulizer, which effectively removes the larger droplets, returning them to the reservoir for recirculation. (Mumford (1986) p. 95).

Advantages of nebulized drug administration:
1. The nebulized drug reaches parts of the airways

it would otherwise not reach by systemic administration. Drugs such as the bronchodilator drug, salbutamol, can be diluted in isotonic saline. The latter has a mucolytic action and aids the expectoration of sputum.
2. The nebulizer can be driven by oxygen or compressed air. In patients with chronic bronchitis, the nebulizer may be driven by compressed air rather than oxygen.
3. Since the drug is administered by inhalation and not systemically, a lower dosage of the drug is required and consequently there is a lower incidence of side-effects.

Instructions for use:
Patients receiving nebulizer therapy should be encouraged to breathe at their normal rate and not to consciously breathe deeply as this affects the drug uptake.

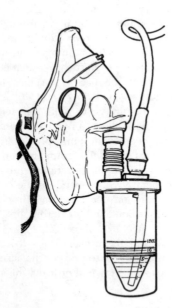

Fig. 13.8   Nebulizer

little as possible when the weather is cold, damp, foggy and windy. They should stop smoking and avoid smoky atmospheres. Patients should take note of the colour of any sputum expectorated. If it becomes green/yellow they should consult their GP as soon as possible in order to receive prompt treatment.
   Nutrition   Abdominal distension is to be avoided as

this interferes with the movement of the diaphragm. Patients should therefore be encouraged to eat several small nutritious well-balanced meals a day instead of three large ones and they should be advised to avoid eating gas-forming foods such as onions, broccoli and cauliflower. If appropriate, a reduction in weight will also aid their breathing.
   Rest and sleep   The house should be warm and they should heat up the bedroom at least 1 hour before retiring into a warm bed.
   Mobilization   The feeling of breathlessness actually does no physical harm but it is a frightening symptom. The patient should be encouraged to mobilize as much as their dyspnoea will allow.
   Work and play   Those patients still in employment should be advised to change their job if possible if the job involves heavy work making them breathless, or if it involves working in a dusty or smoky atmosphere. Patients who have become housebound should be assessed for home help and meals on wheels requirements and organized as appropriate. Loneliness and boredom can be a problem and volunteer visitors to the housebound can provide a useful service.

Infections of the lower respiratory tract

Epidemiology and aetiology

Pneumonia is the commonest infection causing death in the UK (Brunner & Suddarth 1992). It can be de-

Nursing Care Plan 13.1 Care of a breathless patient with a chest infection			
Problem	**Goal**	**Nursing action**	**Rationale**
1. Dyspnoea	To establish a normal breathing pattern	**BREATHING** ❏ Upright position in bed, well supported by pillows	Allows chest expansion and reduces pressure of abdominal contents on the diaphragm
		❏ Help into orthopnoeic position – patient upright, leaning forward on pillow, on bed table	Allows maximal use of accessory muscles of respiration. Pillows help to maintain patient's position
		❏ Approach patient from the side. Do not stand too close to patient	Breathless patients often feel claustrophobic. It is therefore important to increase the patient's personal space rather than invade it
		❏ Nurse in well-ventilated area, use fan near bed area	Gives patient feeling of an airy environment
		❏ Administer oxygen at correct rate, using the correct mask as prescribed	Improves the oxygenation of blood
		❏ Ensure bed linen is not too heavy	Inhibits chest expansion
		❏ Administer prescribed bronchodilator via nebulizer	Reduces bronchospasm in the bronchioles thereby increasing the vital capacity
2. Excessive sputum	Help to expectorate	❏ Physiotherapy, deep breathing exercises and percussion	Breathing exercises improve the vital capacity and improve venous return. Percussion loosens tenacious sputum from the bronchial walls
		❏ Obtain sputum specimen for culture and sensitivity	Will identify causative organism and its sensitivity to antibiotics
		❏ Administer antibiotics as prescribed	Antibiotics will destroy the pathogenic organisms causing the chest infection
		❏ Use postural drainage techniques as appropriate	Positioning and postural drainage uses gravity to help drain sputum from lungs which can then be expectorated
		❏ Provide sputum cups, tissues and disposal bag within the patient's easy reach	Reduces risk of cross-infection and ensures the safe disposal of sputum
		❏ Observe and record amount, colour and consistency of sputum	Monitors the extent of the disease and evaluates the effectiveness of treatment
		❏ Observe and record temperature, pulse, respirations and blood pressure 4 hourly	Monitors patient's response to treatment. Allows recognition and prompt reporting of abnormalities. As antibiotics begin to exert their effect, vital signs should begin to fall towards normal limits
		❏ Observe and report the patient's ability to cough and expectorate	Monitors effectiveness of treatment and identifies any complications arising
		❏ Give regular oral hygiene to remove any remaining sputum	Prevents infection of oral mucosa and removes unpleasant taste which may otherwise spoil appetite
		❏ Encourage hourly drinks of fluid according to patient's preference	A good fluid intake helps keep secretions/sputum less viscous, thereby aiding their expectoration. Allowing patient to choose his drinks helps compliance

Nursing Care Plan 13.1 (*cont'd*)

Problem	Goal	Nursing action	Rationale
3. **Potential respiratory failure**	Detect and report early signs of respiratory failure	❏ Monitor rate, depth, rhythm and effort of respirations	Any abnormality should be reported as it could indicate interference in gaseous exchange
		❏ Monitor patient's mental state	Cerebral anoxia causes confusion, drowsiness and can lead to unconsciousness
MAINTAINING A SAFE ENVIRONMENT			
4. **Patient receiving oxygen therapy**	Ensure safety and comfort of patient	❏ Ensure that oxygen is given at the correct rate via correct mask or nasal cannulae	Too much oxygen may inhibit stimulus to respiration. Too little oxygen will not oxygenate blood to desired level
		❏ Explain necessity of oxygen to patient to gain compliance	Patient is more likely to co-operate with treatment
		❏ Give frequent oral hygiene	Prevents the drying effects of oxygen on oral mucosa. A clean healthy mucosa reduces the risk of infection occurring. A dry mouth makes expectoration more difficult
		❏ Change facemask/nasal cannulae daily and pad around elastic of mask as necessary	Equipment may become contaminated and lead to further infection. Elastic can cause pressure sores around ears
		❏ Explain all the safety precautions required when oxygen is in use to both patient and family: • no smoking whilst oxygen is in use • oil or grease should not be used around any oxygen connections • electrical devices should not be used whilst oxygen is in use • fire extinguisher should be readily available	Oxygen supports combustion. All staff, patients and visitors should be aware of the dangers
		❏ Observe for signs of confusion and adopt protective measures as appropriate	Anoxia may cause confusion. Protective measures taken to prevent patient from harming himself, i.e. use of cot-sides to prevent falling out of bed
5. **Patient receiving bronchodilator and antibiotic therapy**	Monitor for and report desired and unwanted side-effects	❏ Measure and record temperature, pulse, respiration and blood pressure as ordered	Improvement of condition would be reflected in a return of vital signs to normal
		❏ Observe for and report the presence of side-effects of drugs	Allows the appropriate action to be taken promptly
COMMUNICATION			
6. **Admission of anxious patient**	Reduce anxiety of patient	❏ Explain the events which will take place to help patient, in a quiet and confident manner	This should reduce anxiety and remove the fear of the unknown. Anxiety increases oxygen consumption
		❏ Arrange for relatives to be seen by senior staff	Develops a therapeutic relationship and establishes good communication. Will increase confidence in staff, thereby reducing anxiety
		❏ Obtain information for nursing profile from wife as her husband cannot form sentences as he is gasping for breath	Ensures collection of good patient profile and emergency contact number

Nursing Care Plan 13.1 (cont'd)			
Problem	**Goal**	**Nursing action**	**Rationale**
6. (cont'd)		❑ Reassure patient and family regarding effectiveness of treatment	Allays anxiety. Improves morale
7. Potential confusion due to cerebral hypoxia	Prevent from occurring, recognize and treat promptly	❑ Assess mental status hourly	Allows for detection of confusion and disorientation to name, place, date and time
		❑ If confused, orientate patient to name, place date and time at regular intervals	Helps to reorientate patient
		❑ Explain all procedures carefully and with patience	Reduces confusion and anxiety. Orientates patient to his circumstances
		❑ Encourage family visits, photographs of loved ones at bedside	Helps to promote orientation and reduce confusion
8. Difficulty in communicating due to oxygen therapy and dyspnoea	To ensure effective communication	❑ Ensure call bell is within easy reach of the patient and in working order	Allows patient to summon help
		❑ Use closed questions when speaking to patient. Agree signals for yes and no	Allows patient to respond to questions within his ability
		❑ Anticipate patient's needs	Reduce the effort required by the patient to ask for assistance
		❑ Nasal cannulae may be prescribed	Frees the mouth for communication since there is no mask to inhibit communication
DYING			
9. Fear of suffocation	To reduce fear	❑ Sit with patient. Use of touch. Display kindness and empathy. Ensure privacy	Produces an atmosphere conductive to the expression of the patient's fears and concerns
		❑ Encourage patient to express fears and concerns	Once voiced and shared, these fears and concerns usually diminish in magnitude
EATING AND DRINKING			
10. Poor appetite	Ensure adequate nutrition	❑ Offer small appetizing easily swallowed and digested meals	In order to swallow, the patient must stop breathing. Small soft palatable diet is most suitable during acute period as chewing food is tiring and interferes with breathing pattern
		❑ Replace oxygen mask with nasal cannulae at meal times if prescribed	Allows patient to eat and receive an uninterrupted supply of oxygen
		❑ Weigh patient weekly	Helps to assess patient's nutritional status
11. Potential dehydration	Maintain hydration	❑ Give hourly high protein and calorie drinks	Promotes liquification of viscous sputum and promotes healing of damaged lung tissue. Hydrates patient
		❑ Monitor fluid balance accurately	Will indicate any discrepancy in fluid balance
		❑ Administer intravenous fluids and electrolytes via intravenous infusion as prescribed	If patient is unable to maintain desired oral fluid intake due to dyspnoea, intravenous infusion replaces excessive fluid loss and maintains fluid and electrolyte balance

Nursing Care Plan 13.1 (*cont'd*)

Problem	Goal	Nursing action	Rationale
		ELIMINATING	
12. Potential constipation	Prevent and maintain normal bowel habit	❏ Encourage soft fruit and vegetables in diet	Adds fibre to diet
		❏ Encourage hourly drinks	Maintains hydration and prevents constipation and urinary stasis
		❏ Monitor bowel movements	Allows recognition of potential constipation
		❏ Administer mild aperient as prescribed if required	Helps to prevent constipation
		MOBILIZATION	
13. Reluctance to move due to orthopnoea and dyspnoea	Reduce the risks of deep vein thrombosis and pressure sore development	❏ Change position every 2 hours	Relieves pressure and ensures an adequate blood flow bringing oxygen and nutrients to tissues
		❏ Inspect pressure areas for redness and skin breakdown 2 hourly	Ensures early detection of problem and reassessment of care planned as necessary
		❏ Use appropriate pressure-relieving aids	Relieves pressure on pressure areas on an at-risk patient
		❏ Reinforce leg exercises taught by physiotherapist and their importance to patient	Prevents the formation of deep vein thrombosis by using calf muscle pump to encourage venous return back to the heart
		❏ Encourage gentle mobilization as soon as the patient's condition improves	Gentle mobilizing prevents complications of bed rest
		PERSONAL CLEANSING AND DRESSING	
14. Sweating due to pyrexia and increased effort of breathing	Reduce discomfort and prevent skin breakdown	❏ Clean and dry skin as require	Reduces discomfort
		❏ Change linen when damp	Warm, moist, and dark conditions encourage multiplication of bacteria. May predispose to pressure sore formation
		❏ Assist as required with washing and dressing	Patient requires assistance as they will fatigue easily
		❏ Refrain from the overuse of talcum powder	Great care must be taken not to create clouds of talcum dust in the atmosphere as this will cause an increase in dyspnoea and distress
		REST AND SLEEP	
15. Unable to sleep	To promote sleep	❏ Identify cause of sleeplessness. Encourage patient to relax prior to settling down for the night	Patient unable to sleep due to coughing or fear of not waking up again
16. Fatigue, general malaise	To reduce and increase tolerance to activity	❏ Encourage pacing of activities	Allows patient to expend energy in limited amounts without unduly tiring himself
		❏ Ensure rest periods through day, especially after meals	Facilitates recuperation and digestion of meal
		WORK AND PLAY	
17. Boredom	Relieve and restore positive outlook	❏ Encourage involvement in appropriate activities	Reduces the feeling of helplessness and worthlessness
		❏ Use of distraction – television, radio, reading	Programme or interesting reading material will utilize time
		❏ Encourage socializing from staff, other patients, relatives and friends	Helps to relieve boredom and encourages patient to look to the future more positively

scribed as an infection and inflammation of the lung tissue. Those at risk of developing pneumonia are cigarettes smokers, debilitated and immobile patients, immunosuppressed patients, the elderly and patients in intensive care units.

Pneumonia is classified according to the causative organism and can be bacterial, viral or fungal. It can affect one lobe (lobar pneumonia) or more than one lobe or both lungs (bronchopneumonia). The latter is most common and carries a high mortality in the very young and the very old. The incidence is higher in winter and is spread by droplet infection. The affected lobe(s) become consolidated with exudate in the alveoli. When liquefaction of the exudate occurs, the infected material is either absorbed or expectorated.

Pneumonia can also be caused by the aspiration of vomit (aspiration pneumonia). This can occur when the normal defence mechanisms of the respiratory tract are absent or ineffective. This condition can affect the young, the elderly, the debilitated. The aspiration of vomit into the lungs can cause severe damage to the tissue as a result of the action of hydrochloric acid. It has a high mortality rate.

The commonest opportunistic infection (80%) in patients with acquired immunodeficiency syndrome (AIDS) is *Pneumocystis carinii* pneumonia, although it can also be seen in patients who are immunosuppressed due to chemotherapy. It is the most common cause of death in AIDS patients (Pratt 1988).

The incidence of tuberculosis in the western world has fallen due to improvement in housing, environment and nutrition. There are 5000–7000 new cases annually in the UK. However, world-wide tuberculosis continues to be a serious problem with a yearly toll of 3–4 million deaths.

In the UK, those susceptible to the disease are in contact with an infectious patient, are in poor general health, have unfavourable social conditions, are members of the Asian immigrant community who have a low racial resistance to the disease (Davies 1990, Brunner & Suddarth 1992) or have AIDS.

Tuberculosis is caused by the micro-organism *Mycobacterium tuberculosis*. The route of infection is most commonly by inhalation of air containing the tubercle bacilli which have been coughed up or sneezed into the atmosphere by an infectious patient. When infected for the first time, the lesion is known as primary and may heal spontaneously, providing the patient with acquired immunity (see Ch. 4). A healed primary lesion may be reactivated in later years if the patient's general health deteriorates.

Legionnaires' disease was identified in 1976 when a large number of deaths occurred in delegates attend-ing an American Legion conference in Philadelphia. Initially the cause of death was unknown but eventually a new bacterium, *Legionella pneumophilia*, was discovered. It is carried in water and inhaled via showers and air cooling systems. Most patients recover from the disease but the mortality rate in the elderly is about 30% (Davies 1990).

Common symptomatology (for more detail see p. 444)

1. **Dyspnoea.**
2. **Pyrexia and rigors.** Often the onset is sudden with the temperature rising to 40°C within a few hours. Patients with tuberculosis often have an evening pyrexia.
3. **Tachycardia.**
4. **General malaise and lethargy.**
5. **Pleuritic pain.**
6. **Cough.** This varies according to the type of infection present. Patients with tuberculosis usually have a dry irritating cough, patients with pneumonia or *Pneumocystis carinii* initially complain of an unproductive cough which later becomes productive. Patients with aspiration pneumonia have a severe cough which produces purulent sputum.
7. **Weight loss** may be evident, particularly in patients with *Pneumocystis carinii* or tuberculosis.
8. **Confusion** may manifest due to cerebral anoxia.

Significance of nursing role in establishing differential diagnosis

By careful observation and questioning of the patient, the nurse can aid in the diagnosis. By using assessment skills she can determine the character and position of pain, its severity, what relieves it and what makes it worse. By monitoring patients' respiration, the degree of dyspnoea can be identified.

The observation of the amount, colour and consistency of sputum can aid in identification of suspected organisms, for example rusty-coloured sputum usually indicates the presence of pneumococcus. Elderly patients who become uncharacteristically confused or behave oddly should be seen by the medical staff as these may be the first signs of pneumonia.

Range of investigations (for more detail see p. 445)

1. Clinical examination reveals consolidation of the affected part of lung.
2. Chest X-ray confirms the area(s) of the lung involved.

3. Sputum specimen sent for culture and sensitivity to identify pathogenic organism. If tuberculosis is suspected, three consecutive early morning specimens are collected and sent for acid alkali fast bacilli (AAFB) testing. The tubercle is described as acid alkali fast because of the method used in the laboratory to identify them. Where legionnaires' disease is suspected the sputum undergoes specialized staining and culture.

4. Blood specimen sent for culture and sensitivity if rigors are present as this usually indicates bacterial invasion of the blood.

5. Fibreoptic bronchoscopy and biopsy may be required to diagnose *Pneumocystis carinii*. Precautions are taken during and after this procedure to prevent the transmission of human immunodeficiency virus (HIV). (For more detail see Pratt 1988).

Therapeutic management

Antibiotics Patients with lower respiratory tract infections are treated with antibiotics. Until the causative organism is identified, broad spectrum antibiotics are used and then altered as necessary when the microbiology results are available.

Patients with *Pneumocystis carinii* are given high dose antibiotics, initially intravenously, as this disorder carries a 25% mortality rate. In pneumonia there is usually a quick response to antibiotic therapy, with a corresponding improvement in the patient's symptoms. Patients with tuberculosis are treated by using a combination of antimicrobial drugs for considerably longer than the other infections.

A standard therapeutic regimen is rifampicin, isoniazid and ethambutol for 2 months followed by rifampicin and isoniazid for 7 months.

It is important that close contacts of the patient with newly diagnosed tuberculosis are screened in order to control the disease within the community. Screening involves sending sputum specimens for bacterial examination.

Not everyone who inhales the tubercle bacillus will develop tuberculosis. Those contacts with positive results are clinically examined, have a tuberculin skin test (heaf or mantoux) and a chest X-ray. They have a repeat chest X-ray at 6 and 12 months and if these are clear they are discharged. If the positive contacts are Asian or African, they are followed up for 2 years since the prevalence of tuberculosis is higher in these groups (Flenley 1990).

Contacts who were tuberculin negative are re-tested 6 weeks later. If they remain negative, they are given a BCG (Bacille Calmette Guerin – the original strain of non-virulent bacillus developed in 1922) vaccination. A BCG vaccination affords a high degree of protection against subsequent tuberculosis infection. For this reason, those who are in special high risk groups and those working in areas of high risk (nurses, doctors, dentists and school teachers) should be vaccinated (Cole & Mackay 1990).

Hospitalization Patients are usually hospitalized with the exception of the patient with tuberculosis. Treatment depends on whether the patient is only infected or is both infected and infectious.

An infected patient can be cared for in the community under the supervision of the health authorities (it is a notifiable disease) but if the patient is also infectious as shown by acid fast bacilli in his sputum, he must be nursed in isolation until his sputum culture is negative. (For isolation nursing see Pritchard & David 1988.) He can then be discharged and continue his drug therapy at home.

Patients with other lower respiratory tract infections are admitted to allow treatment to be as effective as possible. Patients require bed rest initially. Pain can be relieved by analgesia. Oxygen therapy may be prescribed during the acute stages if the patient appears cyanosed or has signs of cerebral anoxia. Efficient expectoration and chest expansion can be achieved with the aid of physiotherapy.

A complication following bronchopneumonia is bronchiectasis, but fortunately the incidence of this disease has reduced since the advent of antibiotics for the treatment of bronchopneumonia. In bronchiectasis, there is irreversible damage to the bronchial walls and cilia and the patient is predisposed to recurrent chest infections.

Since most patients with bronchiectasis have widespread disease, surgery in the form of a lobectomy is rarely possible. Treatment is aimed at the control of infection by the use of antibiotics and the drainage of sputum. The latter is achieved by the use of postural drainage, which is achieved by placing the patient in a position most suitable for drainage by gravity from the affected area (Fig. 13.9).

Nursing strategies

The nursing care of a patient with a lower respiratory tract infection involves the care of a breathless patient with an infection, as described in Nursing Care Plan 13.1.

Patients with AIDS and *Pneumocystis carinii* require specialist nursing. Their care is planned holistically to meet each patient's individual needs. (For more detail see Pratt 1988.)

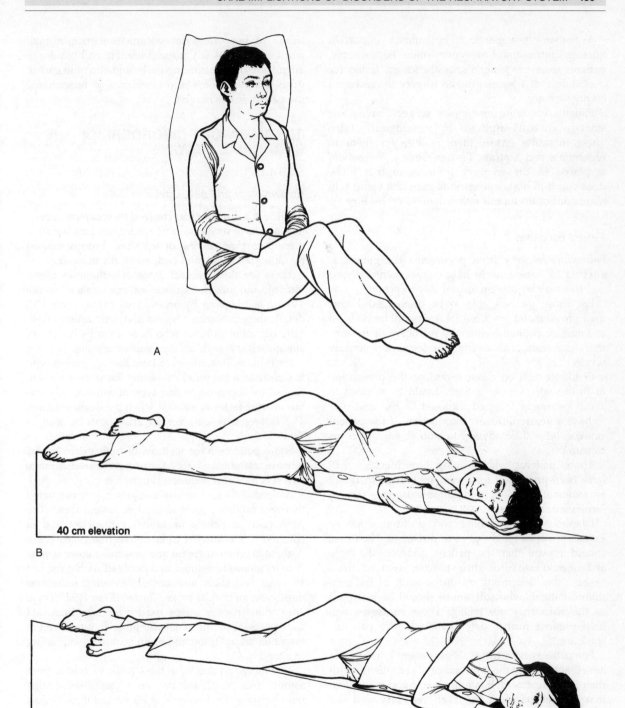

Fig. 13.9 (A) Position used to facilitate removal of secretions from right upper lobe and upper segment of left upper lobe (B) Position used to facilitate removal of secretions from right middle lobe (C) Position used to facilitate removal of secretions from right lower lobe

Aspiration pneumonia. The most important nursing contribution here is prevention. For example, patients receiving general anaesthetics are fasted for a minimum of 4 hours prior to surgery to ensure an empty stomach.

Patients requiring emergency surgery have their stomach contents aspirated by a nasogastric tube. These measures ensure there is little for them to regurgitate and aspirate. Postoperatively, the patient is placed in the recovery position so that if he does vomit in his semiconscious state, the vomit will trickle out of his mouth rather than down his airway.

Patient education

Following recovery from pneumonia the patient is advised to have a fairly long convalescence period and this may require prolonged stay in hospital.

For those patients able to be discharged home, their physical and psychosocial needs will be assessed and met accordingly, either by members of the primary care team or those from the social or voluntary services.

Guidance will be given regarding the prevention of further attacks; the patient should be advised to avoid becoming fatigued, exposed to the cold and to have a yearly influenza vaccination. If the patient smokes, he will be advised to stop or cut down his consumption.

Those patients who develop bronchiectasis will have been prescribed long-term antibiotics, therefore an explanation of their importance is necessary to facilitate compliance.

Diaphragmatic breathing and postural drainage exercises will be taught prior to discharge. The nurse should ensure that the patient understands these and should reinforce their practice two to three times a day depending on the severity of the condition. Patients who still smoke should be informed of the risks they are taking. These measures will help prevent further deterioration in the patient's condition.

For patients with tuberculosis, patient education is aimed at stressing the importance of compliance with their drug treatment. It is impressed upon the patient that the tablets must be taken regularly and the full course completed otherwise he will not be cured – the temptation to stop taking the tablets must be resisted because he is feeling well again. Patients should be warned that rifampicin causes orange staining of body fluids and for this reason they are advised not to wear contact lenses during treatment. During treatment, the patient can continue to work as normal and live a completely normal life. He will require to attend for clinic visits regularly and if at the end of drug treatment there is no evidence of tuberculosis the patient is discharged.

INFLAMMATORY DISORDERS OF THE BRONCHIAL AIRWAYS

Asthma

Epidemiology and aetiology

Asthma is a disease characterized by recurrent reversible attacks of dyspnoea and wheezing. This is due to a temporary narrowing of the small bronchi caused by muscular spasm and oedema of the mucosa.

There are three clinical types of asthma: extrinsic, intrinsic and mixed. Extrinsic asthma implies that the asthma is triggered by an external cause. Table 13.2 details these common triggers. Extrinsic asthma typically occurs in children who have a family history of allergic disease such as hay fever or eczema.

Intrinsic asthma occurs in later life in a person who has neither a personal or family history of disease caused by allergens. In this type of asthma, no obvious allergic factor is isolated when the disease occurs. The factors which trigger an attack can be seen in Table 13.3.

Some patients have features of both extrinsic and intrinsic asthma and are said to have mixed asthma, which is the most common type.

Asthma can occur in any age group. It is estimated that two million people in the UK have asthma. The prevalence of asthma in adults is about 5% and in children it is estimated to be above 10% (Rees 1989). Asthma is on the increase and becoming more severe: 'The incidence of asthma had doubled within the last 15 years and chest physicians are seeing more and more cases of it in its severe forms' (Pinn 1992). There are various reasons suspected for this; the increased use of aerosol products, talcum powder, increased environmental pollution and an increased susceptibility to allergens.

Two thousand people in the UK die each year from asthma, five people per day on average. This is distressing since it is known that 80–90% of these deaths could be preventable with improved management and patient education. Patients with poorly controlled asthma have more absence from school/work and have more difficulty in leading a normal life than those whose condition is well controlled. Patient education aims to equip the patient with the necessary

Table 13.2   Factors which trigger extrinsic asthma

Allergen	Source	Comment
House dust mite's faecal pellets	Mites live off human skin scales and can be found in bedding, soft toys, carpets, furniture. They also thrive in warm, damp conditions	80% of children with asthma are sensitive to house dust mites. It should be noted that the presence of mites does not reflect on the cleanliness of the house. It is impossible to get rid of them completely (Hilton 1984)
Pollen	Grass, trees, weeds, flowers, rape seed crops	Grass pollen seems to be the most troublesome in the UK
Animal danders	Allergens are found in animal fur, hair, body fluids and feathers	
Food	Milk, eggs, nuts, fish, alcohol, sulphur dioxide in fizzy drinks and tartrazine (an artificial food colouring)	Food allergens are the least common of triggers

Table 13.3   Factors which trigger intrinsic asthma

Trigger	Comment
Respiratory tract infection	Common trigger
Exercise	Common trigger. Exercise involving the rapid inspiration of cool air, for example running causes more problems than swimming
Emotion and stress	Both positive and negative emotions and stressors can trigger asthma
Environmental pollutants	Smoke, fumes and sprays can trigger asthma
Some drugs	Some asthmatics are sensitive to aspirin and non-steroidal anti-inflammatory drugs. Beta blocker drugs are contraindicated in asthmatic patients since they provoke asthmatic attacks

knowledge and skills to prevent and treat his own asthma.

People with asthma should learn to live with their condition rather than suffer from it. If children are labelled as suffering from asthma they are often made a special case and treated differently from their peer group. This can hinder their development.

Common symptomatology

There is a history of periodic attacks of dyspnoea and wheezing, especially on expiration. The wheeze can be described as a whistling sound caused by the obstructed airway. It varies during the day and worsens at night or in the early morning on waking. Adults experience a feeling of chest tightness on waking and sometimes during the night.

The onset of an attack of asthma may be extremely quick and can cause great alarm to the patient and their family. The patient will be dyspnoeic, have a tachycardia and may be cyanosed. The patient will adopt an upright leaning forward position and use their accessory muscles of respiration in an attempt to improve expiration. The attack may last several hours, leaving the patient physically and emotionally exhausted. Patients with a continuous asthma attack lasting more than 12 hours are admitted to hospital.

These patients will be severely breathless, wheezy and extremely distressed. There will be signs of hypoxia.

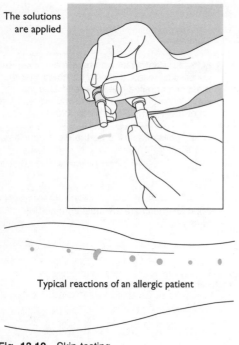

The solutions are applied

The solutions are pricked in

Typical reactions of an allergic patient

Fig. 13.10   Skin testing

Investigations

1. Clinical examination which will include an investigation into the patient's personal and family medical history.

2. Sensitivity tests are performed to identify any allergen. These involve an injection of a small extract of suspected allergic substance into a superficial layer of skin. If a weal develops 10–20 minutes later, the patient is allergic to that substance (Fig. 13.10).

3. During an attack, investigations to measure the increased resistance to airflow may be made, for example, FEV, FVC and PEFR (Table 13.1).

Therapeutic management

Patients who have asthma are advised to avoid all known and common allergens. Drug treatment falls into two categories. Drugs such as sodium cromoglycate (Intal) or beclomethasone (Becotide) are prescribed to be taken on a regular basis to prevent attacks from occurring. The former drug is used particularly in children. Salbutamol (Ventolin) is prescribed to relieve symptoms should they occur.

Patients admitted with severe asthma require nebulized salbutamol to relax bronchial spasm, oxygen therapy to help correct hypoxia and the oedema caused by inflammatory changes can be controlled by the anti-inflammatory effects of steroid therapy. Their anxiety and agitation are managed by nursing measures as sedatives are contraindicated since they increase the risk of the patient developing respiratory failure.

Nursing strategies

The nursing care required by a patient admitted with a severe asthmatic attack is described in Nursing Care Plan 13.2. The use of nebulizer therapy is discussed in Box 13.1.

Patient education

The nurse plays a vital role here. Patients who are well informed about their asthma lead a normal life requiring the minimum of hospital admissions. The more informed a patient is the more likely they are to feel in control of their asthma and comply with the treatment.

The patient should be taught about his disorder, for example, what happens to the airways in asthma, the factors which may trigger it and how their asthma will be managed. Leaflets from the Asthma Society and Chest, Heart and Stroke Association are useful in reinforcing important points. The patient should be informed about how to monitor his respiratory

Nursing Care Plan 13.2 Care of a young adult with an acute asthmatic attack requiring admission to hospital

Problem	Aim	Nursing action	Rationale
		COMMUNICATION	
1. **Anxiety – patient is literally fighting for breath**	To relieve and restore calm, quiet behaviour	❑ Nurse to adopt calm positive professional manner	Instils confidence in patient and reduces anxiety
		❑ Allow patient to adopt position in which he feels most comfortable	Failure to do so will only serve to increase anxiety, fear and anger all of which increase respirations and oxygen consumption
		❑ Approach patient from side rather than face on	Patient will feel less hemmed in and less anxious
		❑ Give patient plenty of space around themselves	During attack the patient's personal space requirements are increased
		❑ Give clear calm explanations, reinforcing information given by medical staff	Increases confidence in the caring team since information is consistent
		❑ Avoid asking open questions whilst patient is acutely ill	Patient will be unable to answer open questions due to breathlessness. Closed questions are more easily answered
		❑ Place call bell within easy reach and ensure it is working	Reduces anxiety knowing that help is immediately available
		❑ Provide patient with comfort and support	Reassuring sensitive nurse can anticipate needs and concerns. Touch and physical presence may be a major factor in improving breathing
		BREATHING	
2. **Dyspnoea**	Decrease respiratory rate and prolong expiratory phase of breathing	❑ Position patient upright, well supported with pillows. Orthopnoeic position	Allows chest expansion and reduces pressure of abdominal contents on diaphragm
		❑ Ensure adequate ventilation of immediate environment – use of fan	Gives patient feeling of an airy environment
		❑ Remove known allergens from environment, i.e. feather pillows, flowers	Allergens would only serve to aggravate patient's condition
		❑ Encourage patient to use deep breathing exercises as taught by physiotherapist	Patient is anxious, therefore his/her concentration and memory will be poorer than normal, so the need to keep reminding him/her deep breathing exercises
		❑ Administer bronchodilators and corticosteroids as prescribed and monitor their effect	Will relieve patient's breathing difficulties. If drugs are not relieving symptoms, medical staff should be informed
		MAINTAINING A SAFE ENVIRONMENT	
3. **Patient receiving oxygen therapy**	Ensure safety and comfort of patient	❑ Ensure that oxygen is given at the correct rate via correct mask or nasal cannulae	Too much oxygen may inhibit stimulus to respiration, too little oxygen will not oxygenate blood to desired level
		❑ Explain necessity of oxygen to patient to gain compliance	Patient is more likely to co-operate with treatment
		❑ Give frequent oral hygiene	Prevents the drying effects of oxygen on oral mucosa
		❑ Change face mask/nasal cannulae daily and pad around elastic of mask as necessary	Equipment may become contaminated and lead to further infection. Elastic can cause pressure sores around ears

Nursing Care Plan 13.2 (*cont'd*)

Problem	Aim	Nursing action	Rationale
3. (cont'd)		❐ Explain all the safety precautions required when oxygen is in use to both patient and family: ● No smoking whilst oxygen is in use ● Oil or grease should not be used around any oxygen connections ● Electrical devices should not be used whilst oxygen is in use ● Fire extinguisher should be readily available	Oxygen supports combustion. All staff, patients and visitors should be aware of the dangers
4. **Presence of sputum which is difficult to expectorate**	To aid expectoration and obtain sample for microbiology	❐ Encourage patient to cough. Assistance given by physiotherapist ❐ Obtain sputum specimen for culture and sensitivity ❐ Administer antibiotics as prescribed	Physiotherapy techniques will aid expectoration of sputum Respiratory tract infection may have triggered attack. Culture and sensitivity of sputum will establish causative organism and its sensitivity to antibiotics These should be effective in destroying organisms causing respiratory tract infection
5. **Potential development of complications**	Monitor progress and detect complications of pneumothorax and respiratory failure promptly	❐ Observe pulse, respirations and blood pressure half hourly and temperature hourly. Report abnormalities promptly	Rising pulse and decreasing dyspnoea may indicate pneumothorax Pulse which disappears on inspiration and becomes fuller on expiration is termed pulsus paradoxus and is a sign of respiratory failure Increasing laboured shallow breathing may indicate respiratory failure. Patients nearing exhaustion will not have the energy to increase their breathing and will breathe at a reduced rate. This should not be mistaken for signs of improvement as it can mean a serious deterioration in the patient's condition. Prompt recognition and reporting of complications allows immediate intervention and treatment
		MOBILIZATION	
6. **Patient exhausted due to condition**	To allow patient to rest as much as possible until acute episode is over	❐ Patient placed on bed rest and encouraged to avoid exertion ❐ Change position 2 hourly ❐ Inspect pressure areas for redness and skin breakdown 2 hourly ❐ Use appropriate pressure-relieving aids ❐ Perform passive leg exercises	Conserves energy for breathing Relieves pressure and ensures an adequate blood flow bringing oxygen and nutrients to tissues Ensures early detection of problem and reassessment of care planned as necessary Relieves pressure on pressure areas on an at-risk patient Prevents the formation of deep vein thrombosis by using calf muscle pump to encourage venous return back to the heart

Nursing Care Plan 13.2 (*cont'd*)			
Problem	**Aim**	**Nursing action**	**Rationale**
6. (cont'd)		❏ Encourage gentle mobilization as soon as the patient's condition improves	Gentle mobilizing prevents complications of bed rest
PERSONAL CLEANSING AND DRESSING			
7. Sweating due to pyrexia and increased effort of breathing	Reduce discomfort and prevent skin breakdown	❏ Clean and dry skin as required ❏ Change linen when damp ❏ Assist as required with washing and dressing ❏ Refrain from the overuse of talcum powder	Reduces discomfort Warm, moist and dark conditions encourage multiplication of bacteria Patient requires assistance as he/she will fatigue easily Great care must be taken not to create clouds of talcum dust in the atmosphere as this will cause an increase in dyspnoea and distress
EATING AND DRINKING			
8. Dehydration due to excessive sweating, dyspnoea	To correct and maintain hydration	❏ Encourage oral fluids as tolerated ❏ Care of intravenous infusion if patient is unable to take oral fluids: • observe for and report redness, swelling, discomfort around infusion site • Regulate, monitor and record intravenous flow rate as per prescription • Check intravenous fluid bags with prescription and with a registered nurse	Adequate fluid intake is essential to maintain hydration As above The presence of these indicates signs of infiltration of tissues. Intravenous infusion will require to be resited by medical staff Helps to prevent over or under hydration Should ensure that the correct fluid is being given to the correct patient at the correct time

status using a 'mini' peak flow meter (Fig. 13.4b) as this will help in identifying any deterioration in the control of his asthma and to prompt him to seek medical advice. The action and side-effects of prescribed drugs should be explained and their correct administration should be taught to ensure the effective use of inhalers. Ellis (1990, p. 78) quotes research findings which state that '80 per cent of cases of inadequately controlled asthma are partly due to poor technique . . . and that only 62 per cent of people with asthma could use a metered dose inhaler (MDI), even after personal tuition. Furthermore, it is possible to lose good technique with time, particularly if it is not checked regularly'. For correct techniques see Box 13.2. Children who have asthma should be actively involved in this education programme as well as their parents.

Guidance on how to prevent asthmatic attacks can be seen in Box 13.3.

Information about the reasons for and method of recording peak flow measurements can be seen in Box 13.4.

Occupational (industrial) lung disease

Epidemiology and aetiology

Exposure to dust, chemicals, powders, gases or fumes at work can lead to the development of acute bronchitis, pulmonary fibrosis, occupational asthma and lung cancer.

Once an occupational disorder has been diagnosed, the individual should be removed from that working environment and alternative employment found for him.

Individuals with occupational disorders are able to claim compensation. Much attention is now paid to the prevention of such disorders, and this has been helped by the Health and Safety at Work Act (1974) and the COSHH Regulations (1988). The work environment must be properly ventilated to avoid workers coming into contact with noxious substances; improved working conditions in coal mines, protective clothing and health and safety regulations when working with hazardous substances such as asbestos.

The occupational health nurse plays an important

Box 13.2   The correct use of inhalers

Diskhalers
1. The lid of the device should be lifted to pierce the blister containing the powdered drug
2. The patient then breathes in through the mouthpiece and inhales the drug
3. The disk should then be rotated to prime the device with the next dose

Turbohaler
1. The device should be held upright
2. The hand grip should be turned either to the right or left and then back again. This primes the device
3. The patient should be instructed to breathe out
4. The patient should then be asked to place their lips around the mouthpiece ensuring a good seal and inhale the drug
5. There is a dose marker on the side of the device which the patient should be taught to check as this gives an indication of how many doses are left within the device

Rotahaler
1. To prime this device, a capsule of dry powdered medication is loaded
2. The device should then be rotated to break open the capsule
3. The patient can then inhale the drug through the mouthpiece

Metered dose inhaler (aerosol)
1. The inhaler should be shaken vigorously to disperse the drug evenly. The cap should then be removed
2. The patient should then be asked to breathe out, with

the inhaler well away from them as otherwise the spray may become blocked with condensation
3. The patient is then asked to place his lips around the mouthpiece ensuring there is a good seal
4. The patient should then be asked to breathe in slowly and deeply through the mouthpiece whilst depressing the canister to release the drug in a fine mist. The patient is advised to continue to breathe in
5. On removal of the inhaler from their mouth the patient should hold their breath for 10 seconds (if possible) before exhaling slowly
6. Patients who are prescribed 2 puffs of the inhaler should be taught to wait at least 1 minute before repeating the procedure for their second puff. The cap should be replaced

Autohaler
1. This device is primed by raising a lever
2. Since the device is designed as a breath-actuated metered-dose aerosol, the patient simply inhales via the mouthpiece and the dose is automatically released
3. The lever should then be returned to its original position

Space saver devices
1. This involves the use of a space saver device in conjunction with an aerosol inhaler
2. The aerosol is depressed to release the drug in the form of a fine mist into the space saver device
3. The patient inhales the fine mist from the device without having to co-ordinate their breathing. This device is useful for the elderly and young children

Adapted from 'Asthma in the family', ASTRA Pharmaceuticals Ltd.

Box 13.3   Guidance on the prevention of asthmatic attacks

1. Adults should stop smoking, children should not start
2. Take regular exercise but avoid exercising outdoors in cold weather
3. Take medication as often as prescribed even when feeling well
4. Avoid taking aspirin or aspirin-containing drugs as these may bring on an attack
5. Take adequate rest and sleep so that the stresses and strains of life can be better coped with. Practice relaxation exercises when feeling tense or stressed
6. Avoid environmental irritants such as tobacco smoke, dust, talcum powder, perfume and sprays
7. Attempt to avoid respiratory infections
8. Avoid known allergens
9. If allergic to the house dust mite:
   a. discard feather pillows for synthetic ones

   b. use a synthetic mattress
   c. vacuum clean mattress weekly especially along the seams
   d. vacuum carpets frequently
   e. children with asthma should avoid having soft toys in bed beside them
   f. children with asthma should not sleep on bottom bunk bed
   g. pets should not be allowed in the bedroom or on soft furnishings
10. Seek early medical advice if:
   a. peak flow readings begin to deteriorate
   b. signs of chest infection develop
   c. if inhaler fails to reverse symptoms
   d. if exercise cannot be taken without getting symptoms
   e. if sufferer wakes up coughing and/or wheezing during the night or in the morning

---

Box 13.4   Peak flow meter recordings

Reasons
- Measures the amount of air which is able to be expelled out of the lungs in one good huff
- Regular measurements can give the patient and the doctor an indication of how well controlled the asthma is
- Allows doctor to make changes to prescription as necessary
- Recording can be used to predict an asthmatic attack and monitor its response to treatment

Method
Patient should be taught to:
- Stand whilst taking recording
- Take a deep breath and hold it
- Put their lips tightly around peak flow meter ensuring a good seal
- Blow out hard in one short sharp breath
- Repeat until three readings are obtained. Record the highest reading
- Establish a habit of recording peak flow measurements on rising, before taking medication and before retiring

---

role in ensuring the maintenance of health and safety policies within the working environment and screening employees regularly.

MALIGNANT TUMOURS OF THE LUNG

Bronchial carcinoma

Epidemiology and aetiology

Lung cancer is the commonest cancer in the western world with the UK having the highest mortality rate. The incidence rates for lung cancer in Scotland are among the highest in the world (Cull 1991). There are 35 000 deaths every year in the UK. The incidence is highest in the urban areas and lower in rural areas. It affects men more than women although the incidence in women is rising as more women are smoking.

In Scotland the commonest cause of death from cancer is now from lung cancer rather than breast cancer (Cull 1991).

Bronchial carcinoma primarily affects the 40–70 year age group and it has a higher incidence in cigarette smokers and those whose occupation exposes them to the inhalation of carcinogens such as asbestos or nickel. Individuals who give up smoking have a reduced risk of developing cancer.

The commonest types of bronchial carcinoma are squamous cell, adenocarcinoma and small (oat) cell carcinoma. The time interval from the initial malignant change to presentation is about 15 years, 8 years and 3 years respectively. The survival rate is therefore poor since the tumour has usually spread to the lymph nodes, liver, brain or bone by the time the patient first presents to the doctor. It is for this reason that bronchial carcinoma is often referred to as the silent killer.

Common symptomatology

There are usually no symptoms until the tumour is extensive. The patient presents most commonly with a cough, haemoptysis, dyspnoea and weight loss. In some instances, the reason the patient seeks medical advice is due to symptoms arising from the metastases.

Investigations

1. **Chest X-ray** (for more detail see p. 447).
2. **Computerized axial tomography** (see Ch. 5) is performed to locate the position, size and spread of the tumour to the mediastinum, lymph nodes and the other lung.
3. **Fibreoptic bronchoscopy and biopsy** (see p. 447) allow the surgeon to visualize the tumour, assess the possibility of surgery and obtain a biopsy of tumour for histological examination.
4. **Sputum specimen** (see p. 446) is sent for microbiological and cytological examination.
5. **Pulmonary function tests** (see p. 447) are performed to estimate lung function and assess whether this would still be adequate following surgery to remove a lobe(s) or a whole lung.
6. **Liver ultrasound scan** and perhaps bone scans are performed to establish the absence or presence of metastases.
7. **Thoracotomy**, an exploratory operation through the chest wall, may be performed to assess the possibility of removing the tumour.

Therapeutic management

For patients with localized tumours and no evidence of metastatic spread, surgery is performed. This accounts for approximately 25% of patients. The operations which may be performed are lobectomy, the removal of a lobe, or pneumonectomy, the removal of a whole lung. Following lobectomy, the patient will return to the ward with two chest drains in situ, one to remove air and a lower one to remove serous fluid to prevent infection and promote lung expansion (Fig. 13.11). Some surgeons apply low

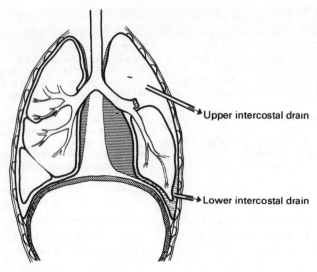

Fig. 13.11 Lobectomy

pressure suction to the upper drain to assist the evacuation of air, thereby increasing the residual lung expansion.

Where surgery is inappropriate, radiotherapy or a combination of cytotoxic drugs and radiotherapy may be indicated to palliatively treat the primary tumour and metastases (see Ch. 4). Palliative radiotherapy is valuable in the treatment of distressing symptoms such as haemoptysis, bone pain and superior vena cava obstruction. Patients who have recurring pleural effusions, which cause them severe dyspnoea, derive benefit from thoracentesis (see p. 448) and the instillation of chemotherapy drugs into the cavity. This sets up an inflammatory response, causing the two pleural layers to adhere together thus preventing further effusions from occurring.

Nursing strategies

Patients undergoing thoracic surgery are admitted a few days prior to surgery to fully prepare them both physically and psychologically for the operation. The pre- and postoperative care of a patient having a lobectomy under general anaesthesia is described in detail in Nursing Care Plans 13.3 and 13.4. For basic pre- and postoperative care see Chapter 4.

The nursing care of the patient following pneumonectomy is similar to that following lobectomy with three exceptions:

1. The space created by the removal of the lung may or may not be drained according to the surgeon's preference. Following a pneumonectomy, most surgeons believe that there is no need for drainage tubes because there is no raw lung tissue remaining on that side to cause air leakage or serous oozing. Before leaving the operating theatre, a negative pressure is introduced on the side of the pneumonectomy to draw the mediastinal contents slightly towards the space and allow full lung expansion.

2. The patient postpneumonectomy is turned from back to affected side only so that no restrictions are placed on the remaining lung on which the patient's respiration depends.

3. Great care is taken not to overload the patient with fluid as the development of pulmonary oedema in a postoperative pneumonectomy patient could be catastrophic. Fluids are therefore restricted to 1–1.5 litres in the first 24 hours. A strictly accurate fluid balance chart is essential to monitor the patient's hydration status.

The nursing care of patients receiving palliative radiotherapy and/or chemotherapy can be found in Chapter 4.

Prognosis

The prognosis of bronchial carcinoma is very poor. Cull (1991) states that the 5 year survival rates remain at less than 10%. These patients and their families face a difficult and uncertain future in which much support can be given by their GP, nurse and medical social worker.

Health education

Since there is no cure for bronchial carcinoma, prevention cannot be stressed strongly enough.

Health education targeted at the prime cause, ciga-

Nursing Care Plan 13.3   Preoperative care of patient undergoing a lobectomy for bronchial carcinoma under general anaesthetic

Problem	Aim	Nursing action	Rationale
		COMMUNICATION	
1. Anxiety regarding forthcoming operation	Prepare patient and family psychologically for surgery	❏ Display kind, caring approach to patient and family	Helps to establish a therapeutic rapport with patient and family
		❏ Encourage patient to vent his/her feelings and concerns and deal with them appropriately	Sharing these should help the patient to feel more relaxed and increase his trust in the team
		❏ Explain operation to patient and family to a level of their understanding	Helps to remove the fear of the unknown
		❏ Explain the need for postoperative equipment such as oxygen, suction, underwater seal drainage system, intravenous infusion	By being forewarned, all equipment is seen as a predictable necessity rather than meaning that something has gone wrong in theatre
		❏ Explain the use of the oxygen saturation monitor	A finger cot probe or ear lobe probe attached to continuously monitor peripheral oxygenation which gives early warning of deterioration. It will alarm when there is an abnormality and also when it becomes dislodged. The latter often occurs
		❏ Explain the use of arterial line	This gives the medical staff ease of access for arterial blood gas estimation. The line can also be used to measure blood pressure
		❏ Arrange visit to postoperative constant care area	A visit to the area may alleviate fears or concerns
		MAINTAINING A SAFE ENVIRONMENT	
2. Patient about to undergo major surgery	Prepare patient physically to ensure optimum postoperative recovery	❏ Prepare patient for preoperative investigations: ● chest X-ray ● electrocardiograph ● pulmonary function tests ● blood sampling ● urinalysis	Physical preparation and explanation of why these investigations will allow patient to understand and gain confidence in that surgery is being planned and carried out meticulously
		❏ Observe and record patient's temperature, pulse respirations and blood pressure 4 hourly	Gives a baseline measurement for postoperative period. Allows for identification of abnormalities prior to surgery
		❏ Encourage patient to have a high calorie, high protein diet and adequate fluid intake (1.5–2 litres daily)	Patient requires to have a good nutritional and hydration status prior to surgery
		❏ Physiotherapist to teach patient: ● deep breathing exercises ● leg exercises ● how to cough postoperatively	Intensive chest physiotherapy helps prevent sputum retention and encourages full chest expansion and prevents the formation of deep vein thrombosis
		❏ Note amount, colour and consistency of sputum expectorated. Report abnormalities promptly	Respiratory tract infections must be treated prior to surgery. If infection is suspected, specimen of sputum can be sent for culture and sensitivity and appropriate antibiotics given

Nursing Care Plan 13.3 (*cont'd*)

Problem	Aim	Nursing action	Rationale
3. Patient to have a general anaesthetic	To prepare patient to ensure his safety prior to during and after anaesthesia	❏ Prepare patient's skin according to unit policy	Purpose of skin preparation is to remove micro-organisms from the surface of the skin to prevent postoperative wound infection
		❏ Fast patient for 4–6 hours prior to operation. Inform patient of reasons and place a fasting sign above bed. Ensure all staff are aware of fasting arrangements	Failure to do so would put the patient at risk of aspiration pneumonia
		❏ Take time to sit and talk to patient about fears or concerns	By allowing patient to express himself any unrelieved anxieties may be discussed
		❏ Administer suppositories as prescribed if the patient has not had a bowel movement this day	If there are faeces in the lower bowel, the patient can be faecally incontinent in theatre due to the action of the muscle relaxant drugs given
		❏ Administer night sedation if prescribed	Helps the patient to relax and hopefully obtain a good night's sleep prior to theatre
		MORNING OF OPERATION ❏ Patient to have shower prior to theatre. Ensure skin, hair, nails and umbilicus are clean	These areas can harbour micro-organisms
		❏ Help dress patient in theatre gown and modesty pants	These are made of cotton. Nylon is not permitted in theatre as it can causes static electricity which would be a hazard since there are anaesthetic gases and oxygen present
		❏ Patient encouraged to rest in clean bed	Reduces further potential skin contamination
		❏ Complete the nursing checklist prior to theatre: • remove any dentures, note crowns or loose teeth	Ensures safety of patient. Dentures could slip backwards and occlude the airway during anaesthesia. Crowns and loose teeth must be reported to anaesthetist so that extra care may be taken to prevent them being accidentally knocked and falling down airway
		• remove contact lenses or glasses	Unless removed contact lenses would dry out on cornea causing problems. Glasses not worn during operation but kept safe on the ward
		• remove all jewellery except wedding ring if worn; ring should be taped to finger using non-allergic tape	Jewellery is removed because; a. it harbours micro-organisms b. if diathermy machine is used in theatre and patient's jewellery comes in contact with metal of table, the electricity may go through their jewellery to get to earth, causing a diathermy burn
		• with patient's permission, deal with their valuables according to hospital policy	Keeps patient's property safe
		• record presence of prostheses not removed, i.e. artificial eye, wig, hearing aid	Theatre staff should be aware that prostheses are still in situ. Hearing aid is particularly important to aid pre- and postoperative communication

Problem	Aim	Nursing action	Rationale
3. (cont'd)		• check patient's identity by asking him/her for his/her full name and date of birth; this information should be checked with identity band on patient's wrist	Asking the patient to identify him/herself ensures correct identification identity band allows correct identification when the patient is unable to respond
		❏ Ask patient to empty his/her bladder approximately 1 hour prior to surgery	Patient's bladder should be empty prior to receiving anaesthesia, as muscle relaxing drugs would allow a full bladder to empty soiling the theatre
		❏ Explain purpose of and administer premedication as prescribed:	Premedication helps to relax patient and reduce anxiety. It also helps facilitate the administration of the anaesthetic
		• warn patient that the drugs may make them drowsy, light headed and produce a dry mouth; patient also warned that he/she should not attempt to get out of bed alone as he/she may fall	Gives patient warning that he/she may feel drowsy and sleepy and not to worry about how he/she is feeling Maintains patient's safety
		• ensure call bell is within easy reach so that he/she can summon help rather than get out of bed himself	
		❏ Continuing to support the patient emotionally accompany patient to theatre with his/her notes and X-rays, according to hospital policy	Maintains the comfort and safety of patient

Nursing Care Plan 13.3 (*cont'd*)

rette smoking, should be continued to make the public aware of the very real risks they are taking when they smoke cigarettes.

Patient education

After surgery, the patient who has an uneventful postoperative recovery will be discharged home after about 7 days following lobectomy and about 10 days following pneumonectomy. Discharge advice given to patients and their family can be seen in Box 13.5.

CYSTIC FIBROSIS

A definition and diagnosis of this fatal disorder can be found on p. 517. The term cystic fibrosis is perhaps confusing, since the disease is one of obstruction caused by thickened secretions (Byers 1989).

Epidemiology and aetiology

Cystic fibrosis predominantly affects north-western Europeans but other races and ethnic groups can be affected. In Great Britain there is a baby born with cystic fibrosis (Maynard 1994) every day. It is estimated that, by the 2000, there will be 6000 affected individuals, with 2000 of those over the age of 18 (Helms 1993).

The life expectancy of patients with cystic fibrosis has improved markedly. In 1938, 80% of children died in their first year of life. By 1966, life expectancy was 7.5 years. In 1975 it was 12.8 years and in the 1990s it is 27 years. It is projected that babies being diagnosed now will live into their 40s (Helms 1993).

The most common cause of death is respiratory failure brought on by repeated lung infections. The vastly improved life expectancy is due to meticulous care provided by medical and paediatric nursing staff and the aggressive treatment of acute and chronic lung infections (Webb & David 1994).

Common symptomatology

Only symptoms related to the respiratory tract will be discussed here (see p. 517 for gastrointestinal symptoms).

Cystic fibrosis causes overproduction of thick

Nursing Care Plan 13.4 Postoperative care of patient undergoing a lobectomy for bronchial carcinoma under general anaesthetic

Problem	Aim	Nursing action	Rationale
		COMMUNICATION	
1. Anxiety, fear, disorientation on recovery from anaesthesia	Reassure patient and explain all procedures at a level of the patient's understanding	❑ Explain all procedures prior to them being performed using terms the patient understands. Repeat explanations as necessary	Continues philosophy of having a well-informed patient. Research has shown that patients who are well informed are more likely to have an uncomplicated and speedy postoperative recovery
		MAINTAINING A SAFE ENVIRONMENT	
2. Potential development of reactionary haemorrhage or postoperative shock	To detect early signs and report promptly	❑ Record blood pressure, pulse, respirations as instructed	Hypovolaemia would be detected by falling blood readings and a rising pulse rate
		❑ Observe the patient's skin and report pale, cold, clammy skin	Indicates the presence of shock
		❑ Observe wound site for signs of oozing or leakage	May require the application of pressure dressing or further attention from surgeon
		❑ Assist patient as necessary during postoperative chest X-rays	Monitors events occurring in the thoracic cavity
3. Potential development of respiratory distress, hypostatic pneumonia	To prevent secretions to accumulate in lung which could lead to obstruction or infection	❑ Once vital signs are stabilized, patient should be assisted into an upright position well supported by pillows and nursed from side to back to side still maintaining upright position	The upright position aids fuller chest expansion and turning encourages ventilation of both lungs
		❑ Ensure patient is pain free	Surgery and the presence of large painful wound will inhibit the patient's breathing and expectoration of sputum
		❑ Encourage patient to expectorate sputum and assist patient by supporting wound, providing sputum carton and tissues	If sputum and secretions are retained they inhibit gaseous exchange and predispose patient to chest infection
		❑ Encourage patient to perform deep breathing hourly as taught preoperatively by physiotherapist	Removes secretions from lungs preventing infection and atelectasis. Increases aeration of remaining lobes of lung
4. Potential hypoxia	To maintain normal oxygenation	❑ Oxygen therapy as prescribed	Additional oxygen will increase level of oxygen available to tissues thus preventing hypoxia
		❑ Record oxygen saturation, monitor readings as ordered	Gives an indication of peripheral oxygenation and allows for abnormalities to be detected and appropriate treatment commenced
		❑ Ensure mask is comfortable and reasons for its use are reinforced to patient	If the mask is uncomfortable it will cause sores and will not be tolerated by patient
		❑ Explain all the safety precautions required when oxygen is in use to both patient and family: ● no smoking whilst oxygen is in use ● oil or grease should not be used around any oxygen connections	Oxygen supports combustion and all staff, patients and visitors should be aware of the dangers

(cont'd)

Nursing Care Plan 13.4 (*cont'd*)			
Problem	**Aim**	**Nursing action**	**Rationale**
4. (cont'd)		• electrical devices should not be used whilst oxygen is in use • fire extinguisher should be readily available ☐ Give regular oral hygiene to prevent oral mucosa becoming dry	Oral mucosa dries quickly when oxygen is used and can soon become sore and infected unless kept moist
5. Postoperative pain due to large wound	To control pain by effective use of analgesia	☐ Give analgesia as prescribed, particularly prior to known painful events, i.e. visit by physiotherapist ☐ Monitor effectiveness of analgesia with the aid of a pain chart	Patient who is pain free will be able to participate with physiotherapist, move around in bed, cough and expectorate more fully. Pain-free patient will also benefit psychologically If analgesia is not controlling pain then medical staff should be asked to review prescription
6. Potential development of chest wound	Prevent infection occurring	☐ Give prophylactic antibiotics as prescribed ☐ Monitor patient's temperature 4 hourly. Note and report pyrexia, confusion and restlessness ☐ Monitor sputum for signs of infection – change to yellow or green colour Send specimen for culture and sensitivity ☐ Observe wound for signs of infection; redness, increased warmth, presence of purulent exudate. Send wound swab for culture and sensitivity if infection is suspected ☐ Encourage patient to support wound when coughing	Greatly reduces the possibility of infection occurring These are signs of infection. Early identification and reporting allows prompt treatment Identifies presence of infection Sputum specimen allows identification of offending organism, allowing appropriate antibiotics to be prescribed Any developing infection must be identified and treated promptly Any increase in stress on the wound could lead to wound breakdown and delayed healing
7. Potential problems of patient with intercostal underwater drainage systems in situ	To maintain patency of underwater seal drainage system and prevent complications	☐ Monitor and record amount and character of drainage, i.e. blood, purulent exudate ☐ Ensure drainage system is working properly: • check tubing for kinking • check for leaks, disconnections • check stopper is secure • check level of sterile water in bottle is correct (300 ml) • check tube is not clamped off unless otherwise directed • ensure no loops in tubing	Blood loss through the drain should not exceed 200–300 ml in any one hour. Excessive blood loss could indicate a loose ligature and necessitate return of patient to theatre Two drains are in situ connected separately to Winchester bottles. Ensures patency of system Allows mainly air to drain from the apical drain and mainly fluid from the basal drain Loops would lead to inefficiency and prevent proper drainage

Nursing Care Plan 13.4 (*cont'd*)			
Problem	**Aim**	**Nursing action**	**Rationale**
7. (cont'd)		• ensure intercostal drainage systems are 'swinging', i.e. fluctuation of the fluid in the drainage bottle, moving up and down the tubing to correspond with patient's respirations	If swinging is not present, it could indicate that the tubing is kinked or the lung has collapsed. In either event prompt action to rectify problem is required
		❒ If drainage system bottles have to be raised, the tubing must be clamped off. Once patient is mobile he/she must be instructed never to lift bottle above waist height. Other staff and visitors must also be aware of this	If the bottle is raised above waist level, the fluid in the bottle will flow back into the lung by a siphon effect
		Release clamp after re-positioning of bottle	If tubing is clamped off it can cause a tension pneumothorax as the build up of air and fluid causes further lung collapse
		❒ Milk tubing as necessary to prevent blockage by blood clots or fibrin	If tubing becomes blocked it could lead to a tension pneumothorax
		❒ Change drainage bottles daily using strict aseptic technique. Ensure tubing is double clamped prior to changing bottles	Aseptic technique should prevent the entry of bacteria into the pleural cavity. If tubing was not clamped off, air would rush in and cause a pneumothorax
		❒ Measure amount of drainage and record on fluid balance chart	Maintains accuracy of fluid balance chart
		EATING AND DRINKING	
8. Potential dehydration	To maintain adequate hydration	❒ Monitor rate and flow of intravenous fluid with a trained member of staff	Important to ensure that the patient receives correct amount of fluid to maintain normal hydration
		❒ Ensure correct fluid is administered to correct patient at the correct time	
		❒ Monitor cannula site for signs of infiltration	If infiltration of the tissues occurs, the medical staff are informed so that they may resite intravenous infusion
		❒ Report signs of overhydration	Increasing dyspnoea, cyanosis, tachycardia and expectorating frothy sputum indicates overhydration causing pulmonary oedema
		❒ 4–5 hours postoperatively offer patient sips of water.	Increases patient's oral comfort. By leaving it this length of time the patient's cough reflex and bowel sounds will have returned as effects of anaesthetic will have worn off
		❒ Introduce diet when fluids are tolerated	Re-establishes normal routine for patient
		PERSONAL CLEANSING AND DRESSING	
9. Patient unable to maintain his own hygiene in the short term	Maintain a good standard of hygiene	❒ On return from theatre once vital signs are stable, patient is given a freshen up and helped into own nightclothes	Helps the patient to feel fresher and more comfortable. If patient moved before their vital signs are stable likely that the movement will cause nausea
		❒ Patient requires bed bath on the first day. Attention paid to all his hygiene needs	Patient too ill to have anything other than a bed bath. Maintains the patient's usual standard

Nursing Care Plan 13.4 (*cont'd*)

Problem	Aim	Nursing action	Rationale
8. (cont'd)		❏ As the patient's condition improves, patient can progress to an immersion bath or preferably a shower	A shower is preferable as there is less risk of infection occurring as the patient is not sitting in potentially contaminated water
		MOBILITY	
9. Patient immobile and prone to complications until he is able to resume full mobility	Prevent the complications of immobility	❏ Prevent the formation of a deep vein thrombosis;	
		• on return from theatre, implement passive leg exercises until such time as the patient is able to exercise his/her legs independently. Encourage deep breathing	Encourages venous return to right side of heart by use of the calf muscle pump. Prevents stasis of blood in deep veins thereby preventing clot formation. Facilitates the removal of anaesthetic gases from lungs, helps to expel air from the pleural cavity and aids the venous return to the heart
		• administer heparin as prescribed	Heparin is an anticoagulant and thus prevents the formation of clots
		• apply antiembolism stockings if prescribed	Aid the venous return from the legs
		• observe calves and report any signs of deep vein thrombosis	Swelling, complaints of calf tenderness or pain, redness, increased heat should be reported promptly
		❏ Prevent the formation of pressure sores;	
		• perform 2 hourly pressure care to coincide with turning regimen. Great care must be taken when turning patient not to pull his/her drainage tubing	Prevents formation of pressure sores There is the real danger of dislodging the tubing
		• use pressure relieving aids as appropriate	Allows regular (2 hourly) evaluation of effectiveness of nursing action and reassessment and planning as required
		ELIMINATION	
10. Potential urinary stasis, infection	Prevent complications occurring	❏ Monitor and record urine output ❏ Report to medical staff if patient has not passed urine 6–8 hours postoperatively	Allows monitoring of fluid balance status Patient may be underhydrated or have retention of urine. Recognition of either allows prompt treatment. Retention of urine can lead to urine infection
		❏ Encourage patient to pass urine regularly	This reduces stasis time in the bladder
		REST AND SLEEP	
11. Potential concern over lack of progress	Keep patient and relatives informed of progress	❏ Once able, patient is encouraged to eat a light diet and drink plenty fluids ❏ Patient is helped to sit out of bed on day 1 or 2 postoperatively ❏ Patient can begin to take a more active part in his personal hygiene as his condition improves ❏ Patient's mobility increased as his/her condition improves ❏ Daily chest X-rays performed to assess re-expansion of lung. Patient informed of results	Once patient is tolerating food and drinking well his/her intravenous infusion can be discontinued Improves morale and enables the patient's lungs to expand more fully Restores a feeling of being more in control of events, thus a positive step towards progress Allows a degree of independence of nursing staff Basal drain usually removed first at about 36 hours postoperatively if drainage is minimal. Apical drain remains in situ until lung re-expands

---

Box 13.5 Discharge advice given to patients and their family following lobectomy or pneumonectomy

1. Stop smoking
2. Make an appointment to see their GP, taking their hospital discharge letter with them
3. Warn them that they will require considerable rest initially but they should gradually build up their exercise tolerance. If they do become breathless, they should stop and rest
4. There is no need to follow any special diet unless directed to do so by the surgeon
5. Should their wound become itchy they should resist the temptation to scratch it. Clothing around the wound should be loose fitting. Any leakage from the wound necessitates medical advice
6. Since they may require assistance getting in and out of a bath for the first couple of weeks, they may find a shower easier
7. At the first sign of the development of a cold or chest infection they must contact their GP
8. Sexual activity should be avoided for 6 weeks postoperatively
9. Driving should be avoided for 6 weeks postoperatively
10. The surgeon will advise the patient when he may return to work. It should be stressed that this depends on the nature of his occupation
11. The patient should refrain from lifting heavy objects and should be warned that household tasks and gardening will be difficult for a couple of weeks. On regaining his strength, the patient should realize for himself what he can and cannot do. In general terms, he should be able to do most everyday activities after 2 months, and after 3 months he should be able to resume normal activities

---

viscous mucus which causes a cough and sputum on a daily basis. These symptoms worsen when a chest infection occurs and are often accompanied by chest pain and haemoptysis. In severe cases the patient will develop cyanosis, tachypnoea and chronic hypoxia leading to cor pulmonale. Over time, this pathological process causes progressive and permanent lung damage.

Therapeutic management and nursing strategies

The cornerstone of management is twice- to thrice-daily physiotherapy and antibiotics for exacerbations of chest infections.

Physiotherapy

The aim is to loosen secretions so that they may be expelled by coughing rather than remaining in the lung as a focus for infection. The combined measures of percussion to loosen the viscous secretions, postural drainage to facilitate drainage of secretions from different areas of lungs (see page 459) and forced expiratory technique are performed in 45-minute sessions twice a day. When the respiratory symptoms are exacerbated by infection, the sessions are performed up to 4 times a day. Many patients receive nebulised salbutamol prior to physiotherapy to enhance its effect. Parents are taught the techniques so that they can perform them at home. As soon as children are old enough, they are taught the forced expiratory technique and encouraged to take responsibility for their own therapy as this can ease problems during adolescence when there is a struggle for independence. The importance of intensive physiotherapy must be stressed as it is required not only to maintain a rea-

sonable quality of life but also quantity of life (Whyte 1992). Exercise also aids clearance of secretions and is therefore encouraged.

Chest infections

Common pathogenic organisms are *Staphylococcus aureas*, *Haemophilus influenzae* and *Pseudomonas aeruginosa*. The latter is the most common. In fact, it is present in the sputum of the majority of adults with cystic fibrosis as it is impossible to eradicate once it has been colonised (Smith & Stableforth 1992). Webb & David (1994) assert that life-long oral antibiotics are prescribed to patients once their lungs are colonised with these organisms, therefore monthly sputum specimens for culture and sensitivity are important. Some doctors prescribe aerosol antibiotics. Prevention of exposure to respiratory bacteria and viruses is vital. Patients are advised to avoid people with colds and to be immunised against influenza, pertussis and measles.

When patients develop exacerbations of chest infections they require intravenous antibiotics but are increasingly being treated with these at home. Although this may increase pressure on home life it is seen as more desirable than hospital admission with the concomitant risk of cross infection. Various devices and implants are used which allow the patient to continue with intravenous antibiotics whilst at school or work. Paediatric community nurses play an important role in education and support.

A recent problem is the emergence of *P. cepacia*. It is effectively resistant to all currently available antibiotics. Some strains seem to be non-pathogenic whilst others cause accelerated lung disease. Treatment at present is focused on the prevention of cross-infection (Webb & David 1994).

Adequate nutrition is important in stabilising respiratory disease. Patients with cystic fibrosis require a high calorie intake because of their raised basal metabolic rate. For those patients unable to eat sufficient calories during the day, overnight enteral feeding is used.

Psychological care

Cystic fibrosis has a profound effect on the individual and the whole family. When parents are first informed of the diagnosis, shock is an overwhelming feeling. They require sensitivity, support and repeated explanations for a lengthy period of time. As the family adjusts to life, anger, denial, depression and anxiety are emotions which can be experienced. Family quarrels are not unknown.

Adolescence can be another period of tension. At this time body image is very important. The individual with cystic fibrosis is often physically underdeveloped, may have finger clubbing and a barrel chest and, if male, may be infertile. In addition, there is the normal fight for independene from parents. It can therefore be a stressful time for all concerned.

Individuals with cystic fibrosis are likely to have friends with the same disease. They therefore will have to cope with the death of friends and their mortality, perhaps much sooner than others of their own age.

Education of the patient and family is paramount. They need to learn about the disease, how to perform physiotherapy, administer antibiotics and maintain adequate nutrition. Without the knowledge and skills, the quality and quantity of life will be reduced (Kendrick 1993, Parcel et al 1994).

What of the future?

With the discovery of the cystic fibrosis gene situated on the long arm of chromosome 7 in 1989, 3 major 3-year pilot studies were commenced in Great Britain to establish a genetic screening programme for cystic fibrosis (Friend 1990).

Research is being conducted into gene therapy whereby genetically engineered cold viruses could carry healthy genes into the airways of individuals with the disease. It is hoped this may lead to a cure (Coutelle et al 1993). Researchers are also investigating the possibility of developing a vaccine against *Pseudomonas* (Kendrick 1993).

Heart and lung transplants are increasingly being performed in patients with cystic fibrosis. This is an easier technique than lung transplant alone, and the healthy heart of the cystic fibrosis may subsequently be used for transplant into another patient. Over 100 patients have had such transplants in the UK, with the probability of survival to 1 year post transplant being 70% (Hodson 1993) and a 2-year survival approaching 65% in some centres (Smith & Stableforth 1992). The first heart lung transplant in the UK was in 1985 and there are patients still alive 8 years later (Helms 1993). As with any transplant, the demand for organs exceeds supply.

DISORDERS AFFECTING THE PLEURA
Pneumothorax

Epidemiology and aetiology

In pneumothorax, air is present in the pleural space, thus preventing normal lung expansion. It may result from chest trauma or occur spontaneously. Spontaneous pneumothorax is the most common type and occurs in otherwise healthy individuals, usually males in their mid twenties to thirties. It is often associated with violent exercise such as squash or underwater diving. It occurs when the rupture of a small airsac, bleb or bullae beneath the surface of the visceral pleural allows air to enter the pleural space.

The collapse of the affected lung can cause displacement of the heart towards the opposite side. The resulting pressure on the opposite lung inhibits expansion. If, as a result of chest trauma, blood is also present in the space, the condition is known as a haemopneumothorax.

A tension pneumothorax is a life-threatening complication of a pneumothorax. In this situation, the way in which the pleura has been damaged allows air to enter into the pleural space but prevents its escape. If left untreated, the remaining lung would collapse, compression on the trachea, great vessels and heart would occur and the patient would die.

Common symptomatology

The patient will present with a sudden onset of pain, breathlessness and chest tightness in the affected side of the chest. Chest expansion of lungs will not be equal. Patients who have suffered trauma and fractural several ribs may exhibit paradoxical breathing. When someone with fractured ribs breathes, the ribs no longer having any anchor point act independently and when the rest of the chest wall moves up and out during inspiration, the damaged area (flail) moves in, and vice versa during expiration. Moderate or severe dyspnoea will occur according to the degree of

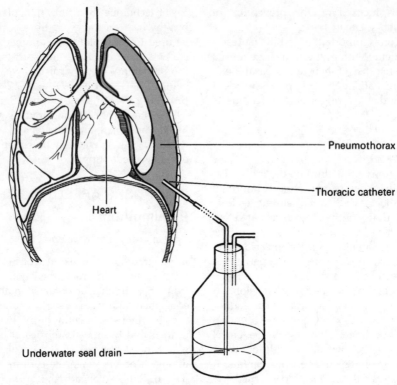

Pneumothorax

Thoracic catheter

Heart

Underwater seal drain

Fig. 13.12 Underwater seal drain

displacement of the heart. If the patient has lost blood he may exhibit signs of hypovolaemic shock (see Ch. 4).

Investigations (see also p. 445)

1. Clinical examination will reveal the absence of breath sounds on the affected side of the chest.

2. Chest X-ray will demonstrate the edge of the collapsed area of lung and the degree of displacement.

Therapeutic management

Treatment is aimed at the re-expansion of the lung by aseptically introducing a thoracic catheter and connecting it to an underwater seal drainage bottle. Air can be removed by placing the catheter in the upper intercostal region (as air rises towards the apex of the lung) but if it is placed lower, air, serosanguinous fluid and blood can be drained from the pleural space (Fig. 13.12). When there is only air present in the pleural space a Heimleich valve (Figs 13.13, 13.14) may be inserted. This type of drainage allows the patient more mobility. Patients who have a haemopneumothorax may require a blood transfusion (see Ch. 14).

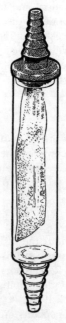

Fig. 13.13 Heimleich valve

Nursing strategies

The nursing care of the patient following insertion of underwater seal drainage is discussed in Nursing Care Plan 13.4, problem 7. After a few days of treatment with intercostal drainage, the affected lung should re-expand and within 5 days the patient is usually discharged home.

Following spontaneous pneumothorax, there is a possibility of recurrence. Recurrent cases are treated initially by reinsertion of underwater seal drainage, but if a further recurrences arises, a pleurodesis or pleurectomy may be performed which prevents further pneumothoraces developing.

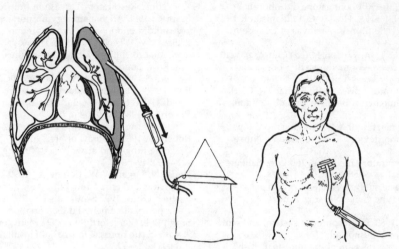

Fig. 13.14   Heimleich valve in use – one-way valve allowing the escape of air from pleural space but preventing its re-entry

---

Suggested assignments

Discussion points

1. Do you think that patients who have serious lung disease caused by their smoking consider that they have a self-inflicted life-threatening condition? Will this put stress on that individual or the relatives? Will it induce anger in the relatives who have tried in vain over the years to persuade their loved one to give up smoking?
2. In the USA there is so much concern about the dangerous effects of passive smoking on children, that the institution of 'child abuse legislation which would prevent parents or adults forcing children to inhale cigarette smoke' (Bysshe 1989) is under consideration. Should this be a strategy in the UK?
3. Why do people continue to smoke despite the obvious and well-known dangers to their health? Do health professionals have a responsibility to act as role models to the general population by giving up smoking?
4. Why do people living in poor housing develop more respiratory disease than those who live in good housing?
5. Are enough measures being taken to control environmental pollution?

Ethical issues

1. The aim of having a well-informed patient is so that he can make an informed choice/decision about his attitudes to his health and life-style. Health educationalists have to respect the rights and autonomy of the individual. The question arises therefore are nurses entitled to tell patients that they should stop smoking? There is an opposing argument from non-smokers; why should they suffer from others' smoking?
2. Consider the ethical issues related to the following:

   We spend £16.5 billon per annum on the NHS.

   We spend £15.8 billion per annum on alcohol and 7 billion on cigarettes and tobacco products.

   In 1985, the health education budget in the UK was under £20 million. In the same year, £650 million was spent advertising alcohol and tobacco. (Thomson et al 1988)
3. Smokers contribute £1000 million to the exchequer every year. The total cost of hospital treatment and sickness benefit related to illnesses caused by smoking is £370 million. This leaves the Government with a profit of £630 million (Bysshe 1989). Is this ethical?
4. Patients who do not comply with treatment are often labelled as bad or unco-operative. Is this acceptable ethically?

REFERENCES AND FURTHER READING

Brunner L S, Suddarth D S 1992 Textbook of adult nursing. Chapman and Hall, London

Byres C 1989 Managing cystic fibrosis. Paediatric Nursing September: 14–19

Bysshe J 1989 Politics in the air. Nursing 3(38): 15–18

Cole R B, Mackay A D 1990 Essentials of respiratory disease, 3rd edn. Churchill Livingstone, Edinburgh

Coutelle C, Caplen N, Hart S, Huxley C, Williamson R 1993 Gene therapy for cystic fibrosis. Archives of Disease in Childhood 68: 437–443

Cull A 1991 Lung cancer. In: Watson M (ed) Cancer patient care. Psychosocial treatment methods. BPS Books and Cambridge University Press, Cambridge, ch 9

Davies R J 1990 Respiratory disease. In: Kumar P J, Clark M L (eds) Clinical medicine. Baillière Tindall, London, ch 12

Ellis P 1990 Asthma: meeting the demand for rapid relief. Drugs and inhalation devices. The Professional Nurse. November: 76–81

Flenley D C 1990 Respiratory medicine, 2nd edn. Baillière Tindall, London

Foss M A 1989 Thoracic surgery. Austen Cornish

Friend B 1990 Tracing the Gene. Nursing Times 86(28): 16–17

Grenville-Mathers R 1983 The respiratory system, 2nd edn. Churchill Livingstone, Edinburgh

Helms P J 1993 Growing up with cystic fibrosis. British Journal of Hospital Medicine 50(6): 326–332

Hilton S 1984 Understanding asthma, 2nd edn. Chest, Heart and Stroke Association, London

Hodson M E 1993 Cystic fibrosis. Update 46(6): 451–462

Johnson N 1989 Lung function tests. Surgery 1641–1645

Kendrick R 1993 Night School. Nursing Times 89(30): 44–45

Luke C 1989 Respiratory investigations. Nursing 3(38): 5–8

Maynard L C 1994 Pediatric heart-lung transplantation for cystic fibrosis. Heary & Lung 23(4): 279–284

Mumford S P 1986 Using jet nebulisers. The Professional Nurse. January: 95–97

Parcel G S, Swank P R, Mariotto M J, Bartholomew L K, Czyzewski D I, Sockrider M M, Seilheimer D K 1994 Self-management of cystic fibrosis: a structural model for educational and behavioural variables. Social Science and Medicine 38(9): 1307–1315

Parrott A 1991 Social drugs: their effects upon health. In: Pitts M, Phillips K (eds) Psychology of health education. Routledge, London

Pinn S 1992 Paediatric asthma – an international consensus meeting. Respiratory Disease In Practice 9(2): 10–11

Pratt R J 1988 AIDS a strategy for nursing care. Edward Arnold, London

Pritchard A P, David J A 1988 The Royal Marsden Hospital manual of clinical nursing procedures, 2nd edn. Harper & Row, London

Redfern S 1989 Pulmonary tuberculosis. Nursing 3(38): 9–11

Rees J 1989 Definition and diagnosis. In: Rees J, Price J (eds) ABC of asthma, 2nd edn. BMA, London

Roberts A 1988 Systems of life. No 163 – Senior systems ageing lungs and airways (1). Nursing Times 84(32): 45–48

Roberts A 1988 Systems of life. No 163 – Senior systems ageing lungs and airways (2). Nursing Times 84(37): 49–52

Roper N, Logan W W, Tierney A J 1990 The elements of nursing, 3rd edn. Churchill Livingstone, Edinburgh

Scottish Office 1992 Scotland's Health. A challenge to us all – a policy statement. HMSO, London

Smith D L, Stableforth D E 1992 Management of adults with cystic fibrosis. Journal of Hospital Medicine 48(11): 713–723

Thomson I E, Melia K M, Boyd K M 1988 Nursing ethics, 2nd edn. Churchill Livingstone, Edinburgh

Walsh M 1989 Asthma: the Orem self care model approach. Nursing 3(38): 19–21

Webb A K, David T J 1994 Clinical management of children and adults with cystic fibrosis. British Medical Journal 308(6926): 459–462

Whyte D A 1992 A family nursing approach to the care of a child with a chronic illness. Journal of Advanced Nursing

Wilson K J W 1990 Ross & Wilson: Anatomy and physiology, 7th edn. Churchill Livingstone, Edinburgh

Woodman J, Robinson C 1990 Asthma education – a different approach. Community Outlook May: 7–8

14

Care implications of disorders of the blood and immune system

Marylyn Stewart

Blood disorders are diverse; they may affect any age group and their treatments demand a wide variety of skills from both nurses and doctors. Some conditions are common to all mankind while some are found in localized communities, for example sickle cell anaemia in African races. The spread of the acquired immune deficiency syndrome (AIDS) has provided a challenge to modern medicine and requires the skills of nurses both in hospital and the community.

ANATOMY AND PHYSIOLOGY

Blood is red, sticky to touch and has a salty taste. In health it is slightly alkaline pH 7.4. For blood volumes and haemoglobin according to age and sex refer to Table 14.1.

Blood consists of three formed elements, the erythrocytes (red blood cells), leucocytes (white blood cells) and thrombocytes (platelets), suspended in a fluid medium – plasma (Fig. 14.1). These cells are continually being destroyed, either because of old age or as a result of their functional activities, and being replaced by newly formed cells. In healthy subjects there is a finely adjusted balance between the rate of

Table 14.1 Blood volumes and haemoglobin estimations		
	Blood volume	Normal haemoglobin
Newborn	85 ml/kg	16.8 g/dl
Adult male	5–6 litres	13.0–18.0 g/dl
Adult female	4–5 litres	11.5–16.5 g/dl

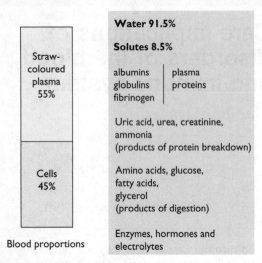

Blood proportions

Fig. 14.1 Contents of plasma

formation and destruction, thus the numbers of each cell remain remarkably constant.

Blood formation

In the fetus all the blood cells develop from cells having their origin in the embryonic connective tissue. Before birth the fetus produces blood cells progressively in the yolk sac, liver and spleen. During the fifth month production decreases at these sites and increases in the bone marrow.

After birth erythrocytes are manufactured primarily and continuously in the red bone marrow of certain bones, especially the vertebrae, sternum, ribs, pelvis and the upper ends of the femur and humerus. This process is known as erythropoiesis.

All blood cells are derived from undifferentiated primitive stem cells in the bone marrow. This cell is the embryonic stem cell which can give rise to both lymphoid cells, erythrocytes, leucocytes and thrombocytes. In the bone marrow the stem cell differentiates

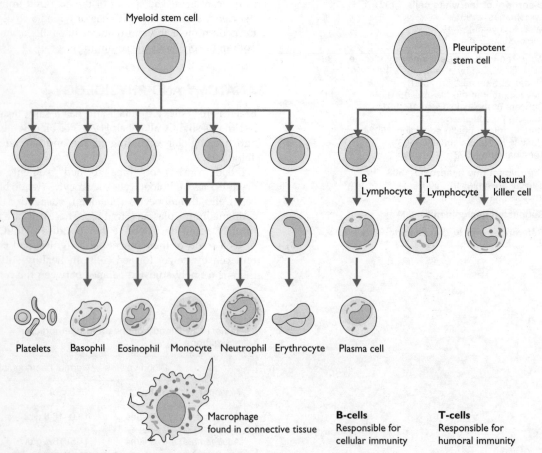

Fig. 14.2 Formation of blood cells

into the multipotent myeloid stem cell which in turn differentiates into the stem cells of each line and their progeny (Fig. 14.2).

Erythrocytes

Erythrocytes are biconcave non-nucleated discs about 7 μm in diameter with a large surface area relative to volume. The biconcave shape of the erythrocyte permits deformity to occur without injury. The life-span of an erythrocyte is 120 days.

Erythrocytes contain a concentration of haemoglobin which provides their red colour. Haemoglobin molecules are composed of protein (globin) and an iron containing pigment (haem). The erythrocytes transport oxygen from the lungs to the tissues and carbon dioxide in the reverse direction back from the tissues to the lungs.

Various nutrients are essential for successful maturation; these include iron, vitamin B complex (especially vitamin B_{12} and folic acid), vitamin C, and also certain hormones including thyroxine and the androgens (Fig. 14.3).

The phase of development of the erythrocyte from the proerythroblast to normoblast is the time when the required number of erythrocytes are formed. The level of haemoglobin is thought to be important at this stage, as low levels will slow down cell division and the cells become increasingly smaller and paler (microcytic and hypochromic). During erythropoieses the nucleus is extruded, leaving the fully developed erythrocyte to enter the circulation.

Thrombocytes (platelets)

Thrombocytes are formed from the cytoplasm of a much larger cell, the megakaryocyte. They are non-nucleated colourless bodies that usually appear as spindles or oval discs, they are about 2–4 μm in diameter. Their life-span is about 10 days. Their functions include blood coagulation and homeostasis related to vasoconstriction and increase in platelet aggregation at the site of injury. Thrombocytes are also thought to have a role in providing nutrition to the endothelial cells of the blood vessels and secreting a growth factor which stimulates proliferation of smooth muscle cells in artery walls.

White blood cells

White blood cells are formed in the red bone marrow from the myeloid stem cell. Refer to Box 14.1.

Various factors such as exercise and emotion change the white blood cell count within normal limits (Table 14.2). Unlike erythrocytes leucocytes are nucleated.

Granulocytes (polymorphonuclear leucocytes)

These cells are easily recognized due to the presence of granules in their cytoplasm and a lobed nucleus. They are 10–14 μm in diameter. There are three cell types:

1. Neutrophils The most numerous of the white cell population. The granules in their cytoplasm contain both digestive and lytic elements.

Functions. Very active during the inflammatory response and in bacterial infection.

2. Eosinophils Mobile phagocytic cells, less active than neutrophils and containing most of the lytic enzymes.

Functions. Eosinophils are involved in immunoglobulin E (IgE) mediated responses; they act as neutralizing agents against such substances as hista-

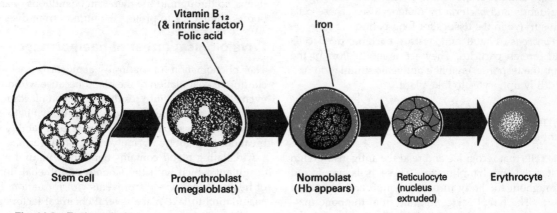

Fig. 14.3 Erythropoiesis

Table 14.2 White cells – size and values

Cell type	Size (μm)	% of total blood volume	Normal values
Leucocytes	10–14	Less than	$4–11 \times 100^9/l$
Neutrophil	10–15	50–70%	$2.5–7.5 \times 100^9/l$
Eosinophil	10–14	1–4%	$0.4–0.4 \times 100^9/l$
Basophil	10	Less than 1%	
Monocyte	10–18	2–8%	$0.2–0.8 \times 100^9/l$
Lymphocytes	8–11	20–40%	Child: $7.0 \pm 1.5 \times 100^9/l$ Adult: $1.5–4.0 \times 100^9/l$

mine and bradykinin released during the inflammatory response. Their numbers increase during allergic response.

3. Basophils Circulating counterparts of tissue mast cells, their granules contain histamine and heparin (Table 14.2).

Heparin is a powerful anticoagulant. In acute hypersensitivity blood clotting is inhibited due to heparin release. The degranulation of basophils attracts eosinophils into the area of antigen-IgE, this interaction causing the release of an eosinophil chemotoxic factor.

Monocytes

These cells contain no granules in their cytoplasm. They are large cells with large oval nuclei. Monocytes are formed in the red bone marrow. Mature monocytes have a half-life of 8 hours in the blood, as they migrate to the tissues they are known as macrophages and move quickly to sites of infection engulfing debris and bacteria by phagocytoses. These cells can survive in the tissues for long periods of time.

Functions Engulf and destroy bacteria, dead cells and foreign particles. They act as modulators of the immune response, enabling antigenic stimulation of T and B lymphocytes to take place.

Lymphocytes (refer to Fig. 14.2 for origin of lymphocytes)

The cells that recognize and read the antigens (foreign materials) are lymphocytes. These cells are found throughout the body in blood, lymph and lymphoid tissue. The lymphocytes migrate from the bone marrow and enter the blood. Some will pass through the

thymus and then into the circulation where they will settle in lymph nodes and spleen. These are known as the T cells. In their journey through the thymus they are slightly altered to acquire specificity, different lymphocytes will recognize different antigens. For example, the T cell may become specific for the polio virus and not affect any other viruses. T cells are classified into several subsets each with a particular function. Some T cells have a regulatory role and stimulate the production of antibody by B cells. The ones that control the immune response are known as T helper cells and those which inhibit them are T suppresser cells. All perform a regulatory role. T cytotoxic cells will destroy any cells in the body which have become infected with a virus. Cytotoxic or killer T cells are mainly responsible for the rejection of tissue and organ transplants.

B cells mature in the lymph nodes and spleen. B cells carry on their surface an antibody molecule which acts as a receptor for antigen. The antibody receptors on each B cell are specific for individual antigens, so throughout life there can be millions of antibodies circulating to protect the human from disease.

Physiological arrest of haemorrhage

The phenomenon of natural haemostasis includes clotting or coagulation of the blood because without it even slight injury could result in a person bleeding to death. In health there is a fine balance drawn between blood clotting capacity and the body's ability to breakdown a clot by fibrinolysis should it form.

Circulating blood contains heparin, a natural anticoagulant which with the smooth endothelial lining of healthy blood vessels prevents clot formation. For coagulation to take place several chemical factors are required. These come from:

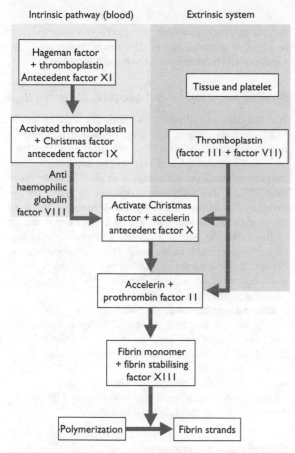

Intrinsic pathway (blood)   Extrinsic system

Fig. 14.4 Blood clotting mechanism

1. The extrinsic pathway – blood vessels and body cells are damaged, releasing tissue and platelet thromboplastin (factor III and factor VII).

2. The intrinsic pathway – platelets adhere to the damaged endothelium releasing contact factors. This increases the stickiness of the platelets and encourages a loose platelet plug to form in the damaged vessel. A sequence of cascade or changes are initiated as one factor activates another (Fig. 14.4).

A loose platelet plug is formed in a fibrin network, which entraps blood cells and stops the bleeding. The clot later retracts if there are adequate numbers of platelets present; it gradually hardens and serum oozes out forming a protective barrier enabling repair of damaged tissue to take place.

Blood groups

It is essential that the blood of a patient receiving a blood transfusion is cross-matched with the donor blood he is about to receive.

ABO blood groups

An individual's blood group is classified by the ABO system. The membrane on the red blood cells and most other cells may contain:

1. antigen A or B, or
2. both antigen A and B, or
3. neither antigen A or B.

Antibodies are found in the plasma, and blood transfused into a patient must not contain an antibody to the patient's cellular antigens, or the patient's antigens will destroy the cells being transfused.

Rhesus factor

About 85% of the people in western populations carry a Rhesus factor in their blood cells and are therefore classified as being Rhesus +ve (positive). Those who lack this factor are called Rhesus –ve (negative).

Although there is no naturally occurring Rhesus antibody, if a Rh –ve person is exposed to Rh +ve cells then antibodies may be formed, once formed they stay in the blood. Exposure may occur through:

1. Transfusion of Rh +ve blood.
2. Pregnancy (Fig. 14.5) when the mother is Rh –ve but her baby has inherited Rh +ve blood from the father. In this situation the mother may form Rhesus antibodies in her blood which then pass via the placenta to the fetus. This results in the destruction

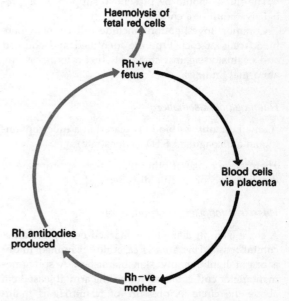

Fig. 14.5 Rhesus antibody production in pregnancy

of the baby's red cells (haemolysis), giving rise to haemolytic disease of the newborn.

Subsequent pregnancies are at greater risk because there is a progressive build up of antibodies (Tortora & Anagnostakos 1990).

INVESTIGATIONS OF BLOOD DISORDERS

History

An accurate medical history should be taken. The doctor may elicit symptoms which may suggest a cause for a blood disorder, for example frequent use of aspirin by the patient causing gastric irritation and blood loss.

General physical examination

This may also reveal signs of disease, an enlarged spleen or purpura.

Examination of the circulating blood

Venepuncture

This is the withdrawal of venous blood from a peripheral vein, usually in the antecubital fossa. Laboratory findings often enable an accurate diagnosis to be made. The correct bottles must be used containing the appropriate anticoagulant. A haematoma may form at the puncture site, but this can be avoided by applying digital pressure and elevation of the arm.

The nurse should be present to support an apprehensive adult or a child.

Common investigations include cell count, where blood cells of each type are identified and counted and evaluated against standard criteria to assess any abnormal findings.

Haemoglobin estimation

A small quantity of blood is placed in a tube containing an anticoagulant ETD (sequestrate).

There are a range of other blood tests appropriate to the diagnosis of specific disorders.

Hess test (capillary resistant test)

A circle 6 cm in diameter is marked out on the antecubital fossa. This area is carefully examined under a bright light for any skin blemishes. A sphygmomanometer cuff is placed round the arm at least 3 cm above the circle. A pressure of 50 mmHg is maintained accurately for a least 10 minutes. After release

of the cuff, the number of small haemorrhages (petechia) appearing within the circle are counted. Up to eight is normal, above that number suggests the capillary characteristics of thrombocytopenia.

Schilling test – test for malabsorption of Vitamin B₁₂

A small dose of radioactive vitamin B_{12} is given orally to the fasting patient, followed by a 1000 µg dose of non-radioactive vitamin B_{12}. All urine for the next 24 hours is collected and sent to the laboratory. Note that complete urine collection is vital. Normally more than 7% of the radioactive dose is secreted in the urine within 24 hours. In pernicious anaemia less than 3% is excreted. If less than 7% of the dose is excreted in the urine the patient is given a capsule containing 60 µg of intrinsic factor and the test repeated as before. If the amount of radioactive vitamin B_{12} now excreted reaches normal levels the diagnosis of pernicious anaemia is confirmed.

Nursing implications Explain to the patient the reason for the test and what will happen during the test. The patient will have to fast for at least 8 hours before the commencement of the test to ensure accuracy of the results. The patient is allowed to drink water during this period. As soon as the patient receives the first intramuscular injection of vitamin B_{12} normal diet and fluids can be resumed.

Sternal marrow puncture

This involves removing a specimen of bone marrow by aspiration. A stout needle is used with an adjustable quard, for example the Salah needle. In adults the sternum and the iliac crests are the preferred sites. The tibia or iliac crests are the sites used for the very young. On extremely rare occasions the vertebral spine is used in very obese people. Laboratory examination is useful for two reasons, diagnosis and monitoring the effect of treatment especially in the leukaemias.

The procedure is carried out under local anaesthetic by a doctor, with a laboratory technician present to collect the specimen in the appropriate container. In the very apprehensive patient light sedation may be given prior to the procedure. The actual removal of the bone marrow is painful.

When the local anaesthetic has worn off analgesia should be administered as prescribed and the patient should be encouraged to rest in bed for at least 2–3 hours.

Complications of the procedure are rare. Infection can be caused by faulty technique. Introducing the needle into the sternum without use of the guard may cause damage to the organs in the mediastinum.

Nursing implications

- To reinforce the information given by the doctor to the patient, thus ensuring patient co-operation.
- Administration of sedation when appropriate.
- Positioning the patient, supine, prone or on his side depending on the site from which marrow is to be extracted.
- Reducing the patient's anxiety throughout the procedure.
- Applying pressure to the puncture site to prevent bruising or the development of a haemotoma.
- Monitoring the patient for development of complications (Pritchard & David 1988).

DISORDERS OF THE RED CELLS

Disorders of the red cells are common worldwide. There may be overproduction or underproduction of cells or abnormality of the cells themselves.

An increase in the number of circulating red cells is known as erythrocytosis occurring in response to hypoxia (Box 14.1). This compensatory response is found in people living in high altitudes, it is also found in children with congenital heart disease and those with chronic respiratory disease. In disease this mechanism can prove beneficial as it increases the oxygen carrying capacity of the blood. A disadvantage is that the blood can become viscous, necessitating withdrawal of an amount of blood by venesection. This causes retention of fluid to maintain blood volume, making the circulating blood less viscous.

Primary disorder polycythaemia

This condition mainly affects people of 40 years or over, and is more common in males than females.

Some patients have no symptoms and the condition can be diagnosed incidentally. Others will present with a variety of symptoms: high colour, suffused conjuctiva, deep red palate and dusky red hands. Other symptoms can include loss of concentration, headaches and symptoms similar to a cerebrovascular accident. The spleen is palpable in 75% of individuals.

Treatment

There are various treatments available depending on the severity of the disease. Venepuncture is the treatment of choice in patients over 60 years of age, up to 50 ml of blood is withdrawn. The treatment can be

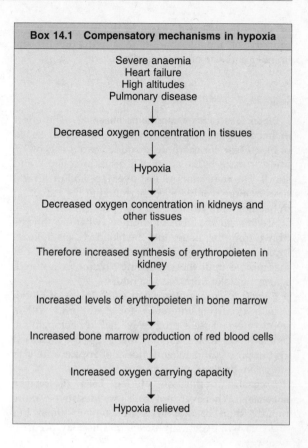

Box 14.1   Compensatory mechanisms in hypoxia

Severe anaemia
Heart failure
High altitudes
Pulmonary disease
↓
Decreased oxygen concentration in tissues
↓
Hypoxia
↓
Decreased oxygen concentration in kidneys and other tissues
↓
Therefore increased synthesis of erythropoieten in kidney
↓
Increased levels of erythropoieten in bone marrow
↓
Increased bone marrow production of red blood cells
↓
Increased oxygen carrying capacity
↓
Hypoxia relieved

repeated within 2 days, the aim of this treatment is to reduce the haemocrit by 45%. If this treatment fails to produce the desired effect, radioactive phosphorous or chemotherapy is used. This treatment has the added risk of the patient developing leukaemia.

Nursing implications

Encourage the patient to have periods of rest alternating with activity to avoid the development of thrombosis. Support any patients receiving chemotherapy. To alleviate anxiety arising from the side-effects, keep the patient well informed about treatment and progress. Encourage the patient to eat small frequent meals rich in iron to reduce the development of anaemia. Evaluate pain control if appropriate. When the patient is discharged explain the importance of keeping follow-up appointments.

Anaemias

The most common group of diseases of the blood is the anaemias. Anaemia can be defined as a condition in which there is a decrease in the oxygen carrying capacity of the blood due to a reduction in the number and size of the red cells.

Causes of anaemia

Blood loss (posthaemorrhagic anaemia) The effect of haemorrhage depends on the volume and speed of blood lost, for example, a sudden rapid loss of 1.5 litres or more in the adult will result in collapse and shock. The same amount lost over a period of several days or more would be less harmful but the reduction in haemoglobin would be similar.

Acute blood loss Haemodilution, whereby fluid is drawn from the tissues into the blood vessels, follows rapid haemorrhage. The degree of anaemia is not measurable until the circulating volume is restored, which can take from 24 to 36 hours.

Chronic blood loss Repeated small losses of blood, usually occurring internally, for example as with a peptic ulcer, cause a progressive fall in haemoglobin. Small blood losses can be made up by increased erythropoiesis and anaemia does not appear until iron stores are depleted.

Excessive destruction of red cells (haemolytic anaemia) Whenever red cells are destroyed more rapidly then haemopoiesis can replace them but anaemia will eventually develop. This may occur in two ways:

1. The red cells are abnormal and therefore are destroyed more easily as in pernicious anaemia and some hereditary diseases such as sickle cell anaemia and thalassaemia.
2. The red cells are normal but their environment is not, as in the presence of infection, such as malaria, toxins or the side-effects of some drugs, for example the drug zidovudine used in the treatment of AIDS. Antibodies can also cause haemolysis for example in haemolytic disease of the newborn (Fig. 14.5).

Iron deficiency anaemia

In iron deficiency anaemia the red cells are small and pale. This is a common form of anaemia worldwide, and all age groups are affected.

Pernicious anaemia (vitamin B_{12} deficiency)

In this type of anaemia the red cells are immature and therefore larger than normal (megaloblastic). Vitamin B_{12} deficiency is always associated with achlorhydria and gastric atrophy.

Causes of pernicious anaemia

1. There may be a dietary deficiency of vitamin B_{12} in those individuals who are on strict vegan diets, which takes many years to develop.
2. Surgical operations, e.g. partial or total gastrectomy.
3. Diseases of the ileum, e.g. Crohn's disease.
4. Loss of vitamin B_{12} during passage through the intestine, e.g. utilised by parasitic worms or bacteria.
5. As pernicious anaemia is also an autoimmune disease, the gastric atrophy is caused by an immune reaction against the parietal cell cytoplasmic constituents and specific antibodies to the intrinsic factor.
6. Familial tendency. The UK incidence in the elderly is about 1:800 in the over 60 age group. Complications if untreated are subacute degeneration of the spinal cord, peripheral neuropathy, atrophy of the vagina causing easily damaged mucosa, anaemia and jaundice.

Folic acid deficiency anaemia

Folic acid is utilized for DNA synthesis with vitamin B_{12}. Folic acid deficiency can be caused by dietary deficiency, lack of green vegetables, cereals, meat, fish and eggs. Increased requirements for folic acid are required during pregnancy (fetal growth), infancy and childhood where there is rapid growth. Some drugs can cause deficiency by utilization block, e.g. for example, chemotherapy agents, anticonvulsants.

Investigations

- haemoglobin estimation
- marrow puncture
- Schilling test
- investigations for underlying disease in chronic blood loss.

Treatment Patient education regarding diet. Giving folic acid orally.

Nursing management of the patient with anaemia

The nursing management will depend on the severity and cause of anaemia. The majority of patients will be cared for in the community with occasional visits to the outpatient department. The patients that are admitted to hospital are very ill. Nursing care is related to the specific needs of the individual. Rest is advised for patients whose haemoglobin level is below 5 g/dl. The patient will require help with all hygiene and personal needs. He will find it more comfortable to sit in an upright position to relieve breathing problems. Care of pressure areas is important due to the vulnerability of the skin. The patient will require support and explanations during the course of the investigative procedures to elicit the cause of his anaemia.

Treatment

Blood transfusion is reserved for the severely anaemic patient. Concentrated blood cells are slowly infused with diuretic cover to prevent cardiac failure. This allows the anaemia to be dealt with promptly.

Oral preparations of iron can also be given. Side-effects can include gastrointestinal upset if the tablets are not taken following main meals. Constipation can be a problem and has to be dealt with. Advising the patient that his stools will be black will reduce anxiety.

Iron is also administered by injection to those individuals who will not accept a blood transfusion on religious grounds, or for patients who are not responding to oral preparations. This type of iron can be administered by intramuscular injection or intravenously. The dose is calculated according to the patient's body weight.

Intravenous iron is given as a test dose initially as anaphylactic reaction can occur. During the infusion the patient is monitored carefully and for an hour following the transfusion. Signs such as flushing, metallic taste, dyspnoea, nausea and vomiting or a fall in blood pressure must be reported immediately, the infusion stopped and antihistamines administered.

Patients whose diet is deficient will require dietary advice, especially individuals who have recently embarked on a strict vegan diet. When dietary advice is being given, consideration must be made of the cost to the patient. Expensive diets encourage non-compliance on the part of the patient.

If adequately treated, and in the absence of any underlying disease, the patient's haemoglobin level should rise by 1% per day which allows the normal level to be reached within 4–8 weeks. Regular appointments will have to be arranged to monitor haemoglobin levels. The patient may feel so well that he stops taking the oral iron, not seeing the importance of continuing the treatment.

For a summary of nursing care refer to Nursing Care Plan 14.1.

Health education in the prevention of iron deficiency anaemia is important. Vulnerable groups should be identified. Medicinal iron should be given in pregnancy and lactation, and if menstruation is heavy. Infants of low birth weight should also be given iron supplements. Teenagers who decide to become vegetarian require advice about diet, as do the elderly who live alone.

Pernicious anaemia: specific nursing problems A blood transfusion of concentrated red cells is given if haemoglobin levels are below 5 g/dl. Replacement of vitamin B_{12} (cobalamin) by intramuscular injection for all patients is necessary as they are unable to absorb the vitamin orally. The preparation is known as hydroxyocobalamin. The dosage is 1000 μg i.m. twice in the first week followed by 1000 μg once per week until levels are returned to normal. There is an improvement in the patient's general condition and they have a feeling of well-being which has been absent for so long. The patient will require a maintenance does of vitamin B_{12} every 3 months for life. The dose is regulated so that the haemoglobin level and blood count remain within normal limits.

If the patient is elderly and housebound, arrangements can be made for the district nurse to visit to monitor the patient's general health and administer the injection on the due date.

Intractable anaemia Patients with intractable anaemia may need to be given a blood transfusion every 3–4 weeks, as a day patient. To minimize the risk of reactions either washed or filtered red cells may be given along with an intravenous injection of a steroid preparation. A diuretic is given to prevent cardiac failure. These patients are tired most of the time and the nurse needs to show understanding and empathy towards them.

COAGULATION DEFICIENCY DISEASES
(Fig. 14.4)

A congenital functional deficiency of factor VIII will cause haemophilia. The production of factor VIII is controlled by a gene on the X chromosome, and in haemophilia the gene is defective. Factor VIII is the product of two genes, one of which is part of the X-linked chromosome and the other is autosomal. It is an inherited defect with the females acting as carriers, the male offspring will be affected as he will have no normal X chromosome and any factor VIII produced will be under the influence of the defective X chromosome.

Haemophilia B (Christmas disease)

This disease is due to a deficiency of factor IX (Christmas factor). This condition is also sex-linked, inherited in a similar fashion as haemophilia, affect-

Nursing Care Plan 14.1 Care plan for a patient with anaemia			
Problem	**Goal**	**Nursing action**	**Rationale**
1. Breathlessness	To improve breathing	☐ Bed rest, oxygen administration only if blood loss is severe ☐ Sit upright	Due to low haemoglobin count
2. Self-care abilities reduced	To improve patient's self-care abilities	☐ Aid the patient with all personal hygiene requirements	Extreme lethargy due to anaemia
3. Development of pressure sores	To reduce the risk of pressure sores	☐ Encourage patient to change position 2 hourly Use of bed aids, risk scales, e.g. Norton scale	Anaemia reduces oxygen to tissues
4. Anorexia	To improve patients appetite	☐ Provision of small attractive meals containing required nutrients	Extreme tiredness due to anaemia reduces ability to eat
5. Constipation	To reduce risk of constipation	☐ Aid patient on to commode/ bedpan. Provide privacy. Give diet containing extra fibre	Poor muscle tone
6. Reduced resistance to infection	To reduce the infection risk	☐ Use aseptic techniques. Frequent oral hygiene. Monitor for urinary tract infection	Due to anaemia
7. Intractable anaemia	To enable both patient and relatives to cope with this chronic condition	☐ Provide support for both patient and family	Due to chronic condition both patient and relatives require support
8. Non-compliance with drug treatment	To monitor the effect of drug therapy	☐ To ensure patient understands the importance of drug therapy	Non-compliance is indicated when there is no improvement in haemoglobin count
9. Anxiety	To relieve anxiety	☐ To explain all treatments and encourage patient to ask questions	Fear of the unknown

ing males only. Clinical features are indistinguishable from true haemophilia. There are other congenital coagulation deficiencies but they are very rare. Haemophilia affects 1 in 10 000 individuals. Although this is a congenital disorder, it is rare for excessive bleeding to occur before the age of 6 months.

Clinical features

The clinical severity of the disease is directly related to the level of factor VIII in the blood (Fig. 14.4). Bleeding can be persistent and excessive as when the clot forms, it breaks down easily, and bleeding continues. In moderate forms of the disease excessive bleeding occurs following dental extraction or minor surgery. In the more severe form spontaneous bleed-

ing can occur especially within joint cavities (haemarthrosis) which, if not treated promptly, will cause progressive joint deterioration.

Bleeding episodes should be treated promptly by raising the factor VIII level. This is administered by intravenous infusion of factor VIII concentrate.

Nursing implications

Patients with haemophilia are treated as outpatients unless they have a severe episode of bleeding. The nursing staff at the clinics develop a special kind of relationship with their patients and their parents. Haemophilia is a subtle disruptive condition which despite treatment can still be life-threatening and handicapping in both its physical and psychological aspects. In the 1990s the use of freeze-dried concentrates improved the lives of these children and adults, by improving pain relief and enabling treatment at home. Life can be made as near normal as possible, with the patients having control of their lives.

The diagnosis of any abnormality is traumatic. Parents suffer from the loss of a normal child and have to reorganize their lives to accommodate frequent hospital visits. At diagnosis the parents will be given an explanation of what the disease is and the future implications for their child. The nurse's role is to encourage parents to participate in their child's treatment. The nurse has a counselling role in helping the mother to cope with her guilt as she is the carrier. The child also has to cope psychologically with being different. The nursing staff will have a role in educating the parents regarding what action to take if the child has a bleed and who to contact. Advice has to be offered as the child becomes older and more independent. Overprotection on the part of the parents can cause rebellion in the adolescent years and further problems in adulthood of total reliance on the parents for support.

Haemophilia and AIDS

Prior to 1985, 60% of haemophiliacs had become infected by the HIV virus. This had a devastating effect on parents of affected children. The parents had to deal with their emotions of fear and anger while they waited to see if their HIV-positive child developed AIDS. The children were ostracised, some being forced to leave school due to the attitudes of both teachers and other parents.

Nurses had to handle their feelings of guilt while providing support for both parents and children. In the UK 1200 people with haemophilia were affected with the HIV virus; 210 have developed AIDS and more than 150 have died. The nightmare still continues.

Deficiency of prothrombin – hypoprothrombinaemia

This can be the result of any process that interferes with the utilization of vitamin K, this vitamin is needed by the liver to synthesize the Prothrombin factors II, VII, IX and X. Hypoprothrombinaemia can occur in preterm babies, when the liver is immature, causing haemorrhagic disease of the newborn. It may also be a complication of obstructive jaundice, and some forms of malabsorption due to failure of the intestine to absorb vitamin K. Injections of vitamin K will cure this condition provided liver function is not impaired. Where liver damage has occurred the missing factor has to be given.

Hypoprothrombinaemia (anticoagulation) can be induced artificially in patients who are at risk of developing thrombi or emboli. Heparin may be used for short-term treatment. It needs to be given by injection. For long-term management, oral anticoagulants are more satisfactory. These have to be commenced at least 36–48 hours before discontinuing heparin.

Patient education

Patients who require to take anticoagulents over a prolonged period of time must be given specific advice to avoid complications. The patient must attend the clinic regularly to have his prothrombin time checked (Box 14.2).

The patient should always inform the dentist or medical practitioner that he is taking anticoagulents.

MYELOFIBROSIS

This is a relatively uncommon progressive disorder of the blood-forming elements in the bone marrow. It usually occurs in the middle aged. Increasingly extensive non-functional fibrous tissue formation takes place in the bone marrow along with considerable enlargement of the spleen and liver in which blood formation also takes place. The disease is eventually fatal as the result of a chronic wasting process (Edwards & Bouchier 1991).

BLOOD TRANSFUSIONS

Blood transfusion was tried around 1492 when a blood transfusion from two healthy Romans to the dying Pope Innocent was attempted. All three died. Many other attempts were made but fatalities were high so the practice was outlawed in 1687.

Box 14.2 Guidelines when taking anticoagulants

- Remember to take the correct dose at the correct time
- Obtain a repeat prescription in time
- Alcohol should be taken only in moderation
- Aspirin and acetyl salicylic acid preparations should not be taken as they increase anticoagulation
- If any sign of bleeding and bruising, medical advice should be sought immediately

In 1900 Karl Landsteiner pioneered the classification of the ABO blood groups which, with the realization in 1914 that sodium citrate prevented clotting, opened the way for extensive use of blood transfusion. Today, blood transfusion is commonplace where both whole blood and separate components are transfused (Table 14.3). Transmission of disease and errors in grouping can be avoided. At Blood Donor Centres careful histories are taken from potential blood donors; for example, recent infections or contact with infection, recent foreign travel and any other relevant factors.

In the laboratory two samples are taken from the donor's blood for:

1. cross-matching
2. testing for the presence of hepatitis and the HIV virus.

Such is the anxiety about infected blood that some individuals are having their own blood stored, especially when travelling abroad where testing is not so stringent as in the UK.

Persons receiving blood have their plasma cross-matched with stored blood to ensure compatibility.

Storage of blood Whole blood can be stored at 4°C for 35 days. Blood should not be taken from the blood bank unless it is going to be transfused within 30 minutes.

Refer to Nursing Care Plan 14.2 for care of a patient receiving a blood transfusion (Contreras 1990).

DISORDERS OF THE WHITE CELLS

White cells are seen in the blood as they migrate to the tissues. The number and type circulating vary with age, lymphocytes being more common in young children than adults. An increase in the number of white cells circulating is known as leucocytosis, and is the normal body response to bacterial invasion.

When there are too few white blood cells, usually granulocytes, this is known as leucopenia. This occurs in response to some specific infections, for example tuberculosis and enteric fever, and further lowering of the body's resistance to other infections.

Agranulocytosis (neutropenia) is a potentially serious disorder in which there is an absence of circulating neutrophils. It can be due to the side-effect of some drugs; for example, chloramphenicol, sulphonamides and phenytoin to name but a few. The drugs should be withdrawn immediately if the patient complains of feeling generally unwell and has a sore

Table 14.3 Blood components given in transfusion	
Blood components	Reason for administration
Whole blood	To replace volume and cells lost during internal and external haemorrhage
Packed red cells	80% plasma removed. Suitable as treatment for anaemia when whole blood volume is intact
Washed cells	7-day-old blood minus white cells and platelets. Minimizes reaction
Plasma	Does not require to be cross matched; can be dried, fresh, frozen or as a plasma protein fraction
Platelets	Extracted from fresh blood and transfused within 24 hours, used to aid clotting
Factor IX	Given in Christmas disease (haemophilia B)
Human immunoglobulin	To confer passive immunity, for example the immunosuppressed patient
Freeze dried concentrates factor VIII	Given in haemophilia
Plasma protein fraction 5% albumin and globulin in saline solution	To treat haemorrhagic shock by replacing clotting factors used up in situations of massive haemorrhage
Prothombin factors II VII and X	To replace clotting factors in patient with haemophilia B or bleeding secondary to severe liver disease

Nursing Care Plan 14.2 Care plan for a patient receiving a blood transfusion

Problem	Goal	Nursing action	Rationale
1. Patient anxiety	To relieve anxiety	❒ Explanation of procedure. Stay with patient while Venflon is being inserted. Patient comfort. Patient's locker and drinks easily accessible. Attention to toilet needs. Ask patient if they are right or left handed. ❒ Baseline observations.	To ensure patient's co-operation and comfort throughout procedure. Needle should be inserted in non-dominant arm to increase independence during transfusion To compare against future observations
2. Burning sensation in arm. Nausea, vomiting. Raised temperature. Raised pulse rate. Difficulty in breathing. Haematuria. Tightness in chest	To ensure patient receives correct blood at correct temperature and rate of transfusion.	❒ Blood checked as per hospital policy. Examine blood for clouding, air bubbles, abnormal colour avoid delay in transfusion. Record on infusion chart T.P.R. and blood pressure every 15 minutes as for first hour ❒ Signs of transfusion reaction. stop infusion, send for medical aid. Keep blood bag for investigation. Monitor urine output	Blood deteriorates rapidly at room temperature Transfusion reaction usually due to incompatible blood transfusion and human error
3. Total circulatory collapse	Continual observation of patient to avoid/ treat complications	❒ Frequent observations throughout transfusion. Resuscitation as necessary	One of the complications of mismatched blood transfusion
4. Pain and swelling round site of infusion	To reduce effects of 'Tissuing' by monitoring position of Venflon and condition of transfusion site	❒ Position arm to achieve maximum patient comfort. Aseptic technique. Re-siting of Venflon as appropriate	Due to misplaced blood entering surrounding tissues
5. Pyrexia rigor. Headache. Loin pain (60–90 min) after commencement of infusion. Dyspnoea. Pulmonary oedema	Careful observation of patient during transfusion to avoid complications	❒ Send for medical aid. Slow down transfusion. Antipyretics given. Steroid in severe reactions. Washed cells given in future transfusions. Set rate of infusion 15–20 drops per minute. Check rate frequently. Send for medical aid. Position patient to aid breathing. Diuretics administered	Due to febrile reaction caused by presence of anti-bodies to white cell or platelet antigens Due to circulatory overload, common in anaemic patients receiving large amounts of blood.

throat. Exposure to some insecticides or other industrial chemicals are also implicated. In rare instances the disease can be inherited. When drugs are not involved the treatment is the same as that for acute leukaemia.

Lymphomas

The lymphomas are a group of malignant neoplasms affecting lymphoid tissue. There are two main types: Hodgkin's lymphoma and non-Hodgkin's lymphoma.

Hodgkin's lymphoma

This is a progressive painless enlargement of lymphoid tissue throughout the body. The male to female ratio is three to one, and it is one of the most common malignancies in young adulthood and in the 45–70 year age group. It is distinguished from non-Hodgkin's lymphoma by the presence of the Reed–Sternberg cells which are present in the affected lymph node tissue. These are thought to be malignant cells.

Clinical features   In early disease the patient

presents with a painless enlargement of the lymph nodes especially in the cervical region. There may also be a pyrexia and later symptoms include general malaise, anaemia, dyspnoea, night sweats, weight loss and a low resistance to infection. The disease is slowly progressive and can be fatal if untreated.

Investigations Staging procedures are used to determine the extent of the disease and also plan treatment. There are four stages. Stage 1 where the disease is confined to one single site to stage 4 where there is widespread involvement.

Investigations used are:

- Full blood count
- blood urea and electrolytes
- biopsy of affected lymph node
- liver function tests
- 24 hour urine collection for Bence Jones protein
- chest X-ray, CT scan
- bone marrow puncture or core biopsy
- ESR.

Treatment Radiotherapy and chemotherapy are used. Advances in the treatment of Hodgkin's diseases have been one of the outstanding successes of cancer treatment of the past two decades.

Non-Hodgkin's lymphoma

In this condition there is malignant proliferation of lymphoid cells, the majority being B cells similar to both lymphoblastic and lymphocytic leukaemias. This group of lymphomas occurs at any age but increases in the older age group. The specific aetiology is unknown although individuals with immunosuppression have been found to be at increased risk.

Clinical features These will depend on the site involved. In many respects this type of lymphoma is similar to Hodgkin's lymphoma, although the effects are usually widespread at the time of diagnosis involving the gastrointestinal tract, lungs, skin, head and neck regions.

Multiple myeloma

This malignant disorder of the plasma cells in the bone marrow is uncommon before the age of 30 years, with a peak incidence between 60 and 70 years. Males are affected more than females and people of central African origin more than Caucasians. The tumour in the bone marrow erodes the bone and may eventually cause a pathological fracture (see Ch. 11). Large amounts of immunoglobulins are produced which cannot function normally.

Clinical features

The most common symptom is bone pain, often in the back caused by a fracture in the vertebrae. Infection is common because of the patient's low resistance. There are also signs of anaemia, neutrapenia and thrombocytopenia due to the changes in the bone marrow. Hypercalcaemia is caused by the release of calcium due to the high level of immunoglobulins.

Investigations:

- X-ray of bone, bone scan
- urea, electrolytes, creatinine
- blood calcium levels
- plasma immunoglobulins
- bleeding time
- blood viscosity
- glomerular filtration rate
- bone marrow aspirate.

Treatment

Chemotherapy is the treatment of choice. Success depends on the stage of the disease when diagnosed.

Leukaemias

This is a group of malignant disorders of the haemopoietic tissues leading to increased numbers of leucocytes. The abnormal leucocytes appearing in the blood collect in the bone marrow, causing disruption of homeopoiesis. The normal production of leucocytes, erythrocytes and platelets ceases, leading to the development of thrombocytopenia and anaemia. The leukaemia cells will proliferate in the bone marrow, spleen, lymph nodes, central nervous system, kidneys and skin.

Leukaemic cells are thought to develop from a single cell mutation; as this cell divides it fails to develop into a normal leucocyte and less normal cells are found in the circulation. The developmental process of leukaemia is given in Box 14.3.

The difference between acute and chronic leukaemia depends on the rapidity of onset. Acute leukaemia has a rapid onset and progression, and is common among children especially young children 2–4 years. Untreated, life expectancy is about 2 months.

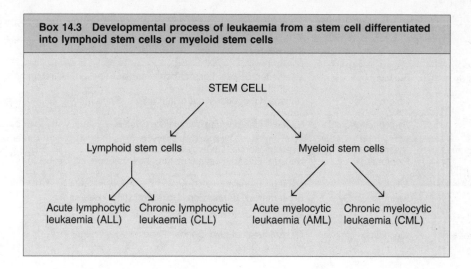

Box 14.3   Developmental process of leukaemia from a stem cell differentiated into lymphoid stem cells or myeloid stem cells

STEM CELL

Lymphoid stem cells

Myeloid stem cells

Acute lymphocytic leukaemia (ALL)

Chronic lymphocytic leukaemia (CLL)

Acute myelocytic leukaemia (AML)

Chronic myelocytic leukaemia (CML)

Chronic leukaemia has a slow onset and development and life expectancy is about 5 years. This rarely affects people under the age of 20 and the incidence increases with age, being most common between 60 and 70 years. Chronic lymphocytic leukaemia is uncommon in persons under 40 years.

The clinical signs of leukaemia are given in Box 14.4.

The precise cause of leukaemia remains a mystery. Research has suggested that certain substances, for example benzene or large doses of radiation, are responsible. Immunological defects and viral infections have also been thought to be responsible.

Diagnostic tests

- Full blood count
- lumbar puncture
- nuclear scanning
- lymphangiography.

Box 14.4 Clinical signs of leukaemia

- Anaemia
- Weight loss
- Epistaxis, bruising, retinal haemorrhage
- Bone and joint pain
- Fatigue
- Fever
- Infection – mouth ulcers, urinary tract infection
- Purpura

Nursing management of malignant disorders of the immune system

Modern treatment is encouraging, producing remissions in the progress of the disease. Some children and a similar number of adults will be cured. For the fortunate few, bone marrow transplant offers a cure for young leukaemic victims; research into these conditions looks promising.

Many of the nursing problems arise as a consequence of treatment with cytotoxic chemotherapy, steroids and antibiotic therapy. Certain conditions require cranial or testicular radiation.

Cytotoxic chemotherapy   These drugs kill rapidly dividing cells by interrupting normal cell synthesis. The drugs do not distinguish between tumours and healthy tissue. Therefore healthy tissues that have rapidly dividing cells, for example hair, mucosal tissue of the gastrointestinal tract, the gonads and the bone marrow, may also be damaged. Cytotoxic agents depress the bone marrow leaving the patient vulnerable to opportunistic commensals. Steroids are also used to suppress lymphopoiesis in patients with certain leukaemias and lymphomas. Table 14.4 indicates some of the cytotoxic agents used.

Some of the side-effects of chemotherapy are:

1. Alopecia – although this is short term, this hair loss can cause great distress.

2. Epistaxis and gastrointestinal bleeding; bruising due to thrombocytopenia may further exacerbate anaemia.

Table 14.4 Some of the drugs used in cytotoxic chemotherapy

Group	Drug	Side-effects
Alkylating agents	Busulphan	Myelosuppression. Loss of bone marrow function. Hyperpigmentation may occur in some patients
	Chlorambucil	Nausea. Gastrointestinal disturbances. Bone marrow depression is less severe
	Cyclophosphamide	Nausea. Haemorrhagic vomiting. Cystitis
Antimetabolites	Cytarabine	Hyperuricaemia. Depression of bone marrow
	Fluorouracil	Nausea. Gastrointestinal disturbance. Leucopenia. Alopecia
Cytotoxic antibiotics	Aclarubicin	Nausea. Vomiting. Leucopenia. Thrombocytopenia
	Actinomycin D	Bone marrow depression. Gastrointestinal disturbance. Stomatitis
Vinca alkaloids	Vincristine	Gastrointestinal disturbance. Constipation. Weight loss. Polyuria. Alopecia

3. Nausea and vomiting – some agents cause diarrhoea, while others cause constipation.

4. Paralytic ileus.

5. Gingivitis and taste changes.

6. Oral ulceration.

Cytotoxic drugs used singly are of little use, but the more aggressive use of a combination of drugs has proved effective. Red cell and platelet transfusions may be given at intervals to maintain the haemoglobin level above 10 g/dl and to control bleeding problems caused by thrombocytopenia.

The patient's problems fall into three distinct areas:

1. The patient's realization that he/she has a life-threatening illness.

2. The side-effects of the treatment and alteration in body image.

3. The need for maintenance therapy involving further admissions to hospital and an uncertain future.

Nurses need to have the skills and knowledge to enable them to plan their nursing management of the patient on an individual basis. The patient is faced with the realization that he may soon die which may precipitate a crisis – the patient will have to go through the stages of the grieving process of shocked disbelief, anger 'why me', and depression, before coming to terms with his condition. Anger is common, and the nurse may well be the focus of this. Knowledge of this behaviour allows the nurse to provide support and involve others such as a religious advisor or counsellor as appropriate. Both the family and the patient may take time to accept the situation,

and over this time nurses can provide support by allowing both parties to express their fears, answering questions honestly about the patient's condition and the treatment. It is important that both medical staff and nursing staff are giving the patient and relatives the same information and are united in putting the needs of the individual and his family first. Family members may find it difficult to put on a brave face when visiting a loved one as they, too, are consumed by anxiety about the future. The nurse can advise about self-help groups that are available where relatives can discuss their fears with others that are undergoing the same difficulties.

Cytotoxic chemotherapy can delay or sometimes cure the disease but the side-effects can cause great distress and discomfort to the patient. To prevent exogenous infection, infection control policies must be strictly adhered to. Special care must be taken by nurses and others involved in the patient's care to prevent cross-infection, hand washing being vitally important. It is important to restrict the number of visitors, and educate relatives, so that no person with an infection visits, including small children who may have been in contact with an infection that can be potentially life-threatening to the patient. Patients undergoing intensive cytotoxic chemotherapy may well require to be in protective isolation because of the effect of the cytotoxic agents depressing the bone marrow. The decision to use isolation is influenced by individual circumstances and available facilities. This can be achieved in several ways:

1. A purpose-built unit which has a filtered air supply. A series of single rooms with integral toilets

and showers. A hatch system allows the transfer of equipment and food without affecting the air pressure.

2. Plastic isolator. A framework erected around a single bed from which a PVC tent is suspended. The tent has an air supply attached to inflate the whole tent. A less-enclosed variation is shown in Figure 14.6.

Isolation of a patient can cause distress to an already ill individual. Careful explanation must be given and access to nursing staff must be easily available. Relatives must also be informed so that they can fully co-operate with the restrictions.

Oral complications are common in patients receiving chemotherapy. Mucositis induced by cytotoxic agents causes mucosal thickening, sloughing and redness leading to ulceration of the mouth. These problems can be further compounded by infection. The most common oral infections are caused by gram-negative bacteria (e.g. pseudomonas, klebsiella, serratia and enterobacter), viruses and fungi (e.g. *Candida albicans*). These infections cause severe pain to the patient who will be reluctant to eat or drink. The nurse's role in assessment of oral status is vital and maintenance of oral hygiene is a nursing responsibility.

The aim of oral hygiene is to keep the oral mucosa clean, soft, moist and intact. The lips should be prevented from becoming dry and cracked. Frequent cleaning and removal of debris using a soft toothbrush or sponge can prevent the development of plaque and development of mouth ulcers. Any oral infection should be identified quickly and treated aggressively. Oral hygiene is an integral part of the patient's care and will improve the quality of his life.

Weight loss and anorexia are common. The patient should be weighed daily. The nutritional needs of the patient require a team approach involving the dietician, nurses and most important of all the patient. The diet should contain all the vital elements but also take into account the likes and dislikes of the patient and the patient's ability to eat.

Fluid and electrolyte balance should be monitored carefully as reduced fluid intake can increase the risk of toxic side-effects on the liver and kidneys.

Diarrhoea and constipation can cause distress and these problems must be identified and treated with the appropriate medications.

Vomiting is also a very distressing side-effect of some cytotoxic agents and can prove very distressing for the patient. Drugs are available to control vomiting. The patient requires a lot of support during these episodes.

If sterility is a cause for concern the availability of sperm banking before commencement of treatment is offered.

Chemotherapy can cause alopecia and these changes in body image can cause great distress. Some of the distress can be alleviated by allowing the patient a choice of wig or hair piece before commencement of treatment. During the course of treatment the patient's image of himself changes – some find their body repugnant due to the disease. They may have excessive reactions towards the side-effects of chemotherapy, but this is often a way of expressing grief at the knowledge of diagnosis. The nurse is usually at the receiving end of this seemingly irrational behaviour and should be able to listen and support the patient through this difficult time. The patient will be very sensitive towards the behaviour of others and relatives should be aware of these difficulties and try not to display shock or distress at the appearance of their loved one. This can cause tremendous stress for relatives and the nurse should be able to comfort and advise relatives and support the patient. The wishes

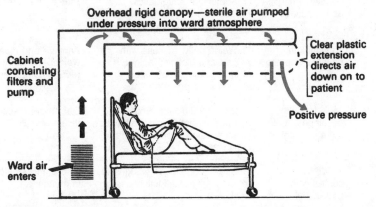

Fig. 14.6 Laminar flow isolation unit

of the patient must always take precedence – if the patient does not want visitors, this should be explained sensitively.

Activity intolerance related to the chemotherapy is a frequent problem. The patient will during the course of treatment feel exhausted and weak. He may also show signs of anaemia. The anaemia can be treated by the administration of red cell and platelet transfusions. The patient should be allowed to rest and sleep for long periods in a quiet and restful environment.

The patient's personal hygiene needs are important and the nurse can assist him with these as appropriate. The patient's skin should be examined at regular intervals for bruising and tissue damage. The use of bed aids will improve comfort and risk charts, for example the Norton scale, can be used to identify potential problems.

The overall aim of treatment is to produce a remission in the disease. Following initial treatment the patient will require maintenance therapy involving further admissions to hospital or treatment at home. If

Nursing Care Plan 14.3 Care plan for a patient with leukaemia			
Problem	**Goal**	**Nursing action**	**Rationale**
1. **Psychological problems**	To support the patient through the grieving process	❏ Provide counselling services for patient and family where appropriate. Explanations about disease ❏ Discuss type of wig before commencement of treatment. ❏ Scalp cooling if doxorubicin is used	Non-acceptance of diagnosis impairs progress Hair loss occurs due to chemotherapy. Raise morale Acts on rapidly dividing cells
2. **Sterility**		❏ Sperm banking arranged before commencement of treatment	Due to chemotherapy, sperm production may not recover after treatment
3. **Infection risk**	Reduce risk of infection	❏ Effective infection control policies. Strict aseptic technique	Due to depressed bone marrow and effects of chemotherapy
4. **Bruising. Bleeding**	To identify bruising episodes and take relevant action	❏ Packed cell and platelet transfusions to correct anaemia. Careful handling and lifting procedures	Due to anaemia, tissues fragile
5. **Dehydration**	To monitor fluid intake	❏ Recording of accurate fluid balance. Knowledge of normal electrolyte values, administration of appropriate supplements	Due to an inadequate fluid intake, some drugs cause toxicity
6. **Nausea and vomiting**	To relieve nausea and vomiting	❏ Administer antiemetics. Frequent oral hygiene. Assess for signs of dehydration	Effects of chemotherapy
7. **Anorexia**	To stimulate patient's appetite	❏ Weigh daily. Discuss with patient and dietician a light nutritional diet. Administer vitamin supplements	Achieve and maintain suitable body weight and nutritional status to reduce complications
8. **Mouth ulceration and infection**	To reduce the development of mouth ulceration	❏ Use of antibiotics. Encourage use of soft toothbrush, antiseptic mouthwashes, topical agents. Limit visitors	Due to depressed bone marrow, tissues fragile
9. **Pain**	To identify and control pain as necessary	❏ Use of continuous analgesia (pump). Assess effectiveness of analgesia	Due to mouth ulceration. Bone pain in myeloma

there is a recurrence of the problem this can cause deep depression. The nurse has an important role in providing support for both the patient and his/her relatives in these circumstances. Many of the patients are well known to the nursing staff in these units and a bond is formed between patients, relatives and nurse. The nurses find themselves sharing in both the joys and sorrows of the families in their care. A summary of nursing care is shown in Nursing Care Plan 14.3.

ACQUIRED IMMUNE DEFICIENCY SYNDROME

As recently as 10 years ago it was widely believed that infectious disease was no longer a threat in the developed world. Immunization programmes were going well; smallpox had been successfully eradicated worldwide in 1979. The remaining challenges were thought to be cancer, degenerative conditions and heart disease. However this confidence was soon shattered in the early 1980s by the advent of a killer disease known as the Acquired Immune Deficiency Syndrome (AIDS). The first cases occurred in the summer of 1981 in the USA. Reports began to appear of *Pneumocystis carinii* (a pneumonia) and Kaposi's sarcoma in young men who were homosexual and immunocompromised. At this time although the condition was recognized as acquired immune deficiency syndrome, the cause and method of transmission was unknown. The virus responsible was not identified until 1983. Despite the shock the scientific community responded quickly. The new virus was classified as the human immunodeficiency virus (HIV), viral targets were identified, and a blood test was formulated in 1984.

Ten years on, it is clear that this virus continues to outpace science. No cure or vaccine has yet been found, though present research looks more promising – maybe by the end of the decade a cure will be found.

What initially was thought to be an epidemic has now turned out to be a pandemic. In 1991 the World Health Organization (WHO) estimated that 40 million men, women and children will be infected with HIV, while the cumulative total of people suffering from full-blown AIDS will be 10 million by the year 2000 (Fig. 14.7). In Africa the virus has affected most of the continent. It is now recognized that cases of AIDS were first seen in the late 1970s. WHO has predicted that around 10 million children will become orphans because of AIDS deaths, and the extended family will

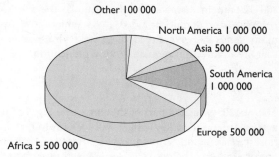

Fig. 14.7 Estimated adult HIV infections – 1991. (Source: WHO/GPA, Geneva)

no longer be there to protect them. Communities already affected by the effects of drought, famine and abject poverty will require both financial and social aid to enable them to survive. The main burden will fall on WHO and the western world to provide these resources. The situation in western countries has now reached epidemic proportions. The first documented death from AIDS in the UK occurred in late 1981.

AIDS is caused by a retrovirus

The retrovirus and its potential for causing cancer is not new. At the beginning of the century several investigators identified transmissible agents in animals that caused leukaemia. In 1980 the first human retrovirus was identified – the human T lymphotrophic virus or HTL-1 – which causes a highly malignant cancer called adult T cell leukaemia (ATL) that is endemic in Japan, Africa and the Caribbean.

What is so special about a retrovirus? Like other viruses the retrovirus cannot replicate without taking over the biosynthesis of the host cell and exploiting it for its own survival. The unique behaviour of a retrovirus allows it to reverse the flow of genetic information. The genetic material contained within the virus is RNA, there is no DNA. However, the enzyme reverse transcriptase uses the viral RNA for a template for making DNA. This DNA can integrate itself into the genome of the host, having taken up residence among the host's genes, the viral DNA will remain latent until the DNA is triggered into the production of new viral particles which will then go on to infect other cells. This latent DNA can also initiate a process that leads to tumour formation.

Special characteristics of the AIDS virus

The virus is icosahedral in shape (Fig. 14.8) and about

100–120 nm in diameter. The genome of the HIV is composed of double-stranded RNA which contains many genes that give directions to make viral proteins that are involved in regulating viral replication.

Pathophysiology

The gp120, (which is part of the virus (see Fig. 14.8)), acts as an antigenic key which will lock on to certain host cell receptors known as CD_4 receptors which are present on T helper cells, some macrophages and glial cells of the brain. HIV is known as a lymphotrophic virus due to its affinity to T cells.

The next stage involves the virus becoming bound to the host cell via the CD_4 receptors; it gains entry into the host cell either by endocytosis or, once the gp120 of the virus becomes locked on to the host cell, it becomes fused with the host cell's membrane and quickly enters the cytoplasm. Once inside the host the virus sheds its outer coat, and implants the RNA and its enzyme reverse transcriptase. Using this enzyme the viral genome copies itself from RNA to DNA. The new DNA then enters the host cell and incorporates itself into the hosts DNA becoming an integral part of the host cell. A latent period ensues.

The virus has now become a latent provirus which is sitting in the nucleus awaiting a signal. The trigger may be an infection causing reproduction of the host cell – the scene is now set. The host cell, now repro-grammed by the provirus, starts manufacturing more viruses. The host cell eventually explodes, releasing the viral material already programmed to attack healthy cells. This mechanism causes the host cell to die. The new viruses surround themselves with protein and lipid coats which they have 'stolen' from the host cell's cytoplasm. Once released, the viruses start searching for new target cells with CD_4 locks and the cycle begins again.

Modes of transmission

- Sexual transmission
- blood transfusion
- transplacental and prenatal transmission
- organ transplantation
- artificial insemination
- substance misuse – intravenous drug users.

Sexual transmission

Casual unprotected sex puts people at risk, whether they be homosexual, bisexual or heterosexual. Providing information, advice and education using the popular press, media coverage and targeting groups of all ages has to some extent made people more aware of the dangers of casual relationships without protection.

Blood transfusion

In the UK blood donors are screened before donating blood. The blood components are heated or chemically treated before transfusion. The risks of receiving infected blood abroad is still possible, some individuals travelling abroad now carry their own stored blood in case of accident.

Transplacental and prenatal transmission

Infection may be contracted in utero, during delivery and in the neonatal period. HIV infection in children was first reported in 1982, and since then the numbers have greatly increased worldwide, with the discovery of large numbers of infected children in Rumania.

Organ transplantation or artificial insemination by donor semen

Routine screening of potential donors is now accepted practice in the UK; however, this is not the case in

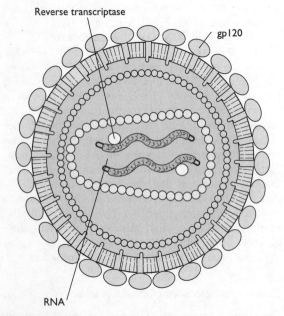

Reverse transcriptase

gp120

RNA

Fig. 14.8 Diagram of the HIV virus

other countries. People who think they are at risk should exclude themselves from becoming donors which will improve the present situation.

Substance misuse

Intravenous drug users are at risk from aquiring HIV infection from contaminated blood from shared needles and syringes. In some areas successful needle exchange schemes have been set up. This can work very well if the service is run from a local shop, is non-judgemental and is available 24 hours per day.

Development of the disease

Initial infection

Some but not all individuals develop an acute illness characterized by joint pains, diarrhoea and a maculo-papular rash. Some develop a non-septic meningitis or a generalized swelling of the lymph nodes. These symptoms can take up to 3 months to develop.

At this point the individual will start producing antibodies to HIV, this is known as seroconversion. Some infections are so slight they go unrecognized by the individual. Once seroconversion takes place the individual may remain symptomless for a prolonged period up to 11 years. It is currently not known how many people are in this category. Testing would have to be mandatory to know the true number of people infected, and even this would not give the true picture.

Stage 2: persistent generalized lymphadenopathy

This can present with palpable lymph node enlargement, with axillary and cervical lymph nodes most affected. Herpes zoster commonly develops and this is thought to be a poor prognostic sign.

Stage 3: AIDS-related complex

The great reduction in the individual's T cell population makes him more vulnerable to opportunistic infection, for example oral candidiasis. Other symptoms include intermittent or persistent diarrhoea, exhaustion, loss of weight, night sweats, fever, hairy leukoplakia and splenomegaly.

Stage 4: AIDS

Development of major opportunistic infection and cancer.

Only a few of the conditions will be mentioned here:

- *Pneumocystis carinii* – pneumonia
- *Mycobacterium tuberculosis* – tuberculosis.

This situation is becoming progressively more serious. It is estimated that three million people had dual infection in 1990, 78% in Africa.

Cancers (neoplastic disease)

About 5% of individuals develop neoplastic disease, the most common being the B cell lymphomas, CNS space-occupying tumours and Kaposi's sarcoma.

Neuropsychiatric syndromes

Medical treatment is primarily palliative, though recent advances suggest that the progress of the disease can be slowed down once stage 3 is reached with drug therapy. Commonly used drugs and their effects are shown in Table 14.5.

Nursing perspectives

Epidemics in the past have shown that the usual human behaviour is to apportion blame and endeavour to isolate or quarantine the afflicted. This may have been appropriate in diseases such as smallpox or plague where transmission was through casual contact. AIDS is not spread in this way but by deliberate human behaviour, especially sexual intercourse. Discrimination leads to secrecy in those who are or suspect they are infected; they may avoid contact with health and social services. AIDS threatens everyone. No one will be spared the effects even if they and their loved ones are never directly affected by the disease.

Table 14.5 Commonly used drugs for palliative management in stage 3 AIDS		
Drug name	Use	Side-effects
Ganciclovir	Effective against a wide range of human herpes viruses including cytomegalovirus	Neutropenia
Zidovudine	Stage 3 AIDS specific	Anaemia
Pentamidine	Pneumocystis carinii pneumonia	

Nurses need to be aware of the cause of AIDS, the behaviour of the virus and the way in which it is transmitted, to enable them to give factual information to the public if asked, diffusing popular myths. Patients suffering from AIDS-related disorders can be admitted to any general or psychiatric ward and the nurse working in all these areas should be able to care for the patient using a non-judgemental approach.

Assessment, planning individualized care and maintenance of confidentiality is every patient's right regardless of colour, race, creed, sexual persuasion or clinical condition.

Certain guidelines must be followed when nursing a patient with a potentially infectious condition. Many of these principles should be accepted practice whether the patient is infected or not. The guidelines outlined in Box 14.5 should allow all patients posing a risk of infection from HIV to be nursed in an open ward. Source isolation would only be instituted when there is external bleeding, for example haematemesis, melaena, or an uncontrolled loss of body fluids, as with uncontrolled diarrhoea. Some of these patients suffer from severe continuous diarrhoea where litres of fluid are lost at any one time.

Nurse's role in health education

Aims

To educate sexually active people to avoid and stop the spread of HIV This can be carried out by school nurses, health visitors and as part of the health board's remit to provide education in schools, youth groups and voluntary groups. Several of the schemes now in action are successfully raising awareness of the dangers of heterosexual spread. Very early on

in the epidemic the homosexual community was in the forefront of providing information about AIDS. Health education will also cover such aspects as safe sexual practices, use of condoms and avoiding multiple sexual partners. The media has been putting across this message for some time.

To stop the spread of AIDS amongst drug users One method in operation is the provision of a service for needle exchange in a non-threatening environment. This has been successful when carried out from a local shop within an area frequented by drug users. Another area has a nurse who is available to give advice to both prostitutes and drug users during unsocial hours, such as during the night.

To educate the general public about AIDS and routes of transmission This can be carried out by the media or nurses talking to groups. This allows some of the myths to be destroyed. Discrimination against people violates their basic human rights. What is needed is a united front in order to defeat the social effects of this disease and have in place community-based helplines.

Counselling and testing

No individual can be tested for HIV without giving their informed consent. Nurses are involved in counselling as part of their remit in clinics and special units.

Nurses counsel both in the pretest and post-test period. They may become involved in counselling on a professional or voluntary basis. They must understand why the test is being carried out. HIV testing is not an emergency situation so time can be given to the client to read the information about the advantages and disadvantages of being tested. If the client gives permission for the test to be carried out, the waiting period for the result can be very traumatic and counselling must be available at this time.

If previous behaviour has put the person in the risk category the test gives an opportunity to receive individual counselling and health education. If the test proves negative there is a chance to alter behaviour. If the test proves to be positive the client has the advantage of close monitoring of health status and opportunistic infections can be treated vigorously. Immunization can be offered against hepatitis B, pneumonia, influenza, which should be done while the immune system is still capable of responding to therapy. Drug therapy can be commenced in an effort to slow down the progression of the disease. For women a positive test can influence various decisions, such as whether to have children or to breast feed.

Box 14.5 Guidelines to prevent cross-infection when caring for an HIV infected person

- Cover cuts and skin abrasions on both patients and staff with a waterproof dressing
- Wear disposable gloves and plastic aprons when carrying out care that might involve skin contamination with body fluids, e.g. venepuncture, mouth care, haematemesis, vomiting or assisting with toilet needs
- Wash hands after delivering care, avoid eating or drinking where there is a potential for infection
- Take care to avoid situations where a patient's body fluids come into contact with skin, nose and mouth

Confidentiality is of the utmost importance, if test results become known to others, the individual could face rejection by friends, colleagues and family. There has been some publicity to ensure that people who have been tested for HIV are not penalized. Insurance companies have now stated that a healthy person who is tested negative for HIV with no added risk factors will not be discriminated against when applying for standard rate insurance.

Nursing in the community

Today it is possible that all members of the primary health care team will become involved in the nursing management of people with AIDS. When the time comes to discharge a patient from hospital it is in the client's best interests to have a support network set up to enable him to remain at home for as long as possible. The client must give permission for his diagnosis to be made known to the GP, failure to give this permission is fraught with difficulties for the client.

There is no reason why clients with AIDS and AIDS-related disorders cannot live at home with their families. The nurse is in the ideal position to give advice and support to the family with regard to health education. There is no risk of transmission as long as acceptable standards of hygiene are maintained in the home. Visits to pubs, restaurants, cinemas and public baths are quite permissible. Children who are infected should be allowed to attend school without discrimination.

Terminal care

Many clients with AIDS may require terminal care at home. This can be difficult if there is neurological dysfunction and lack of nursing support. The needs of the patient are the same as for any terminally ill patient, with attention to symptom control and the services of a twilight or night nursing input.

Some health boards employ a specialist district nurse to act as an expert resource for colleagues.

Hospices and special units

Many individuals suffering from AIDS prefer to be nursed in a special ward or unit within a general hospital or a hospice dealing exclusively with AIDS-related disease. Many patients feel more secure within these units because special care strategies have been developed to meet the complex psychosocial medical issues seen in these patients. The staff have been specially recruited and trained to enable them to deal with the complex issues associated with the disease. There is usually a counselling service within the unit for the staff to enable them to discuss their feelings and reduce their stress. The atmosphere is relaxed and in some hospices uniforms are not worn. There is usually an outpatient facility attached to the hospice so the patients can be cared for both within and outwith the hospice. The Lighthouse in London is a good example of Hospice Care.

Many services have appeared in recent years both in the voluntary sector, for example Milestone House Edinburgh, and within the Health Service (Adler 1987).

Examples of these are listed below:

- Action for AIDS, London
- Terrence Higgins Trust
- Body Positive UK
- Action on AIDS
- Harm Reduction Team Edinburgh
- Needle Exchange.

CHRONIC FATIGUE SYNDROME

Chronic fatigue syndrome has had many names in the past, including Royal Free disease, Iceland disease, myalgic encephalomyelitis and today postviral fatigue syndrome, and 'Yuppie' flu.

Numerous outbreaks of this condition have been reported over the past 50 years. The early symptoms suggested poliomyelitis but no muscle wasting occurred, and the polio virus was never isolated. It was called a new clinical entity and the condition known as benign myalgic encephalitis. No organic basis was found for the disease and the causes of chronic fatigue syndrome are poorly understood.

Clinical presentation

The patient is usually a previously healthy adult in the age group teens to early forties, with females predominating. The patient has a history of a viral illness, sore throat, pyrexia or gastrointestinal upset, but instead of recovering they continue to feel generally unwell and want to sleep all the time. Minimal physical exercise leaves them exhausted, loss of short-term memory and concentration are all features. The patient has periods of recovery followed by periods of complete exhaustion. As the fatigue increases, the performance of tasks involving fine movements become clumsy. There may be an alteration in thermoregulatory control with insensitivity to temperature extremes. These symptoms tend to be chronic and vary in severity from day to day. The symptoms can remain for a prolonged period of time from 6 months to 2 years.

Due to the lack of knowledge about the condition patients have found that many doctors have been less than sympathetic towards them. In some instances the patient is labelled a malingerer, or a hysteric. Chronic fatigue syndrome is difficult to diagnose because the symptoms can be similar to those of other illnesses, such as myasthenia gravis, depression, hypothyroidism and systemic lupus erythematosis to name but a few.

Failure to make the diagnosis may result in insufficient support from social services and DHSS.

Implications for management

The patient requires a lot of support during the period of his illness. Although the individual may not be admitted to hospital, help will be required at home, especially if he is living alone. An understanding of the condition and a supportive GP make the patient feel that he is legitimately ill. Visits from the district nurse and help from the social services may be appropriate to encourage patients to have a positive attitude towards their illness, helping them to focus on what they can do and engendering a belief that they will recover.

Psychoanalysis can sometimes benefit the patient and joining a counselling self-help group is useful in providing a supportive environment in which the patient can share his experiences with others. Relatives require support so that they can fully understand that the patient is genuinely ill, which is often hard to accept when the individual has been fit and active.

Suggested assignments

1. Plan a diet suitable for an adolescent suffering from iron deficiency anaemia. What factors would you take into account?
2. Find out where the self-help groups are in your area to help patients suffering from leukaemia, AIDS and chronic fatigue syndrome.
3. Discuss the implications of a diagnosis of haemophilia on an individual's personal life, work and leisure pursuits.

REFERNCES AND FURTHER READING

Adler M W (ed) 1987 ABC of AIDS. British Medical Journal, London

Aggleton P et el 1992 AIDS Rights, Risk and Reason. Falmer Press

Anthony D Chronic fatigue syndrome: Signs of a new approach. British Journal of Hospital Medicine. Mar. 1991, Vol. 45, No. 3 p 158–163

Belcher A E 1993 Blood disorder. Clinical nursing series. Mosby, St Louis

Contreras M (ed) 1990 ABC of blood transfusion. British Medical Journal, London

Cusack L, Singh S 1994 HIV and AIDS Care. Chapman Hall

Dale S Understanding myalgic encephalomyelitis. Professional Nurse. Mar. 1991, Vol. 6 No. 6 p. 339–340

Edwards R W C, Bouchier I A B (eds) 1991 Davidson's principles and practice of medicine, 16th edn. Churchill Livingstone, Edinburgh

Goodnick P J, Klimas N G 1993 Chronic Fatigue and Related Immune Deficiency Syndromes. American Psychiatric Press Inc. Chapter 1, 2 & 3

Gould P 1993 The slow plague. Blackwell, Oxford

Haak–Flaskerud J, Unguarski P J 1992 HIV/AIDS. A guide to nursing care, 2nd edn. W B Saunders Co.

Jamieson E M, McCall J M, Blythe R 1992 Guidelines for clinical nursing practices, 2nd edn. Churchill Livingstone, Edinburgh

Kirkwood E, Lewis C 1989 Understanding Medical Immunology, 2nd edn. John Wiley & Sons. Section C

Pratt R 1991 AIDS: a strategy for nursing care, 3rd edn. Hodder & Stoughton, New York

Pritchard A P, David J A 1988 The Royal Marsden Hospital Manual of clinical nursing procedures, 2nd edn. Harper Collins, New York

Reamer F G (ed) 1991 AIDS and ethics. Columbia University Press, New York

Shepherd C Myalgic encephalomyelistis – is it a real disease? Practitioner 8th Jan, 1989 p 41

Tiffany R, Webb P 1998 Oncology for Nurses and Health Care Professionals, 2nd edn. Vol. 2 Care and Support

Tortora G J, Anagnostakos P 1990 Principles of anatomy and physiology, 6th edn. Harper Collins, New York

Trounce J 1990 Clinical pharmacology for nurses, 13th edn. Churchill Livingstone, New York

15

Care implications of disorders of the gastrointestinal system

Dorothy Horsburgh

INTRODUCTION

The attitudes which any society has in relation to the ingestion of food and drink and the elimination of waste will be conveyed to its members at a very early age and subsequently reinforced throughout their life-span. These attitudes thus have a potentially powerful influence. If an individual suffers from a disorder which affects their ability to eat, drink or eliminate in a manner which is considered to be acceptable by the society in which they live, then this is likely to have psychosocial, in addition to physical, consequences. The implications for those who care for people suffering from disorders of the gastrointestinal system therefore involve a knowledge not only of the physical processes involved and the physical care required, but also a knowledge of the social and behavioural sciences. (See also Chs 1 and 2.)

ANATOMY AND PHYSIOLOGY

The gastrointestinal tract is a muscular tube about 9 m in length, into which secretions from accessory organs drain (Fig. 15.1). Food and fluids which are ingested into the mouth are reduced in size by the action of the teeth, tongue and the muscles of the jaw and cheek. This chewing action stimulates the salivary glands to increase secretion of saliva, which contains the enzyme salivary amylase. The saliva acts as a lubricant, thus facilitating swallowing and, once food is in the stomach, the minor part which salivary amylase plays in carbohydrate breakdown begins.

From the mouth the food passes through the cricopharyngeal sphincter into the oesophagus and into the stomach by means of peristalsis.

Food enters the stomach via the lower oesophageal (cardiac) sphincter, which prevents regurgitation of stomach contents into the oesophagus.

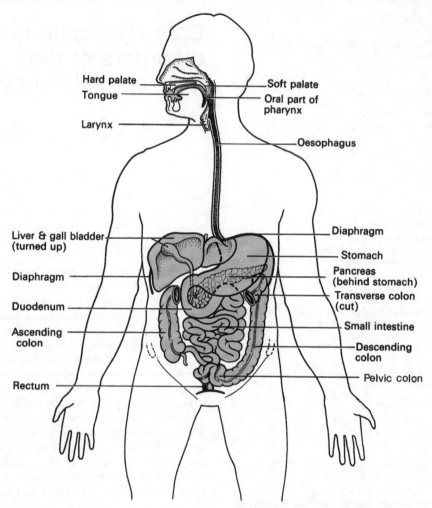

Fig. 15.1 The digestive tract and associated organs. (Reproduced with permission from Wilson 1990, p. 162)

The stomach acts as a reservoir for food and fluids and continues the mechanical breakdown of food by means of muscular contraction into a semi-solid substance called chyme. The sight, smell and taste of food causes the vagus nerve to stimulate gastric secretions and when food reaches the pyloric antrum which forms the lower end of the stomach, the hormone gastrin is secreted which has a stimulatory effect on gastric secretion in the body of the stomach.

Pepsinogen is released from peptic cells, activated into the proteolytic enzyme pepsin by hydrochloric acid (secreted by oxyntic cells), and commences chemical protein breakdown. Intrinsic factor (a glycoprotein) is also secreted, the presence of which is necessary for absorption of vitamin B_{12} in the small in-testine. Hydrochloric acid has the additional function of destruction of some potentially harmful bacteria which may be present in ingested food and fluid.

The latter portion of the stomach, the antrum, secretes alkaline mucus which reduces the acidity of stomach contents prior to their passage into the small intestine. This progression occurs at a controlled rate through the pyloric sphincter. The mucous layer of the stomach contains bicarbonate ions, which provides a protective barrier from the potentially damaging acidity of hydrochloric acid.

Both the small and large intestine are under autonomic nervous system control and have a broadly similar basic structure (Fig. 15.2), the anatomy of each section being related to its specific function. Epithelial

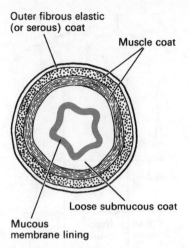

Outer fibrous elastic
(or serous) coat

Muscle coat

Loose submucous coat

Mucous
membrane lining

Fig. 15.2   Cross-section of gastrointestinal tract

cells in the gastrointestinal tract are rapidly removed and replaced; for example, in the small intestine this occurs every 48 hours. Desquamated cells are digested and recyclable components reabsorbed.

The entry of food into the duodenum triggers the

release of the hormone secretin, which stimulates pancreatic exocrine secretions – bicarbonate and the enzymes amylase, lipase and proteolytic enzymes. The hormone cholecystokinin is also released, which stimulates contraction of the gallbladder and the release of bile (secreted by the liver and concentrated and stored in the gallbladder). Bile enters the duodenum via the ampulla of Vater (Fig. 15.3) and plays a vital role in the breakdown of dietary fats.

Enteric hormones stimulate the release of succus entericus within the small intestine, which contains bicarbonate and additional digestive enzymes. The chyme mixes with the bicarbonate, bile and enzymes and as it progresses by means of peristalsis through the duodenum, jejunum and ileum digestion of protein, carbohydrate and fat continues. Following digestion of food components, absorption of the chemicals and nutrients takes place across the villi walls into the bloodstream and lymphatic system.

The residue passes from the small intestine via the ileo-caecal valve into the large intestine. During its progression through the caecum and ascending colon large quantities of water are absorbed from the contents and this process continues to a lesser extent

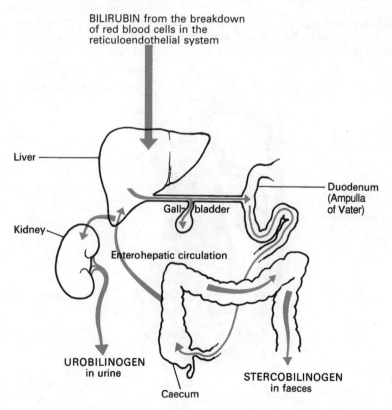

BILIRUBIN from the breakdown
of red blood cells in the
reticuloendothelial system

Liver

Duodenum
(Ampulla
of Vater)

Gall-bladder

Kidney

Enterohepatic circulation

UROBILINOGEN
in urine

STERCOBILINOGEN
in faeces

Caecum

Fig. 15.3   The formation and excretion of bile

during its progression through the transverse, descending and sigmoid (or pelvic) colon. The longer the residue remains in the large intestine the greater the amount of water absorbed from it and the more solid the faecal material becomes.

When faeces enter the rectum, stretch receptors stimulate a desire to defaecate and the internal anal sphincter relaxes. With maturation of the central nervous system the external anal sphincter comes under voluntary control and defaecation may be initiated or suppressed.

The stomach, small and large intestine, liver, pancreas and gallbladder are contained within the abdominal cavity. The abdomen is anatomically identified as having nine distinct regions (Fig. 15.4). The peritoneum, a two-layered serous membrane, lines the abdominal cavity, providing a covering and support for the organs within it (Fig. 15.5). Thickened folds of peritoneum (the mesentery, transverse and pelvic mesocolon) support the blood vessels and nerves which supply the organs. The large anterior fold of peritoneum is called the omentum. This provides a support for blood and lymphatic vessels and, in the event of peritonitis, may confine and localize infection.

The gastrointestinal tract and organs receive additional support from the muscles of the anterior abdominal wall, the pelvic muscles and the diaphragm.

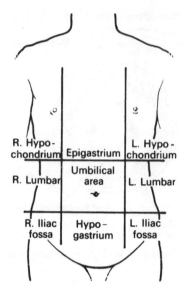

Fig. 15.4 Regions of the abdomen

The physiological effects of ageing upon the gastrointestinal system

As people age, their taste buds, especially those responsible for the appreciation of sweet and salt tastes, reduce in size and number. The chewing force exerted by the jaw and cheek muscles may also

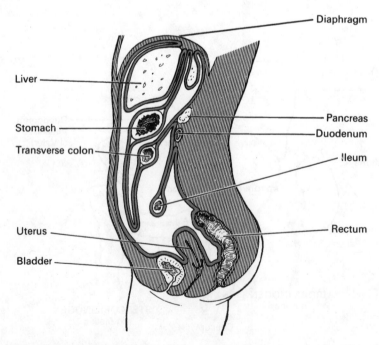

Fig. 15.5 The peritoneum

reduce and, additionally, the person may require to have some or all of their teeth removed as a result of tooth decay or gum disease.

Lower oesophageal (cardiac) sphincter pressure is reduced and this may result in oesophageal reflux of gastric contents. Gastric and pancreatic secretions reduce, but without significant reduction in digestive ability. Hepatic metabolism of drugs is also reduced.

Peristaltic movement may become less vigorous and this, if coupled with reduced mobility, may increase the time taken for the contents of the tract to progress.

EPIDEMIOLOGY AND AETIOLOGY

Epidemiology and aetiology are diverse and detail will be given in discussion relating to specific disorders. There are however, certain factors which may exert an influence on the gastrointestinal system.

Diet

Dietary imbalance may result from either an inappropriate nutritional intake, or from an inability to absorb ingested nutrients.

The ingestion of alcohol in excessive amounts may cause inflammation of the tract, an inability to absorb certain nutrients, or damage to associated organs, for example the liver and the pancreas.

Food and personal hygiene

Social deprivation, overcrowding, poor sanitation, lack of relevant health education or laxity in standards of cleanliness may result in disease. Infectious disorders of the gastrointestinal system may be spread by the faecal–oral route, or by inappropriate storage or preparation of food. Those at particular risk of developing severe illness as a result of infection are infants, elderly people, or those who have a compromised immune system.

Psychosocial factors

Emotional factors, such as anxiety, may influence the functioning of the gastrointestinal tract and may cause nausea, vomiting and/or diarrhoea.

GENERAL FEATURES OF DISORDER

It is important to obtain the patient's account of their signs and symptoms, including the location and duration of these and any precipitating or relieving factors.

There may be more than one cause of many of the features and clinical investigations may have to be undertaken before a diagnosis can be made.

Pain

Pain is a common symptom and may be caused by:

- Abnormally strong smooth muscle contractions which cause colic, either within the tract or within accessory organs such as the gallbladder.
- Erosion of the lining of the tract, causing inflammation and possible ulceration.
- Perforation of an organ, resulting in inflammation and probable infection of the peritoneum, i.e. peritonitis.
- Swelling of an organ due to stretching of its capsule, e.g. the liver in hepatitis.

Pain may occur at the site of origin of a disorder or may be referred to, and experienced in, another area.

Alteration in eating habits

This may take the form of loss of appetite (anorexia), or the avoidance of certain foods/fluids which aggravate the person's signs and symptoms.

Waterbrash

This is due to a sudden overactivity of the salivary glands and is a reflex reponse to a number of upper gastrointestinal problems. It may also occur as a prelude to vomiting.

Nausea/vomiting

These common signs and symptoms have many causes, both physical and emotional.

Heartburn

This is the sensation of burning retrosternal pain or discomfort and may be caused for example by inflammation of the oesophagus (oesophagitis).

Regurgitation

This may be caused by an obstruction within the oesophagus (e.g. tumour), or may be the result of reflux of gastric contents. If due to the latter the person will complain of a bitter, acid taste in the mouth when the regurgitation occurs.

Dysphagia

This term denotes difficulty or pain when swallowing and may be due to obstruction either within the oesophagus itself or from adjacent structures (e.g. tumour in the respiratory tract).

Flatulence

Air which is ingested will usually be eructated from the oesophagus or stomach. If there is a gastric outlet obstruction, for example pyloric stenosis, the person may complain of excessive eructation, which may additionally be foul smelling. Gas which accumulates in the large intestine, whether due to air ingestion or digestive processes, will be passed as flatus per rectum.

Following general anaesthesia individuals may be unable to eructate ingested air, which may then accumulate in excessive amounts in the intestine. The person may then be unable to pass this per rectum until they become mobile, which is one of the reasons why early postoperative mobilization is beneficial.

Alteration in bowel habit

Bowel habit varies greatly from one individual to another; this means that the 'normal' pattern of defaecation is considered to range from passage of stool once per day to three times per week. If the stool is hard and difficult to pass then the person is defined as being constipated, regardless of the frequency of defaecation. If the stool is liquid or semi-formed this is likewise regarded as abnormal, regardless of the frequency with which it occurs.

Bowel habit may be greatly influenced by dietary intake. Foods which contain a high fibre content, especially if taken in conjunction with a high fluid intake, will promote the formation of a soft, bulky stool, whereas a low intake of dietary fibre and a low fluid intake will result in formation of a harder, drier stool.

Other factors which may affect bowel habit are exercise; physical immobility tends to reduce peristaltic activity within the gastrointestinal tract, thus predisposing to constipation. The length of time taken for food to pass through the tract additionally influences the amount of water reabsorption which occurs from the faecal mass through the walls of the large intestine, a longer transit time equalling increased fluid reabsorption.

As bile plays a vital role in the digestion of fats any reduction in, or absence of, bile flow due to obstruction within the biliary system will result in incom-

plete fat digestion and absorption. Partially digested, or undigested, fat will therefore be present in the faeces (steatorrhoea). Faeces will be pale (stercobilinogen, a bile pigment, provides faeces with their characteristic colour). The presence of fat will cause the faeces to be bulky in appearance, foul smelling and difficult to flush from the lavatory bowl. Certain vitamins, including vitamin K, are fat soluble and an inability to absorb fat may lead to a deficiency in these vitamins. (See Ch. 4 for details of the roles played by fat-soluble vitamins.)

As was stated earlier, with maturation of the central nervous system, control of the external anal sphincter is gained and this results in the ability to resist the desire to defaecate. This suppression of the desire to defaecate results in reabsorption of increased amounts of fluid from the unpassed stool and, as the desire to defaecate is unlikely to recur for several hours, the stool will subsequently prove more difficult to expel.

As can be seen from the above, the variations in bowel habits from one individual to another make it vitally important that a history of the person's dietary habits, 'normal' bowel habits and defaecation patterns is obtained, in order to help identify any abnormality.

Alteration in an individual's normal bowel habit may be symptomatic of serious bowel disorder, for example carcinoma of the colon, and thus always requires further investigation.

Diarrhoea

This refers to the passage of liquid or very loosely formed faeces, which usually occurs more than once per day.

Acute diarrhoea may be caused by dietary indiscretion, particularly of foods which have a high fat content, excessive intake of alcohol, particularly of beer, or gastrointestinal infection.

Chronic diarrhoea is a symptom of several disorders; one example is ulcerative colitis.

Constipation

Acute constipation is usually organic in origin resulting, for example, from intestinal obstruction.
Chronic constipation may be caused by the predisposing factors outlined earlier in this section.

Intestinal haemorrhage

Bleeding in the upper gastrointestinal tract may cause haematemesis, that is vomiting of blood. If the blood remains within the stomach for even a relatively short time, partial digestion will occur, and the vomitus will be brown in colour and granular; this is referred to as 'coffee ground vomit'. Bleeding which occurs further down the tract may cause melaena, resulting in the passage of a stool which is black and sticky.

Severe bleeding within the tract may cause both haematemesis and melaena. If the bleeding is rapid or severe its appearance in the stool may be little altered and may be bright red. (Bright red bleeding in small or moderate amounts per rectum may also however indicate the presence of haemorrhoids.)

Chronic, slow bleeding may result in anaemia over a period of time, but may not be macroscopically visible in the stool. The presence of occult blood in the faeces can be detected by the use of clinical reagents.

Weight loss

This may be caused by a reduced dietary intake, for example in a person desiring to lose weight.

Weight loss is frequently a symptom in individuals who are unable to ingest or retain food due to nausea, vomiting or loss of appetite, or who avoid certain foods which they identify as being causative of symptoms such as pain, heartburn or dysphagia. Weight loss may also be a result of malabsorption of nutrients in the small intestine, or protein loss from a diseased colon. Carcinoma is also a common gastrointestinal cause of weight loss.

INVESTIGATIONS OF DISORDER

Gastrointestinal investigations may be lengthy, exhausting and perceived by the patient as being undignified and even humiliating. The person undergoing such investigations may feel physically unwell as a result of their underlying disorder and psychologically anxious as to the possible causes of their signs and symptoms.

It is important that, prior to any investigation being carried out, its purpose is explained carefully to the patient, as well as what is entailed for the patient and what is expected of them whilst it is being carried out. Any physical preparation which is required in order to carry out the investigation must also be explained. The patient should additionally be invited to ask any questions which they may have.

Prior to certain investigative procedures the patient's informed consent is required; it is the responsibility of the medical staff to obtain this. Investigations may be carried out on people who are outpatients, or who are hospitalized.

During investigations to which the nurse accompanies the patient her role is the provision of physical and psychological support. The latter role includes ensuring maximum maintenance of the patient's privacy and dignity, providing reinforcement of previous explanations and acting as the patient's advocate if necessary (see Ch. 3).

Following investigation the patient should be made physically comfortable and any further queries should be answered. Findings, and the implications of these, should be explained as soon as these become available. The patient may require additional psychological support, as may their significant others, at this time.

Information relating to some of the investigations which are discussed in the following sections may also be found in Chapter 4.

Initial investigations

This includes discussion with the patient in order to obtain a medical and nursing history. The latter differs from the former in that its focus is not the disease process, but the patient's actual or potential physical and psychosocial problems. Once these have been identified nursing goals may be set, with the aim of alleviating or preventing the occurrence of problems. Nursing actions are then identified, which are necessary for goal achievement. Evaluation of the effectiveness, or otherwise, of the nursing actions is carried out by an experienced nurse at regular intervals throughout the patient's stay in hospital. (See Ch. 3 for a detailed description of the nursing process and models of nursing.)

Medical staff will carry out a physical examination of the patient, which will include inspection, palpation, percussion and auscultation of the gastrointestinal and other body systems. Digital examination of the patient's rectum may also be carried out as an aid to diagnosis.

Nursing staff will obtain recordings of the patient's temperature, pulse, respirations and blood pressure. In addition to identifying any abnormalities of these on admission, the recordings are used to provide a baseline for comparison with subsequent recordings.

Examination of faeces may be carried out. The presence of occult blood may be detected using clinical reagents, or specimens may be sent for laboratory analysis to ascertain for example whether bacteria or other organisms are present. It may be necessary for some specimens to be maintained at body temperature from the time of collection and during transit to the laboratory. This is achieved by the use of a special flask ('hot stool' specimen).

It may also be necessary to collect all stools passed by the patient for a period of several days in order to carry out faecal fat estimation.

Radiological examination

Plain radiographs

Abdominal X-rays will illustrate soft tissue shadows of the liver, spleen, kidneys and the presence of any abnormal shadows. Opacities caused by calculi or calcification of organs may also be demonstrated. Gas within the gastrointestinal tract acts as a contrast medium and can help to identify the position of the intestine within the abdominal cavity. Fluid levels within the tract may also be identified; these may be clearly visible, for example, in patients who have intestinal obstruction.

Chest X-rays will illustrate the diaphragm. If gas is present under the diaphragm, this may indicate that perforation of the gastrointestinal tract has taken place. Possible thoracic origins of pain referred to the abdomen may also be identified.

Barium studies

Barium is a radio-opaque substance which may be ingested orally or instilled rectally. It is used to identify abnormalities of the gut mucosa and gut motility and irregularities in organ outlines.

Although barium may be artificially flavoured in order to minimize the unpleasantness of its intrinsic taste, it is likely that it will prove mildly unpleasant for the patient who is required to ingest it. As barium has a constipating effect it may be necessary for the patient to be prescribed an oral aperient or rectal enema following the studies, whether these have been conducted orally or rectally. A high roughage diet, accompanied by an increased fluid intake, may alternatively be recommended.

Barium swallow/barium meal

Prior to barium swallow/meal it is necessary for the patient to fast, usually for approximately 6–8 hours, in order to ensure that the upper gastrointestinal tract is empty.

This investigation will demonstrate abnormalities of the oesophagus and stomach. In order to enhance the image of the stomach on the film a double contrast may be achieved by utilization of a small amount of barium in conjunction with introduction of gas to the stomach in order to distend it.

Barium follow-through involves repeat X-rays being taken at regular intervals for several hours following ingestion of barium in order to follow its progress through the small intestine and identify any existing abnormalities.

Barium enema

Prior to this investigation it is necessary to ensure that the large intestine is cleared of faeces. This may be achieved by the oral administration of laxatives and by the ingestion of a low roughage diet for several days prior to the examination. (The patient should be warned that the laxatives may cause diarrhoea and urgency.) Alternatively an enema or colonic lavage may be required.

It is usually unnecessary for the patient to fast immediately prior to the barium enema and a light meal and fluids may be given.

Instillation of barium, which takes place in the X-ray department, may cause the patient physical discomfort, and emotional distress at the possibility that they may be unable to retain the barium and may be 'incontinent'. Reassurance can be given that, although this does sometimes occur, it is not faeces that will be expelled but only barium. Given that society considers that adult failure to control bowel function is demeaning and socially unacceptable the patient may, despite reassurance, feel embarrassment and humiliation if this does occur. Following the taking of X-ray films the patient should be offered the opportunity to evacuate the barium in the lavatory prior to leaving the radiology department.

During all barium studies the patient may be tilted on the X-ray table in order to ensure the uptake of barium by as much of the organ and tract mucosa as possible and this may be physically uncomfortable for the patient.

Imaging studies

Computerized tomography (CT) and magnetic resonance imaging (MRI)

These investigations are painless, but the positions which the patient undergoing them is required to assume may cause them discomfort. CT and MRI are of particular value in visualization of organs and regions which are inaccessible to investigation by other means. Examples of their use are in the diagnosis of pancreatic disease, such as acute pancreatitis and carcinoma of the pancreas. They are also used in the assessment of tumour spread to adjacent or distant organs.

Ultrasound

The presence of cysts and abcesses may be identified by this means. If the organ to be examined is the gallbladder the patient will require to fast before the examination in order to prevent its stimulation.

Radionuclide screening

This provides diagnostic information about the liver and spleen and can also be utilized to locate the approximate site of haemorrhage.

Endoscopy

Endoscopy is the examination, under direct vision, of the lining of a tube or organ, by means of an instrument which has a light at the distal end. This instrument may be a rigid or flexible tube which is warmed and lubricated prior to use. Examination of the oesophagus, rectum and lower third of the sigmoid colon are usually carried out using rigid instruments, whereas for endoscopy of the stomach, duodenum and large intestine a flexible instrument is used. During endoscopy samples of secretions and/or tissue may be obtained.

Physical risks to the patient during endoscopy are that perforation of the area which is under examination, or through which the tube is being passed, may occur. During endoscopy inhalation of secretions may occur, or cardiac arrhythmias or arrest may be stimulated. There is also the risk of infection transmission, either as a result of inadequate cleansing of equipment between patients, or by transmission of infection from one area of the person's body to another by means of the tube. These complications are rare provided that care is taken to minimize the potential risks, but the patient must be observed both during, and subsequent to, the procedure in order to identify complications should they occur.

Endoscopy of the upper gastrointestinal tract

The patient is fasted for 12 hours prior to this procedure. Several minutes before the tube is passed the patient's pharynx is anaesthetized, using for example lignocaine spray, and the patient is given intravenous sedation. This is sufficient to cause drowsiness and allay anxiety, but does not cause unconsciousness and the patient will be able to swallow when requested to do so in order to pass the instrument.

The patient will be unable to speak during the procedure and it is therefore important that they have some means of communicating distress. This may for example be achieved by prior arrangement with the patient to hold the nurse's hand during the procedure and to squeeze it if they are in distress. It is also important that the procedure is re-explained to the patient whilst it is taking place. This should provide reassurance and should additionally reinforce to the patient the fact that someone is with him and that they as an individual are the focus of attention.

Dependent upon the sedative used, the patient may experience retrograde amnesia, that is they will subsequently be able to remember little or nothing of the procedure.

The effect of the local anaesthesia may interfere with the patient's swallow reflex for approximately 4 hours following its administration and it is vital that this has returned prior to the patient ingesting food or fluids. The patient should be asked to swallow and the exterior of their throat observed for the rise and fall of the laryngeal cartilage which accompanies successful swallowing. To confirm the patient's ability to swallow only small sips of water should initially be given. If these are tolerated food and fluids may be given, as allowed by the patient's physical condition.

Oesophagoscopy In addition to investigation of disorder, oesophagoscopy may be undertaken in order to dilate a stricture. This is known as **bouginage** and, as there is the possibility that trauma will be caused to the oesophagus, aftercare of the patient is of great importance. Frequent regular recordings are made of temperature, pulse and blood pressure for approximately 12 hours following the procedure. Any abnormalities of these, or complaints of pain by the patient, must be reported to senior staff immediately. The patient may be given sips of fluid, or ice to suck, after approximately 6 hours, following which they should be asked to report any feelings of pain or discomfort to the nursing staff.

Other endoscopic examinations of the upper gastrointestinal tract are those of the stomach, **gastroscopy**, of the duodenum, **duodenoscopy** (Fig. 15.6), and of the pancreatic and biliary ducts, **endoscopic retrograde cholangio-pancreatography (ERCP)**. This latter investigation involves cannulation of the ampulla of Vater during duodenoscopy by means of a fine-bore catheter. Radio-opaque dye is then injected into the biliary and pancreatic ducts and the findings may aid diagnosis of biliary or pancreatic disorder. Calculi removal from the biliary tract may be possible during this procedure.

Endoscopy of the lower gastrointestinal tract

Proctoscopy and sigmoidoscopy Proctoscopy (ex-

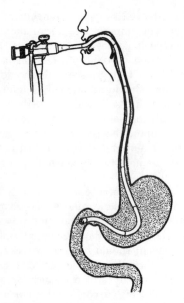

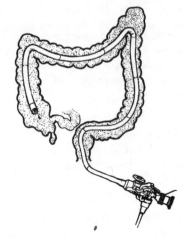

Fig. 15.7   Colonoscopy

Fig. 15.6   Oesophago-gastroduodenoscope in use

amination of the anus and rectum) may be used to confirm the presence of haemorrhoids and may also be used, in conjunction with anaesthesia, for the injection of these with sclerosing agents. Sigmoidoscopy (examination of the rectum and lower sigmoid colon) is used to confirm diagnosis when the presence of rectal polyps, malignancy, proctitis or ulcerative colitis is suspected.

Physical preparation of the patient for these procedures varies; those for whom inflammatory bowel disease is not a possible diagnosis may be given an enema in order to clear the rectum of faecal material, if necessary. If the patient is known to have, or suspected of having, an inflammatory bowel disorder, bowel preparation is usually omitted, due to the risk that the inflamed colon may perforate.

The investigation is carried out with the patient in the left lateral position for proctoscopy and the knee–chest or left lateral position for sigmoidoscopy. Although the examination may not cause pain, it is likely to be an uncomfortable and possibly embarrassing experience for the patient. During sigmoidoscopy air may be pumped into the colon in order to distend the lumen and thereby improve vision of the mucosa. This may cause an increase in discomfort and possibly pain and syncope.

The nurse's role is to support the patient, to observe them for evidence of distress during the procedure and to report any such distress to the medical staff carrying out the investigation. The patient may find

that deep breathing may aid relaxation as much as is possible during these investigations.

Colonoscopy   This examination provides vision of the entirety of the large intestine by means of a flexible fibreoptic colonoscope (Fig. 15.7). Bowel preparation is usually carried out by means of dietary restriction, laxatives and/or colonic lavage, in order to ensure removal of all faecal material.

Colonoscopy may be carried out under general anaesthesia as it is lengthy and likely to cause considerable discomfort.

Biopsy

As discussed under the section on endoscopy, tissue samples may be obtained during these investigations. Obtaining tissue from certain areas of the tract requires use of different techniques.

Jejunal biopsy

If malabsorption is suspected a tissue sample from the jejunum is obtained by means of a **Crosby capsule**. This is a small hollow capsule attached to a length of thin radio-opaque tubing. Within the capsule is contained a circular, spring-loaded blade. Once the capsule is observed by means of X-ray to be positioned correctly, application of suction to the proximal end of the tubing draws the mucosa into a small aperture situated on the side of the capsule. The negative pressure created by the suction is also responsible for firing the blade which severs the mucosa.

There is a slight risk of haemorrhage associated

with this investigation and the patient's platelet count and prothrombin time are therefore ascertained as being within normal levels before the procedure is carried out. This is necessary because an abnormally low platelet count would increase the risk of haemorrhage following the biopsy and a lengthy prothrombin time would increase the time taken for any bleeding to cease.

The patient is fasted overnight prior to the investigation and is asked to swallow the capsule. This is facilitated by the patient sitting upright. The patient may be prescribed a peristaltic stimulant, for example metoclopramide, which encourages progression of the capsule and additionally minimizes nausea. Following removal of the tube from the body a check is carried out to ensure that the apparatus is intact.

Liver biopsy

This investigation may be undertaken to confirm diagnosis of chronic hepatitis or cirrhosis. It may be carried out in the clinical area, using strict aseptic technique. Due to the significant risk of haemorrhage following this procedure the patient's prothrombin time and platelet count are ascertained to be normal before it takes place. (The reason for this is explained in the preceding section on jejunal biopsy.)

The specimen of liver tissue is obtained using a special needle inserted through an intercostal space, following cleansing and anaesthetization of the skin. As the patient has to be able to hold their breath whilst the biopsy is being taken, it is important that the medical staff are informed if there is any doubt about the patient's ability to do so. It is necessary for the patient to remain in bed for 12–24 hours following the procedure, during which time observations of the biopsy site and the patient's pulse and blood pressure are made regularly and frequently.

Possible complications which may occur, other than haemorrhage, are the onset of severe pain which may be symptomatic of bile leakage into the peritoneum (causing peritonitis), or breathlessness due to pneumothorax (entry of air into the pleural space – in this instance as a result of accidental biopsy needle puncture). Any complaints of pain, or deterioration in the patient's condition, should be reported immediately.

As the patient is bed bound during this period he will require assistance with personal hygiene, the provision of facilities for elimination, the means to summon the nursing staff should he require assistance and the opportunity for discussion with staff.

Other investigations

Pentagastrin test

This is an investigation of gastric secretion. If the patient is prescribed H_2-receptor antagonist drugs (e.g. cimetidine, ranitidine) these should not be taken for at least 48 hours prior to the test. (An explanation of the action of these drugs is provided on p. 516.)

The patient fasts overnight and a nasogastric tube is passed in the morning (see Ch. 4). This is an unpleasant procedure for the patient, but once the tube is in the stomach physical discomfort should be minimal. The contents of the stomach are aspirated and the volume measured, subsequent to which stomach secretions are collected continuously for 1 hour. The patient is then given a subcutaneous dose of pentagastrin. This is a synthetic substance which has the biological effects of the hormone gastrin (i.e. it stimulates secretions in the body of the stomach). Following this, the patient's stomach secretions are collected for a further hour.

The results of this test may demonstrate that the patient has abnormally high levels of fasting secretions, which may indicate a gastric outlet obstruction. It will also identify achlorhydria (absence of gastric acid) or high acid secretion levels.

Liver function tests

This is a collective term used to describe a number of biochemical investigations which help in the diagnosis of liver disorder, including an indication of the area and extent of damage. They may also be used in monitoring the patient's reponse to treatment.

THERAPEUTIC MANAGEMENT

Therapeutic management of the patient who has a gastrointestinal disorder may comprise or include prescription of drug therapy. It is important that the nurse acquires knowledge of the action and potential side-effects of drugs as, in addition to their administration, she is then in a position to ensure that the patient receives explanation of the purpose of the therapy. She is also able to observe the patient's reaction, therapeutic or adverse, to it.

Drugs which are commonly prescribed in the treatment of patients who have gastrointestinal disorders are antacids, antibiotics, analgesics and steroids. The action of these is outlined in Chapter 4, with additional information in relation to steroids being given in Chapter 16.

Drugs which may be prescribed in the treatment of

peptic ulceration are histamine H_2-receptor antagonists. Their action is to block histamine receptor cells situated on, or near, the parietal cells in the stomach, the desired result being a decrease in gastric secretion. Examples of H_2-receptor antagonists are ranitidine and cimetidine, both of which are effective in healing at least 80% of duodenal ulcers and 70% of gastric ulcers over a 4 week period. They have proven safety records, both in short- and long-term usage, although cimetidine may impair the metabolism of certain other drugs (such as warfarin and phenytoin) and may occasionally cause confusion in elderly people.

Surgical intervention is required in the treatment of a variety of disorders of the gastrointestinal system, for example those which are inflammatory in nature (such as ulcerative colitis) or malignant.

NURSING STRATEGIES

The role of the nurse is the subject material of Chapter 3 and it is assumed in the following discussion of nursing strategies that the reader will be familiar with the concepts discussed within it. The philosophy of the nursing process and the framework which it provides for the use of nursing models, or for primary nursing, is the starting point for any discussion of nursing strategies. The nursing models used in this chapter to illustrate examples of the approach to, and methods of, care are based on those of Roper et al (1990) and Orem (1991).

Nursing strategies or actions will be discussed under headings which relate to specific types of disorder (e.g. inflammatory, infective) from which patients may suffer. Potential or actual problems which may be experienced by the patient will be identified and nursing goals formulated and strategies identified in relation to the prevention or alleviation of these. The rationale for each nursing strategy will be given.

Although no column headed 'Evaluation' will be listed in the care plans in this chapter because of their hypothetical nature, evaluation of nursing strategies in order to determine their effectiveness, or otherwise, must be carried out regularly and frequently within the clinical setting.

NURSING STRATEGIES IN RELATION TO THE PATIENT WHO HAS A CONGENITAL DISORDER

Features of these disorders usually present in the first few weeks or months following birth. Parents of the child may understandably be extremely anxious, not only in relation to their child's immediate welfare, but also in relation to the implications which the disorder may have in the long term, for both the child and carers. In addition to being given explanations about the investigations and treatment which their child receives, parents must additionally be given the opportunity to ask questions and to voice their fears, anxieties and discuss possible problems.

Parents are now actively encouraged to spend as much time as is possible with hospitalized children and may, when appropriate, be involved in their physical care. Facilities are available within some paediatric units to enable parents to reside within the unit for the duration of their child's stay.

When disorders have a genetic association it is additionally important that parents receive genetic counselling to enable them to establish the likelihood that other children which they already have, or contemplate having in the future, may suffer from the same disorder. Siblings of the affected child may require investigation in order to determine whether they too suffer from the disorder.

Parents may experience feelings of guilt (however misplaced these may be) when they realize that their genetic contribution to their child has predisposed, or caused, development of disorder. They may require encouragement to discuss their feelings and expert counselling in order to come to terms with these.

Infants or children who are ill may derive inestimable reassurance from the presence of a parent or significant other. Children who are admitted to hospital find themselves within an unfamiliar environment and, especially if they are too young to understand the reasons why this change is necessary, or are deprived of contact with people with whom they are familiar, they may experience great emotional distress. Frequently the reason for their admission means that they are feeling ill or are in pain and during their stay it is necessary for them to undergo investigations and procedures which may be physically unpleasant and emotionally distressing. They require simple explanations of any investigations and physical and psychological reassurance from the nurse.

Pyloric stenosis

There is a familial tendency to develop this disorder. Male children are affected more frequently than females.

Spasmodic contractions of the pyloric sphincter muscle lead to hypertrophy of the stomach muscle in the pyloric antrum in an effort to overcome sphincter resistance to the onward passage of food and fluids. Pyloric obstruction results from this within 2–3 weeks, the initial symptom being vomiting which is often projectile in nature. As a result of inability to absorb fluids and nutrients the infant will fail to thrive and will rapidly develop the signs and symptoms of dehydration (see Ch. 4).

The aim of initial therapeutic intervention is to rehydrate the infant intravenously and to aspirate stomach contents in order to alleviate distension. Investigations include barium meal and endoscopy in order to confirm the diagnosis. Cure of the condition necessitates surgical treatment.

Hirschsprung's disease

This is a congenital condition caused by abnormal nerve fibres and the absence of ganglion cells in the wall of the large intestine. The distal end of the rectum is invariably involved and the area affected extends proximally for varying lengths, in some people involving the entirety of the large intestine. It results in an inability to maintain peristalsis in the affected area. Colonic contents are unable to pass through and this causes distension of the unaffected area.

The condition is first noticed by the absence or delay in passage of meconium shortly after birth and in loose stools during the early weeks of life. During the first year of life there is abdominal distension and severe constipation with the passage of small, ribbon-like stools. The condition may be sufficiently severe to cause anorexia, vomiting and intestinal obstruction.

Investigations carried out to confirm the diagnosis include barium enema, rectal examination, manometry (measurement of gases) and examination of rectal and colonic biopsies in order to determine the level at which normal nerve cells are present.

If the infant develops intestinal obstruction, surgery is required, possibly within days of birth. A temporary colostomy is formed and fluid and electrolyte balance maintained by intravenous infusion via a scalp vein for approximately 24 hours following surgery. An accurate recording must be made of fluid intake and output and faecal output.

The colostomy remains until the child is approximately 18 months old, when major surgery is carried out in order to remove the affected segment of intestine and reconnect the unaffected areas. The need for the temporary colostomy must be explained to the child's carers, as must the care which the child will require in relation to it. It may prove helpful and reassuring to the child's parents if a meeting can be arranged with the parents of a child who has previously had a temporary colostomy. The stoma therapist should also be contacted, as should the community interdisciplinary team, in order to provide continued support for the parents and child following discharge home. An explanation of the nursing strategies which are required in relation to the care of a stoma is given in Nursing Care Plan 15.4.

If the condition is less severe the infant will not require surgery. The problems of constipation and abdominal distension can be alleviated by the taking of a high fluid and roughage content in the diet and by possible prescription of aperients and enemas if required.

It is important that the child's parents receive advice on, and support with, the care that their child will require, particularly in relation to dietary advice and the observations which should be made of the child's faecal output. Regular health and developmental assessments are carried out by a paediatrician, but the child's carers should additionally have a person, for example a health visitor, whom they can contact for advice should they require it.

Cystic fibrosis

This is an autosomal recessive disorder which causes pancreatic insufficiency and respiratory failure as a result of generalized dysfunction of all exocrine glands. Mucus secreted by pancreatic and respiratory cells is thick and viscid, causing cystic changes in the pancreas and lungs and bronchiectasis in the latter. (See also Ch. 13.)

The disorder usually presents in early life, when the infant 'fails to thrive'. Defective pancreatic enzyme secretion results in incomplete digestion and subsequent malabsorption of fat. The infant's stools are therefore bulky, pale and foul smelling and the infant is usually underweight. Blockage within the respiratory system causes recurrent chest infections.

The disorder is diagnosed by means of a **sweat test** (Shearman and Crean 1991). The purpose of the test is to obtain an estimation of the concentration of sodium in sweat. The amount is found to be above normal in 95% of children who have cystic fibrosis.

The investigation, and its purpose, is explained to the child (in a manner appropriate to his level of comprehension) and to the parent(s). The test is painless, although a mild tingling sensation may be experienced and the skin used may subsequently be pink for a short period. An explanation beforehand should help to alleviate anxiety and ensure co-operation. Babies and small children may require the constant presence of a nurse while the test is in progress.

The two areas of skin which are to be used are carefully cleansed with distilled water and dried using filter papers and possibly a hairdrier. A swab which has been soaked in a pilocarpine solution (the purpose of which is to stimulate sweat production) is applied to one of the areas and is covered by a positive electrode from an iontophoresis apparatus. A magnesium sulphate-soaked swab is applied to the other area of skin and is covered by a negative electrode. The electrodes are then connected to the power supply for 4 minutes, having first ensured that no part of either metal plate is in contact with the child's skin. The electrodes, plates and swabs are then removed and the underlying skin washed and dried in the same manner as before.

Using forceps, a piece of filter paper from the weighed sweat test bottle (obtained from biochemistry) is applied to the area of skin which had been covered by the pilocarpine-soaked swab. This is covered by polythene and secured by four pieces of waterproof tape. A fifth piece of tape is secured diagonally across the polythene to ensure contact between the filter paper and the skin.

The filter paper is left in situ for a minimum period of 1 hour, following which the process is reversed and the filter paper removed from the skin using forceps. The paper is then placed into the weighed bottle and despatched (with the appropriate form) to the laboratory. It is vital that contamination of the specimen, or evaporation of sweat from it, is avoided throughout the procedure.

If cystic fibrosis is undiagnosed in childhood and investigations are carried out during adolescence, sweat test results may be difficult to interpret and the diagnosis is then made on the evidence of pancreatic insufficiency, chronic respiratory infections and pulmonary damage and a family history of the disorder.

There is at present no cure for cystic fibrosis. Therapeutic management includes oral pancreatic enzyme replacements, prevention and control of respiratory infections by means of breathing exercises, frequent chest physiotherapy and antibiotic therapy. Please see Chapter 13 for details of therapeutic management and nursing strategies.

NURSING STRATEGIES IN RELATION TO THE PATIENT WHO HAS AN INFLAMMATORY DISORDER

Inflammation affecting the gastrointestinal system and associated organs (i.e. the liver, gallbladder and pancreas) may be caused by varied pathophysiology.

Inflammation may additionally be associated with infection, either as its cause, or as its result.

Inflammation of the oral cavity

Stomatitis is a general term denoting inflammation of the mouth and **glossitis** refers to inflammation of the tongue. If acute, glossitis gives the tongue a red, raw appearance and painful surface. If chronic, the tongue is moist and has an abnormally 'clean' appearance due to atrophy of papillae. These conditions may be caused by infection (see section on 'Nursing strategies in relation to the patient who has an infective disorder', below), or by nutritional deficiency of vitamins, in particular niacin, riboflavin, folate and vitamin B_{12}. (See Ch. 4 for details of the action of these vitamins). Stomatitis may also be caused by an allergic reaction to chemicals in drugs, foodstuffs or dental preparations.

Aphthous ulcers are painful, superficial ulcers which may be multiple and may recur. The person is usually otherwise healthy and outbreaks may be associated with a specific phase of the menstrual cycle, or with emotional stress. They may also exist in a chronic form in people who have Crohn's disease, ulcerative colitis or coeliac disease.

Leukoplakia is a chronic condition in which white patches appear on the sides of the tongue and the roof of the mouth. This may be asymptomatic in the early stages, but the later development of fissures usually causes tenderness of the affected areas. The identification of leukoplakia is important, as it may be a precursor of carcinoma and it is therefore important that, when any patient is admitted, the nursing staff carry out physical examination of the patient's mouth as part of their overall initial assessment.

Nursing strategies

The aim of therapeutic intervention for patients who have an inflammatory disorder affecting the mouth is identification of the cause in order that appropriate treatment may be commenced. The patient's problem in relation to an inflammatory disorder of the mouth is usually pain or discomfort, possibly causing anorexia or an aversion to particular foods or fluids which are identified by the patient as exacerbating the condition.

Nursing strategies to relieve pain and discomfort include provision of facilities for the patient to carry out frequent and regular (usually 2 hourly) oral hygiene, including the use of mouthwashes. A solution of sodium bicarbonate may provide some symptomatic relief, or alternatively specific mouthwashes or lozenges may be prescribed, apthous ulceration for example being treated by use of hydrocortisone hemisuccinate lozenges.

Some patients who suffer from a painful mouth may be too debilitated to carry out their own oral hygiene, in which case they will require assistance. If the mucosa is tender, use of oral hygiene sponges may be unsuitable and a gloved finger, covered by a soft gauze swab dipped in mouthwash solution, may be used. This is obviously inadvisable if the patient is confused or unco-operative in which case individualized alternative strategies will need to be identified.

Oesophagitis and hiatus hernia

Inflammation of the oesophagus may be caused by the ingestion of irritant substances, but the most common cause is reflux of gastric contents into the lower end of the oesophagus as a result of **hiatus hernia.**

An increase in abdominal pressure, or alteration to the oblique angle at which the oesophagus enters the stomach, may override the ability of the lower oesophageal sphincter to prevent reflux of stomach contents. This causes acid-pepsin digestion of the oesophageal mucosa, leading to ulceration and spasm and, if untreated, scar tissue formation may cause oesophageal stricture and dysphagia.

Aetiology

Reflux oesophagitis and hiatus hernia most commonly occur in middle-aged and elderly women, although hormonal influences in pregnancy may lead to their earlier development. Obesity is a predisposing factor.

Diagnosis

Diagnosis of the disorder is by means of the patient's history of signs and symptoms and by barium swallow/meal and endoscopy.

Treatment

For an outline of nursing strategies and their rationale please refer to Nursing Care Plan 15.1.

Surgical repair of hiatus hernia may be necessary if the measures outlined in Nursing Care Plan 15.1 are ineffective.

If the person has developed a stricture they may suffer from dysphagia and will therefore require a liquid or semi-liquid diet prior to bouginage to dilate the affected area.

Gastritis

Inflammation of the stomach mucosa may be acute, caused by ingestion of gastric irritants, for example anti-inflammatory drugs or alcohol. The person may be asymptomatic, or may suffer anorexia, nausea, epigastric pain and heartburn. Use of antacids may provide symptomatic relief and the patient should be advised to avoid causative factors (which may entail alteration to their current drug therapy). If alcohol is the cause the patient may, if a habitual abuser, have other concommitant problems. Nursing strategies which may be used in caring for people who abuse alcohol are discussed in Chapter 9.

Gastritis may alternatively be chronic, resulting in peptic ulceration, carcinoma or pernicious anaemia. The cause may be identified by reference to the patient's signs and symptoms and investigation of these by barium studies and endoscopy.

Peptic ulceration

This term refers to the presence of an ulcer in the lower oesophagus, stomach or duodenum. Ulcers in the stomach or duodenum may be acute or chronic, the latter being associated with local fibrosis (due to formation of scar tissue).

Epidemiology and aetiology

The immediate cause of ulceration is mucosal digestion by the acid and pepsin in gastric juice but, as the normal stomach has the capacity to resist the potentially damaging action of its own secretions, there are obviously other factors involved.

Physiologically, any factor which causes an increase in the secretion of hydrochloric acid or pepsin, or which reduces the resistance of the mucosa to these substances, may result in mucosal ulceration. Certain conditions, such as the Zollinger–Ellison syndrome (see Ch. 16), cause hypersecretion of gastric acid. Alternatively the mucosal resistance may be decreased by, for example, the ingestion of non-steroidal anti-inflammatory drugs.

Following major trauma an individual may develop **stress ulcers**, so called because their cause is severe physical stress. In the event of head injury these may be a result of gastric acid hypersecretion. Following severe burns, major surgery or septicaemia their cause is probably a combination of bile reflux into the stomach and mucosal ischaemia.

The incidence of peptic ulceration is decreasing in many western countries, but is still quite common, affecting males more frequently than females and

Nursing Care Plan 15.1 Care for a person who has oesophageal reflux/hiatus hernia			
Problem (actual/ potential)	**Goal**	**Actions**	**Rationale**
Pain/discomfort: –retrosternal — burning sensation	To alleviate pain/ discomfort	❒ Administration of medication as prescribed, for example: ● antacid agents ● H$_2$-receptor antagonists, e.g. cimetidine, ranitidine ● metoclopramide ❒ Advise patient to eat small volumes of food at frequent intervals ❒ Advise patient to avoid foods which have a high fat content ❒ Advise patient to lose weight if they are overweight/obese ❒ Advise patient to avoid bending from the waist ❒ Advise patient to sleep in an upright position, i. e. use of pillows, backrest, blocks to elevate the head of the bed ❒ Advise patient to stop smoking, if applicable	Counteract effect of acidity on oesophageal mucosa Reduce gastric secretions Increase contraction of lower oesophageal sphincter Promote gastric emptying Large amounts of food may overfill the stomach and encourage reflux These promote reflux and delay gastric emptying Correction of obesity will alleviate symptoms Waist bending facilitates reflux These measures help to prevent reflux Smoking reduces lower oesophageal sphincter pressure (facilitates reflux)

existing in approximately 10% of males at some time in their lives. Variations in incidence occur between countries and in different parts of the same country, the incidence of duodenal ulcers in Scotland for example is considerably higher than that in southern England (Shearman and Crean 1991).

Heredity is an established predisposing factor, sufferers frequently having a family history of the same disorder. There is additionally a higher than average incidence of peptic ulceration in those who are of blood group O, particularly in conjunction with an absence of AB antigens in saliva.

There is growing evidence that cigarette smoking may be a contributing factor in peptic ulcer formation and that it may prevent healing of existing ulceration.

Emotional factors (i.e. the experience of psychological stress, particularly if sustained) may possibly contribute to ulcer formation by causing hypersecretion of gastric juice, but there has been no incontrovertible evidence to confirm this.

Clinical features of peptic ulceration

The individual may complain of having had chronic, episodic pain or discomfort for months or years prior to diagnosis of ulceration. They may have sought advice from their GP and undergone investigations and treatment as an outpatient. Hospitalization may possibly only occur if the person develops a complica-

tion of the disorder, such as haemorrhage as a result of blood vessel erosion or peritonitis caused by perforation of the ulcerated area. Complications of peptic ulceration may also arise without any prior history of ulcer symptoms.

The pain caused by peptic ulceration can usually be pinpointed by the patient as being localized in the epigastrium (Fig. 15.4). It is described as gnawing or burning in nature and may be relieved by antacids, by vomiting or by food.

Investigation by means of barium meal is usually sufficient to establish the diagnosis.

Therapeutic management and nursing strategies

Several drugs may be prescribed in the treatment of peptic ulceration, but those most commonly used are antacids and H$_2$-receptor antagonists.

Antacid therapy If an antacid is prescribed (e.g. aluminium hydroxide), the person should be given advice on the frequency and quantity of administration as excessive use may lead to fluid or electrolyte disturbance (see also Ch. 4).

H$_2$-receptor antagonist therapy The effect of H$_2$-receptor antagonist drugs (e.g. ranitidine, cimetidine) is to reduce gastric secretions (see p. 516 for further details). Following commencement of therapy the patient is usually symptom free within 2–7 days, but the medication must be continued as prescribed, usually for a period of 4 weeks. It is therefore essential that the patient appreciates the importance of this, as ulcer recurrence may otherwise result.

The patient may experience future episodes of ulceration, necessitating further courses of therapy or, if relapses are frequent, the use of low dosage maintenance therapy.

Other drugs which it is proposed can be used in first-line ulcer therapy have been developed, for example those aimed at the eradication of *Helicobacter pylori*. This organism is found asymptomatically in a minority of the general population, but is present in almost all people who have duodenal ulceration. Eradication of *H. pylori* appears to reduce significantly the incidence of ulcer relapse but this involves the use of a combination of drugs (triple therapy). Clinical trials of *H. pylori* eradication regimens are currently being undertaken and evaluated (Pounder 1994).

Surgery may be required if there is continued evidence of ulceration following several courses of H_2-receptor antagonists, or during maintenance therapy. The aim of surgery is to reduce stimulation of gastric secretions by means of severance of some of the branches of the vagus nerve (highly selective vagotomy) (Fig. 15.8) which innervate the parietal cells in the stomach. A care plan for a person undergoing gastric surgery is given in Nursing Care Plan 15.2.

In addition to drug therapy it is reasonable to advise the person who has a peptic ulcer to reduce their exposure to physical and psychological stressors until the acute exacerbation of the ulcerated area has resolved i.e. until H_2-receptor antagonist therapy has been underway for 1–2 weeks.

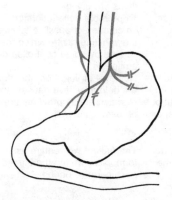

Fig. 15.8 Highly selective vagotomy

As the patient is unlikely to be hospitalized for more than a few days (unless they have the complications associated with peptic ulceration or are hospitalized for some other reason), patient education is important and the following aspects should be discussed with the patient, ensuring that he/she has the opportunity to ask questions or voice anxieties.

If the patient smokes, the advisability of stopping should be emphasized, given that the research evidence at present available indicates that smoking may delay ulcer healing, or be causative of further ulceration.

The patient must be informed about the harmful effects which aspirin and other anti-inflammatory drugs may have and should be given information about, and possible prescription of, acceptable alternatives, should these be required.

Whilst alcohol in small or moderate amounts is not contraindicated unless it causes exacerbation of the person's symptoms, advice should be given about the recommended limits which it is advisable to impose upon intake. As there is currently no evidence that avoidance of, or ingestion of, specific foods affects ulcer healing, advice on diet is normally restricted to avoidance of foods which the patient finds cause him/her discomfort.

Complications of peptic ulceration

Haemorrhage Peptic ulceration may cause erosion of blood vessels and bleeding (see p. 528 for details). If severe the patient will display the clinical features of shock (see Ch. 4). Therapeutic management and nursing strategies will be tailored to the needs of the individual patient, but will include rapid adequate blood replacement. An intravenous infusion is commenced and a plasma-expander such as dextran may be used until cross-matching has been carried out and a blood transfusion is available.

The patient's pulse and blood pressure are recorded frequently, possibly half hourly. An intravenous line may be inserted in order to measure central venous pressure (see Ch. 12). Vomitus and faecal output are tested for the presence of blood by use of clinical reagents. A nasogastric tube may be passed and aspirated as necessary to remove stomach contents. The patient will have nil orally and will require almost total assistance with the activities of daily living until his/her condition improves.

Perforation A peptic ulcer may perforate through its organ of origin into the peritoneal cavity. This will cause leakage of the organ contents into the peritoneal space and irritation (peritonitis), accom-

Nursing Care Plan 15.2 Care for a patient who has undergone gastric surgery

Problem (actual/ potential)	Goal	Actions	Rationale
1. Pain	To prevent/alleviate pain/discomfort	❐ Controlled drug analgesia to be given regularly for approx. 48 hours postoperatively; analgesia as prescribed thereafter	Freedom from pain will help to: • promote the patient's psychological well-being • ensure that pain does not preclude adequate lung ventilation
		❐ Possible administration of analgesia via a controlled-rate infusion pump	Provides a consistent level of pain relief
		❐ Possible administration of analgesia via a patient-actuated pump	Enables patient to control administration of analgesia
		❐ Encourage the patient to adopt a semirecumbent position initially and upright position when able: provide support for the patient with backrest and pillows	To ensure support to, and drainage from, the wound site
		❐ Explain all procedures prior to implementation. Provide the patient with the opportunity to ask questions and voice anxieties	To minimize patient anxiety. To ensure patient co-operation To promote the patient's psychological well-being
2. Haemorrhage	To identify promptly evidence of haemorrhage	❐ Observation of wound, wound drainage for blood loss, record pulse and blood pressure: ½ hourly for 2 hours if satisfactory: hourly for 4 hours 2 hourly for 4 hours 4 hourly thereafter Observation of patient's skin temperature and skin colour	Recognition of excessive blood loss will enable initiation of measures to stop bleeding and enable replacement of blood/fluid loss visible bleeding tachycardia weak, thready pulse } may indicate hypotension } haemorrhage pale, cold clammy skin
3. Inability to ensure own hydration and nutrition	To ensure that patient's hydration and nutrition needs are met	❐ Care of i.v. infusion, possible total parenteral nutrition, provision of oral fluids and diet once this is possible	Patient is initially unable to tolerate oral fluids/diet
		❐ Record fluid balance	In order to monitor fluid balance
4. Nausea/vomiting	To prevent/alleviate nausea	❐ Avoidance of oral fluids until bowel sounds return	Absence of peristaltic activity will result in nausea/vomiting if oral fluids are given
		❐ Possible administration of an antiemetic drug, e.g. cyclizine	To promote patient comfort. To counteract possible stimulation of the vomiting centre which may be caused by some controlled drug analgesia
		❐ Aspiration of nasogastric tube if present: aspiration may be continuous, i.e. by attachment of the tube to low-grade suction, or intermittent, e.g. hourly	Removal of fluid from the stomach will help to relieve nausea. Keeping stomach empty prevents pressure on gastric sutures
5. Inability to attend to elimination needs unaided	To assist the patient until he/she is able to self-care	❐ Provision of toilet facilities at the patient's bedside: assist the patient to get out of bed	The patient will require assistance to mobilize during the immediate postoperative period

Nursing Care Plan 15.2 *(cont'd)*			
Problem (actual/ potential)	Goal	Actions	Rationale
6. Infection	To prevent development of infection	❑ Ensure strict aseptic technique whilst caring for the patient's wound site and during removal of drains and sutures	This will help to prevent entry of micro-organisms into wound site
	To identify infection promptly should it occur	❑ Record patient's temperature 2 hourly during the immediate postoperative period. If satisfactory, 4 hourly thereafter	Pyrexia may indicate the presence of infection
		❑ Observe wound site for: • excessive redness • excessive swelling • purulent exudate	These may indicate the presence of infection
7. Problems associated with reduced mobility, i.e. pressure sores, chest infection, deep venous thrombosis	To prevent/minimize the possibility of their occurrence	❑ Assist patient to change their position every 2–4 hours. Observation of skin over sites which are subjected to pressure. Possible use of pressure-relieving devices, e.g. Spenco mattress	To prevent development of pressure sores Prompt identification of areas of redness Relief of pressure
		❑ Encourage patient to breathe deeply and ensure that they are painfree (see 'Pain')	To maximize lung expansion and prevent development of chest infection
		Encourage patient to move their legs and feet whilst in bed. Encourage early mobilization. Possible fitting of patient with thromboembolic deterrent stockings. Administration of subcutaneous heparin if prescribed	In order to prevent development of deep venous thrombosis
8. Inability to attend to own personal hygiene needs	To assist the patient with these until they are able to self-care	❑ Assist patient to wash in bed and later in shower until they are able to self-care	Ensure patient comfort and hygiene. Showering is preferable to bathing; it reduces the risk of wound infection
		❑ Assist patient to implement oral hygiene 2–4 hourly until they are able to tolerate oral fluids/diet. Assist them as required thereafter	To ensure patient comfort and hygiene

panied possibly by infection. This condition is also known as **acute abdomen**. The patient experiences a sudden onset of severe pain, which is made worse by movement, and may be accompanied by vomiting. The pain may radiate to the shoulder tip as a result of diaphagmatic irritation. The patient will lie as still as is possible and will display the clinical features of shock (see Ch. 4). The patient's abdomen is rigid and intestinal sounds are absent.

Therapeutic management, following diagnosis of acute abdomen, involves surgical intervention in order to repair the perforation. Nursing strategies therefore are directed at preparing the patient, physically and psychologically, for emergency surgery and in caring for them during the postoperative period. The principles of pre- and postoperative care are outlined in Chapter 4. A care plan for a patient who has undergone major abdominal surgery is given in Nursing Care Plan 15.2.

Inflammatory bowel disease

This term is used to denote either Crohn's disease or ulcerative colitis.

Crohn's disease (regional enteritis)

This is a non-specific inflammatory disorder, which causes thickening of the submucosa and ulceration and hypertrophy of the muscle wall. This narrows the intestinal lumen. Clefts and fissures form and these may lead to **fistula** formation. Crohn's disease may affect any area between the mouth and anus, although the ileum is the most commonly affected. In addition to the other clinical features involvement of the ileum causes interference with normal absorption of fat and protein.

Aetiology Crohn's disease may occur at any age, but the incidence is highest between the ages of 20 and 40 years. It occurs in equal numbers in both sexes and may take the form of an acute or chronic illness.

Clinical features These vary. Some patients may require emergency admission suffering from acute abdominal pain or intestinal obstruction, whilst others have a history of general ill health, weight loss and anaemia. Intermittent colicky pain accompanied by diarrhoea may occur three or four times daily. Faeces may contain mucus, pus and undigested food. The person may present with problems associated with fistula formation.

Investigation is by means of barium meal and follow-through. This identifies the areas of the small intestine which are affected. Barium enema is also carried out in order to assess colonic involvement.

Therapeutic management Crohn's is a chronic debilitating disease, which may necessitate repeated hospital admissions for the sufferer during acute exacerbations of the condition. Complications such as intestinal obstruction, and abcess or fistula formation will require surgical intervention, but surgery is not otherwise indicated.

The general aim of treatment is to reduce inflammation, for example by the use of corticosteroid drugs. Antibiotic therapy is prescribed when infection is present.

Nursing strategies These are aimed at improving the person's quality of life and in assisting them to undertake the activities of daily living during acute exacerbations of the disorder. Nursing strategies are also needed to enable the patient to come to terms with the physical and psychological implications of suffering from a life-long disorder for which there is no cure. Patients should be given opportunities to discuss their feelings, along with specific fears or anxieties which they may have.

Patient education will be required in relation to medication (see Ch. 16 for an outline of the advice which should be given to patients who are prescribed long-term steroid therapy).

Advice will be necessary on diet and the dietician should be involved in this. Foods which have a low roughage content will reduce the frequency of intesti-

nal colic. Steatorrhoea (see p. 510) can be minimized by a diet that is low in fat. The person's diet should be high in protein and carbohydrate. (It should be ascertained that the person understands which foods are entailed and in what quantities; if they do not, then details should be provided.) Vitamin and mineral supplements may also be required.

If these measures are insufficient to maintain the patient's nutritional status, enteral feeding to supplement or replace normal oral intake may be required. This may be achieved by means of gastrostomy. Using an aseptic technique (see Ch. 4) an opening is made into the person's stomach via the abdominal wall. A tube is inserted, which is secured to the skin surface, usually by means of a suture. The patient's nutritional requirements are individually assessed and instillation of prepared nutrients takes place by means of a syringe for intermittent (bolus) feeding or tubing for continuous feeding.

The patient may, if sufficiently healthy, be discharged home with the gastrostomy tube in situ. The patient, or their carer, will require education in care of the gastrostomy and in relation to the feeding regimen. Points which require emphasis relate to skin care. The enzymatic action of the gastric juice is excoriative to skin. The risk of infection of the skin and subcutaneous tissues around the gastrostomy entry site must also be emphasized and advice given on how these problems may be avoided.

It should also be appreciated that the patient may develop psychosocial problems related to their altered body image, or to the fact that they are unable to ingest food in the manner considered normal by society (see Ch. 4). The patient should be given the opportunity to voice their feelings and may require counselling.

Occasionally patients who have Crohn's disease may require total parenteral nutrition (see Ch. 4).

Long-term support may be required for the patient and the need for this must be assessed, in conjunction with the patient, prior to discharge from hospital. Societies such as the National Association for Colitis and Crohn's Disease may provide peer group and other support and the patient should be informed of their existence and how to contact them.

Ulcerative colitis

This is an inflammatory disease affecting the mucosa and submucosa of some or all of the large intestine. The mucosa is oedematous and bleeds easily, following which ulceration develops. The disorder is chronic, with the person experiencing relapses and remissions.

Aetiology This is unknown, but it is thought that

it may be due to an abnormal immune response and that a familial tendency may exist. Stressful experiences may sometimes appear to precipitate exacerbations, but psychological factors are not otherwise considered to be important. Some patients may be anxious and depressed, but these features are a consequence of the disease rather than its cause and improve or disappear during remissions.

Ulcerative colitis may occur at any age, but is most common between the ages of 20 and 40 years.

Clinical features   The main symptom is diarrhoea. The stools contain blood, pus and mucus and defaecation may be accompanied by abdominal discomfort. The frequency and severity of diarrhoea depend upon the severity of the disease.

There is an increased incidence of colonic carcinoma in people who have suffered from ulcerative colitis compared with the general population and it is therefore important that the person's colonic mucosa is checked at specified intervals.

Investigations   Proctoscopy and sigmoidoscopy are performed, during which biopsies are obtained. Barium enema may help to assess the severity of ulceration. Blood samples are analysed to identify the existence of anaemia and to assess the extent of protein loss and electrolye imbalance.

Therapeutic management   The patient will require to be hospitalized during acute exacerbations. They may require total parenteral nutrition (see Ch. 4) if they are thin and malnourished. Dehydration and electrolyte imbalances will also require correction. If infection is present antibiotic therapy is prescribed. Antidiarrhoeal drugs such as loperamide or codeine may be prescribed.

Corticosteroid drugs may be effective in inducing remission. These may be given locally (i.e. rectally) or systemically. Sulphasalazine may be used once remission is achieved, as it reduces the likelihood of relapse. Azothiaprine is being increasingly utilised in order to sustain remission (Mayberry et al 1994).

Failure of conservative measures to control exacerbations may necessitate surgical intervention. The operative procedure varies. An ileo-anal pouch may be formed following excision of the colon (restorative proctocolectomy). When this is carried out a temporary ileostomy is usually performed in order to allow the **anatamoses** to heal. Once healing has taken place the ileostomy is reversed and the small intestine anastamosed to the pouch. The person will thereafter continue to evacuate excreta per anus, although they will require to do so approximately every 4–6 hours. As the excreta is directly from the small intestine its consistency is fluid and as it contains enzymes the danger of skin excoriation is high.

The alternative surgery is proctocolectomy and formation of a permanent ileostomy. Care plans for patients following restorative proctocolectomy and following stoma formation are given at the end of this section in Nursing Care Plans 15.3 and 15.4.

The decision to undergo surgery as treatment for ulcerative colitis is one which should be determined by the patient, in conjunction with advice from the physician and surgeon. The patient may feel that his/her quality of life is so diminished by the effects of the disease that surgery, which will eradicate the symptoms, is a viable and desirable alternative. The implications of surgery, and of the different types of intervention available, should be explained to the patient, in order that he may make an informed choice.

Nursing strategies   During acute exacerbations of ulcerative colitis the patient will require assistance to undertake the activities of daily living. Of particular physical importance is care of the patient's peri-anal area, which is at risk of excoriation due to frequent diarrhoea. Barrier creams may be useful, in addition to careful washing and drying of the area following defaecation.

The patient may feel embarrassed about their symptoms and anxious about the long-term implications of the disease. Psychological care of the patient includes providing explanations of investigations and procedures and in spending time with the patient in order to encourage then to express their feelings. Problems and potential problems may then be identified and strategies proposed in order to overcome these.

Case Report to accompany Nursing Care Plan 15.3 for Steven, who has undergone restorative proctocolectomy

Steven is 25 years old. He was diagnosed as having ulcerative colitis when he was 19 and has required many hospital admissions since then. The periods of time when he is in remission are infrequent, despite anti-inflammatory drug therapy. He feels generally unwell, is thin and feels socially limited because of his frequent bouts of diarrhoea.

He lives alone in a flat, but has a girlfriend and several close friends. He maintains close contact with his parents and married brother and sister, seeing them approximately once a week.

He is employed in an insurance office, but is quite frequently absent due to illness, which he feels has hindered his chances of promotion.

Following discussions with his physician and a surgeon to whom he had been referred, Steven decided to undergo restorative proctocolectomy with formation of a temporary ileostomy.

His postoperative care is provided in Nursing Care Plan 15.3

Nursing Care Plan 15.3 Care for Steven during 48–72 hours following restorative proctocolectomy			
Problem (actual/ potential)	**Goal**	**Actions**	**Rationale**

1. Airway obstruction due to anaesthesia	To ensure maintenance of a clear airway	❐ Prone, semiprone or extended lateral positioning until Steven is fully conscious
		
		❐ Observation of respirations ½ hourly for 2 hours if satisfactory:
		    hourly for 4 hours
		    2 hourly for 4 hours
		    4 hourly thereafter
			These positions should ensure maintenance of a clear airway. Should vomiting occur risk of vomitus inhalation is minimized
			To monitor rate, depth and quality of respirations and to ensure that airway is unobstructed

2. Pain	To prevent/minimize pain	❐ Administration of prescribed analgesia (initially controlled drug by i.m. or i.v. route, possibly by continuous infusion) ❐ Teach Steven to support his wound whilst moving. Maintain correct positioning of drainage tubes ❐ Repetition of preoperative explanations regarding postoperative care ❐ Observe for non-verbal indications that Steven is in pain, e.g. restlessness, tachycardia, raised blood pressure, pallor, facial expression. Ask Steven to report any experience of pain	Postoperative pain may be severe To minimize traction on wound sites To alleviate Steven's possible anxieties; anxiety may increase his perception of pain Steven may be reluctant to complain of pain

3. Haemorrhage (internal or external)	To prevent if possible, or identify promptly should it occur	❐ Observation of:
		● Wound drainage (usually two abdominal suction drains and a latex drain in ano)
		● wound sites
		● record pulse rate
		● blood pressure
		● skin colour
		● skin temperature
		½ hourly for 2 hours if satisfactory:
		    hourly for 4 hours
		    2 hourly for 4 hours
		    4 hourly thereafter
			Recognition of excess blood loss will enable replacement and initiation of measures to stop bleeding
			
			● tachycardia
			● weak, thready pulse } may indicate
			● hypotension haemorrhage
			● pallor
			● cold, clammy skin

4. Infection	To prevent if possible, or identify promptly should it occur	❐ Use of aseptic technique whilst caring for wound and drainage sites. Removal of drainage tubes and abdominal wound dressing after 48–72 hours. Irrigation of anal pouch as directed, e.g. 50 ml 0.9% saline instilled 4 hourly via anal catheter; catheter usually removed after 24–48 hours. Urinary catheter hygiene 2–4 hourly until its removal; approximately 5 days postoperatively	To minimize entry of micro-organisms and development of infection

Nursing Care Plan 15.3 *(cont'd)*

Problem (actual/potential)	Goal	Actions	Rationale
4. (cont'd)		❏ Observe skin around wound and drainage sites. Observe nature of exudate ❏ Record temperature 2 hourly during the immediate postoperative period. If satisfactory 4 hourly thereafter	Red, inflamed skin and/or purulent discharge may indicate the presence of infection Pyrexia may indicate the presence of infection
5. Inability to attend to own nutrition and hydration needs	To ensure that nutritional needs are met	❏ Care of i.v. infusion and possible total parenteral nutrition (TPN) ❏ Care of nasogastric tube if applicable and possible aspiration of this ❏ Oral fluids, light diet when bowel sounds return. Record oral/i.v. intake	Oral food/fluids would not be tolerated initially due to absence or diminution of peristalsis If a temporary ileostomy has been formed, food and fluids may recommence orally: if not, ileo-anal anastamosis requires time to heal prior to commencement of oral intake
6. Limited mobility	To prevent the complications associated with reduced mobility	❏ Assist Steven to change his position every 2–4 hours. Possible use of pressure-relieving aids, e.g. Spenco mattress ❏ Encourage Steven to breathe deeply. Encourage an upright position in bed supported by backrest and pillows ❏ Encourage Steven to move his legs and feet. Possible use of thromboembolic deterrent stockings. Administration of subcutaneous heparin if prescribed. Early mobilization ❏ Administration of analgesia as prescribed	To prevent development of pressure sores To prevent development of a chest infection To promote venous return and prevent deep venous thrombosis formation Minimization of pain will encourage mobilization
7. Inability to attend to own personal hygiene needs	To assist Steven to maintain his personal hygiene	❏ Bedbath Steven and assist him to wash as required ❏ Provide assistance to carry out oral hygiene 2–4 hourly ❏ Encourage Steven to assist as able	To promote comfort and to reduce risk of infection Oral mucosa will become dry due to lack of oral intake Promote independence and maintenance of self-esteem
8. Inability to attend to own elimination needs unaided	To ensure Steven's elimination needs are met	❏ Care of Steven's urinary catheter, measure urine volume and fluid balance ❏ Observe colour, consistency, odour ❏ Care of temporary loop ileostomy (if applicable) and encourage Steven to watch/participate whilst care is carried out ❏ Care of the skin surrounding the ileostomy: ensure its protection from excreta	To ensure that bladder remains empty: bladder filling may cause trauma to the anal pouch Observe for visual abnormalities To monitor stoma output To prepare Steven to care for the stoma himself Effluent from the small intestine will excoriate skin

Nursing Care Plan 15.3 (*cont'd*)

Problem (actual/ potential)	Goal	Actions	Rationale
9. Altered body image due to surgery and formation of temporary ileostomy (if present)	To assist Steven to come to terms with this	❏ Encourage Steven to observe, and participate in, stoma care ❏ Ensure that the verbal and non-verbal communication on the part of the nursing staff is appropriate ❏ Encourage Steven to discuss his feelings, and possible anxieties, in relation to his altered body image	To encourage his acceptance of the stoma and to prepare him for self-care Positive verbal communication and avoidance of non-verbal expressions of distaste or repugnance may assist him in acceptance of the stoma Discussion of feelings may encourage acceptance of altered body image. Identification of anxieties can enable staff and Steven to formulate strategies to overcome these

Nursing Care Plan 15.4   Care for a patient who has had formation of a stoma

Problem (actual/ potential)	Goal	Actions	Rationale
1. Pain	To prevent/alleviate pain/discomfort	❏ Controlled drug analgesia to be given regularly for approx. 48 hours postoperatively. Oral analgesia as prescribed thereafter ❏ Possible administration of analgesia via a controlled-rate infusion pump ❏ Possible administration of analgesia via a patient-actuated pump ❏ Encourage the patient to adopt a semirecumbent position initially and upright position when able: provide support for the patient with backrest and pillows ❏ Explain all procedures prior to implementation. Provide the patient with the opportunity to ask questions and voice anxieties	Freedom from pain will help to: ● promote the patient's psychological well-being ● ensure that pain does not preclude adequate lung ventilation Provides a consistent level of pain relief Enables patient to control administration of analgesia To ensure support to, and drainage from, the wound site To minimize patient anxiety. To ensure patient co-operation. To promote the patient's psychological well-being

2. Haemorrhage	To identify promptly evidence of haemorrhage	❏ Observation of wound, wound drainage and stoma drainage – for blood loss. Record pulse and blood pressure ½ hourly for 2 hours
		if satisfactory:
		   2 hourly for 4 hours
		   2 hourly for 4 hours
		   4 hourly thereafter
		Observation of patient's skin temperature and skin colour
			Recognition of excessive blood loss will enable initiation of measures to stop bleeding and enable replacement of blood/fluid loss
			
			● visible bleeding
			● tachycardia
			● weak, thready pulse ⎫ may indicate
			● hypotension ⎬ haemorrhage
			● pale, cold clammy skin ⎭

Nursing Care Plan 15.4 (*cont'd*)

Problem (actual/potential)	Goal	Actions	Rationale
3. **Inability to ensure own hydration and nutrition**	To ensure that patient's hydration and nutrition needs are met	❒ Care of i.v. infusion, possible total parenteral nutrition, provision of oral fluids and diet once this is possible (usually when bowel sounds return) record fluid balance	Patient is initially unable to tolerate oral fluids/diet. In order to monitor fluid balance
4. **Nausea/Vomiting**	To prevent/alleviate nausea	❒ Avoidance of oral fluids until bowel sounds return ❒ Possible administration of an antiemetic drug, e.g. cyclizine	Absence of peristaltic activity will result in nausea/vomiting if oral fluids are given To promote patient comfort. To counteract possible stimulation of the vomiting centre which may be caused by some controlled drug analgesia
5. **Infection**	To prevent development of infection To identify infection promptly should it occur	❒ Ensure strict aseptic technique whilst caring for the patient's wound site(s) and during removal of drains and sutures ❒ Record patient's temperature 2 hourly during the immediate postoperative period, if satisfactory, 4 hourly thereafter ❒ Observe wound site(s) and stoma for: excessive redness, excessive swelling, purulent exudate	This will help to prevent entry of micro-organisms into wound sites Pyrexia may indicate the presence of infection These may indicate the presence of infection
6. **Problems associated with reduced mobility, i.e pressure sores, chest infection, deep venous thrombosis**	To prevent/minimize the possibility of their occurrence	❒ Assist the patient to change their position every 2–4 hours. Observation of skin over sites which are subjected to pressure. Possible use of pressure-relieving devices, e.g. Spenco mattress ❒ Encourage the patient to breathe deeply and ensure that they are painfree (see 'Pain') ❒ Encourage the patient to move their legs and feet whilst in bed. Encourage early mobilization. Possible fitting of patient with thromboembolic deterrent stockings. Administration of subcutaneous heparin if prescribed	To prevent development of pressure sores. Prompt identification of areas of redness. Relief of pressure To maximize lung expansion and prevent development of chest infection In order to prevent development of deep venous thrombosis
7. **Inability to attend to own personal hygiene needs**	To assist the patient with these until they are able to self-care	❒ Assist the patient to wash in bed and later in shower until they are able to self-care ❒ Assist patient to implement oral hygiene 2–4 hourly until they are able to tolerate oral fluids/diet. Assist them as required thereafter	To ensure patient comfort and hygiene. Showering is preferable to bathing; it reduces the risk of wound infection To ensure patient comfort and hygiene

Nursing Care Plan 15.4 (*cont'd*)

Problem (actual/ potential)	Goal	Actions	Rationale
7. (cont'd)		❏ Carry out gentle cleansing of the stoma as required, using warm water, disposable wipes and disposal bag	To ensure patient comfort and hygiene
		❏ Encourage the patient to observe implementation of stoma care and to ask questions. Encourage the patient to assume responsibility (initially with nursing guidance) for stoma care as soon as possible	To promote the patient's acceptance of the stoma and to increase their confidence in caring for it
8. **Inability to attend to elimination needs**	To assist the patient until he/she is able to self-care	❏ Use of transparent, drainable stoma bags during the immediate postoperative period. Observation and recording of stoma output: • volume • consistency • colour • odour	To enable observation of stoma drainage. Exudate will initially be fluid: Use of drainable bag reduces the number of bag changes (which might cause discomfort to the patient during the immediate postoperative period)
		❏ Report any bleeding from *within* the stoma	This may indicate haemorrhage
		❏ Reinforce preoperative explanations in relation to the stoma output and changes in stoma appearance, e.g. oedema will subside. Encourage the patient to ask questions and voice anxieties	To provide reassurance and to promote the patient's psychological well-being
		❏ Assist the patient to the commode to pass urine, or to use a urinal	The patient will require assistance to mobilize
		❏ A urinary catheter may be in situ during the immediate postoperative period	To provide an accurate recording of urine output To minimize patient discomfort
		❏ Ensure that catheter care is carried out 2 hourly	To minimize the possibility of urinary tract infection
		❏ Record urine output	To monitor urine output and fluid balance
9. **Excoriation of skin surrounding the stoma: this is a particular risk if the patient has an ileostomy as digestive enzymes in the effluent will cause excoriation**	To prevent excoriation. To educate the patient in relation to skin care	❏ Use of well-fitting appliances in order to ensure that effluent does not contact skin	A well-fitting appliance will prevent contact between the effluent and the skin
		❏ If contact between skin and effluent occurs whilst changing bags, ensure that skin is thoroughly washed and dried: use of a barrier cream may be indicated	To minimize the skin damage which may be caused by effluent
		❏ Provide advice to the patient in relation to skin care and appliance sizing/fitting. Provide advice regarding action to be taken should skin excoriation occur	Patient education is necessary in order to ensure maintenance of skin care following discharge home

Nursing Care Plan 15.4 (*cont'd*)			
Problem (actual/ potential)	**Goal**	**Actions**	**Rationale**
10. **Altered body image as a result of stoma formation**	To enable patient to achieve acceptance of this	❑ Reinforcement of preoperative explanations and discussions, provide the patient with opportunities to ventilate their feelings and to ask questions. Involvement of significant others in these discussions if patient so wishes	To enable the patient to come to terms with their altered body image
		❑ Provision of support for the patient following his/her discharge home, e.g. stoma therapist, hospital, ostomy societies, written information	To provide continuing support and to prevent feelings of isolation

Preoperative preparation If surgery has been decided upon, psychological preparation of the patient is of vital importance as the major surgery involved and the formation of a stoma will cause an alteration in body image (see Ch. 4). Successful preparation of the patient may play a considerable part in assisting them to come to terms with this alteration.

Time is spent with the patient in order to explain what the surgery will entail and to discuss its implications, both in the immediate postoperative period and in the long term. The use of diagrams, photographs and written material may be helpful. A stoma care nurse should be involved at this stage, as he has specialist knowledge of all aspects of stoma care. The patient may also find it helpful to meet with a patient who has had successful ileostomy and discuss surgery and its aftermath with them. The patient should be encouraged to ask questions and express any fears and anxieties which he may have.

Physical preparation of the patient includes preparation of the bowel. The form which this takes will depend upon the patient's condition, as inflamed sections of intestine may be at risk of perforation if certain types of preparation are used.

General principles of preoperative and postoperative care are provided in Chapter 4. An outline of the specific care which the patient will require following restorative proctocolectomy or proctocolectomy and stoma formation is provided in Nursing Care Plans 15.3 and 15.4.

Coeliac disease

The gluten component of wheat causes a mucosal abnormality of the small intestine in some individuals. Barley, oats and rye may also be responsible. The disorder is usually diagnosed during the first 3 years of life. The child fails to thrive, has abdominal distension, anaemia and passes voluminous pale stools. Diagnosis is by means of intestinal biopsy (see p. 514). The damage to the mucosa is thought to be due to an inappropriate immunological process and is reversible when gluten is eradicated from the diet.

Nursing strategies

The child's parents will require careful explanations about the disorder and the measures necessary to ensure that it is not exacerbated. When the child is old enough to understand, he must also be given clear, simple explanations about what they can and cannot eat and why the restrictions are necessary.

The person who has coeliac disease must adhere to a gluten-free diet indefinitely. This means the total exclusion of any foods which contain wheat, barley, oats and rye. Restrictions upon foods which the person may eat are therefore considerable. The child's parents, and the child when appropriate, require dietary advice and details of which foods contain gluten and where gluten-free products may be obtained. The Coeliac Society in the UK provides diet sheets, recipes and advice and the family should be informed of their existence. Regular follow-up appointments are arranged in order to monitor the child's health and these may be used to discuss areas of concern which the parent or child may have.

Irritable bowel syndrome

Epidemiology and aetiology

This is one of the commonest disorders of the gastrointestinal tract. It consists of disturbance of an individual's bowel habit over a long period, for which no organic cause can be found. The disturbance may take the form of diarrhoea, constipation, or alternating periods of each.

Irritable bowel syndrome most commonly affects women between the ages of 20 and 40 years. It has been found that many who are affected are psychologically tense and conscientious people (Shearman and Crean 1991). Some individuals relate the onset of symptoms to a bout of infective diarrhoea, or find that certain types of food cause exacerbation of symptoms.

The commonest symptom which the individual experiences is abdominal pain, frequently sited in the right or left iliac fossa or hypogastrium (Fig. 15.4). This may be relieved by defaecation and exacerbated by food. Diarrhoea, when present, occurs most frequently during the early part of the day and may also follow meals. Abdominal distension may also be a feature, as may an increase in bowel sounds and in the amount of flatus passed. Non-specific symptoms, such as tiredness, nausea and headaches, may also be present.

Investigation

Sigmoidoscopy and barium enema may be carried out in order to exclude the possibility of an organic basis for the individual's symptoms.

Therapeutic management and nursing strategies

Following exclusion of organic disease as a cause of symptoms reassurance can be given to the individual, who may have been worried that they had, for example, malignant disease.

As anxiety and stress may exacerbate symptoms, the alleviation of these may help to reduce symptoms. The person is advised that stress reduction will be beneficial. For some people avoidance of excessive stress may be possible. For others stress reduction may be achieved by utilization of coping strategies. These may include relaxation techniques and discussion should take place with the patient in order to identify areas of stress and measures which may be appropriate to alleviate it.

If constipation is a symptom an increase in the consumption of roughage and possible prescription of a stool-bulking agent may be prescribed. Laxatives however should not be taken.

The symptoms of pain and diarrhoea may be treated by prescription of an antispasmodic or anticholinergic drug which will help to reduce excess peristalsis. Diarrhoea which is painless may be alleviated by use of loperamide or codeine phosphate in emergencies, and by avoidance of foods likely to cause diarrhoea, for example fresh fruit.

Diverticular disease

A diverticulum is a herniation of mucosa through the muscle wall (Fig. 15.9). The term diverticulosis denotes the presence of diverticula at any point in the gastrointestinal tract, although they most commonly occur in the colon.

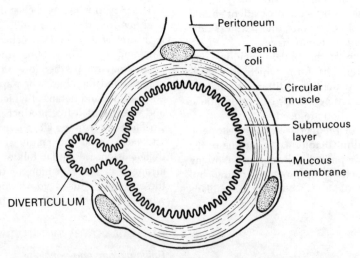

Fig. 15.9 Intestinal diverticula: cross-section of bowel showing one diverticulum. (Reproduced with permission from Wilson 1990, p. 203)

Aetiology

Diverticula are most commonly found in the colon of individuals who are middle aged or elderly. Some research findings indicate that as many as 50% of people in western populations may have some degree of diverticular disease by the age of 70.

Dietary factors are thought to be at least partially responsible, as diverticular disease is rarely found in areas of the world in which people eat a high roughage diet. The incidence is increasing in western countries in which food refinement involves removal of roughage.

Diverticula may become inflamed (**diverticulitis**), the cause of which is unclear, but is possibly due to faecal material becoming trapped within diverticula. Diverticulitis may resolve spontaneously or the inflamed diverticula may rupture, resulting in peritonitis. Repeated attacks of diverticulitis cause thickening of the bowel wall and narrowing of the intestinal lumen. If severe this may lead to intestinal obstruction.

Common symptoms

Discomfort or pain, which may be severe, is usually sited in the left iliac fossa (Fig. 15.4). Signs and symptoms associated with peritonitis (see pp. 521–522) or intestinal obstruction may be present. The person may experience alteration in bowel habit, possibly accompanied by rectal bleeding which may be severe.

Investigation

Sigmoidoscopy and possibly colonoscopy may be carried out, in order to exclude the presence of malignancy.

Radiological examination following barium enema is usually sufficient to establish the diagnosis.

Therapeutic management and nursing strategies

During an acute attack of diverticulitis the person will require to rest as much as possible and bed rest is recommended, the person getting up only for toilet purposes. Antibiotic therapy may be prescribed. Fluids may be given orally, but if the attack is severe intravenous fluids and nil orally may be necessary.

The majority of patients will then recover, but occasionally emergency surgery may be required, with the formation of a temporary colostomy. For an outline of the care which the patient will require in relation to the colostomy see Nursing Care Plan 15.4. Elective surgery in order to remove areas of the colon which are affected and to resect these may be recommended for some patients, following resolution of the acute attack.

The ingestion of a high fibre diet, with the possible prescription of a bulk laxative such as methylcellulose, will help to prevent constipation. The person will therefore require explanations about the disorder and advice on the dietary measures which may help to prevent exacerbations.

Intestinal obstruction

The contents of the gastrointestinal tract may be unable to progress onwards for a variety of reasons. Following surgery or inflammatory bowel disease adhesions may form between portions of the tract and other organs. Alternatively an obstruction may occur within the tract. This may be caused for example by a large bolus of food, a large gallstone or a tumour. Other causes are strangulation of a hernia (see p. 550), or intussusception, in which one part of the intestine slips into the section located beyond it. Alternatively the intestine may twist upon itself (volvulus), causing obstruction of the lumen and possible necrosis, perforation and peritonitis. Severe pain or trauma (including handling of the intestine during surgery) may cause disruption to peristalsis. This is known as paralytic ileus.

Common symptoms

Distension of the intestine proximal to the obstruction is caused by the accumulation of swallowed air and bacterial decomposition of stagnant intestinal contents. The intestine reacts to obstruction (other than that caused by paralytic ileus) by increasing the strength and frequency of peristalsis. This causes colicky abdominal pain. If the obstruction is in the large intestine this colic occurs every 10–20 minutes, whereas obstruction in the small intestine causes colic every 2–3 minutes.

Intestinal distension causes vomiting. Vomitus initially comprises stomach contents, but is later bile stained and, if the condition remains untreated, faeculent. In the initial stages of hyperperistalsis diarrhoea may occur, but when the muscle becomes exhausted and adynamic (i.e. peristalsis ceases) complete constipation and absence of bowel sounds and flatus will occur.

As intestinal obstruction prevents the absorption of fluids and electrolyes the patient will become dehydrated. In addition to the other symptoms, they are likely to be apprehensive or fearful as to the cause of their illness.

If untreated the patient's condition would deteriorate rapidly, severe dehydration and electrolyte imbalance leading to cardiovascular complications. The affected section of intestine would be at risk of necrosis or perforation (with resultant peritonitis).

Investigations

Initially auscultation of the patient's abdomen may reveal hyperperistalsis. Later, or from the outset in patients whose obstruction is due to paralytic ileus, there will be total absence of bowel sounds.

Abdominal X-rays of the patient in the supine and erect positions will demonstrate the accumulation of gas and fluid levels.

Therapeutic management and nursing strategies

The patient requires an explanation of what intestinal obstruction involves and of the measures which will be taken to alleviate it and to investigate its cause. As the patient is acutely ill, the use of closed questions may be appropriate in order to reduce the effort required of the patient in replying.

The patient is given nil orally. A nasogastric tube is passed (see Ch. 4) and is attached to low-grade suction in order to keep the stomach free of fluid. This will help to alleviate nausea and vomiting. The amount, colour and consistency of the aspirate is recorded. Intravenous replacement of fluid and electrolytes is commenced. Emergency surgical intervention may be required in order to remove the cause of obstruction. Resection may be possible at that time, or formation of a temporary colostomy may be carried out, followed by resection at a later date. Nursing Care Plan 15.4 outlines the care which the patient may require if they have undergone colostomy formation.

The patient who has intestinal obstruction will require almost total assistance with the activities of living. Personal hygiene, including cleansing of the nasal cavity around the nasogastric tube, is carried out for the patient. The patient's debilitated state renders them at high risk of pressure sore development and they therefore require assistance to change position 2 hourly, at which time pressure areas should be examined for evidence of damage to skin integrity. Oral hygiene is given frequently (usually 2 hourly) as the patient's mouth will be dry because of having nil orally and being dehydrated.

Appendicitis

This is an inflammatory condition of the appendix. The incidence has decreased considerably during the past 40 years and it is thought that this may be related to improved sanitation and food cleanliness. Those affected are usually in their teens or twenties. The cause is thought to be obstruction of the lumen by swelling of lymphoid tissue and/or by a faecolith (i.e. a dry hardened lump of faecal material). Perforation and subsequent peritonitis may occur.

Clinical features

The patient experiences abdominal pain, which subsequently localizes between the umbilicus and right ileum. The pain is accompanied by anorexia, nausea and vomiting and possibly a mild pyrexia. If untreated abcess formation and possible perforation of the appendix may result.

Investigations

Abdominal palpation and rectal examination. These reveal guarding and tenderness.

Therapeutic management and nursing strategies

Surgical removal of the appendix (appendicectomy) is carried out. The patient therefore requires explanations and preoperative preparation. Antibiotic therapy is usually given. If surgery is uncomplicated the patient will be allowed oral fluids if bowel sounds are present. They will be encouraged to mobilize and self-care and are normally discharged home within 2–3 days. If a surgical drain has been inserted into the wound site the amount, colour and consistency of exudate is recorded and the drain is usually removed within 48–72 hours following surgery. A dry dressing is then applied over the drain site. Wound sutures are usually absorbable. The general principles of preoperative and postoperative care are outlined in Chapter 4.

Prior to discharge the patient is given advice about wound hygiene and the observations which should be made to identify the presence of wound infection. A follow-up appointment is arranged and advice is given about any restrictions in the activities of daily living, for example in relation to lifting.

Pancreatitis

Pancreatitis may be acute or chronic. Inflammation of

the organ leads to autodigestion of pancreatic tissue and possible damage to adjacent organs. Pancreatic enzymes may also travel in the bloodstream and cause pulmonary damage. The endocrine function of the pancreas may be impaired, resulting in glycosuria (see Ch. 16).

Acute pancreatitis

Aetiology   Within the UK 50% of individuals who develop acute pancreatitis do so as a result of biliary disease. For 20% the association is with alcohol abuse and in the remaining number the cause is unknown. There is known to be an association with certain infections, for example mumps, or drugs, for example azothiaprine.

Clinical features   The person experiences a sudden onset of acute pain, located in the epigastric or right hyponchondrial regions (Fig. 15.4). It is constant and may radiate to the back, shoulders or abdomen. The onset of pain is frequently within the 12–24 hours following a large meal and consumption of alcohol. Nausea and vomiting occur. If the pancreatitis is severe the clinical features of shock may be present (see Ch. 4).

Investigations   Blood samples are taken to assess amylase levels, which rise within 2–12 hours following the onset of symptoms. Blood glucose levels rise above normal limits and blood calcium levels are decreased. Abdominal X-rays are carried out, as are CT and ultrasound scanning.

Therapeutic management and nursing strategies Treatment of shock, if present, is a priority, as is treatment of respiratory problems. Pain relief is provided by controlled drug analgesia, usually pethidine. (Morphine is contraindicated, as it stimulates spasm of the sphincter of Oddi.) The patient's physical condition is monitored closely by estimation of arterial blood gas levels and possibly central venous pressure recording (see Ch. 12).

Fluids are provided intravenously, the patient is given nil orally and a nasogastric tube is inserted and aspirated either intermittently or continuously. Urine output is measured and catheterization may be necessary. Shock may lead to development of paralytic ileus (see p. 533). When the pancreatitis is severe it may be necessary for the patient to be nursed in an intensive care area. The patient is acutely ill and will require almost total assistance with the activities of daily living.

Clear and concise explanations of investigative procedures and of treatment are required. These should also be provided for the patient's significant others, who may require considerable psychological support and who should be given the opportunity to ask questions and to voice anxieties.

Chronic pancreatitis

Aetiology   Within the UK the majority of people who develop this disorder do so as a result of long-term alchohol abuse. It most commonly affects males between the ages of 35 and 45 years.

Clinical features   The person experiences abdominal pain, which may have a gradual onset, and which is less severe than that of acute pancreatitis. They may have anorexia and weight loss, with the possibility that the pancreatic damage may have caused diabetes mellitus, malabsorption, steatorrhoea or jaundice.

Investigations   Abdominal X-rays, CT, ultrasound scanning and tests of pancreatic function are carried out in order to assess the extent of pancreatic damage.

Therapeutic management and nursing strategies The patient who has chronic pancreatitis is unlikely to make a full recovery as the damage is usually extensive. Pancreatic enzyme replacement may be given orally. This reduces abdominal pain and discomfort and enables improved fat digestion to take place. H_2-receptor antagonists may also be prescribed; their action is outlined on page 520. Analgesia may additionally be required in order to achieve pain relief.

Alcohol abuse is the most common cause of chronic pancreatitis and therefore other physical and psychological problems co-exist. Individual assessment of the patient's physical and psychosocial status is vital in order to develop a suitable care plan. A favourable prognosis for patients who have chronic pancreatitis is closely linked with cessation of alcohol ingestion. It is important that this is made clear to the patient and that all available help is given to aid the patient to stop drinking alcohol. (See p. 315 for discussion of nursing strategies for the care of those suffering from alchohol abuse).

Cirrhosis of the liver

Necrosis of liver cells may occur for a number of reasons. In cirrhosis this necrosis is accompanied and succeeded by fibrosis and nodular overgrowth of the remaining hepatocytes. Cirrhosis affects cells throughout the liver.

Aetiology

There are many causes. Cirrhosis may follow viral

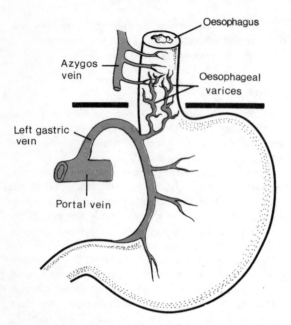

Fig. 15.10 Oesophageal varices. (Reproduced with permission from Wilson 1990, p. 196)

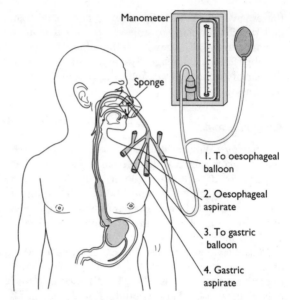

Fig. 15.11 Application of pressure to bleeding oesophageal varices by means of oesophageal-gastric tube

hepatitis, prolonged biliary obstruction and certain long-term drug regimens, for example methyldopa. It may also be caused by long-term alcohol abuse.

Common symptoms

The patient may have no symptoms, or may complain of weakness, fatigue or weight loss. Anorexia, nausea, vomiting and upper abdominal discomfort may be present. Males may develop gynaecomastia. Pre-menopausal women may have an irregular menstrual cycle or amenorrhoea. Loss of libido occurs in both sexes. Spider naevi may be visible in the skin. These comprise a central arteriole, from which small vessels radiate. The most common sites for these are the upper chest, face, necklace area of the neck, forearms and dorsum of the hands.

The patient may have hypertension of the portal circulation. This leads to the development of a collateral blood circulation. Distended veins (varices) may be present in the distal oesophagus (Fig. 15.10). The risk is that these may rupture and bleed; such bleeding may be severe and acute or, less commonly, slow and chronic.

For details of the therapeutic management and nursing strategies used when caring for people who have gastrointestinal bleeding please see page 521. One emergency measure which may be taken is the insertion of an oesophago-gastric tube, for example Sengstaken tube (Fig. 15.11). Once the tube is in situ the balloons are inflated; the rationale is that the sustained pressure will cause the bleeding to cease. Vasopressin or other drug therapy may be administered intravenously in order to reduce portal venous pressure.

Endoscopy may be carried out, during which sclerosing agents may be injected into the varices in order to prevent further bleeding. Alternatively, surgical formation of a shunt may be undertaken in order to reduce the pressure.

If liver failure is present in addition to cirrhosis the patient may develop ascites (the accumulation of excess fluid in the peritoneal cavity). This causes progressive distension of the abdomen and an alternation in body image. The patient may also suffer from symptoms caused by pressure from the fluid, for example breathlessness as lung expansion is impeded.

The patient who has ascites will require hospitalization for treatment. Nursing Care Plan 15.5 illustrates a care plan for such a person.

Cholelithiasis

The presence of gallstones is known as **cholelithiasis**. The person who has gallstones may be asymptomatic whilst the stones remain within the gallbladder. They will however experience symptoms if the calculi

| Nursing Care Plan 15.5   Care of a person who has cirrhosis of the liver accompanied by severe ascites ||||

Problem (actual/ potential)	Goal	Actions	Rationale
1. Dyspnoea/ abdominal discomfort (caused by pressure from ascitic fluid)	To alleviate dyspnoea, discomfort	❏ Bedrest	Reduces metabolic demands of tissues. Alleviates patient's feelings of tiredness and dyspnoea
		❏ Upright position; patient well supported by backrest and pillows	Facilitates lung expansion, gravity will alleviate pressure of ascitic fluid on lungs
		❏ Advise patient to avoid foods which have a high salt content, e.g. ham, bacon, and to avoid adding salt to cooked food. Emphasize the importance of this and possibly involve dietician in discussion of suitable and unsuitable foods	Reduction in salt intake will help to reduce fluid retention
		❏ Fluid restriction of 1 litre/day: explain importance of this to the patient	Fluid restriction will inhibit the formation of ascitic fluid
		❏ Possible administration of diuretic drugs	To facilitate excretion of ascitic fluid
		❏ Possible abdominal paracentesis (removal of excess ascitic fluid using a strict aseptic technique)	Symptomatic relief. Prevention of infection
		❏ Possible insertion of a LeVeen shunt if other measures are ineffective	To divert ascitic fluid from peritoneum to central veins
		❏ Weigh patient daily	Monitor effectiveness of therapy (i.e. aim is to achieve weight reduction of 0.5–1 kg/day)
		❏ Daily blood samples to ascertain urea and electrolyte levels	Identify and treat any abnormalities
		❏ Record patient's respiratory rate 2–4 hourly	Monitor dyspnoea
2. Potential problem: poor nutritional status	To improve nutritional status	❏ When ascites has diminished a high protein (80–100 g/day) and high calorie (3000/day) intake is encouraged	A high protein and calorie intake will improve the patient's general health
		❏ Vitamin supplements may initially be required	
		❏ Discussion with patient to identify suitable and unsuitable foods	
3. Altered body image due to abdominal distension	To alleviate psychological distress	❏ Explanation of ascites and of aims of treatment, i.e. elimination of ascitic fluid. Encourage patient to voice feelings and express fears/anxieties	To provide reassurance that treatment will alleviate abdominal distension
		❏ Possible measurements of abdominal girth	To monitor the patient's response to treatment
4. Those associated with immobility, i.e. pressure sores, chest infection, deep venous thrombosis	To prevent/ minimize the possibility of their occurrence	❏ Assist the patient to change their position every 2–4 hours. Possible use of pressure-relieving aids, e.g. Spenco mattress	To prevent development of pressure sores
		❏ Encourage the patient to breathe deeply	To ensure maximum lung expansion and to prevent development of chest infection
		❏ Encourage the patient to move their legs and feet. Possible use of thromboembolic deterrent stockings	To prevent development of a deep venous thrombosis

Nursing Care Plan 15.5 (*cont'd*)			
Problem (actual/ potential)	**Goal**	**Actions**	**Rationale**
5. Inability to attend to personal hygiene needs unaided	To assist the patient with these as required	❏ Assist the patient to wash in bed until he/she is mobile and is able to self-care ❏ Assist the patient to implement oral hygiene	To promote patient comfort and hygiene To promote patient comfort and hygiene
6. Inability to attend to elimination needs unaided	To assist the patient whilst they are unable to self-care	❏ Provision of toilet facilities at the patient's bedside, e.g. urinal, commode: wheel the patient to the toilet area if possible ❏ Monitor urine and faecal output ❏ Ensure the patient's privacy	To promote patient comfort To identify fluid imbalance and abnormality of bowel habit To minimize the patient's embarrassment and to promote their self-esteem
7. Possible abnormality of temperature, pulse, blood pressure	To identify and report any abnormalities	❏ Record the patient's temperature, pulse and blood pressure 4 hourly, or more frequently if indicated	To identify abnormalities To monitor the patient's progress
8. Tendency to bleed/bruise easily due to interference with liver function **Bleeding from oesophageal varices**	To identify bleeding	❏ Observe the patient's excreta. Observe the patient's skin for visible bruising. Improve patient's nutritional status. Vitamin supplements may be required, e.g. vitamin K (see also p. 537)	Haematuria/melaena/haematemesis may indicate internal haemorrhage. This may indicate that clotting mechanisms are deficient. Adequate nutrition may enhance the patient's clotting mechanisms
9. Underlying cause of cirrhosis	To identify underlying causes and minimize damage caused	❏ Patient education if required in relation to the need to abstain from alcohol. See Chapter 9 for further information relating to the care of people who have alcohol-related problems	Abstention from alcohol will prevent further liver damage

move into the bile duct. Figure 15.12 illustrates sites of biliary tract obstruction. The bile duct muscle becomes hyperactive, causing severe pain (biliary colic). Alternatively, inflammation of the gallbladder may cause **cholecystitis**.

Epidemiology and aetiology

Within the UK the adult incidence of gallstones is estimated to be between 15% and 20%. In those who are over 60 years the incidence is 40%. In adults under the age of 40 there is a three to one female to male ratio, whereas in elderly people the ratios are almost equal.

Gallstones occur more frequently in 'developed' countries and in these the incidence has increased during the past 30 years and occurs at an earlier age than previously. The majority of sufferers in devel-oped countries have stones whose main component is cholesterol, pigment stones being less common.

Certain factors may predispose people to gallstone formation, for example obesity, multiple pregnancies or the long-term use of oral contraceptives.

Common symptoms

Spasm of the gallbladder or cystic duct will cause biliary colic. The person experiences severe, spasmodic pain which radiates from the right upper quadrant of the abdomen to the right shoulder-tip. Acute cholecystitis may cause pain, pyrexia, nausea and vomiting. Pain may follow food ingestion. A care plan for a patient who is suffering from acute cholecystitis is given in Nursing Care Plan 15.6.

If a stone becomes impacted in the common bile duct the patient may develop obstructive jaundice.

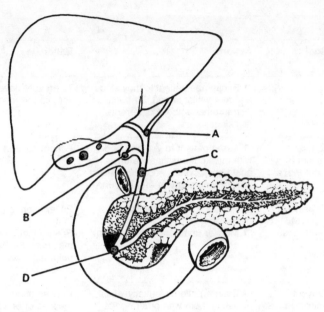

Fig. 15.12   Sites of biliary tract obstruction due to gall-stones. (A) Hepatic duct. (B) Cystic duct. (C) Bile duct. (D) Sphincter of Oddi

Nursing Care Plan 15.6 Care for a person who has cholecystitis			
Problem (actual/ potential)	**Goal**	**Actions**	**Rationale**
1. Pain due to spasm of gall bladder muscle (biliary colic). Pain exacerbated by deep inspiration	Alleviate patient's pain and discomfort	❒ Administration of controlled drug analgesia, e.g. pethidine i.m. ❒ If pain is very severe morphine i.m. may be required ❒ Atropine i.m.	To relieve pain Morphine provides a higher degree of pain relief To counteract increased tone sphincter of Oddi caused by morphine
2. Nausea/vomiting	To prevent/ alleviate nausea/ vomiting	❒ Administration of antiemetic drug, e.g. cyclizine i.m. ❒ Light diet, low fat content, encourage oral fluids if able to tolerate these ❒ If unable to tolerate oral fluids, c/o i.v. infusion ❒ Nasogastric tube if nausea/ vomiting severe ❒ Record fluid balance ❒ Ensure that patient rests, i.e. bed rest, up only to commode	Pain may cause nausea If biliary obstruction present ingestion of fat may cause nausea/vomiting due to effect of cholecystokinin on gall bladder To ensure that patient does not become dehydrated To rest gastrointestinal tract To ensure that patient's fluid balance is maintained Reduce metabolic demands of body tissues
3. Complications of immobility, i.e. pressure sores, chest infection, deep venous thrombosis	To prevent occurrence of complications of immobility	❒ Assist patient to change their position every 2–4 hours, possible use of pressure-relieving aids ❒ Encourage patient to breathe deeply	To prevent development of pressure sores To ensure maximum lung expansion and prevent development of chest infection

Nursing Care Plan 15.6 (cont'd)

Problem (actual/ potential)	Goal	Actions	Rationale
3. (cont'd)		❒ Encourage patient to move legs and feet whilst in bed. Fit patient with thromboembolic deterrent stockings	To prevent development of a deep venous thrombosis
4. Inability to attended to own personal hygiene needs	To assist patient to meet these	❒ Assist patient to wash in bed with maximum assistance until acute cholecystitis subsides. Assist patient to implement oral hygiene	Patient comfort and hygiene
5. Inability to attend to own elimination needs	To assist patient to meet these	❒ Provision of toilet facilities at bedside ❒ Monitor urine and faecal output	Patient comfort and hygiene Ensure that patient's fluid balance is maintained. Observe faecal output: pale, fatty stools may indicate biliary obstruction
6. Loss of dignity and autonomy	Prevent /minimize loss of these	❒ Ensure patient's privacy whilst assisting them with other needs ❒ Include patient in care planning and decision making	Prevent/minimize patient's possible feelings of embarrassment Promote patient's self-esteem and feelings of self-control
7. Infection	To identify presence of infection	❒ Record patient's temperature and pulse 4 hourly	Pyrexia and/or tachycardia may indicate infection
8. Jaundice (if biliary obstruction present)	To identify and monitor	❒ Observe colour of patient's skin and mucous membranes	To monitor progression/subsidence of jaundice
9. Pruritus	To alleviate pruritis	❒ Ensure patient's skin is clean and dry. Use of creams to reduce itch. Administer drugs, if prescribed, to reduce itch	Alleviation of discomfort of pruritis
10. Altered body image due to jaundice	To provide reassurance	❒ Explanations of why jaundice has occurred and that it will subside once biliary obstruction has been relieved	To provide reassurance to patient that jaundice will soon subside

Jaundice occurs because the excretion of bilirubin is blocked; this substance therefore circulates within the bloodstream. The patients urine becomes very dark due to excess bilirubin excretion by this route. The stools on the other hand become pale and fatty due to lack of bile pigment and fat malabsorption.

Inability to absorb fat may result in malabsorption also of fat-soluble vitamins, including vitamin K. This may cause coagulation defects.

Investigations

Examination of urine and faeces is made both at ward level and in the laboratory in order to confirm bilirubinuria and the presence of faecal fat. Ultrasound examination and endoscopic retrograde cholangiopancreatography (ERCP) may be used to determine the presence and position of gallstones and it may be possible to remove these during ERCP.

Therapeutic management and nursing intervention

If the patient has an adequately functioning gallbladder and the stones are of the cholesterol type it may be possible to dissolve them by means of oral

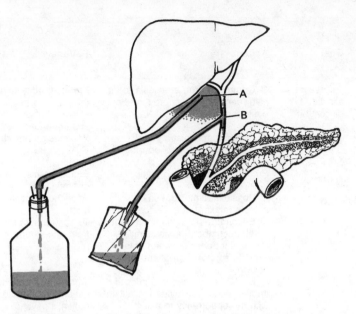

Fig. 15.13 Tube drainage following open cholecystectomy

medication. The process of dissolution is slow (6 months to 2 years) and is only suitable for approximately 30% of patients who have gallstones.

As stated under 'Investigations', above, stone removal during ERCP may be possible.

Lithotripsy may be suitable for some patients. Shock waves are directed at the calculi (whilst the patient is anaesthetized) and these waves fragment the stones, following which the residue may progress down the bile duct for excretion in faeces.

Cholecystectomy

The most satisfactory treatment of gallstones is removal of the gallbladder (cholecystectomy) and of any stones which are present. This operation may be carried out by means of 'open' surgery. The gallbladder is removed via a large abdominal incision and a drain is inserted into the area from which it has been removed. It may also be necessary to explore the bile duct in order to remove calculi. As handling the bile duct causes it to become inflamed and oedematous it is necessary to insert a T-tube drain (Fig. 15.13) for a period of 7–10 days following surgery in order to ensure maintenance of bile flow.

Nursing Care Plan 15.7 illustrates a care plan for a person who has undergone this type of cholecystectomy.

Laparoscopic cholecystectomy Removal of the gallbladder by laparoscopic means is now being carried out by an increasing number of surgeons. The patient is given general anaesthesia and four abdominal incisions are made. These are used for insertion of the laparoscope, for insertion of gas into the peritoneal cavity (which enables the surgeon to have clear vision of, and access to, the gallbladder) and for removal of the gallbladder.

It is of particular importance that, prior to laparoscopic cholecystectomy, the patient fully empties their bladder. This is a precaution against the possibility of bladder perforation during surgery.

When the necessity for surgery has been agreed, it must be explained to the patient that laparoscopic removal of the gallbladder is sometimes impossible, for example if the patient has abdominal adhesions. If this is the case they may require an open cholecystectomy and a basic outline of what they will then experience on return from surgery should be given. As is the case prior to any procedure the patient must, in addition to explanations, be given the opportunity to ask questions and voice any fears or anxieties which they may have. For an outline of the general principles of care for patients prior to surgery under general anaesthesia, please see Chapter 4.

An outline of the differentiation between open and laparoscopic cholecystectomy, and the implications of each for the patient, is given in Table 15.1. As this illustrates, laparoscopic surgery is preferable whenever it is possible. The patient suffers minimal discomfort postoperatively, in comparison to the patient

Nursing Care Plan 15.7   Care for a patient who has had an open cholecystectomy

Problem (actual/ potential)	Goal	Actions	Rationale
1. Pain	To prevent/ alleviate discomfort	❑ Controlled drug analgesia to be given regularly for approx. 48 hours postoperatively	Freedom from pain will help to promote the patient's psychological well-being. Ensure that pain does not preclude adequate lung ventilation
		❑ Possible administration of analgesia via a controlled-rate infusion	Provides a consistent level of pain-relief
		Pump/patient-actuated pump	Enables patient to control administration of analgesia
		❑ Possible administration of muscle relaxant, e.g. Buscopan	To reduce muscle spasm within bile duct
		❑ Encourage the patient to adopt a semirecumbent position initially and upright position when able. Provide support for patient with backrest and pillows	To ensure support to, and drainage from, the wound site
		❑ Explain all procedures prior to implementation. Provide the patient with the opportunity to ask questions and voice anxieties	To minimize patient anxiety. To ensure patient co-operation. To promote patient's psychological well-being
		❑ Ensure provision of controlled drug analgesia prior to removal of the T-tube (if T-tube is in situ)	Removal is painful for the patient and may cause spasm of the bile duct
		❑ Care of the T-tube (if one is in situ) to prevent blockage or to identify this promptly if it occurs	T-tube ensures unobstructed bile flow. Pain may indicate that T-tube has become blocked
		❑ T-tube may be clamped for periods approximately 5 days post-operatively	Clamping encourages bile flow into duodenum (instead of into drainage bag); this enables fat digestion.
		❑ Report promptly any evidence that the tube may be blocked, e.g. patient pain, reduced/absent drainage when tube is not clamped	Enables action to be taken to overcome blockage, e.g. irrigation of the tube by medical staff
		❑ Ensure that bile does not come into contact with the patient's skin: if this occurs ensure that skin is cleansed promptly and thoroughly	Bile is excoriative to skin and will cause patient pain
2. Haemorrhage: potential problem	To identify evidence that haemorrhage has occurred	❑ Observation of wound drainage and wound site + record pulse and blood pressure: ½ hourly for 2 hours if satisfactory: hourly for 4 hours 2 hourly for 4 hours 4 hourly thereafter Observation of patient's skin colour and temperature	Recognition of excessive blood loss will enable replacement + initiation of measures to stop bleeding • tachycardia • weak, thready pulse • hypotension • pallor • cold, clammy skin } may indicate haemorrhage
3. Dehydration: (potential problem)	To ensure that patient's hydration needs are met	❑ c/o i.v. infusion + provision of adequate volumes of oral fluid once this is possible (i.e. when bowel sounds have returned)	Patient may initially be unable to tolerate oral fluids
4. Nausea/vomiting	To prevent/ alleviate nausea	❑ Avoidance of oral fluids until peristalsis returns ❑ Possible administration of an antiemetic drug	Absence of peristalsis will result in nausea/vomiting if oral fluids are given Promote patient comfort and possibly counter stimulation of vomiting centre which may be caused by some controlled drug analgesia

Problem (actual/ potential)	Goal	Actions	Rationale
5. Infection	To prevent development of infection To identify infection promptly should it be present	❏ Ensure strict aseptic technique whilst caring for the patient's wound site ❏ Record patient's temperature 2 hourly in the immediate postoperative period; if satisfactory 4 hourly thereafter ❏ Observe wound site for excessive redness, excessive swelling, purulent exudate	Will help to prevent entry of micro-organisms Pyrexia may indicate the presence of infection These may indicate that infection is present
6. Potential problems: those associated with immobility, i.e. pressure sores, chest infection, deep venous thrombosis	To prevent/ minimize the possibility of their occurrence	❏ Assist the patient to change their position every 2–4 hours ❏ Encourage the patient to breathe deeply and ensure that they are pain free (pain may inhibit adequate lung expansion) ❏ Encourage the patient to move legs and feet and encourage early mobility. Prior to surgery fit patient with thromboembolic deterrent stockings. Administer subcutaneous heparin injections if prescribed	To prevent development of pressure sores To maximize lung expansion and prevent development of a chest infection To prevent development of a deep venous thrombosis
7. Inability to attend to personal hygiene needs	To assist patient	❏ Assist the patient to wash in bed or in shower until patient is able to self-care. Assist patient to implement oral hygiene	Ensure patient comfort and hygiene
8. Inability to attend to elimination needs unaided	To assist patient	❏ Assist patient to get out of bed to use commode at bedside, or to be wheeled through to toilet area. Assist patient to mobilize	Patient will require assistance to mobilize for approximately 48–72 hours postoperatively
9. Loss of dignity and autonomy	To maintain patient's dignity and autonomy	❏ Ensure the patient's privacy whilst assisting them with other needs ❏ Include patient in care planning and decision making	Prevent/minimize patient's possible feelings of embarrassment Promote patient's self-esteem and feelings of self-control

undergoing open cholecystectomy, and is fully mobile and discharged home on the day following surgery. The occurrence of the complications which can result from postoperative reduction of mobility is therefore minimized. Activities of daily living may be rapidly resumed following discharge from hospital. A follow-up appointment is arranged 4–6 weeks following surgery.

Nursing Care Plan 15.8 illustrates a care plan for a patient who has undergone laparoscopic chole-cystectomy.

Methods of removal of gallbladder calculi without cholecystectomy are also being pioneered. A small ab-dominal incision is made under general anaesthesia. A needle is inserted into the gallbladder and calculi

are removed. This procedure may be suitable for patients whose calculi are not deemed likely to recur, or for those for whom general anaesthesia is contraindicated.

CARE OF THE PATIENT WHO HAS AN INFECTIVE DISORDER OF THE GASTROINTESTINAL SYSTEM

Oral infections

Oral infections may be caused by poor attention to oral hygiene. Persons particularly at risk are those suffering from general debility due to illness, or who have a compromised immune system. It is therefore a

Table 15.1 Comparison between open and laparoscopic cholecystectomy: implications for the patient

	Open cholecystectomy	Laparoscopic cholecystectomy
Surgical wounds	Long subcostal incision + drainage sites: 1 penrose drain (in situ for 48 hours) + possibly T-tube drain (in situ approx. 8–10 days)	Four abdominal incisions 0.5–1.5 cm long, no drainage required
Mobility	Gradual: not fully mobile for 7–10 days following surgery	Fully mobile on the day following surgery
Pain/discomfort	Considerable: will require controlled drug analgesia for several days + oral analgesia for several days thereafter	Controlled drug analgesia on day of surgery; may require oral analgesia for 24–48 hours thereafter
Nutrition/hydration	i.v. infusion: fluids and normal diet upon return of bowel sounds (may require restriction of dietary fat if T-tube is in situ)	Oral fluids and normal diet as soon as possible
Discharge from hospital	8–12 days following surgery	Usually on the day following surgery
Resumption of all activities of daily living	Gradual; restrictions imposed by wound, e.g. no heavy lifting for 6 weeks	As soon as possible
Return to work	4–6 weeks following surgery	2–3 weeks following surgery

Nursing Care Plan 15.8 Care for a patient who has undergone a laparoscopic cholecystectomy

Problem (actual/ potential)	Goal	Actions	Rationale
1. Pain/Discomfort (Feelings of abdominal distension and shoulder tip pain. This is caused by the presence of air in the peritoneal cavity: inserted during laparoscopy to aid vision)	To prevent/ minimize patient's pain/ discomfort	❐ Controlled drug analgesia, e.g. papaveretum i.m. during the immediate postoperative period	Pain may be quite severe initially
		❐ Possible antiemetic drug, e.g. cyclizine i.m.	Papaveretum may cause nausea. Postoperative discomfort may cause nausea
		❐ Oral analgesia, e.g. co-proxamol if required thereafter	
		❐ Reinforcement of the explanations given to the patient prior to surgery	Air will be reabsorbed over a period of several days
		❐ Reassurance that pain/discomfort will be transient	Explanation may help to reduce anxiety
		❐ Report any complaints of severe pain	Severe persistent pain may indicate a biliary leak into the peritoneum
		❐ Advise patient prior to discharge that an increase in the severity of pain, or its continuation for more than a few days, should be reported to their GP or to the hospital	As above
2. Haemorrhage (potential problem)	To identify this promptly should it occur	❐ Observation of any exudate from wound sites and record pulse and blood pressure: ½ hourly for 2 hours if satisfactory: hourly for 4 hours 2 hourly for 4 hours 4–6 hourly thereafter	Recognition of blood loss, external or internal. Tachycardia or hypotension may indicate haemorrhage

Nursing Care Plan 15.8 *(cont'd)*			
Problem (actual/ potential)	**Goal**	**Actions**	**Rationale**
3. Deep venous thrombosis/ pulmonary embolus (potential problem)	To prevent this	❐ Prior to surgery fit patient with thromboembolic deterrent stockings	To encourage venous return
		❐ Administer subcutaneous heparin if prescribed	Inhibit thrombus formation
		❐ Early, full mobilization, i.e. morning following surgery	To encourage venous return
4. Infection (potential problem)	To prevent infection entering wounds	❐ Educate patient re wound care, i.e. keep wound sites clean. Sutures are subcutaneous and dispersible	Minimize possibility of wound infection
	To identify infection should it occur	❐ Record temp. 6 hourly in postoperatively period	Pyrexia may indicate infection
		❐ Advise patient that if wound sites become inflamed and swollen, painful or discharge, they should contact their GP or the hospital	This may indicate infection

potential problem in patients who have disorders such as leukaemia (see Ch. 14 for further details), those who are receiving cytotoxic therapy as treatment for malignant disease (see Ch. 4) immunosuppressant drugs (see Ch. 16), or those who are suffering from AIDS (see Ch. 14).

Infection may arise because particles of food which remain in the mouth may cause proliferation of harmful bacteria if oral hygiene is not implemented. Infection may spread from the oral cavity into the parotid glands (parotitis). The parotid glands become swollen and painful to the patient and the condition requires treatment with antibiotic therapy. Parotitis may be prevented by careful assessment of the person's oral status and of their ability to self-care in relation to oral hygiene. Those who are unable to self-care will require assistance.

Those whose immune system is compromised are at particular risk of developing infection as a result of overgrowth of the fungus *Candida albicans*. This is found as a commensal organism in the mouths of healthy people, but its proliferation (known as thrush) causes white patches to appear on the tongue and buccal mucosa. This causes the patient discomfort, which may be made worse by eating, or drinking hot fluids.

In addition to meticulous attention to the patient's oral hygiene, treatment is by administration of nystatin lozenges or lotion. These are given following meals and the patient is encouraged to allow the lozenges to dissolve slowly, or to retain the lotion within the mouth for as long as possible, in order to maximize its effect. Although the risk of transmission of thrush is not high (unless mouth-to-mouth contact occurs), it is advisable that the person uses disposable plates, cutlery and drinking utensils until the infection has been eradicated.

Certain disorders which affect the gastrointestinal system may be transmitted from one person to another. The route of spread may be faecal/oral, whereby faecal micro-organisms bearing disease from the carrier are ingested by another person or persons. Faecal micro-organisms on the hands of the carrier may be transmitted onto food, which is then ingested by others. Alternatively, contamination of drinking water may take place and cause disease transmission. Examples of disorders which may be transmitted in this way are salmonella and shigella (dysentery).

Although poor sanitation may facilitate spread of these diseases, their transmission in the UK is virtually always a result of poor personal hygiene, such as inadequate handwashing following defaecation. The nurse, both in hospitals and the community, therefore has an important role to play in educating people into an appreciation of how gastrointestinal infections may be transmitted and thereby how their spread may be avoided.

Other infections, for example viral hepatitis, may additionally be spread in blood and other bodily secretions. The care that a patient who has viral hepatitis will require, including the precautions which must be taken in order to prevent spread of disease, is discussed later in this section. Chapter 4 outlines the principles which require to be followed in order to prevent disease transmission.

Many patients who have infectious disorders of the gastrointestinal system will not require to be hospitalized. As most infective disorders cause vomiting and/or diarrhoea, there is a possibility that the patient may become dehydrated: this is a particular risk for babies and small children. Replacement of lost fluids is vital and if this is impossible due to nausea or vomiting, medical assistance should be sought, as hospitalization and intravenous fluid replacement may be required.

Viral hepatitis

Liver cells become inflamed and unable to conjugate and excrete bile. An excess of unconjugated bilirubin circulates in the blood and causes jaundice. Viral hepatitis is classed as being either infective/type A hepatitis or serum/type B hepatitis. There are additionally other, more rare, types.

Infective hepatitis/type A

The virus is contained in the blood and faeces of an already infected person, or in an otherwise healthy carrier of the disease. The incubation period is 10–40 days.

Aetiology Hepatitis type A is the most common liver disease in the UK and is transmitted by ingestion of contaminated food or water. Incidence of the disease is highest among children who have to live in overcrowded and insanitary conditions. Also affected are people returning from areas abroad in which hepatitis A is endemic. A vaccine has now been developed which provides immunity to hepatitis A and this may be given to those who are at particular risk of contracting the disease.

Clinical features The person who has been infected feels generally unwell and anorexic for a period of up to 7 days. They may have a mild pyrexia. Following this initial period the person becomes jaundiced and may experience troublesome skin pruritis. Pale stools and dark urine are excreted. The person's liver is tender and may be enlarged. Their prothrombin time may be prolonged, which may predispose them to bruise easily. This stage of the illness lasts 3–6 weeks and is almost always followed by complete recovery.

Investigations Blood samples are taken to identify the disease and to monitor the levels of bilirubin.

Therapeutic management and nursing strategies Hospitalization is usually unnecessary, but rest is required until serum bilirubin levels subside. Dietary restrictions are not required, although adequate amounts of glucose and protein should be taken. Alcohol should be avoided completely during the acute phase of the disease. The patient may be advised to abstain from alcohol for 6 months following illness, although it is now thought that complete abstension may be unnecessary. The person should be able to undertake their normal activities approximately 3 weeks following the resolution of jaundice.

Prevention of spread of the infection is important. Advice should be given about the nature of the disease and the mode of spread. Guidance should be provided about the importance of handwashing prior to the preparation and ingestion of food and following defaecation. This advice should be adhered to not only by the sufferer, but by all those who share accommodation with him/her.

Serum hepatitis/type B

This is less common but more severe than infective hepatitis. The incubation period is approximately 3 months and the disease is transmitted by infected serum. It is thought that transmission may also occur via bodily secretions such as saliva, vaginal and seminal fluid and serous exudate. Close personal contact appears to be necessary in order for transmission to occur, for example sexual intercourse, or the sharing of needles by infected intravenous drug abusers. It may also be transmitted by accidental needle-stick injury and for this reason vaccination against the virus is offered to personnel who are deemed to be at high risk, for example, nurses.

Clinical features These are similar to, but more severe than, those for infective/type A hepatitis. The patient may become acutely and severely ill and may require the support of intensive care nursing.

Therapeutic management and nursing strategies Patients who are severely and acutely ill require to be barrier nursed in an intensive care environment. Therapy is supportive and individually tailored to the patient's condition. The prognosis depends upon the virulence of the virus, the age of the patient and the existence of any underlying disease. Complete recovery may follow the acute phase of the illness, or chronic hepatitis or liver scarring may result.

As the severity of the disease is so variable, nursing strategies will be devised following assessment of the individual needs of the patient. It is necessary to take measures to ensure the safe disposal of the patient's excretions and the disposal or sterilization of objects which have come into contact with the patient's excreta or other bodily secretions.

Psychological support is vital for the patient who,

in addition to feeling extremely unwell and debilitated, may feel isolated or unclean as a result of the precautions taken to prevent the transmission of infection to others. Those who visit the patient will require to be given explanations and advice about the isolation procedures and may also require psychological support.

Following recovery the patient will receive counselling prior to discharge in order to minimize the possibility that they may transmit the infection to others. The patient's blood will be tested at regular intervals in order to determine whether he remains a carrier of the virus. Some people may remain an asymptomatic carrier for an indefinite period of time.

The routes of infection are explained and measures identified in order to ensure that transmission to others will not occur. If the patient is an intravenous drug abuser a needle-exchange system may be offered and the importance of not sharing needles with others will be emphasized. The importance of using barrier methods of protection during sexual intercourse is similarly emphasized. The patient should be asked if they have any questions and should be given the opportunity to air their possible anxieties and fears. Counselling will be required should the patient wish to have children, as it is possible not only to infect one's sexual partner, but also to transmit the virus to the fetus.

CARE OF THE PATIENT WHO HAS A MALIGNANT DISORDER OF THE GASTROINTESTINAL SYSTEM

The physical and psychological needs of the patient who has a malignant disorder will vary considerably and be determined by many factors. Despite the fact that many cancers are treatable, the perception which is held by the public still tends to be that cancer is a disease from which few people make a full recovery. This may have a deleterious psychological effect upon the patient.

Activities of living which may be problematic for the person who has a malignant disorder of the gastrointestinal tract are those of nutrition, hydration and elimination. Depending upon the severity of their illness, or its stage of progression, they may additionally experience difficulties relating to other activities of living. As was discussed at the beginning of this chapter, the inability to eat, drink and eliminate in a manner which society regards as 'normal' and 'acceptable' may have a profound psychosocial effect upon the individual. Malignancy may also

cause, either as a result of the disease process, or of its treatment, an alteration in the person's body image. The concept of body image, and the factors which may interfere with it, are discussed in Chapter 9.

Patients for whom excision of tumour is possible require both physical and psychological preparation for the major surgery involved. The care which the person requires before and after surgery will depend upon the nature of the operation which they undergo. For a discussion of the general principles of preoperative and postoperative care please see Chapter 4.

It is of great importance that the patient is given clear explanations of what they should expect, both in the immediate postoperative period and in the long term. In addition to explanations the patient must also be given opportunities to ask questions and to voice their anxieties. They may wish their significant others to be involved in these discussions.

The above considerations are of equal importance when the treatment which the patient receives is palliative and not curative. Explanations must be given to enable them to understand that the primary purpose of such treatment is to alleviate present and future symptoms of the disorder and not to effect a cure. The patient and their significant others may require considerable psychological support in coming to terms with the terminal nature of their illness.

Implications of suffering from malignancy affecting the upper gastrointestinal tract

Malignancy affecting the upper gastrointestinal tract usually affects the person's ability to ingest food in a form or manner which society regards as 'normal'. Cancer of the oesophagus may cause dysphagia or regurgitation of food. Cancer of the stomach, if treatable by gastrectomy, will reduce the volume of food which the patient is able to ingest and also the form in which the food may be taken – solid foods may cause abdominal discomfort. The patient who has malignancy of the upper tract will therefore lose some of the social contact which is associated with communal eating.

Cancer of the oesophagus

Epidemiology and aetiology

The incidence of oesophageal cancer varies considerably in different parts of the word. In western societies it is linked with excessive alcohol ingestion and cigarette smoking.

Common symptoms

The patient's symptoms arise because the tumour causes a partial or total obstruction to the passage of food. Symptoms frequently occur for the first time in people between the ages of 60 and 70 years of age. The patient experiences intermittent dysphagia when eating solid food. The dysphagia is progressive and the patient eventually has difficulty in swallowing even fluids. This leads to weight loss and dehydration. The patient may also present with the symptoms of metastatic spread to the lymph nodes, liver or mediastinum.

Investigations

A barium swallow (see p. 512) will usually illustrate obstruction and narrowing of the oesophagus in the location of the tumour. Oesophagoscopy and biopsy will confirm the diagnosis. Investigations may also be carried out in order to determine whether metastatic spread has occurred.

Therapeutic management

Cure is only possible for approximately 10% of patients and entails either removal of the oesophagus and stomach (oesophagogastrectomy) or radiotherapy, or a combination of both. Prior to surgery the patient may require restoration of fluid and electrolyte and nutritional balance intravenously. If the tumour is extensive, palliative, as opposed to curative, treatment may be indicated. This involves the endoscopic insertion of a permanent tube into the oesophagus which enables the patient to swallow liquids.

Carcinoma of the stomach

Epidemiology and aetiology

The geographical incidence of stomach cancer varies, being high in Japan but relatively uncommon in the USA and UK. There is a possibility that environmental factors may be one cause, for example ingestion of trace elements in water. The incidence is high in people who have pernicious anaemia and in those who have undergone partial gastrectomy, but the reason for this is not yet certain.

Common symptoms

The onset is usually in middle age. Early symptoms are anorexia, mild nausea and abdominal discomfort after eating. This leads to weight loss and possible anaemia (as a result of poor nutrition and of bleeding from the tumour). As the symptoms are not very specific the person may not consult their doctor for some time, by which stage the cancer is well advanced. Ascites (see p. 536) may be present, as may evidence of metastatic spread to the liver or lymph glands.

Investigations

A double-contrast barium meal (see p. 512) may indicate the presence of a tumour. Gastroscopy and biopsy confirm the diagnosis. Investigations may also be carried out for evidence of spread to other organs.

Therapeutic management

Laparotomy may be carried out, in order to determine whether gastrectomy (the only hope of cure) is possible. Prior to surgery the person may require correction of electrolyte, fluid and nutritional imbalances caused by the patient's symptoms. Treatment of anaemia is also necessary. Cytotoxic drug therapy may achieve remission for some people, but the prognosis for most people who have gastric cancer is poor (Deakin and Elder 1994).

Cancer of the pancreas

Epidemiology and aetiology

Cancer of the pancreas is more common in males than females and occurs most frequently when the person is in their sixties. Its development is linked with cigarette smoking, exposure to industrial pollutants and a high intake of dietary fat.

Common symptoms

Some tumours may cause jaundice at an early stage, but most people are asymptomatic until the disease is advanced. The patient may experience epigastric pain or discomfort, anorexia, nausea and possible vomiting and weight loss.

Investigations

Pancreatic function tests and a barium meal may demonstrate abnormalities. Ultrasound or CT scanning (see pp. 512–513) is carried out and biopsy may also be required to confirm the diagnosis.

Therapeutic intervention

Surgical excision of the head of the pancreas and duodenum may be possible, but the prognosis for most people is poor.

Nursing strategies in caring for people who have cancer of the upper gastrointestinal tract

General approaches are outlined at the beginning of this chapter and this section.

The symptoms which the patient may suffer by the time they are admitted to hospital include those associated with malnutrition and anaemia. The patient may thus be in a weakened and emaciated state and require assistance with many of the activities of living.

The implications of suffering from malignancy affecting the lower gastrointestinal tract

Malignancy affecting the lower gastrointestinal tract may affect the patient's ability to excrete faeces in a manner which society regards as 'normal'. Formation of a permanent or temporary colostomy will cause an alteration in body image. A positive attitude displayed by the nurse when caring for the patient who excretes faeces via a stoma is vital in helping the patient to come to terms with it.

Carcinoma of the colon and rectum

Epidemiology and aetiology

There is a wide variation in the incidence of carcinoma of the colon and rectum. In countries such as Africa and Asia it is virtually unknown, whereas in the UK it is the most common form of malignancy in the gastrointestinal system.

Much research has been undertaken in an effort to identify factors which may predispose to the development of, or provide protection against, this form of cancer. Evidence suggests that a diet which has a high roughage content and thus promotes the formation of bulky, soft faeces may provide some protection against carcinoma of the colon and rectum, whereas a diet which has a low roughage content and produces a constipated stool may be linked with its development.

People who have had ulcerative colitis have an increased risk of development of malignancy of the colon and rectum.

Common symptoms

These vary, depending on the location of the malig-nancy. Common to most are a change in bowel habit, bleeding (which may be occult or visible) and which gives rise to the signs and symptoms of anaemia. The person may develop intestinal obstruction if the tumour is located in the descending colon or rectum, due to the fact that faecal material is by then semi-formed. Rectal cancer may cause early bleeding and mucous discharge. The person may have the sensation that they are unable to completely empty their rectum on defaecation.

Investigations

Rectal digital examination, barium enema, endoscopy and biopsy are carried out. For a discussion of these investigations, and the role of the nurse whilst the patient is undergoing them, please see pages 511–515. Investigations will also be carried out in order to ascertain if the tumour has metastasized.

Therapeutic management

If possible the area of bowel affected by the tumour is excised and the remaining bowel anastamosed. If this is impossible it may be necessary to remove the affected length of colon and rectum and create a permanent colostomy by bringing the lumen of the large intestine onto the abdominal surface.

Preoperative counselling is vital for the patient and for their significant others, in order that they may begin to come to terms with the life changes which this surgery will entail. It is important that this is undertaken by a nurse who has expertise in caring for patients who have undergone stoma formation. In addition to alteration of body image the surgery may, for some patients, cause interference with their sexual ability – it may cause an inability to have an erection in some men and dyspareunia in some women. This must be discussed with the patient if it is felt that it may be a side-effect of surgery.

The nature of the proposed surgery and the site of the stoma and consistency of faeces which it will excrete must also be discussed. A stoma formed from the ascending or transverse colon will excrete liquid faeces, whereas one lower down in the tract (i.e. descending or pelvic colon) will excrete faeces similar in consistency to that excreted normally per rectum.

The type of appliances which may be used are shown to the patient, with the opportunity to discuss the advantages and disadvantages of each. A suitable site for the stoma is selected. It is vital that siting of the stoma is carried out prior to surgery, with the patient standing, sitting and bending. This is to ensure that the patient's movements will not cause obstruction of the stoma and that skin folds will not interfere with the patency of the equipment.

Following selection of a stoma site the patient is encouraged to wear an appliance for a 24 hour period in order to confirm the suitability of the site.

The patient should be given the opportunity to meet with someone who has successfully undergone stoma formation in the past if they so wish. Most hospitals provide information booklets for people who are to undergo colostomy formation and this provides a useful reference for the patient. Booklets should however be regarded as a supplement to oral information and discussion and not a substitute for it.

The Colostomy Association of Great Britain provides support and wide-ranging information booklets to ostomists. These deal with all aspects of colostomy management and its implications. The patient should also have an identified contact person, such as a stoma nurse, who will provide support and advice to the patient following discharge. Stoma equipment is obtainable by prescription following discharge and the patient is entitled to exemption from charges. Information must also be given about disposal of used appliances.

Prior to surgery the patient may require bowel preparation in order to ensure that faecal content is removed. This may be achieved for example by administration of oral laxatives and a diet which is low in roughage and is confined to clear liquids in the immediate preoperative period. In order to minimize the bacterial content of the bowel oral antibiotic therapy may be given.

In order to promote venous return whilst the patient is in the operating theatre and during the postoperative period thromboembolic deterrent stockings may be fitted. For a discussion of the general principles of preoperative and postoperative care, see Chapter 4.

Nursing Care Plan 15.4 illustrates the care which the patient will require following the formation of a permanent colostomy.

CARE OF THE PATIENT WHO HAS HERNIATION OR PROLAPSE OF THE GASTROINTESTINAL TRACT

Care of the patient who has a hernia

A hernia is the protrusion of an organ from its own cavity. Herniation of the anterior abdominal wall may result from a congenital weakness of the supporting

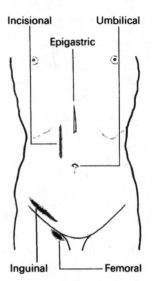

Fig. 15.14 Common sites of herniation of the anterior abdominal wall

muscles. Alternatively it may occur following physical strain, for example heavy lifting, chronic coughing, straining at stool. Common sites of herniation of the anterior abdominal wall are shown in Figure 15.14. These include sites at which the musculature of the anterior abdominal wall has been weakened by previous surgical intervention.

If the organ can be returned to its cavity of origin it is described as being reducible; if this is not possible it is termed irreducible. A herniated organ may become trapped by surrounding musculature and its blood supply impaired (strangulated hernia), which constitutes a surgical emergency as it may cause necrosis of the organ.

Common symptoms

The person, or the carer of a small child, may notice a swelling at the site of the hernia. This may enlarge when the person coughs, strains or lifts heavy objects and may be accompanied by local discomfort which is alleviated by lying flat. The person whose hernia becomes strangulated will experience pain and the symptoms associated with intestinal obstruction (see p. 533).

The person who has a rectal prolapse usually experiences symptoms following defaecation, particularly if this has involved straining at stool. The prolapse may return spontaneously when the person lies down, but frequently requires manual replacement.

Investigation

This is by clinical examination, in conjunction with the patient's history.

Therapeutic management and nursing strategies

Surgical repair of the hernia is carried out. This provides not only symptomatic relief, but also prevents the occurrence of strangulation. For a discussion of general principles of pre- and postoperative care please see Chapter 4.

For some patients surgical repair may be carried out in a day bed area, whilst others may be admitted on the day prior to surgery and are usually able to be discharged home within 48 hours of surgery, unless the repair has been extensive or has been carried out as emergency treatment of a strangulated hernia.

The patient must be given advice in relation to support of the wound site whilst coughing, sneezing laughing or defaecating. Heavy lifting should be avoided for a variable period, dependent upon the location and size of herniation.

Care of the patient who has haemorrhoids

Dilatations of the veins which lie in the submucosa of the anal canal are referred to as haemorrhoids. They may project into the lumen of the anal canal, or may prolapse and be visible outwith the anus.

Epidemiology and aetiology

Haemorrhoids affect men and women equally. Factors which inhibit haemorrhoidal venous drainage, for example chronic constipation or pregnancy, are predisposing factors.

Common symptoms

Haemorrhoids may cause local pain or discomfort, anal pruritis, bleeding during defaecation (bright red blood) and possible prolapse. Strangulation of pro-lapsed haemorrhoids may occur, which is extremely painful and usually renders the patient unable to walk or to sit down.

Investigations

Digital examination of the anal canal and rectum and proctoscopy are usually sufficient to confirm the diagnosis.

Therapeutic intervention and nursing strategies

This depends upon the severity of the haemorrhoids and the symptoms suffered by the individual. If the haemorrhoids do not cause severe symptoms, dietary advice may be sufficient. The patient is recommended to ensure that food which has a high roughage content is taken and is accompanied by a high fluid intake. This will avoid the necessity of straining at stool. Pruritis may be minimized by careful attention to personal hygiene and by use of creams such as Anusol, which also help to alleviate discomfort.

Haemorrhoids which give rise to severe symptoms may be treated by either sclerotherapy or surgery. Sclerotherapy involves injection of the haemorrhoids with a substance which causes shrinkage of the dilated veins.

Surgery involves excision and ligation of the haemorrhoids. For a discussion of the general principles of pre- and postoperative care, please see Chapter 4.

Particular points of note when caring for a patient who has had a haemorrhoidectomy are that pain may be severe; pain relief involves administration of analgesia and assistance in finding a comfortable position. Haemorrhage may also occur and wound site checks must be carried out frequently and regularly during the immediate postoperative period. The patient who has haemorrhoids may feel embarrassment and the nurse should take measures to minimize this.

Whichever method of therapeutic intervention is decided upon, dietary advice is important, as continued constipation and straining at stool is otherwise likely to lead to haemorrhoid recurrence.

Suggested assignments

Discussion topics

1. Anne Kingsley is a 22-year-old intravenous drug user who has recovered from a serum hepatitis/type B viral infection. Blood results indicate that she remains a carrier of the infection.

   Compile a patient education programme for Anne to enable her to avoid transmitting the disease to others. Compare the programme which you have devised with that of other students. Discuss with them the most suitable way in which to implement the programme.

2. Mrs Ambrose, who is 78 years old, has recovered from an episode of acute diverticulitis.

   Discuss the dietary advice which she should receive in order to avoid future recurrence of her problem.

3. Imagine that you have been told that you require to have formation of a permanent stoma.

   Compile a list of the anxieties/fears which you think that you might experience on being given this information.
   Compare this list with that of fellow students.

Either:
   a. Identify, and as a group discuss, possible nursing strategies aimed at the goal of alleviation of these anxieties/fears.

or:
   b. Carry out a role play in which one student adopts the role of the person who is to undergo stoma formation. Another student adopts the role of the nurse.
   The purpose of the dialogue is for the 'nurse' to encourage the 'patient' to express his/her anxieties and to discuss these. The purpose of the discussion is alleviation of the 'patient's' anxieties.
   It is useful if this role play can be videotaped, in order that the participants can identify to what extent the discussion has achieved its aim and the factors which contributed to this. Alternatively a third person (or more) may witness the role play as an observer, their function being to attempt an objective assessment to aid analysis and discussion following completion of the role play.

REFERENCES AND FURTHER READING

Bouchier I et al 1991 Davidson's principles and practice of medicine, 16th edn. Churchill Livingstone, Edinburgh

Brunner L S, Suddarth D S 1989 The Lippincott manual of medical-surgical nursing, 2nd edn. Harper and Row, Philadelphia

Brunner L S, Suddarth D S 1992 The textbook of adult nursing, 6th edn. Adapted for the UK from Gilchrist B et al The Lippincott textbook of medical-surgical nursing. Chapman and Hall, London

Craft M J 1990 Nursing interventions for infants and children. Saunders, Philadelphia

Deakin M, Elder J B 1994 Gastric cancer. Medicine International, UK edn. Vol 22, 6 June 1994

Foster R L R, Hunsberger M M, Anderson J J T 1989 Family-centred nursing care of children. Saunders, Philadelphia

Mayberry J F, Rhodes J, Williams G T 1994 Ulcerative colitis. Medicine International, UK edn. Vol 22, 8 August 1994

Orem D E 1991 Nursing: concepts of practice, 4th edn. Mosby Year Book, St Louis

Pounder R 1994 Peptic ulceration. Medicine International: UK edn. Vol 22, 6 June 1994

Roper N, Logan W W, Tierney A J 1990 Elements of nursing, 3rd edn. Churchill Livingstone, Edinburgh

Shearman D J C, Crean G P 1991 In Bouchier I A D, Edwards C R W (eds) 1991 Davidson's principles and practice of medicine, 16th edn. Churchill Livingstone, Edinburgh

Wilson K J W 1990 Ross & Wilson's anatomy and physiology in health and illness, 7th edn. Churchill Livingstone, Edinburgh

16

Care implications of disorders of the endocrine system

Margaret B. Thomson

THE ENDOCRINE SYSTEM AS A CONTROLLING SYSTEM

The body's physiological processes are influenced by two controlling systems. These are the nervous system (see Ch. 5) and the endocrine system, which although anatomically separate, complement each other functionally in the maintenance of a stable internal environment, i.e. homeostasis (Hinchliff & Montague 1988) (see Ch. 4). The controlling systems respond to body needs through monitoring mechanisms situated throughout the body, and, by means of a negative feedback system (see Ch. 4), imbalances in the internal environment are corrected.

The reaction of each system in response to body needs varies in relation to speed of action. The nervous system is fast acting through the transmission of nerve impulses which, although they stimulate organs to respond within milliseconds, are short lasting in their effect. In contrast, the endocrine system acts by slow release of hormones into the arterial circulation from a series of endocrine glands, and the responses they evoke are more prolonged than the responses of the nervous system.

Hormones (*hormon* meaning to excite) are chemical messengers which act to stimulate and co-ordinate the activities of different tissues within the body. The stimulated structures are known as target glands or target tissues and are sited some distance from the hormone secretion.

Hormones are specific in action and each endocrine gland exerts its effect upon a specific target area. Cells of target areas contain receptor sites which recognize specific hormones, and although the hormones circulate systemically, they are active only when recognized by specific receptors.

Hormones have two main modes of action. They may enter the cell and stimulate the production of a second messenger adenosine monophosphate (AMP), or they may pass through the nuclear membrane to initiate the formation of proteins. In each process, enzymes are produced which dictate cell production.

Hormones can be proteins, composed of amino acid-based molecules, or they can be steroids synthesized from cholesterol. On completion of their activities within the target cells, hormones are inactivated by the liver before being excreted. Some hormones have a very short half-life, while others may be effective for some time. Measurable amounts of hormones or their metabolites can be found in urine and this can be helpful for diagnostic purposes.

Some hormones are secreted by cells which are not part of the endocrine system, for example gastrointestinal hormones (see Ch. 15) and prostaglandins which are hormones secreted by most cells of the body and have local action.

ORGANIZATION OF THE ENDOCRINE SYSTEM

The glands which comprise the endocrine system are anatomically discrete and situated throughout the body (Fig. 16.1). Although each gland is specific in

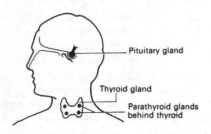

Pituitary gland

Thyroid gland

Parathyroid glands behind thyroid

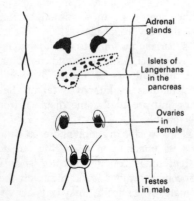

Adrenal glands

Islets of Langerhans in the pancreas

Ovaries in female

Testes in male

Fig. 16.1 Diagram of the positions in the body of the endocrine glands. (Reproduced with permission from Wilson 1990, p. 311)

action, all are interdependent and malfunctioning of one gland tends to affect the whole system.

Each gland is supplied by a fine, dense capillary network, an arrangement whereby the gland can pass its secretion directly into the extracellular space and then into the arterial bloodstream. The endocrine glands are therefore without ducts and are described as the ductless glands.

Release of hormones from the endocrine glands is in response to body needs and follows a series of sensory communications whereby information related to specific needs is fed back to the appropriate gland and hormone levels are maintained within physiological limits. Because of this communication system, the endocrine system is able to carry out its functions of controlling cellular metabolism, growth and development, and responding to sudden body demands created by changes in body fluids, extremes of temperature and stressful situations, both mental and physical. Its role in the functions of reproduction, parturition and lactation is indispensable.

The endocrine glands to be discussed in this chapter are:

- hypothalamus
- pituitary gland
- thyroid gland
- parathyroid glands
- adrenal glands
- pancreas
- thymus gland
- pineal gland.

Disorders affecting these glands lead to undersecretion or oversecretion of their respective hormones.

INVESTIGATIONS IN DISORDERS OF THE ENDOCRINE SYSTEM

These include:

- patient's history to identify symptoms
- general physical assessment
- radioimmunoassays of hormone levels
- 24-hour urine collections
- investigation of faeces
- X-ray examination
- CT scans
- estimation of antibodies.

The responsibilities of the nurse include preparation of the patient for the test, ensuring accuracy in the collections, and education of the patient. A patient who understands the purpose of tests will be more relaxed and thus the results more reliable.

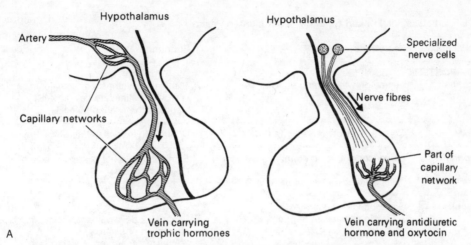

Fig. 16.2 The pituitary gland. (A) Relationship of anterior pituitary to hypothalamus. A portal venous system carries releasing and inhibiting factors from the hypothalamus to the anterior pituitary, stimulating or inhibiting its release of trophic hormones into the bloodstream.
(B) Relationship of posterior pituitary to hypothalamus. Oxytocin and antidiuretic hormones are produced by special cells in the hypothalamus, travel along nerve fibres, are stored and released by the posterior pituitary into the bloodstream.

The communication enhances mutual trust and understanding.

STRUCTURE AND FUNCTION OF THE HYPOTHALAMUS

The hypothalamus, which is considered to be part of the endocrine system because of its synthesis of hormones, works closely with the pituitary gland in controlling most of the endocrine glands, exceptions being the parathyroid glands and the pancreas. It is part of the diencephalon and is situated above the brain stem. It is connected anatomically to the pituitary gland by means of the pituitary stalk, forming the hypothalamic–pituitary pathway which provides the route for hypothalamic hormones to reach the pituitary gland. The hypothalamus synthesizes and secretes hormone releasing factors which stimulate the production of trophic hormones from the anterior pituitary gland. Trophic hormones (*trop* means to turn or change) regulate the output of hormones from target glands or tissues. The hypothalamus also synthesizes antidiuretic hormone and oxytocin which are passed via the pituitary stalk to the posterior pituitary gland for storage.

The hypothalamus has a direct communication with the limbic system (see Ch. 5), a system of neurone networks spread widely throughout the forebrain and which is affected by emotions. Through these connections, external factors can influence pituitary secretions.

The hypothalamus therefore exerts an influence over both anterior and posterior pituitary glands.

The anatomical relationship between the hypothalamus and the pituitary gland is illustrated in Figure 16.2.

PITUITARY GLAND (HYPOPHYSIS)

This essential gland is situated in the grooved sella turcica of the sphenoid bone, an arrangement which provides protection for the gland.

The pituitary gland is in fact two glands, the anterior and posterior pituitary glands, joined as a composite whole. The anterior pituitary gland is derived from an upward growth of pharyngeal tissue, hence its alternative name of adenohypophysis, while the posterior pituitary gland is derived from downward growth of neural tissue from the hypothalamus giving it the alternative name of neurohypophysis.

The anterior pituitary gland manufactures and secretes trophic hormones which act on target glands, stimulating them to act. The posterior pituitary gland stores and secretes two hormones which are manufactured in the hypothalamus and which act directly on specific tissues (Table 16.1).

The target areas for anterior and posterior pituitary gland secretions are illustrated in Figure 16.3.

Table 16.1   Cell classification and function in the pituitary gland

Cell classification	Secretions	Functions
ANTERIOR POSTERIOR GLAND		
Somatotrophs	Human growth hormone (GH)	Stimulates synthesis of somatomedins in the liver which stimulate cell growth Opposes the actions of insulin
Thyrotrophs	Thyroid stimulating hormone (TSH)	Controls thyroid gland activity
Corticotrophs	Adrenocorticotrophic hormones (ACTH)	Stimulates adrenal cortex to secrete glucocorticocoids
	Melanocyte stimulating hormone (MSH)	Increases skin pigmentation
Gonadotrophs	Gonadotrophic hormones Follicle stimulating hormone (FSH)	Stimulates development of ovarian follicle with production of oestrogen Stimulates spermatogenesis
	Luteinising hormone (LH)	Stimulates development of corpus luteum Stimulates production of testosterone
Lactotrophs	Prolactin	Initiates milk production
POSTERIOR PITUITARY GLAND		
Pituicytes	Oxytocin	Stimulates uterine contractions at term inducing labour Facilitates milk ejection during lactation
	Antidiuretic hormone (ADH)	Conserves body water by increasing the reabsorption of water from the renal tubules

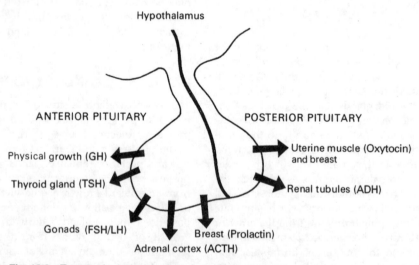

Fig. 16.3   Targets of principal groups of pituitary hormones

Damage can occur in any or all of these cells giving rise to specific signs and symptoms related to undersecretion (hypopituitarism) or oversecretion (hyperpituitarism) of their hormones. Damage can arise through trauma, infection, tumours, or it can be idiopathic. Because of the location of the gland, there is little facility within the site for enlargement of the gland tissue, and a tumour can cause pressure on the optic chiasma (see Ch. 5) which is situated above the gland. Problems affecting vision are an early symptom of pituitary tumour.

Disorders of the anterior pituitary gland

Hypopituitarism

Undersecretion of growth hormone (somatotrophin) Secretion of growth hormone is controlled by two hypothalamic hormones. These are growth hormone releasing factor which stimulates release of growth hormone, and growth hormone release-inhibiting factor (somatostatin) which inhibits the release of growth hormone. In childhood, undersecretion of growth hormone leads to small stature, but the child grows proportionately. It is important that affected children are recognized early so that therapy can be instituted using a biosynthetic human growth hormone called somatrophin. Treatment is long term involving regular injections, usually nightly, and the child/young person requires much support and understanding, as do the parents, to continue with the treatment.

Nurses, particularly in the field of paediatric care, should be very aware of growth and development parameters in children and seek advice where there is concern. It is important to consider parental stature as the child's stature is genetically determined.

Undersecretion of growth hormone may also be accompanied by deficiency in secretion of other trophic hormones. Normal growth and sexual development may be arrested and the child develops characteristics associated with premature ageing.

There is no evidence of undersecretion of growth hormone causing disorder in adults, although it is thought by some authorities that premature visible signs of ageing may be attributed to reduced somatotrophin activity.

Undersecretion of all anterior pituitary hormones (Simmond's disease) If the hypopituitarism arises from a tumour or cyst destroying anterior pituitary cells, or from sudden reduction in blood flow to the gland, as in haemorrhage, then all trophic hormones are affected. Target glands will atrophy because of reduced stimulation and secretions diminish. The clinical effects of inactive target glands will become apparent.

Treatment will include hormone replacement therapy. A tumour or cyst will be removed.

Nursing care of the patient should involve a problem-solving approach, attention being paid to the patient's compliance in adhering to the schedule for the correct administration of medication. Diet is important because of muscle wasting, and encouragement should be given to the patient to eat well-balanced, vitamin-enriched meals. Adequate fluid intake is important because of homeostatic imbalance arising from lack of controlling hormones. Physical inactivity leads to problems of immobility which must be addressed.

Untreated hypopituitarism can lead to coma if the existing situation is exacerbated by injury or infection. The effects of adrenal insufficiency will be present. The nurse should be aware of these effects which are in the section on disorders of the adrenal glands discussed on p. 567.

Hyperpituitarism

Oversecretion of growth hormone Growth hormone acts on most body tissues, but particularly in the liver which is stimulated by growth hormone to produce somatomedins. Somatomedins stimulate cell growth, especially in bone, cartilage, muscle and other soft tissues. Thus hypersecretion of growth hormone will result in clinical manifestations of overgrowth of these tissues with implications for nursing practice. It is usually caused by a benign tumour of the anterior pituitary gland.

Gigantism Oversecretion of growth hormone in the young, prior to closure of the epiphyses, leads to the condition of gigantism where the young adult grows excessively, and during this period of growth, bones enlarge both in length and width. The young person may reach a height of 7 feet or more.

Acromegaly Oversecretion in adults leads to the condition of acromegaly. Because epiphyseal fusion has taken place in the adult, bones enlarge transversely and the patient develops very distinctive coarse heavy features. Increase in the size of hands and feet may be the patient's first indication of disordered growth. In many patients, joints are affected leading to osteoarthritis. Areas which are particularly affected are the small joints of the hands and wrists, and the knee joint. The spine may also be affected, and kyphosis may develop.

The skeletal features of acromegaly cannot be reversed and persist following treatment of the disorder. They can, however, be arrested.

Changes in muscle and other soft tissues lead to enlargement of internal organs – visceromegaly. This enlargement leads to overworked muscle, and cardiac failure can develop. The patient is lethargic and weak.

Tissue changes affect the size of the tongue and lips, affecting speech, and eating problems can arise. Increase in the size of the vocal cords leads to deepening of the voice.

Increase in the growth of glandular tissue, both

exocrine and endocrine, leads to oversecretion. Excess thyroid production increases the metabolic rate and sweating and sebum production are increased. Gonadal function may be increased, but if the pituitary tumour destroys or compresses gonadotrophs, then libido is lost, impotence develops in men and oligomenorrhoea or amenorrhoea in women.

Visual disturbances arise because of pressure of the tumour on the optic chiasma.

Metabolic disturbances arise because growth hormone is an insulin antagonist and as such is diabetogenic in effect. Clinical diabetes is a characteristic of acromegaly.

Pressure on the brain tissue by the expanding pituitary tumour may cause severe and persistent headaches.

All of these developments arising from overgrowth of body tissues have implications for nursing care. The nurse must be vigilant in her observation of the patient, nursing management must be evaluated with care and the patient must be treated with sensitivity and understanding. The patient's psychological status may be disturbed because of appearance and he must be able to discuss any fears and worries.

Treatment of gigantism and acromegaly may be by surgical or medical methods.

Surgical intervention involves removal or ablation of the affected pituitary tissue. This can be done by implantation of yttrium-90, by external irradiation, by trans-sphenoidal hypophysectomy, or by removal of the anterior pituitary gland by craniotomy.

Following trans-sphenoidal hypophysectomy, specific observations include those for signs of haemorrhage and leakage of cerebrospinal fluid, indications of which are clear nasal drip and constant swallowing.

Care of the patient following craniotomy is described in Chapter 5.

Without secretion of trophic hormones, target glands will become inactive and will atrophy. When the source of all pituitary trophic hormones has been removed, replacement therapy for corticosteroids and thyroid hormone will be for life.

Medical treatment of acromegaly includes hormone therapy.

Somatostatin, synthesized in the hypothalamus, inhibits the secretion of growth hormone. An analogue of somatostatin, called octreotide, has been used with considerable success in treating patients with acromegaly. The medication is given by subcutaneous injection, usually three times daily. Growth hormone levels fall with the administration of octreotide. The patient will need encouragement to maintain this stressful schedule of drug administration (Edwards & Bouchier 1991).

Other manifestations of anterior hyperpituitarism These include oversecretion of the trophic hormones adrenocorticotrophic hormone (ACTH), thyroid stimulating hormone (TSH) and gonadotrophic hormones. The effects of oversecretion of ACTH and TSH are discussed in later sections of this chapter, while disorders of gonadotrophic hormones are discussed in Chapter 17.

Posterior pituitary gland

The function of the posterior pituitary gland is to store and secrete antidiuretic hormone and oxytocin. Synthesis of these hormones takes place in the hypothalamus.

Undersecretion or absence of antidiuretic hormone ADH

Removal of the posterior pituitary gland may necessitate administration of vasopressin (ADH replacement) therapy because of the danger of fluid and electrolyte imbalance for a few weeks following surgery, but is not usually required thereafter as the hypothalamus synthesizes antidiuretic hormone.

Failure of synthesis of antidiuretic hormone leads to a condition known as diabetes insipidus. Primary diabetes insipidus is not common, but the condition can follow brain injury, other trauma, or can be idiopathic.

In this condition, the kidneys cannot concentrate urine in the distal tubules (see Ch. 17) and large amounts of fluid are lost from the body. The patient has an insatiable thirst (polydipsia), weakness and weight loss. If the fluid loss cannot be balanced by fluid intake, then electrolyte loss, severe dehydration and shock will follow. Figure 16.4 illustrates the effects of ADH on fluid balance in the body.

Treatment of diabetes insipidus consists of replacement therapy. A synthetic analogue of the hormone (desmopresin) can be administered intranasally when it is absorbed into the nasal mucosa. The patient is instructed to take the medication during episodes of polydipsia or polyuria. If the patient requires surgery, the medication must be given by injection during the postoperative period, or if the patient should ever be unconscious.

THYROID GLAND

Structure and function of the thyroid gland

The thyroid gland is situated in the neck just below the larynx. It consists of two lobes, one on each side of

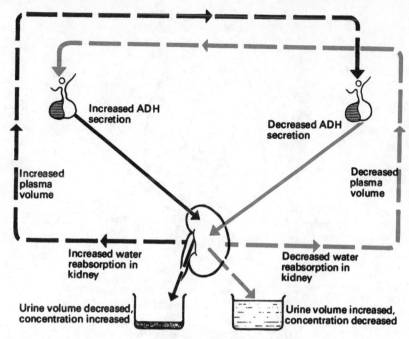

Fig. 16.4 Role of ADH in maintaining water balance

the trachea. The lobes are joined by a band of thyroid tissue, the isthmus, situated just below the cricoid cartilage. Thyroid tissue is composed of follicles, each follicle having a wall of follicular cells with some parafollicular cells spaced at intervals between the layer of follicular cells and the basement membrane of the follicle. The lumen of the follicle contains colloid in which thyroid hormones are stored as thyroglobulin (Fig. 16.5).

The functions of the thyroid gland are:

1. To produce thyroid hormones:
   a. tetra-iodothyronine (thyroxine) referred to as T4 because the molecule contains four atoms of iodine, and
   b. tri-iodothyronine, referred to as T3 because the molecule contains three atoms of iodine.
2. To store the hormones.
3. To release the hormones according to body demand.

Iodine from the chest is necessary for the production of thyroid hormones.

These regulate body metabolism by controlling basal metabolic rate. They are secreted when metabolic rate has to be accelerated. This means a corresponding increase in oxygen uptake. It therefore has an effect on most of the body tissues, and is involved with growth hormone in growth, maintenance and repair of body tissues. It reactivates the nervous system.

A byproduct of metabolism is heat, and thyroid hormone is accordingly termed a 'calorigenic hormone'. The thyroid gland functions less efficiently in the elderly, and the resulting reduced metabolism is one of the reasons why the elderly feel the cold so readily.

Regulation of thyroid hormone secretion is by negative feedback mechanism of hormonal control via the hypothalamic–pituitary pathway. Understanding of this feedback mechanism leads to understanding of thyroid disorders and diagnostic techniques.

Parafollicular cells manufacture and secrete the hormone calcitonin. Calcitonin and parathormone from the parathyroid glands maintain calcium homeostasis in the body by the following process:

- Calcitonin lowers blood calcium levels by aiding the entry of calcium into bone tissue.
- Parathormone raises blood calcium by mobilizing stored calcium from bone tissue for secretion into the blood.

The secretion of calcitonin and parathormone are controlled by calcium levels in the blood – humoral negative feedback mechanism.

Disorders of the thyroid gland

Disorders of this gland can result in either:

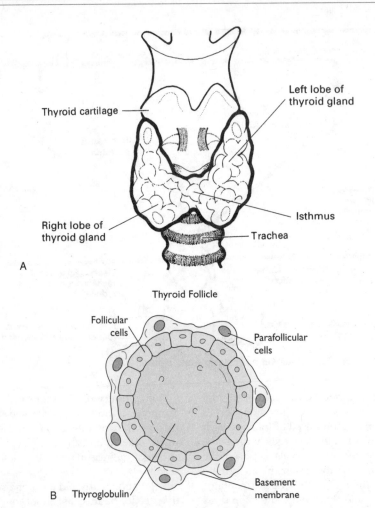

Fig. 16.5 (A) Anterior view of thyroid gland. (B) Thyroid follicle. (Reproduced with permission from McKenna & Callander 1990, p. 167)

1. Hypersecretion of thyroid hormones leading to hyperthyroidism, where basal metabolic rate, therefore cell metabolism, is greatly increased. This affects all body systems.

or:

2. Hyposecretion of thyroid hormones leading to hypothyroidism, where basal metabolic rate, therefore cell metabolism, is lowered. This affects all body systems (Table 16.2).

Aetiology of hyperthyroidism

Most cases of hyperthyroidism (over 90%) are of Graves' disease where the production of antibodies, directed against follicular cells, stimulates increased production and secretion of thyroid hormones. The cause is unknown but in genetically predisposed indi-

viduals the stimulating factors could be viral or bacterial infection, inflammation, emotional disturbance or stress.

Investigations

Diagnosis is made by the patient's history, appearance (which can frequently be very informative) and biochemical assays of circulating hormones. The raised circulating levels of the thyroid hormones T4 and T3 in hyperthyroidism will, because of hormonal feedback mechanism, inhibit the secretion of TSH.

A radioactive iodine uptake test may be performed to diagnose thyroid disease. The follicular cells of the thyroid gland extract the iodine from the bloodstream and its presence in the cells can be detected on scanning. In hyperthyroidism, the uptake of radio-

Table 16.2 Clinical features of thyroid disorder

Hyperthyroidism	Hypothyroidism
Goitre	Puffiness around eyes
Exophthalmus	
Weight loss	Weight gain despite loss of appetite
Hyperdefaecation	Constipation
Diarrhoea	
Tachycardia	Bradycardia
Palpitations	Anaemia
Atrial fibrillation	
Dyspnoea	
Nervousness	Lethargy
Emotional lability	Dull facial expression
Fatigue	Impairment of memory
Weakness	Hoarseness
Tremor	
Sleep disturbance	Somnolence
Menstrual disturbances	Menstrual disturbances
Heat intolerance	Sensitivity to cold
Increased sweating	Dry skin and hair
	Alopecia

active iodine will be increased, and the amount detected on scanning aids in diagnosis.

The nurse's role in the investigations is to aid the patient's understanding of the test and to ensure that pretest requirements such as written instructions for outpatients, and correct timing arrangements, are met.

Care of the patient with thyrotoxicosis

Treatment may be with antithyroid drugs, radioactive iodine or surgery.

Antithyroid drugs

Carbimazole This drug reduces the synthesis of new thyroid hormone. It also has some immunosuppressive action, thereby reducing antibody activity. The patient will be asked to report any development of unusual symptoms, especially sore throat, as agranulocytosis can be a complication of the drug.

Propanolol This is a non-selective beta-blocking drug which reduces cardiac output and therefore reduces the heart rate. It may be given where rapid reduction of thyrotoxic symptoms is required. It may also be given as preoperative preparation in rendering the patient euthyroid.

Potassium iodide This drug is given as preoperative preparation. Its action is to reduce vascularity of the gland and inhibit the release of thyroid hormones thereby reducing circulating levels.

Radioactive iodine The follicular cells of the thyroid gland take up iodine from the bloodstream. This ability allows the gland to concentrate the drug in the follicular cells. In doing so, the cells are destroyed.

In addition to drug therapy, supportive care should include the following recommendations:

1. Rest appropriate to the patient's condition will be advised and the reduced physical activity should aid in lowering the patient's metabolic rate.

2. Diet should include ample protein to correct weight loss and carbohydrate to supply energy. Carbohydrate acts as a protein sparer and prevents the breakdown of body tissue as a source of energy.

3. Vitamin supplements should be prescribed.

4. Caffeine-containing drinks should be avoided because of their stimulant effect.

5. Emotional support will help the patient regain confidence, and family and friends should be helped to understand the patient's emotional lability. The advantages of a calm environment should be explained to all.

The efficacy of treatment will be assessed by hormone assays and monitoring of the parameters of weight, blood pressure, pulse rate and anxiety levels. Stabilization of these measurements will indicate improvement in the patient's condition.

Surgery

Subtotal thyroidectomy The patient must be euthyroid prior to surgery. Antithyroid drugs will be discontinued approximately 2 weeks prior to surgery and replaced with potassium iodide orally.

About two-thirds of the gland is removed, thus leaving sufficient thyroid tissue to produce hormones. Specific preoperative preparation includes:

1. Electrocardiogram to assess cardiac action.

2. Explanation to the patient of postoperative positioning, how to support his neck following surgery, and exercises which will aid movement and respiratory function and decrease postoperative anxiety.

3. Because of the proximity of the recurrent laryngeal nerve to the thyroid gland, there is a danger, albeit remote, of damage to this nerve during surgery. The patient will have voice tests before and following surgery. Vocal cords will be inspected by laryngoscopy.

4. Explanation of wound closure and drains will be given.

5. An assurance that the scar will be in a natural

fold of the skin of the neck will re-assure the patient of a good cosmetic result.

Postoperatively, the patient will be observed carefully. Pain control is important not only for the relief of pain, but also to reduce anxiety. Blood pressure, temperature, pulse and respiratory rates will be recorded at 15 minute intervals initially, the intervals increasing as the patient's condition improves. Altered breathing must be reported to medical staff without delay as this could indicate respiratory distress due to pressure on the trachea.

A vacuum-type drain will be removed 24 hours following surgery if the wound is satisfactory.

Wound dressing should be observed for evidence of bleeding. As blood will trickle along the line of least resistance, the sides of the dressing, the back of the patient's neck and the pillows should also be checked. If bleeding occurs, the swollen tissues will put pressure on the trachea causing respiratory embarrassment to the patient. This pressure should be relieved by releasing the accumulated blood. Equipment to do this should be readily available and will be appropriate to the type of wound closure.

External wound closure such as stitches or clips will be removed after 48–72 hours. Early removal of stitches or clips gives a better cosmetic result.

Following recovery from anaesthetic, and if the patient's condition is satisfactory, he will be placed in a more upright position well supported with pillows. The patient's head and neck should be supported during movement, and until he is self-sufficient when moving. Speaking and coughing are encouraged as soon as the patient rouses, as are deep breathing exercises. Drinks are encouraged as soon as the patient is able to tolerate fluids. Soft food may be given on the evening of surgery.

On the day following surgery the diet will be increased and the patient encouraged to chew.

Voice tests are repeated to assess postoperative voice status. If hoarseness or sore throat are present, a moist inhalation containing Friar's Balsam will provide some comfort.

Ambulation is started the evening of surgery when the patient is allowed to sit in a chair for a short time, great care being taken to support his head and neck. Analgesics will be prescribed as required.

Providing the patient's postoperative condition is uncomplicated he may be discharged 2–3 days following surgery.

Emphasis must be placed on the importance of follow-up visits, and the patient made aware of the first appointment as an outpatient. The patient's hormone levels will be assessed regularly following surgery because of the potential danger of hypothyroidism.

Total thyroidectomy, performed for cancer of the thyroid gland, will require the patient to have life-long replacement therapy with thyroxine.

A very rare complication of thyroidectomy is tetany arising from inadvertent removal of the parathyroid glands. These glands, while not part of the thyroid gland, are in very close proximity to it posteriorly. Emergency treatment of tetany consists of intravenous administration of calcium gluconate. (See 'Parathyroid disorders' below.)

Thyroid crisis

The condition is rare but, when it occurs, is life-threatening. The patient would exhibit exaggerated symptoms of thyrotoxicosis, which may be the presenting features of thyroid disease. The high standard of preoperative care given to patients undergoing thyroid surgery normally prevents this complication postoperatively when it is due to excessive handling of the thyroid gland, an ill-prepared gland, or infection.

Immediate treatment consists of rehydration and the appropriate administration of antibiotics, carbimazole and propanolol.

Hypothyroidism (myxoedema)

Patients with hypothyroidism may present at varying stages of the condition, and some are detected when presenting with minor or non-specific symptoms. Many elderly people suffer from decreased thyroid production, and the elderly should be encouraged to attend GP's clinics regularly so that detection is made early.

Hypothyroidism can be treated on an outpatient basis.

Diagnosis is made by hormone assay which will show raised TSH levels and low levels of thyroid hormones, showing that the thyroid gland cannot be stimulated to greater production.

Thyroxine is the only treatment for hypothyroidism.

Improvement is noticed in the patient's condition within 2–3 weeks and physical improvement a few weeks later. Biochemical assay will then show reduction in levels of TSH (because of hormonal feedback mechanism).

The patient should be monitored closely, especially at the start of therapy, to ensure that he is responding appropriately to the dosage prescribed. The patient may require much encouragement to attend clinics, but continued compliance is essential for his well-being.

Supportive therapy for the patient with hypo-thyroidism includes:

- supervision of medications
- skin care with lotions which will help combat dryness
- a warm environment
- prevention of constipation by high fibre diet, adequate fluid intake and exercise
- promotion of good nutritional status and weight control
- observation of patient for effects and side-effects of medications.

Hypothyroidism in children

In children this is known as **cretinism**. Maternal hormones supply a baby's needs for up to 3 months after birth, then, if the baby is hypothyroid, features due to deficiency begin to appear. These are associated with a general stunting of mental and physical growth. If left untreated, the child becomes a mentally retarded dwarf with coarse facial features. Early detection and administration of the deficient hormone leads to great improvement in physical growth and, in some children, mental development. In others, some mental retardation persists.

STRUCTURE AND FUNCTION OF PARATHYROID GLANDS

The four parathyroids lie behind the thyroid gland (Fig. 16.5); branches of the thyroid arteries provide their blood supply.

In the embryo, the parathyroids occasionally migrate elsewhere, for example to the mediastinum. Their number can also vary. They secrete **parathormone**, which maintains plasma calcium levels within a narrow range despite the large daily exchanges of calcium between intestines, bloodstream, kidneys and bones.

Parathormone secretion is not regulated by the anterior pituitary but varies inversely with plasma concentration. Plasma phosphate concentration is inversely related to that of calcium.

The main functions of parathormone are:

1. To mobilize calcium and phosphate from bones into blood.
2. To reduce renal excretion of calcium.
3. To promote intestinal absorption of calcium

aided by vitamin D. (These actions raise the plasma calcium.)

4. To reduce phosphorus reabsorption by the kidneys, thus promoting its excretion and lowering plasma phosphate. This is necessary, since calcium and phosphate together tend to precipitate out of solution and could thus damage tissues and especially arterial walls.

PARATHYROID DISORDERS

Hyperparathyroidism

This term denotes excessive parathyroid activity; the condition is uncommon, the highest incidence being among females and between the ages of 30 and 50 years. The disease may be familial.

Primary hyperparathyroidism   The cause is usually a benign adenoma or adenomas (90% of cases), occasionally hyperplasia and more rarely cancer. There is oversecretion of parathormone, regardless of plasma calcium concentration. Calcium and phosphorus are mobilized from bone, renal absorption of calcium is increased, plasma calcium levels rise and urinary phosphate excretion is increased.

Secondary hyperparathyroidism   In some diseases where there is depression of the plasma calcium, there is compensatory enlargement of the parathyroids. The underlying disease may be intestinal, causing malabsorption of vitamin D and calcium, or renal, where there is excess calcium excretion.

Clinical features of primary hyperparathyroidism

A raised plasma calcium level causes lethargy and anorexia. It weakens and eventually paralyses muscles. The paralysing effects of excess calcium on the gut wall may cause abdominal pain and constipation. Polyuria occurs, since the kidneys are filtering and excreting excess mineral salts. The nauseated patient may be reluctant to drink, but he should be encouraged to do so to prevent dehydration and formation of renal stones. Renal disorders are common, with formation of calcium-containing kidney stones due to high urinary calcium. Calcium-depleted bones become brittle. Osteitis fibrosa (replacement of bone by fibrous tissue) causes vague pains, which may be mistaken for rheumatism and can lead to bone deformities. Cyst formation in bones adds swelling to deformity. Calcium 'ring' deposits can occur in the cornea, and effects on nervous tissue may cause agitation, confusion or depression.

Nurses should ensure that patients whose bones are so fragile are protected from accidents.

Investigations

1. **Measurement of plasma calcium** with the patient at rest and fasting. (Calcium absorption following meals would affect the readings.) Plasma calcium is raised and plasma phosphorus reduced in primary hyperparathyroidism.

2. **Measurement of parathormone levels** by radio-immunoassay when possible.

3. **Bone X-rays**. These may reveal cysts and low bone density.

4. **Bone biopsy**. This may show reabsorption of trabeculae by osteoclasts and replacement by fibrous tissue (oesteitis fibrosa).

5. **Intravenous urogram**. This may demonstrate calcium deposits in the renal tract.

6. **Urinary calcium**, measured on a normal diet, is increased because the increase in the amount filtered overwhelms the effect of renal reabsorption under the influence of parathormone.

Treatment

Secondary hyperparathyroidism Oral vitamin D will raise plasma calcium levels by enhancing absorption and so remove the stimulus to parathyroid hyperplasia. Operative treatment is seldom indicated.

Primary hyperparathyroidism is treated by surgical removal of abnormal parathyroid tissue. If hyperplasia of all four glands exists, three and a half are removed.

Preparation for operation Preoperatively, the patient may be infused with methylene blue to facilitate recognition of parathyroid tissue. This procedure causes skin and mucous membrane to develop a greenish tinge. The patient and relatives should be warned about this beforehand and assured that the colour will disappear quickly. Ward staff without experience of this operation should also be prepared for this change in appearance.

Postoperative observations Hypoparathyroidism occurs if too much parathyroid tissue is removed and because calcium-depleted bones take up free calcium. Plasma calcium levels are monitored by:

1. Taking blood samples.
2. Frequent observation of the patient for signs of latent tetany, using Chvostek's and Trousseau's signs (see p. 565) and noting any tingling sensations in the limbs.

Should signs of hypocalcaemia develop, an intravenous injection of 10% calcium gluconate is given. Dihydrotachysterol (DHT), an analogue of vitamin D, is sometimes given in large doses postoperatively (8 mg daily for 2 days). As they act more slowly than DHT, vitamin D preparations are less satisfactory for immediate postoperative management. Aluminium hydroxide may be given orally with meals to reduce phosphorus absorption. (Since blood calcium levels are now reduced phosphorus levels rise). Later, a high calcium diet is given, the calcium usually consisting of calcium salts, because these patients often have renal disorders and milk is inadvisable because of its high protein and phosphorus content.

Postoperative complications These are similar to those which may follow thyroidectomy, for example a slipped blood vessel ligature resulting in a haematoma which compresses the trachea. Clip or stitch removers should be available for such an eventuality, so that pressure on the trachea may be relieved. If the surgeon has explored the mediastinum chest complications may arise.

Rehabilitation

Maintenance therapy with DHT is continued, with outpatient supervision of dosage, until bone healing occurs. If hypocalcaemia persists, the patient may require life-long calcium supplements and vitamin D_2. Existing stones do not dissolve so renal function may be impaired permanently.

Hypoparathyroidism

Hypoparathyroidism may either arise spontaneously or follow disease or injury, but more often it results from accidental removal of the parathyroids during thyroidectomy.

Clinical features

1. **Tetany** develops when plasma calcium falls significantly below the normal 2.12–2.62 mmol/l. There is increased excitability of nerves and muscles. Motor and sensory nerve impulses fire off spontaneously. Abnormal sensory impulses cause tingling sensations (paraesthesiae), while the motor impulses cause involuntary muscle twitches. These twitches are most obvious in the muscles of the inner forearm and hand supplied by the ulnar nerve. There is flexion of wrist and knuckles with extension of the fingers (Fig. 16.6). As a result of defective muscular control, the patient is more liable to fall and requires careful observation. Two signs of latent tetany are:

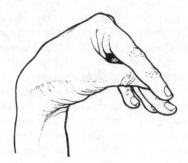

Fig. 16.6 Carpal spasm

Chvostek's sign. Tapping the facial nerve at the jaw angle produces twitching of facial muscles.

Trousseau's sign. Applying a blood pressure cuff to the arm causes muscular spasm of forearm and hand.

2. **Laryngospasm** may be severe enough to obstruct the airway.

3. **Epileptic convulsions**, due to increased excitability of nerve cells in the brain, may be the first symptom.

4. **Psychological disturbances** may range from minor disorders to major psychoses.

Investigations

These are carried out when the patient's condition permits. They include the following:

1. Fasting plasma calcium.
2. Serum inorganic phosphate.
3. Renal phosphate clearance.
4. 24-hour urine collection to measure urinary calcium excretion. Nurses must explain to the patient the importance of an accurate 24-hour urine collection and of fasting before certain blood specimens are taken. It may also be necessary to collect faeces. Some investigations may make it imperative that the calcium intake is known and, if this is so, a special diet will be supplied.
5. Electrocardiograph may demonstrate variations in cardiac function.

Treatment

Emergency treatment Calcium salts such as 10 ml of 10% calcium gluconate are given intravenously to raise the plasma calcium level when symptoms are severe and require urgent relief. If epileptic convulsions occur, the patient must be protected from injury.

ADRENAL GLANDS

Structure and function

The adrenal glands sit one on top of each kidney. Although they are in close proximity to the kidneys, there is no anatomical attachment. Each gland consists of two discrete parts, the cortex and the medulla, which have developed from separate embryonic layers. Figure 16.7 illustrates a cross-section of an adrenal gland identifying cortex and medulla.

The cortex is derived from the epithelial cells of the mesoderm, which is also the origin of the gonads. Structurally, the cortex consists of three layers, each producing specific hormones. The outermost layer secretes mineralocorticoids, the middle layer glucocorticoids, and the innermost layer secretes gonadocorticoids, primarily androgens.

The medulla is derived from the ectoderm and comprises neural tissue. The medulla secretes adrenaline and noradrenaline (epinephrine and nor-epinephrine).

The main mineralocorticoid is aldosterone, the body's predominant sodium-retaining hormone. Secretion of aldosterone is not under hypothalamic–pituitary control, but under the control of the renin–angiotensin mechanism (see Ch. 17). When body sodium is depleted, as in fluid loss or insufficient intake, then aldosterone is secreted. It acts on the distal tubule of the nephron and sodium is retained.

The glucocorticoids comprise cortisol (hydrocortisone), corticosterone and cortisone. The most abundant is cortisol. Glucocorticoids are essential to life, and their functions are many. In summary, the glucocorticoids:

- promote normal metabolism
- promote glycolysis

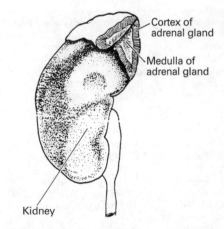

Fig. 16.7 Section of adrenal gland

- promote glycogenesis
- combat stress by increasing resistance
- increase sensitivity to blood chemicals which constrict blood vessels
- are anti-inflammatory and anti-allergenic.

It is their activity in the stress response which makes the glucocorticoids essential to life. When there is a lack of these hormones, even a minor stressful situation, such as a common cold, could be fatal. For this reason, patients receiving corticosteroid therapy are educated in its dosage, effects and administration.

Natural secretion of glucocorticoids in the body is related to the circadian cycle – the secretion is highest in the early morning and reduces throughout the day until it is lowest around midnight. This fact is reflected in the timing of corticosteroid medication when the larger dose is given in the morning and the smaller dose in the early evening.

Nurses working night duty invariably feel at their lowest ebb at around 02.00 hours. This is related to the cyclical secretion of glucocorticoids.

Secretion of glucocorticoids is under the influence of the hypothalamic–pituitary pathway.

The glucocorticoids have some mineralocorticoid effect, albeit small. Glucocorticoid replacement therapy therefore also compensates for lost mineralocorticoids in most cases.

The gonadocorticoid hormones from the adrenal cortex consist of both androgens and oestrogens. These hormones are the only active sex hormones prior to puberty, and the balanced nature of output explains why young children are not greatly differentiated physically, except for genitalia. It is the onset of puberty with the erratic production of the ovarian/testicular hormones that creates the physical and emotional changes of puberty and adolescence.

The medulla secretes adrenaline and noradrenaline from its neural tissue. It is under the control of the autonomic nervous system (see Ch. 5).

The adrenal glands present an example within one gland of the differing time reactions of the body's controlling systems to meet body needs – the medulla acts instantly and has short-term effects, while the secretions from the cortex are blood borne and slower to act but with longer-lasting effects.

Disorders of the adrenal glands

Aetiology

Disorders of the adrenal glands arise from over- or undersecretion of specific hormones. Table 16.3 summarizes conditions which arise from oversecretion and undersecretion of these hormones.

In conditions leading to oversecretion of adrenal hormones, the cause must be removed. Glucocorticoid excess may be of pituitary origin, when ACTH production will be high, or arise from adrenal tumour or hyperplasia when cortisol levels will be high.

Adrenalin oversecretion is of medullary origin.

Removal of the offending tissue may be by partial or total adrenalectomy, or by removal of pituitary tumour or pituitary ablation.

Care of the patient undergoing pituitary surgery is discussed in Chapter 5.

Removal of adrenal tissue

The patient undergoing adrenal surgery requires very

Table 16.3 Conditions arising from disordered adrenal secretion and the resulting clinical effects		
Hormone	Condition arising	Effects
Oversecretion of cortical hormones		
Aldosterone	Hyperaldosteronism	Hypertension, hyperkalaemia, muscle weakness
Glucocorticoids	Cushing's syndrome	Obesity, bruising, striae, hypertension, moonface, muscle weakness, plethora, hirsutism, disordered gonadal function
Oversecretion of medullary hormones		
Catecholamines	Phaeochromocytoma	Hypertension, headache, palpitations, sweating, anxiety, weight loss, glucose intolerance
Undersecretion of cortical hormones (adrenocortical insufficiency)		
Glucocorticoids	Addison's disease	Weight loss, malaise, weakness, anorexia,
Mineralocorticoids		gastrointestinal disturbances, hypotension,
Adrenal androgens		hypoglycaemia, skin pigmentation, loss of body hair

careful and very accurate monitoring both pre- and postoperatively.

Preoperatively, specific care involves the administration of hydrocortisone by intravenous infusion 6 hourly for 24 four hours prior to operation. This action will prevent adrenal insufficiency (when the stress response would be absent) immediately following removal of the adrenal glands. Oversecretion of adrenal cortical hormones creates imbalance in serum electrolyte levels. Excess aldosterone causes sodium retention (therefore fluid retention) and potassium depletion. Blood pressure is elevated because of the fluid retention, and weakness occurs because of potassium loss. Serum electrolytes therefore will be monitored, and a careful record kept of fluid intake and output. Blood pressure will be recorded at regular prescribed intervals.

Specific postoperative observations include attention to blood pressure as hypotension may occur following removal of the glands.

Blood pressure recordings should be made at 15 minute intervals for the first 4–6 hours, then with decreasing, but regular, frequency as the patient's condition stabilizes. Pulse recordings follow a similar pattern. Fluid balance should be accurately monitored. Hydrocortisone will be administered intravenously until the patient is stabilized on oral medication. Intravenous infusion of glucose continues until after withdrawal of intravenous hydrocortisone. The nurse must be aware of the dangers of too little or too much corticoid medication.

Symptoms of adrenal insufficiency include vomiting, weakness, dehydration, hypotension.

Phaeocromocytoma is a rare tumour of the adrenal medulla which secretes large quantities of catecholamines. It is treated by surgical removal. Preoperative reduction and control of blood pressure is of paramount importance. Blood pressure recordings will continue on a frequent basis for up to 48 hours at intervals of perhaps ½ hour to 1 hour. The reason for this frequency is that during surgery a release of catecholamines is possible, causing a surge in blood pressure which must receive instant attention.

The patient undergoing adrenal surgery requires close supervision postoperatively at all times and should never be left unattended during critical periods.

If adrenalectomy is bilateral, then the patient will require corticosteroid replacement for life. Fludrocortisone (a mineralocorticoid) may also be necessary, but the mineralocorticoid effect of corticosteroids may be sufficient.

If adrenalectomy is unilateral, it may take a considerable time, over a period of months, for the remaining gland and the hypothalamic–pituitary pathway to recover. Any sudden episode of stress may create increased need which the remaining gland cannot meet initially. The patient, therefore, should be advised to avoid overtiredness, extremes of temperature, especially cold, infections and emotional disturbances.

Any indication of weakness, fever, nausea or vomiting should not be neglected, and the patient should contact his medical adviser. Corticosteroid supplement may be required. A careful follow-up regimen is essential and the importance of compliance in attendance at clinics must be emphasized to the patient.

Corticosteroid replacement is given when glands are removed or are non-functioning, as in Addison's disease.

Patient education is of the essence and family members should be included in the programme (see Box 16.1).

Box 16.1   Advice to the patient following adrenalectomy

- The need to maintain medication as prescribed – never miss a dose.
- The need to increase medication during illness – in this respect the patient should keep in touch with his medical adviser.
- If vomiting occurs, then hospitalization will be necessary as hydrocortisone will require to be given intravenously.
- The need to avoid infection.
- The need to avoid extremes of temperature, especially cold.
- The need to avoid stressful situations.
- The desirability of carrying a card with details of medication, timing of medication, and name of doctor.
- The wearing of an appropriately engraved bracelet is advised.

Therapeutic use of corticosteroids

Corticosteroids are given as replacement therapy when the dosage is physiological and are also given therapeutically in the management of some non-endocrine disorders such as asthma and allergic conditions which produce an inflammatory response. In the latter conditions, therapeutic dosages, larger than physiological doses, are given to counteract the inflammatory and allergic responses.

Oral administration of corticosteroids reduces ACTH secretion through the hormonal negative feedback mechanism. This is turn results in reduced secretion from the adrenal glands which may atrophy. Medication in these situations must not be stopped abruptly, but should be withdrawn gradually over a period of time to allow the target gland time to recommence production and secretion of hormones.

The main side-effects of corticosteroid therapy are:

- moon face
- hirsutism
- hyperglycaemia
- hypertension
- susceptibility to infection
- peptic ulceration
- euphoria
- truncal obesity
- acne; striae; delayed wound healing
- impotence
- menstrual irregularities.

DISORDERS OF THE PANCREAS

The pancreas is a gland composed of acinar and endocrine tissue giving it both acinar and endocrine functions. The exocrine functions are essential for chemical digestion of foodstuffs (see Ch. 15). The endocrine functions regulate blood glucose levels maintaining blood glucose homeostasis. Adequate levels of blood glucose must be maintained to provide energy for cell metabolism. The nervous system is unable to store glucose and therefore requires a constant supply from the bloodstream.

Pancreatic endocrine hormones are secreted from specialized groups of cells scattered throughout pancreatic tissue. These groups of cells are the Islets of Langerhans and comprise alpha cells which secrete the hormone glucagon, the actions of which raise blood glucose levels, and beta cells which secrete insulin, the actions of which lower blood glucose levels.

Insulin is a protein (polypeptide) substance and is ineffective if taken orally as digestive processes would reduce the insulin molecule to basic amino acids.

Secretion of insulin and glucagon is stimulated by the level of glucose in the bloodstream, recognition of which is made in the pancreas from circulating blood – humoral feedback control – and not via the hypothalamic–pituitary pathway.

Actions of insulin

1. Aids the transport of glucose across cell membranes.
2. Aids the entry of amino acids into cells and the synthesis of proteins.
3. Glycogenesis.
4. Lipogenesis from glucose.
5. Decreases glycogenolysis.
6. Slows gluconeogenesis.
7. Promotes cellular potassium uptake.

Aetiology of diabetes mellitus

Diabetes mellitus is a condition which develops due to lack or absence of insulin. This is a disorder of carbohydrate metabolism with subsequent disturbance of fat and protein metabolism.

Diabetes is a chronic disease affecting metabolism throughout the 24-hour span and affects the patient for life. Its incidence in the UK is 1–2% of the population and it affects all age groups from infancy (although rare) onwards. It is the most common of all the endocrine disorders.

Care of the patient with diabetes requires a multidisciplinary approach both in hospital and in the community. It involves medical and nursing staff, dietician, podiatrist, possibly social worker, and liaison between hospital and community is essential for the patient's well-being.

The aetiology of diabetes is uncertain, but the interaction of environmental factors with genetic predisposition determines development of the disease. Viral infections, autoimmune response, obesity and stress may be implicated in the development of the disease.

These theories apply to primary diabetes, but secondary diabetes can occur following pancreatitis, pancreatic carcinoma, Cushing's syndrome, or it can develop iatrogenically when medication for other disorders, for example hydrocortisone, raises blood glucose levels to a point where insulin production is insufficient to cope with demands.

It will develop following removal of the pancreas. It is important to monitor blood glucose levels and perform urinalysis regularly and conscientiously in a patient at risk of developing secondary diabetes.

Investigations to diagnose diabetes mellitus

Investigations which are carried out to ascertain the diagnosis of diabetes mellitus are

1. Urinalysis to test for glycosuria and ketonuria.
2. Random blood glucose sampling.
3. Oral glucose tolerance test. The procedure for this test is explained in Box 16.2.

Diabetes is classified as insulin-dependent diabetes mellitus (IDDM) or non-insulin-dependent diabetes mellitus (NIDDM). Approximately 20% of diabetics

---

Box 16.2 Diagnostic investigations in diabetes mellitus

Urine tests
Glycosuria suggests diabetes

Blood glucose tests
High blood glucose levels (over 8.3 mmol/l) indicate diabetes in anyone displaying other classical symptoms of the disease. Most people need no other tests

Oral glucose tolerance tests (OGTT)
Glucose 75 g is given orally to the fasting patient and blood samples are taken half hourly for 2 hours. A fasting venous blood glucose level of 7 mmol/l or more and a 2 hour level of more than 10 mmol/l are diagnostic of diabetes mellitus. Nurses must ensure that the glucose is properly dissolved and diluted to the same strength since the concentration affects the absorption rate. The mixture is more palatable when flavoured with pure lemon juice and chilled. The patient must drink all of the mixture and he should not reduce his carbohydrate intake in the days prior to OGTT since the test should reflect insulin response under normal dietary conditions. He should also refrain from smoking and remain at rest throughout the test as smoking and exercise will influence blood glucose levels. Urine may be tested hourly during OGTT but little extra information is gained

---

Table 16.4 Characteristics of IDDM and NIDDM

	IDDM	NIDDM
Age at onset	Under 40 years	Over 50 years
Duration of symptoms	Weeks	Months/years
Body weight	Normal or low	Obese
Ketonuria	Yes	No
Rapid death without treatment with insulin	Yes	No
Autoantibodies	Yes	No
Diabetic complications at diagnosis	No	10–20%
Other autoimmune disease	Yes	No

are IDDM. Table 16.4 compares the salient features of the two types.

Pathology of diabetes mellitus

All cells require energy to carry out their metabolic processes (see Ch. 4). This energy is derived from the biochemical breakdown within the cells of molecules of digested foodstuffs, mainly carbohydrate as glucose and fats as fatty acids. The end result of these chemical reactions is the formation of energy in the form of adenosine triphosphate (ATP) and heat as a byproduct of metabolism. Water and carbon dioxide are formed as waste products – metabolic water. Cell metabolism is described in Chapter 4.

While fatty acids can pass through cell membranes, glucose requires insulin to facilitate its entry. In the absence of insulin, glucose cannot enter the cell and remains in the bloodstream following its absorption from the gastrointestinal tract. There follows a sequence of events shown in Box 16.3.

Other features are weakness and fatigue caused by the body's inability to meet its energy requirements, and pruritis vulvae caused by the irritating effect of glycosuria.

In the IDDM patient the above events take place over a short period of time. In the older, obese patient with NIDDM the development of symptoms takes place over a longer period of time and is initially insidious. In fact, in the older patient, it may be some complication of the disease which makes him seek medical advice.

Management of diabetes mellitus

Whatever the type of diabetes, the approach to management is the same for each.

The overall aim of patient management is to achieve and maintain satisfactory blood glucose levels and the maintenance of desirable weight by implementing a programme of education which will enable the patient (and his family/significant others) to understand the condition, and to accept and manage the patient's altered health status to achieve a lifestyle as near normality as possible. Good metabolic control will delay or prevent the onset of complications associated with the condition.

Achieving and maintaining satisfactory blood glucose levels

Stabilization of blood glucose levels is managed on an outpatient basis except in an emergency or where the patient has to travel some distance to the clinic.

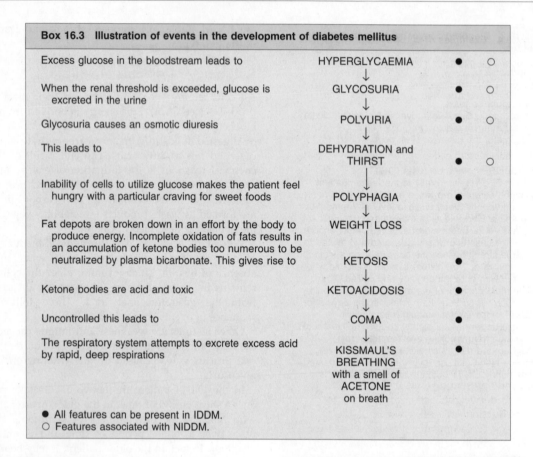

Box 16.3 Illustration of events in the development of diabetes mellitus

Excess glucose in the bloodstream leads to	HYPERGLYCAEMIA ↓	● ○
When the renal threshold is exceeded, glucose is excreted in the urine	GLYCOSURIA ↓	● ○
Glycosuria causes an osmotic diuresis	POLYURIA ↓	● ○
This leads to	DEHYDRATION and THIRST ↓	● ○
Inability of cells to utilize glucose makes the patient feel hungry with a particular craving for sweet foods	POLYPHAGIA ↓	●
Fat depots are broken down in an effort by the body to produce energy. Incomplete oxidation of fats results in an accumulation of ketone bodies too numerous to be neutralized by plasma bicarbonate. This gives rise to	WEIGHT LOSS ↓ KETOSIS ↓	●
Ketone bodies are acid and toxic	KETOACIDOSIS ↓	●
Uncontrolled this leads to	COMA ↓	●
The respiratory system attempts to excrete excess acid by rapid, deep respirations	KISSMAUL'S BREATHING with a smell of ACETONE on breath	●

● All features can be present in IDDM.
○ Features associated with NIDDM.

Diabetic patients cannot be adequately prepared for daily living within the confines of a hospital ward, and this fact should be explained.

The method of controlling blood glucose is dictated by the type of diabetes and stage of the disease. Control may be achieved by dietary control alone, by dietary control and oral hypoglycaemic agents (OHAs), or by insulin administration and dietary control. Regular planned monitoring of glycaemic levels will assess the efficacy of the planned approach.

Dietary control is essential in all diabetic care, and the principles of the necessary management are applicable for all patients. Many diabetics are surprised to know the range of foods available to them.

The patient's energy requirements are calculated according to stature, age, sex, occupation, with the aim being to achieve the standard desirable weight.

The dietician features prominently in the patient's care. Approximately 50% of the diet should consist of carbohydrate, and this is taken as exchanges, each exchange being the equivalent of 10 grams of carbohydrate. Table 16.5 illustrates the construction of the diet.

Table 16.5 Construction of a weight maintenance diet

Exchanges	Carbohydrate (g)	Energy (kcal)
21 carbohydrate	210	1050
2/3rd pint milk	20	260
4 protein	—	280
2 fat	—	220
Total	230	1810

1. The diet contains approximately 1800 kcal (7560 kJ) with 230 g carbohydrate, 72 g protein, 66 g fat providing 51%, 16% and 33% of calories respectively.
2. The 23 carbohydrate and 4 protein exchanges are distributed throughout the day according to the eating habits and daily routine of the patient.

Adapted from Edwards & Bouchier 1991, table 13.24, p. 671

The dietary proportions entered in Box 16.4 are those recommended by the British Diabetic Association (BDA) as a starting guide for dietary control.

Box 16.4   Examples of carbohydrate exchanges

Each item on this list = 1 carbohydrate exchange = 10 g carbohydrate

- ½ slice bread from a large loaf
- 1 large digestive biscuit
- 2 cream crackers
- ⅓ teacup natural unsweetened orange or grapefruit juice
- 1 medium-sized eating apple or orange
- 10 grapes
- 1 small banana
- ⅓ pint (200 ml) milk
- 1 teacup cooked porridge
- 1 teacup cream or tinned soup
- ⅔ teacup cornflakes
- 1 small packet crisps
- 1 small potato

Reproduced with permission from Edwards & Bouchier 1991, p. 671.

Dietary prescription, however, is based on individual requirements and may vary considerably. Variables to be considered are based on the patient's age, sex, work, and presenting nutritional status such as over- or underweight.

The reduction of refined carbohydrate in the diet and its replacement with high fibre foods is a well-recognized benefit in diabetic care. Refined carbohydrate contains glucose which, as a basic carbohydrate molecule, is ready for immediate absorption. Fibre in food delays the digestion and absorption of glucose from the gastrointestinal tract and reduces the sudden demand for insulin, thus giving a better control of blood glucose levels.

So-called 'diabetic foods' are not a necessary inclusion in the diabetic patient's diet and should be avoided as routine purchases. As an occasional treat, their use should be inhibited rather than prohibited. They are very expensive and it comes as a surprise to patients to know that such foods have to be counted among the exchanges.

Protein is not restricted, but should comprise approximately 15% of the diet.

Recommendations are made in relation to fat intake. All diabetics should reduce their intake of animal fats and dairy produce. These foods predispose to the formation of atheroma.

Dietary advice and education will, in most centres, be given by specialist dieticians, but nurses caring for diabetic patients have a professional responsibility to become knowledgeable about dietary principles (Davis 1991).

Dietary control alone may be effective for the mature overweight patient. Dietary intake will be discussed with the patient, and will aim for weight reduction as well as blood glucose control. Such patients do produce insulin but the insulin output from the pancreas (about 50 units daily in health) will have been insufficient to cope with metabolic demands imposed by dietary indiscretions. When the diet and weight are corrected then the patient's condition will improve, although this does not signal the end of dietary control which must continue.

NIDDM patients may require, in addition to dietary control, administration of oral hypoglycaemic agents (OHAs). The main OHAs given are from the sulphonylurea range, for example tolbutamide, chlorpropamide. These drugs appear to stimulate functioning Islet of Langerhans to produce more insulin. The biguanides, much less commonly used because of side-effects, act by increasing uptake of glucose by cells, but their precise mechanism of action is not known. One of the group, metformin, may be given to overweight patients.

Patients receiving OHAs must be aware that their medication has to be taken exactly as prescribed and that they must monitor their blood glucose levels and urinalysis regularly, although not as frequently as patients taking insulin. Frequency will be prescribed; commonly two to four times weekly, when the patient is well. It is preferable to sample fasting blood glucose levels, but occasional postprandial sampling may be indicated.

Hypoglycaemia can occur in patients taking OHAs, a fact not universally realized, and patients must be educated to recognize when it is occurring.

It may be necessary on occasion to administer insulin to patients being controlled on OHAs, for example during acute illness, or when surgical intervention is required. Following the episode, the patient should be able to resume the previous regimen of medication.

Patient self-monitoring of blood glucose estimation is done by testing capillary blood. Urinalysis may also be carried out. Blood glucose analysis is more accurate and it also shows true glucose levels earlier than those indicated by urinalysis.

A number of devices are available for monitoring blood glucose levels, but the nurse must be fully aware of their use and follow manufacturers' instructions carefully before attempting patient teaching. Patients must be instructed in the protocol advised by the clinic. Many patients are apprehensive about capillary testing, but with help and reassurance they will gain confidence in their ability to carry it out with accuracy.

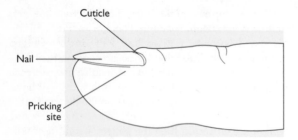

Fig. 16.8 Finger pricking site

While finger-tip pricking has been, and may still be used (Cradock 1989), the finger-tip is not the best site. In diabetics who develop complications, peripheral neuropathy is common, and sensation is impaired. It would be possible for the patient to damage the finger-tip without being aware of doing so. Healing is slow in diabetic tissue because of microangiopathy and because glucose in the tissues creates an excellent medium for growth of micro-organisms.

A more suitable area from which to obtain the sample is demonstrated in Figure 16.8. This area is less likely to be damaged than the finger-tip.

Insulin dosage is calculated according to the patient's carbohydrate requirements. It is planned to provide release of insulin throughout 24 hours and to prevent hypoglycaemia. How this is done varies, but usually involves a combination of rapid onset (unmodified) and delayed onset (modified) insulins. Unmodified (rapid onset, short acting) insulins are effective from about 30 minutes after subcutaneous injection and last approximately 6 hours. They should be administered no more than 20–30 minutes prior to a meal. Unmodified insulins are used when an instant response is required when they would be given intravenously. Table 16.6 identifies insulins in common use and their sources.

In health, the pancreas, on average, secretes about 50 international units (i.u.) of insulin over 24 hours but patients vary in their requirements.

Some patients are resistant to insulin and may require large doses (e.g. 200 i.u.). Blood glucose levels are affected by a number of factors, including growth hormone and glucagon levels. It has been noted that some diabetics have high levels of glucagon which mobilize stored glycogen, thus raising blood glucose levels. Glucocorticoid hormones also raise blood glucose levels.

Table 16.6 Insulin preparations in common use			
Type	Proprietary preparations*	Species	Approximate duration (hours)
Unmodified Clear solutions Rapid onset Short action	Actrapid (Novo-Nordisk) Velosulin (Novo-Nordisk) Humulin S (Lilly) Hypurin Neutral (CP Pharm)	Human Human Porcine Human Bovine	6
Modified (depot) Cloudy solutions Delayed onset Prolonged action	Monotard (Novo-Nordisk) Insulatard (Novo-Nordisk) Humulin I (Lilly) Hypurin isophane (CP Pharm) Ultratard (NOVO) Humulin Zn (Lilly) Hypurin Protamine (CP Pharm)	Human Human Porcine Human Bovine Human Human Bovine	12 24

*In Britain and the USA all these insulin preparations are available only in 100 i.u./ml strength for routine clinical use. In other parts of the world insulins are also available in 40 and 80 i.u./ml strength.
Pre-mixed insulin preparations, containing a wide range of fixed ratios of unmodified and intermediate depot, are also available.

Reproduced with permission from Edwards & Bouchier 1991, table 13.26, p. 674.

While nearly all IDDM patients are controlled with a combination of both types of insulin, unmodified insulin will be used during episodes of acute illness or in newly diagnosed patients in the early stages of the condition. Illness makes erratic demands on the body, and the rapid action of unmodified insulin gives ease of control in unstable situations.

Insulin is dispensed in a strength of 100 i.u./ml. An insulin syringe is calibrated in units with each line representing 1 unit of insulin, so that, for example, 6 units of insulin would occupy six marks on an insulin syringe. This strength is used in Britain, North America, New Zealand and Australia, but in other parts of the world 40 and 80 i.u./ml strengths are still in use, an important point for diabetics travelling abroad in relation to supply and calculation.

Patients should be taught and encouraged to give their first injection as soon as possible. It is false kindness to delay the patient's participation in giving his own injections, and there is an argument in favour of leaving the theory of injection technique until after the patient has practised a few injections under full supervision. The theory may be very stressful and inhibiting for some patients and do little to instil confidence in their ability.

Patients now have access to disposable syringes on prescription and these come fitted with subcutaneous needles. The angle at which the needle should be inserted has been the subject of debate, but the Professional Advisory Committee of the British Diabetic Association (BDA) advises that the current practice of inserting the needle at an angle of 90 degrees should continue with some modification. This angle makes for a less painful injection because fewer sensory nerve endings are stimulated. The amount of subcutaneous fat present affects the injection technique. If the patient is lean or thin, then it is recommended that the skin is 'pinched up' prior to injection. This prevents the injection becoming an intramuscular one, and as the intramuscular route gives faster absorption, such injections could result in erratic control of blood glucose (Sykes 1991).

The patient should be given a chart illustrating injection sites. These are the lower parts of the abdomen, upper outer quadrants of the thigh, upper arm and buttocks. Vigorous cleansing of the skin with alcohol-based products has been shown to be unnecessary and even harmful to the skin, and it is sufficient that the skin is clean and dry. Absorption rates vary with the sites, being faster in the arm and slowest in the thigh. The patient should be taught to vary the injection site. Figure 16.9 demonstrates injection sites.

Correct storage of insulin is important. Unopened vials are kept in a (domestic) refrigerator. Once opened, the vial need not be refrigerated, but should be dated and discarded after 1 month irrespective of how it has been stored during that time or the amount left unused.

A number of pen-type devices are available for the administration of insulin. These deliver metered doses of insulin and are extremely useful when travelling. They are not available on NHS prescription.

The IDDM patient must be aware of the need for regular and frequent monitoring of blood glucose levels. Capillary blood testing should be carried out approximately six times per week and should coincide with such times as the peak action times of insulin and fasting blood glucose. Monitoring does not control blood glucose levels, but it gives a picture of events. This record is also beneficial for the patient who is taught to regulate his insulin intake to meet changes in his daily activities such as increased exercise.

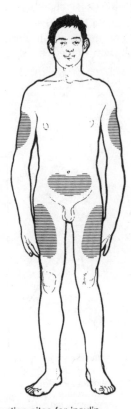

Fig. 16.9 Injection sites for insulin

IDDM patients must understand the action to be taken during illness. Insulin must never be omitted during illness. Energy is required to combat infection or illness, and this places extra demand on body metabolism. Any illness creates stress, the physiological effects of which raise blood glucose levels. It is understandable that an unwell person feels disinclined to eat, but the food should be replaced with suitable drinks to meet exchange requirements. If vomiting develops and cannot be controlled, then the patient should be removed to hospital immediately. A usually well-controlled diabetic can become a critically ill patient in a very short space of time.

Figure 16.10 indicates situations in which insulin must be adjusted.

Diabetes and pregnancy

Pregnancy is not contraindicated in the diabetic patient whose condition is well controlled and who is otherwise healthy. Good control of blood glucose levels is imperative before and during the pregnancy for the health of the mother and baby. Pregnancy makes heavy demands on the mother's body metabolism, altering energy needs. The reader should refer to a textbook specializing in this field.

Glycosuria is not uncommon in normal pregnancy because of a reduction in the renal threshold for glucose, but its presence will always be investigated. The situation is temporary.

A condition known as gestational diabetes can occur in women who have a genetic predisposition to the development of diabetes. Pregnancy can act as a triggering factor in this development. The hyperglycaemia associated with gestational diabetes may or may not disappear following delivery. During pregnancy, the patient's hyperglycaemia may be controlled by dietary measures alone or with insulin administration. Control of maternal hyperglycaemia reduces fetal risk. The patient will require regular monitoring for some time thereafter, and the development of overt diabetes during a subsequent pregnancy or in later life is a strong possibility.

The diabetic patient requiring surgery

A patient who is to have elective surgery requires full assessment by the diabetologist. It may be possible to have this done on an outpatient basis, or the patient may be admitted in advance of the operation date for this purpose. The dietician will arrange the patient's dietary requirements. Specifically, the patient will have an intravenous infusion started on the morning of, or evening prior to, surgery, and insulin prescribed by the diabetologist will be given via a controlled intravenous pump. Unmodified insulin

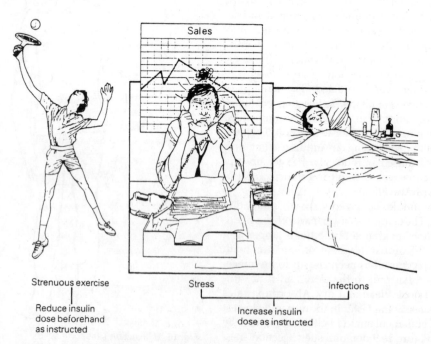

Strenuous exercise

Reduce insulin dose beforehand as instructed

Stress

Infections

Increase insulin dose as instructed

Fig. 16.10 Stressors affecting insulin requirements

will be given during the immediate pre- and post-operative period until the patient's usual regimen can be resumed.

Regular monitoring of blood glucose levels at ward level and in the biochemical laboratory will be carried out. Urinalysis will be done regularly, for example four times in 24 hours.

Other parameters to be monitored carefully include electrolyte balance, cardiac function (ECG recordings), conscious level, temperature, pulse and blood pressure.

The patient should recommence oral intake of food and fluid as soon as his condition allows. Intravenous hydration may continue for a time following re-commencement of oral intake, but it is likely that by then insulin will be given by subcutaneous injection. The patient's previous insulin-dietary regimen will be re-established prior to his discharge home.

The diabetic patient admitted as a surgical emergency will present with many problems, both actual and potential. Stabilization of blood glucose levels has to be achieved prior to surgery. Thereafter the care will be as for elective surgery.

NIDDM patients controlled with OHAs will have their medication discontinued and replaced with un-modified insulin when undergoing major surgery. Care of the patient will be the same as for IDDM patients pre- and postoperatively. The usual regimen will, hopefully, be reintroduced prior to discharge. If the surgery is of a minor nature, it may be sufficient to monitor the patient's blood glucose frequently and observe him closely.

The diabetic patient with sight problems

The diabetic patient who is partially sighted or blind merits specific mention.

Community nursing services and the social work department will be very involved in their care, and if the patient lives alone and is elderly, it may be necessary for insulin to be given by community nursing staff. Syringes are available which deliver metered doses of insulin and give auditory signals. There are also urine-testing devices which give auditory signals relative to the level of glycosuria. If the patient is controlled with OHAs this should be less problematical in administration than insulin, but regular monitoring of the patient's ability to be independent with medication is required none the less.

Social work departments will arrange help in the home for the blind diabetic patient living alone, and such helpers become indispensable to the patient. They can be taught to help the patient with administration of medication, and how to deal with emergencies.

Paediatric patients

Children, because of their growth requirements, and their understandable difficulty in coming to terms with their altered health status, require singular care and monitoring. As the care of children is a specialized area, the reader should refer to a paediatric nursing textbook which will identify the particular difficulties associated with the care of the diabetic child.

Complications of diabetes mellitus

Diabetes is for life, and the diabetic patient should be seen at regular intervals by staff who are specialized in their care. Regular assessment of the patient's condition and appropriate action will help to keep the patient's disease well controlled, this is the cornerstone of care and minimizes complications.

Complications can be considered as acute or long term. The former include hypoglycaemia and keto-acidosis, while the latter include diabetic retinopathy, nephropathy, cardiopathy, neuropathy, and circulatory problems, particularly those affecting the feet (diabetic foot).

The nurse caring for diabetics either in a hospital ward or in the community should have a knowledge of these complications.

Hypoglycaemia

Hypoglycaemia can occur in NIDDM as well as IDDM patients, particularly in those taking the OHA chlorpropamide. Hypoglycaemia can arise because of late or missed meals, or when the balance between insulin and dietary intake is disturbed; for example, unplanned or unaccustomed exercise, or too few carbohydrate exchanges.

The symptoms are:

- weakness
- hunger
- sweating
- diplopia and blurring of vision
- mental confusion
- abnormal behaviour leading to coma.

In children, there could be:

- lassitude or irritability
- somnolence
- neuromuscular signs
- vomiting.

Diabetic patients are introduced to the experience of hypoglycaemia prior to discharge from hospital or in the diabetic clinic. It can be induced by withholding, under strict supervision, a lunchtime meal until the patient recognizes the early symptoms. No patient education is complete without this exercise.

Nursing staff on night duty should be aware of the symptoms of hypoglycaemia and be vigilant in their observation of diabetic patients. Sweating is a common early symptom and it is justifiable to disturb the patient to assess the situation. The nurse should always be aware of the need for immediate action, and glucose drinks should be readily available.

Diabetic patients are advised to carry dextrose tablets at all times. While delayed meals should be avoided, unplanned situations can happen. Dextrose is a simple glucose, and as such requires no further digestion, therefore it is easily absorbed through the gastric mucosa, but it should not be regarded as a substitute for a meal.

If the patient becomes stuporose, then he should be given an intramuscular injection of glucagon followed by a glucose drink on arousal. The nursing staff should instruct the patient's relatives in this procedure.

Diabetic ketoacidosis (DKA)

Diabetic ketoacidosis is a medical emergency.

In established diabetes, it can arise as a result of misuse of insulin, dietary abuse, or illness when the need for energy is increased and metabolic processes are intensified. The physical stress of illness stimulates the secretion of glucocorticoids and adrenalin, glycogen is mobilized as glucose thus raising blood glucose levels. Fat is also broken down for energy resulting in ketosis.

In the undiagnosed diabetic, lack of treatment in the early stages of development of the disease leads to ketoacidosis, but the majority of these emergencies occur in patients with established diabetes.

Depending on the severity of the patient's condition on admission, his neurological state may vary from drowsiness to a state of unconsciousness and shock.

The aims of immediate treatment are:

- to replace lost fluid
- to control hypoglycaemia and ketoacidosis
- to correct electrolyte imbalance
- to search for and treat the cause, e.g. infection, as control will not be achieved while the cause remains.

All of these aims are undertaken simultaneously.

Care and attention must be given to anxious relatives/friends who are likely to be distressed. This will be difficult in the urgency of the situation, but efforts should be made to communicate with them and to establish trust.

Intravenous hydration will be commenced for the patient immediately on arrival in the emergency department. He is likely to be severely dehydrated.

The critically ill patient is likely to have his haemodynamic status assessed by monitoring of central venous pressure.

Rehydration commences with isotonic (0.9%) saline solution as extracellular fluid is lost before intracellular fluid. A large amount of replacement fluid may be required. In cases of severe dehydration as much as 3 litres in 3 hours may have to be given. Constant monitoring of the haemodynamic state is essential. This includes central venous pressure measurements, cardiac function, blood pressure and pulse measurements. Accurate measurement of urine output is essential and catheterization will usually be prescribed.

The nurse should recognize responses to rehydration in improved blood pressure readings, pulse rate, respiratory rate and warming of the extremities. Mucous membranes become moist, and urine output increases with increased kidney perfusion and glomerular filtration.

Unmodified insulin is administered initially as a bolus dose of 10–20 units intravenously or intramuscularly, followed by 4–6 units per hour via a constant rate intravenous pump. When the blood glucose level returns to 10 mmol/l then insulin dosage will be reduced. Intravenous glucose will be given to prevent hypoglycaemia. The intravenous fluid regimen will include glucose/saline, glucose, and isotonic saline solutions. Blood glucose and serum electrolyte levels will be monitored by biochemcal assessment. Additionally, blood glucose estimation by capillary blood testing and urinalysis to assess ketone levels will be carried out at ward level.

Neurological observations will be made and recorded.

If ketoacidosis is the result of infection, antibiotic therapy will be given. It is difficult to control ketoacidosis while the causative factor remains untreated.

As the patient improves, the aim will be to establish or re-establish the insulin/dietary regimen. Oral food and fluids will be introduced as soon as possible.

Monitoring of blood glucose levels will continue on a regular basis but with less frequency, and the patient will be encouraged to participate in his/her own care.

Discharge from the ward and referral to the out-patient department will be a priority arrangement.

Response to treatment of ketoacidosis is usually rapid, and the essential factor following recovery from the acute episode is holistic assessment of the patient and re-education where appropriate.

Diabetic retinopathy

This complication arises from microangiopathic changes. Retinopathy can now be treated effectively at an early stage using retinal photocoagulation. Care of the patient undergoing this treatment is discussed in Chapter 6.

Regular attendance at clinics is to be emphasized. Ophthalmoscopy will be a regular investigation enabling early detection of the condition.

Diabetic nephropathy

An early indicator of nephropathy is microalbumin-uria. This can be detected by regular urinalysis. Blood pressure monitoring and control is essential.

Diabetic cardiopathy

Atheroma is common is diabetes and this can lead to cardio- and peripheral-vascular complications. Dietary advice will be aimed at the prevention of such complications.

Diabetic neuropathy

This common complication occurs early in the diabetic patient. The majority of patients with this complication are symptomless.

Neuropathy causes loss of sensation peripherally, and great care is required in caring for the patients and when advising them. Reference has already been made to finger sites for capillary blood testing, and patients should be advised to protect limb extremities. No direct heat should be applied, and extreme care taken of the feet as damage may be ignored because of impaired sensation.

Any cuts should be treated with care as healing is slow in diabetic tissues. The presence of glucose in the tissues acts as an excellent medium for bacterial growth.

Any damage to the foot must receive instant medical attention as neglect may ultimately lead to gangrene of the extremity.

Circulatory problems affecting the feet (diabetic foot)

The reader is referred to Box 16.5 listing instructions on care of the feet.

It should be noted that the presence of warmth and pulsation in a diabetic patient's feet is not neces-sarily an indication that all is well, and should be considered together with other parameters.

Further advice for patients

Vehicle driving Diabetics need not stop driving but they must notify the Driving Vehicle Licensing Authority at Swansea of their condition. Patients who are prone to hypoglycaemic reactions should take especial care with timing of their meals and insulin dosage. Long journeys should be planned with frequent stops and an adequate food and fluid supply should be carried.

Irregular working hours This is very relevant to nursing staff. It is always advisable to contact the diabetic care staff for advice regarding change of routine affecting working hours and uncertain mealtimes. Insulin timing will be changed and extra monitoring required to assess the blood glucose level, but unless there is evidence of previous instability irregular working hours are not contraindicated.

Stress It is right that diabetic patients should be advised to avoid stressful situations but this is not practical in real terms. Stress is present in everyday activities and cannot be avoided. It can be pointed out to the patient that stress raises blood glucose level, and where possible the patient should be helped to deal with stressful situations.

The diabetic on holiday The ability to meet dietary needs while on holiday, particularly abroad, should be considered before setting out (Piper & Lewin 1990). Sufficient insulin and syringes should be taken and appropriate storage conditions for insulin observed.

It may be necessary for the patient to take medical certification, particularly when carrying syringes through customs. It is essential that a card is carried, stating that the person is diabetic. An example of such a card is illustrated in Figure 16.11.

British Diabetic Association This Association is of great benefit to patients and families. The Association advises members over a wide range of problems, and their monthly magazine provides good information on recent research findings. Patients will find the magazine recipes very welcome.

While diabetes cannot be cured, good control of the disease will delay the onset of complications. Research into approaches to treatment is producing some encouraging findings.

Box 16.5   Guidelines for care of the feet in patients with diabetes

Although most people with diabetes are not likely to have serious problems with their feet, foot care is extremely important to the diabetic and you should follow the advice given below

FOOTWEAR
1. Wear well-fitting shoes with soft uppers. Lace-up shoes are recommended because they hold your heel firmly in place and prevent your foot from sliding forward. They also leave plenty of room for your toes. If you must wear unlaced shoes, do so only for short periods. New shoes should at first be worn for a short period only each day.
2. It is important that your shoe fitting is correct, so never buy shoes that the fitter does not recommend and always ask for your feet to be measured when you buy new shoes.
3. Although it is hard in these days of stretch garments to find socks and stockings long enough for your feet, try to wear those which will not cramp your toes.
4. Avoid wearing garters as these will interfere with your circulation.
5. Do not walk about barefoot.

HEAT AND COLD
Awareness of heat and cold may also be diminished and circulation may be less efficient than in an non-diabetic. Because of this, strict attention should be paid to the following points:

1. Avoid overheated baths. The water should not be heated to more than 43 degrees Centigrade or 110 degrees Fahrenheit.
2. Do not sit too close to fires or heaters.
3. Before you get into bed, remove bed heaters, such as hot water bottles, and switch off electric blankets.
4. Woollen bedsocks should not be worn unless they are loose fitting.
5. Wet feet should be dried before putting on dry socks, stockings, tights or shoes.
6. Do not use hot poultices.

CORNS AND CALLOUSES
1. Do not cut them yourself or allow friends to do it for you.
2. Corn paints and corn plasters contain acids, which can be very dangerous – so do not use them.
3. If you develop any corns, callouses, ingrowing toenails or any other foot troubles, make an appointment at the Diabetic Foot Clinic.

HYGIENE
Wash your feet daily in tepid water, using a good mild toilet soap. Rinse the skin well after washing and dry carefully especially between the toes.

If your toes overlap, separate them with a wisp of cotton wool or piece of gauze. Change to clean socks or stockings daily.
If your skin is dry, after bathing your feet, apply a little cream such as E45 cream.
If your skin is moist, use a swab of cotton wool to wipe your feet (especially between the toes) with surgical spirit. When the spirit is dry, dust your feet with a fine talcum powder such as baby powder. Do not use talcum powder between toes as this can result in irritation.

Awareness of pain may be diminished or absent and minor injuries to the foot can take place without your knowledge. It is thus important that careful examination of your feet should be made after washing. If you are unable to see well or get down to your feet easily, then you should ensure that someone else examines your feet.

NAIL CUTTING
Cut your toe nails after a bath when the nails are soft. They should be cut straight across and not too short. Consult the Diabetic Foot Clinic if your nails are painful or difficult to cut. It is unwise to use a sharp instrument to clean the free edge of the nail or the nail grooves.

FIRST AID MEASURES
1. Any minor cuts should be covered with sterile gauze, or apply a modern antiseptic such as Savlon in conjunction with a loosely applied gauze dressing. Do not bandage or apply constricting adhesive dressings to toes.
2. Do not apply adhesive strapping directly to the foot, without first covering the wound with a gauze dressing.
3. Do not prick blisters but leave them to dry up on their own or cover them with a dressing. If they burst and discharge their fluid, apply an antiseptic dressing.
4. Never use strong medicines like Iodine.
5. If minor injuries do not respond to your own treatment, attend your own GP or phone the Diabetic Foot Clinic for advice.

SIGNS OF UNHEALTHY FEET
As even mild infections can upset your diabetes, consult your doctor or the Clinic immediately if:

1. You notice a colour change in any part of the foot or leg.
2. You notice a discharge coming from a break in the skin, from a corn or under a toenail.
3. There is any troublesome pain, throbbing, swelling or itching.

(Reproduced with kind permission from the Dept of Diabetes, Royal Infirmary of Edinburgh NHS Trust.)

THYMUS GLAND

The thymus gland is situated in the mediastinum behind the sternum. It is large in infancy. Growth ceases at puberty and by old age the gland has been replaced with fibrous tissue. It is composed of epithelial cells called thymocytes which secrete the hormones thymosin and thymopoietin. These hormones play an important role in the develop-

I am a diabetic

If I am found ill or fainting please

read the instructions overleaf . . . .

I am a diabetic

If I am found ill or fainting please give me two tablespoonfuls of sugar in water. If this does not revive me please call a doctor or an ambulance immediately.

Name

Address

Telephone No.

Name of Doctor or Hospital

Address

Telephone No.

My usual dose of insulin is   units of

(type of insulin)

brand

given at

(time(s) of day)

Fig. 16.11 An example of a diabetic card

ment of the immune system by promoting maturation of lymphocytes. Because of this function, the thymus gland is considered as part of the lymphatic system, but it is its role in hormone production and secretion which classifies it as an endocrine organ.

Disorders of the thymus gland

Disorders in children result in reduced resistance to infection.

Myasthenia gravis is a rare neuromuscular condition which affects mainly young adults. It is characterized by muscle weakness and fatigue. Ptosis of the eyelids and diplopia are also factors.

The cause of the condition is not known but genetic and autoimmune factors are thought to be implicated. Abnormalities of the thymus gland resulting in increased antibody formation are associated with the condition.

Thymectomy may be considered as the treatment of choice.

THE PINEAL GLAND (PINEAL BODY)

This small gland is located within the diencephalon, suspended from the roof of the third ventricle. The gland is composed of neuroglial and secretory cells which are called pinealocytes. The gland secretes the hormone melatonin, and although it alters in structure after puberty, it continues to secrete.

The pineal gland responds to a diurnal cycle with highest levels of melatonin in the blood during the night, in contrast to adrenal secretions which have their lowest levels during the night.

Melatonin is thought to have an antigonadotrophic effect which appears to control the onset of puberty and inhibit precocious sexual development. This belief is based on findings that children who have secreting pineal tumours have delayed puberty, while those who have destructive lesions show precocious puberty.

Pineal function is thought to be associated with 'jet-lag', the disturbance to the diurnal cycle caused by travelling through time zones.

IMPLICATIONS FOR NURSING PATIENTS WITH ENDOCRINE DISORDERS

Endocrine disorders are invariably long-term conditions. Some disorders are treated medically by the administration of hormones for therapeutic purposes where the treatment will be limited, or for replacement purposes where treatment is life long. Some disorders are treated by surgery which may effect a cure or may result in the alleviation of symptoms with the need for replacement therapy.

The patient requiring long-term or life-long therapy requires much support, and continuity of care is of prime consideration. Establishment of rapport between patient and carers is an early requirement so that trust and mutual confidence can develop. Only in such an environment will a patient feel able and comfortable to discuss his problems.

The majority of patients with endocrine disorders are treated on an outpatient basis and require admission to hospital only during spells of acute illness or planned medical/surgical intervention. Where education and other communication systems are effective, then emergencies should be infrequent.

Family involvement or involvement of significant others is highly desirable so that those around the patient can be helped to understand the situation and can, in turn, help him to pursue as satisfying a life-style as is possible.

Encouragement to attend outpatient clinics as instructed may be needed and also support to maintain morale in cases of long-term conditions. The patient should be assured that he has access to the clinic staff at any time should advice be required.

ADVICE TO THE PATIENT RECEIVING LONG-TERM MEDICATION

The effect of long-term medication can be disheartening to many patients and this fact should be uppermost in the nurse's mind. Patients may need encouragement to continue with medication and an assurance of its efficacy, in particular once the initial treatment has removed symptoms and they feel well. The importance of timing of medications and self-managed tests should be stressed and a warning given that on no account should the medication be stopped. Effects and side-effects of medication should be discussed.

A simple explanation of the negative feedback mechanism can be given so that the patient can understand the reason for instructions.

Patients receiving hormone therapy should carry a card stating the medication, dose, time/s of administration, and a telephone number to contact. Such a card is of great value in an emergency and could prove to be life-saving.

Management of care

Care of the patient can be guided using the nursing process where assessment will identify the patient's problems, and planning of care can be achieved using an appropriate nursing model. As most patients will be treated on an outpatient basis, then a model incorporating patient participation should be employed. An example is Orem's model.

Planning of care should involve the patient and his/her wishes should be considered. Frequent supervision in the early stages of the patient's care should be observed, but as treatment progresses the aim of staff and patient should be the establishment of patient independence through mutual trust.

Suggested assignments

1. Patients having long-term hormonal replacement therapy may, from time to time, experience problems.

Explain how in the case of (a) thyroid hormone replacement and (b) cortisone replacement these problems can be detected early.
How should patients be helped to recognize the early symptoms?
2. A diabetic must be knowledgeable about his condition if he is to lead a normal and active life. Investigate the education of diabetics in your hospital, in particular:
   a. which personnel are involved?
   b. what is taught to diabetics?
   c. how are allowances made for patients of differing abilities to understand what is being taught?
3. What associations for diabetics are available in your locality? As an exercise, find out how such an organization endeavours to meet the special needs of diabetics.
4. Thyroid disease is manifested by symptoms which may be confused with other conditions.

Discuss the differential diagnosis, the role of the nurse in determining the correct diagnosis, and the implications for other patients and family/carers during the early stages of treatment.

REFERENCES AND FURTHER READING

Bloom S R, Polak J M 1987 Somatostatin Regular Review 295(1): 288–289
Burton S 1989 Corticosterone therapy. Nursing 3(41): 17–19
Chilman A, Thomas M (eds) 1988 Understanding nursing care, 3rd edn. Churchill Livingstone, Edinburgh
Cradock S 1989 Blood glucose monitoring – why test? Diabetic Nursing 1(2): 5–6
Davis R 1991 Diabetes education – the professional issues. Diabetic Nursing 2(3): 11–12
Edwards C R W, Bouchier I A D (eds) 1991 Davidson's Principles and Practice of Medicine, 16th edn. Churchill Livingstone, London
Harkness Hood G, Dincher J R 1992 Total patient care – foundations and practice of adult health nursing, 8th edn. Mosby-Year-Book, St Louis
Hinchliff S, Montague S (eds) 1988 Physiology for nursing practice, 1st edn. Baillière Tindall, London
Marieb E M 1992 Human anatomy and physiology, 2nd edn. Benjamin-Cummings, California
McKenna & Callander 1990 Illustrated physiology, 5th edn. Churchill Livingstone, Edinburgh
Milne C 1989 The endocrine system – the pituitary gland. Nursing Standard 2(50): 16–17

Milne C 1988 The endocrine system – the pancreas. Nursing Standard 2(51): 26–27
Piper L D, Lewin I 1990 Basic diabetes care in general practice 2 – meeting the educational needs of the diabetic patient. Diabetic Nursing 1(3): 7–9
Richmond J 1991 Injections – diabetes. Diabetic Nursing 2(July): 6–7
Wilson K J W 1990 Ross & Wilson anatomy and physiology, 7th edn. Churchill Livingstone, Edinburgh
Royle J, Walsh M (eds) 1992 Watson's medical-surgical nursing and related physiology, 4th edn. Baillière Tindall, London
Sykes J 1991 Insulin injections – injections diabetes. Diabetic Nursing 2(1): 3–4
Tortora G J, Grabowski S R 1993 Principles of anatomy and physiology, 7th edn. Harper Collins, New York
Weetman A P 1991 Investigations and management of pituitary tumours. Update 42(11): 1039–1048
Weetman A P 1991 Management of adrenal disease. Update 43(1): 17–25
Wheeler M H 1988 Investigation of the thyroid. Surgery (62): 1477–1479

17

Care implications of disorders of the genitourinary and reproductive systems

Shirley Gregor

STRUCTURE AND FUNCTIONS OF THE URINARY SYSTEM

The urinary system is made up of two kidneys, two ureters, one urinary bladder and a urethra (Fig. 17.1). The primary function of the system is to help keep the homeostatic balance of the body by controlling the composition and volume of body fluids. In health the kidneys carry out this function by the formation of urine.

The two kidneys lie retroperitoneally on the posterior abdominal wall. They are located at the levels of the last thoracic and third lumbar vertebrae. The right kidney is situated slightly lower than the left due to the space taken up by the liver.

Each kidney is composed of approximately one million nephrons (Fig. 17.2) which are responsible for the formation of urine by the processes of filtration and selective reabsorption. Once urine is formed it drains from the pelvis of the kidneys into the ureters and is carried by peristalsis to the bladder. Each ureter extends 25–30 cm from the pelvis of the kidney to the bladder.

The urinary bladder is a hollow muscular organ in the pelvic cavity and acts as a resevoir for urine. In the male it lies anteriorly to the rectum. In the female it is anterior to the vagina and inferior to the uterus (Tortora 1989).

The urethra is a small tube which extends from the floor of the bladder to the exterior of the body.

INFECTIVE DISORDERS OF THE URINARY TRACT

URINARY TRACT INFECTION
Epidemiology and aetiology

Urinary tract infections may affect any part of the

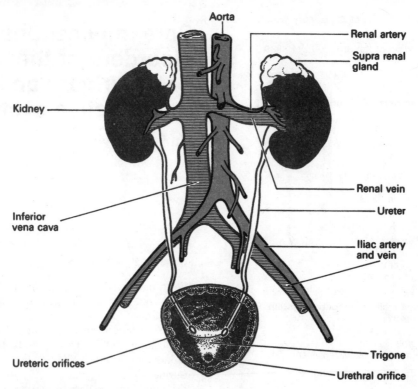

Fig. 17.1 Kidneys, ureters and bladder: relationships

urinary tract. They are most commonly due to organisms gaining access via the urethra and ascending the urinary tract. The most common causative organism is *Escherichia coli*, but gram-negative organisms such as proteus and pseudomonas occur particularly after instrumentation or in the presence of obstruction. Predisposing factors include any structrual abnormality (e.g. urinary tract obstruction, neurogenic bladder or vesico-ureteric reflux), foreign bodies (e.g. calculi or catheters) or invasive procedures such as cystoscopy or catheterization. Infection is also common during pregnancy due to stasis of urine, caused by the relaxing effects of progesterone on the ureters.

Acute pyelonephritis

Pyelonephritis is an inflammation of the renal parenchyma most commonly due to bacterial infection.

Clinical features

The patient complains of loin pain and tenderness. This is usually accompanied by symptoms of systemic infection such as pyrexia, rigors, nausea and general malaise. There may or may not be urinary symptoms

such as frequency of micturition and urgency. The urine may appear cloudy and have an unpleasant smell.

Investigations

A midstream specimen of urine should be obtained to identify the causative organism and for antibiotic sensitivity testing.

Therapeutic management

An appropriate antibiotic will be prescribed according to the organisms found on culture. Analgesia may be prescribed to relieve loin pain and the patient's fluid intake should be increased to more than 3 litres in 24 hours.

Nursing strategies

All urine should be observed for abnormalities, such as cloudy appearance, offensive smell or pus deposits. Assessment should be made for level and type of pain and when the pain occurs.

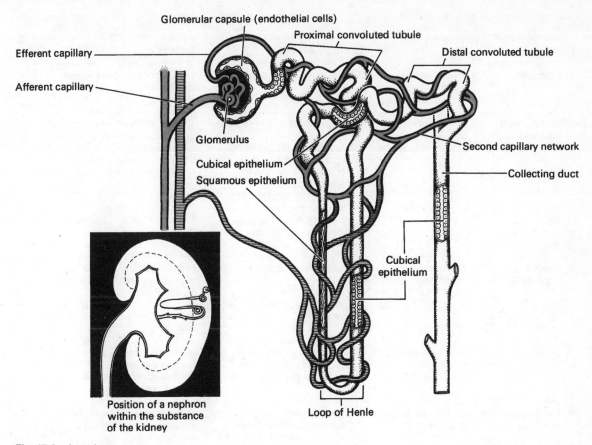

Glomerular capsule (endothelial cells)

Proximal convoluted tubule

Efferent capillary

Distal convoluted tubule

Afferent capillary

Glomerulus

Second capillary network

Cubical epithelium

Squamous epithelium

Collecting duct

Cubical epithelium

Position of a nephron within the substance of the kidney

Loop of Henle

Fig. 17.2 A nephron

The nurse should ensure that the patient takes the antibiotics as prescribed. A high fluid intake is essential to increase renal blood flow and dilute the number of bacteria. Analgesics and antipyretics are given as prescribed when required. All care as required during a febrile illness should be given. (See Nursing Care Plan 17.1 for a patient with acute pyelonephritis.)

Chronic pyelonephritis

In chronic pyelonephritis there is gross scarring of the kidneys which may be much reduced in size. This is usually due to recurrent infection caused by obstruction in the urinary tract or vesicoureteric reflux.

Clinical features

The patient may present with recurrent urinary tract infections, the early symptoms of chronic renal failure (see p. 598) or with persistent loin pain.

Therapeutic management

Appropriate antibiotics are either repeated or given long term. Any obstruction in the urinary tract is relieved and chronic renal failure treated appropriately.

Cystitis

Cystitis is an inflammation of the bladder mucosa. It is more common in women because of a female's anatomical vulnerability to bacterial invasion and is usually an ascending infection, with *E. coli* being the most common causative organism.

Clinical features

The patient complains of passing only small amounts of urine frequently. This is accompanied by burning on micturition. There may also be suprapubic pain or bladder spasm. The urine usually smells offensive.

Nursing Care Plan 17.1   Care plan for a patient with pyelonephritis

Problem	Goal	Nursing intervention	Rationale
1. Loin pain	To alleviate pain due to inflammation of renal tissue	❐ Give analgesia as prescribed	Ensures patient comfort and co-operation
2. Urinary tract infection	To treat infection effectively and prevent recurrence	❐ Give antibiotics as prescribed ❐ Encourage a fluid intake of more than 3 litres per day ❐ Record accurate fluid intake/output ❐ Test urine for protein, blood and specific gravity ❐ Obtain midstream specimens of urine every 3 days for culture and sensitivity	To treat infection with appropriate antibiotic as soon as possible Increases urinary output to flush debris from urinary tract Allows assessment of fluid balance Monitors kidney function Monitors effects of treatment
3. Frequency/urgency	To achieve normal pattern of voiding	❐ Give antispasmodic as prescribed ❐ Ensure easy access to toilet or commode	Helps to reduce bladder spasm if infection involves bladder as well as upper tract Reduce anxiety about incontinence from not being able to get to toilet in time
4. Dysuria	To relieve voiding discomfort	❐ Give alkalis as prescribed, e.g. mixture of potassium citrate ❐ Encourage high fluid intake	Neutralizes acidity and reduces burning sensation Increases urinary output and dilutes urine
5. Nausea and vomiting	To alleviate nausea and vomiting	❐ Give antiemetics as prescribed ❐ Offer frequent mouthwashes ❐ Encourage sips of iced water	Relieves patient discomfort Relieves unpleasant taste Helps to relieve nausea and also cool febrile patient
6. Fever and general malaise	To reduce fever and minimize discomfort	❐ Give antipyretic as prescribed ❐ Record temperature regularly ❐ Encourage bed rest while febrile ❐ Give regular changes of bedlinen and night clothing ❐ Use electric fan as necessary ❐ Give cool fluids hourly	Assists in reduction of body temperature Monitors effect of treatment Rest promotes tissue repair Encourages loss of heat and provides comfort Encourages loss of heat Replaces fluid loss by sweating and assists in reduction of body temperature
7. Anxiety		❐ Explain present illness and reasons for treatment ❐ Give ongoing information as to effect of treatment ❐ Allow patient to talk about anxieties	Assists patient's understanding of illness and promotes co-operation in treatment Reassures patient and enables planning for discharge Assists nurse to identify causes of anxiety so that appropriate help can be given

Investigations

Urine culture is necessary to isolate the causative organism and for antibiotic sensitivity testing.

Therapeutic management

The appropriate antibiotic will be prescribed according to culture and sensitivity testing. Analgesics and antispasmodics may be required. Alkalis can be helpful in alleviating burning on micturition. Fluid intake should be increased to at least 3 litres in 24 hours.

Nursing strategies

Women who have recurrent cystitis should be advised about the measures they can take to prevent cystitis or to alleviate symptoms if it does occur:

1. Perineal hygiene to prevent bacterial contamination:
   a. shower instead of immersion bath
   b. careful washing from front to back after defaecation
   c. avoid external irritants such as bubble bath, vaginal deodorants, creams and talcum powders
   d. cotton underwear should be worn.
2. Avoid irritants such as coffee, tea and alcohol.
3. Frequent voiding and a high urine flow rate will lower the concentration of bacteria in urine. The bladder should be emptied at least every 3 hours and at least 3 litres of fluid should be taken daily.
4. Sexually active women, who are prone to cystitis, and their partners should be encouraged to wash before intercourse. The women should void before and after intercourse. Use of a lubricant, such as KY Jelly, will help to lessen the risk of urethral trauma.
5. If cystitis does occur, symptoms can be alleviated by drinking bland liquids every 20 minutes. This will dilute the urine and help to flush out infection. Alkalis, e.g. sodium bicarbonate, can be taken to reduce the acidity of urine and reduce burning. Mild analgesics can be taken if necessary (Kilmartin 1979).

RENAL CALCULI

Stones may develop anywhere in the urinary tract and are formed from deposits of crystalline substances found in urine. They can vary in size from small particles like sand to round bladder stones the size of an orange (Fig. 17.3) and large irregular shaped staghorn calculi that fill the pelvis of a kidney (Fig. 17.4).

Aetiology

Since the constituents of calculi are found in normal urine, any condition which increases urinary concentration or causes urinary stasis predisposes to calculus formation. Other conditions favourable to stone formation are hyperparathyriodism, gout and urinary tract infection.

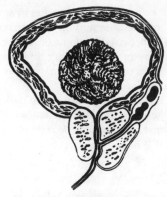

Fig. 17.3 Large bladder calculus showing rough spiky surface

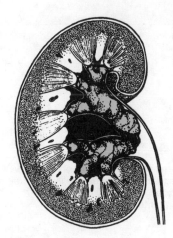

Fig. 17.4 Staghorn calculus

Clinical features

Symptoms of renal and ureteric calculi depend on the site of the stone, the degree of obstruction, extent of mucosal irritation and whether or not infection is present. Therefore the presenting features could be any of the following:

Loin pain: a constant dull ache in the renal area is due to irritation of the tissues by movement of the stone or back-pressure and fluid accumulation from a degree of obstruction.

Haematuria: results from injury to the membranous lining of the pelvis of the kidney or ureter.

Urinary tract infection: infection is often associated with stones and if present may cause fever and dysuria.

RENAL COLIC

If a small stone blocks the pelvi-ureteric junction or

ureter, renal colic results. This is due to severe spasm of smooth muscle attempting to overcome the obstruction. The patient complains of sudden agonizing pain starting in the loin shooting down to the groin. This is usually accompanied by nausea, vomiting and signs of shock and collapse.

This is a medical emergency as the patient requires strong analgesia. A high fluid intake is necessary and an intravenous infusion may be required, particularly if the patient is nauseated.

Investigations

Once the pain has been controlled an intravenous urogram is performed to locate the site of the stone. Urine is collected every 24 hours for elevated levels of constituents which predispose to stone formation. A midstream specimen of urine is sent for culture to detect the presence of infection.

Nursing strategies

Nursing Care Plan 17.2 outlines a care plan for a patient with renal colic.

Therapeutic management

This is dictated by the size, shape and composition

Nursing Care Plan 17.2 Care plan for management of a patient with renal colic			
Problem	**Goal**	**Nursing intervention**	**Rationale**
1. Pain	To relieve pain	❏ Give analgesia as prescribed	The pain of renal colic is very severe and normally narcotic analgesia will be required
		❏ Give antispasmodic as prescribed	Antispasmodics will reduce the severity of ureteric spasm which intensifies the pain
		❏ Monitor effectiveness of analgesia	Allows evaluation of effectiveness of dosage and type of analgesia given
2. Potential for passage of abnormal constituents	To monitor abnormalities in urinary output	❏ Sieve *all* urine and send any fragments for analysis	Very small pieces of stone may be passed without the patient's knowledge; chemical analysis of stone will assist in future prevention
		❏ Encourage a high fluid intake of more than 3 litres per 24 hours	A good diuresis may assist in moving stone through ureter
		❏ Measure and record accurate intake and output	To monitor that intake is greater than 3 litres per day and that diuresis is adequate
		❏ Obtain urine specimens – for urinalysis – for culture and sensitivity	Patients with stones frequently have infected urine
		❏ Obtain continuous 24 hour urine collections	Determines total excretion of substances over a 24 hour period
3. Potential for nausea and vomiting	To alleviate nausea and vomiting	❏ Give antiemetics as required as prescribed	To minimize nausea or vomiting
		❏ Intravenous fluids may be necessary	To ensure a high fluid intake
		❏ Offer frequent mouth care	To minimize unpleasant taste after vomiting
4. Potential for anxiety	Reduce levels of anxiety	❏ Explain necessity of all tests and X-rays	Assists patient's understanding and therefore promotes co-operation
		❏ Allow patient to discuss anxieties	Assists nurse so that appropriate help can be given
5. Knowledge deficit	To ensure understanding of disorder and follow-up care	❏ Explain to patient necessity of follow-up care	To reduce the possibility of future recurrence
		❏ Specific treatment for prevention of further stones should be explained	
		❏ Ensure patient understands necessity for continuing to take a high fluid intake	

of the stones. A high fluid intake is encouraged to prevent urinary stasis and concentration. Frequent specimens of urine should be sent for culture and sensitivity to eliminate infection. X-rays are taken to check the location of stone(s). If the composition of the stones is known, appropriate drug and diet regimens can be given; for example, for calcium stones dairy products are restricted, or for uric acid stones allopurinol is prescribed.

Interventional methods of stone management

Stone destruction

1. *Percutaneous lithotripsy.* Under X-ray screening a tract is established through the renal parenchyma. A nephroscope is used to visualize the stones, then an ultrasonic probe is used to shatter large stones and the debris is removed by continuous suction.

2. *Extracorporeal shock-wave lithotripsy.* This is a non-invasive form of treatment. The lithotripter uses low frequency sound waves transmitted through water to disintegrate kidney stones (Fig. 17.5).

Endoscopic procedures

1. *Percutaneous nephrolithotomy.* Under X-ray screening a tract is made through the renal parenchyma and a catheter placed in the renal pelvis. After 24 hours the tract can be dilated and a nephroscope used to visualize the stones. Small stones and fragments can be retrieved by forceps or stone basket (Fig. 17.6).

2. *Dormia basket.* Stones in the lower third of the ureter can be removed with the use of a dormia basket. A cystoscope is used to visualize the ureteric orifice and the catheter is inserted past the stone. The basket is then opened and the stone lifted out (Fig. 17.7).

3. *Litholapaxy.* A lithotrite is passed urethrally into the bladder and crushes the stone. The fragments can then be washed out (Fig. 17.8).

Surgical procedures

For the various surgical procedures see Figures 17.9–17.11.

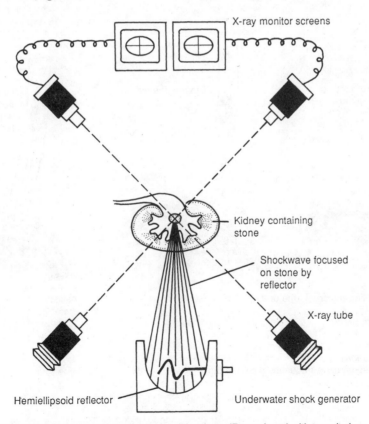

Fig. 17.5 Extracorporeal shockwave lithotripsy. (Reproduced with permission from Bullock et al 1989, Fig. 10.8)

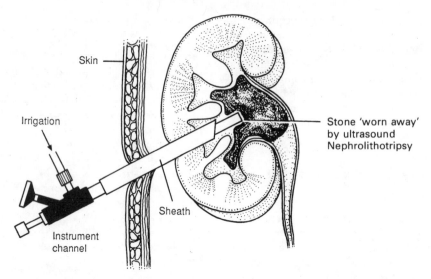

Fig. 17.6 Percutaneous stone removal. (Reproduced with permission from Bullock et al 1989, Fig. 10.7)

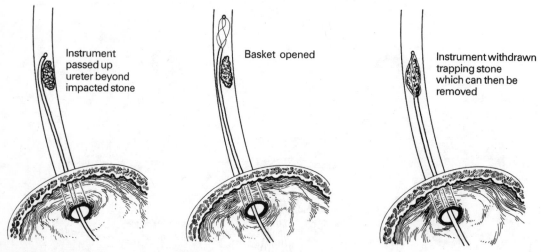

Fig. 17.7 Basketing a stone in the ureter
Disorder
Stone impacted in ureter
Operation
Removal of stone using a 'wire' basket
Possible complications
Haematuria – observe urine frequently for 48 hours

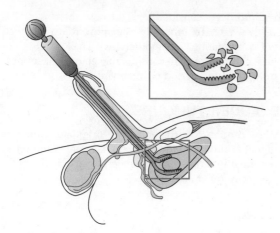

Fig. 17.8 Litholapaxy.

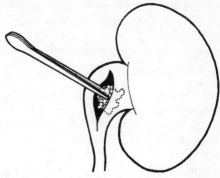

Fig. 17.10
Disorder
Large stone lodged in renal pelvis
Operation
Pyelolithotomy
Description
The stone is removed via an incision in the renal pelvis
Complications
Haemorrhage, urinary leakage, ureteric obstruction, UTI, renal failure, urinary fistula

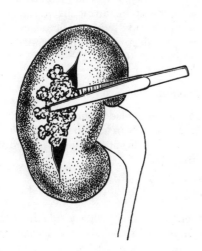

Fig. 17.9
Disorder
Staghorn calculus in calyces of the kidney
Operation
Nephrolithotomy
Description
Calculus is removed from the body of the kidney
Special complications
Haemorrhage (especially secondary), infection, urinary leakage, renal fistula, renal failure – anuria, UTI

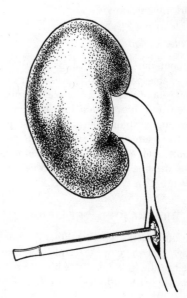

Fig. 17.11
Disorder
Stone impacted in ureter
Operation
Ureterolithotomy
Description
Removal of stone via incision in the ureter
Special complications
Haemorrhage, leakage of urine, stricture of ureter

NEOPLASTIC DISORDERS OF THE URINARY TRACT

KIDNEY TUMOURS

Renal cell carcinoma is the most common malignant renal tumour and occurs most frequently in men between the ages of 50 and 60 years. It metastasizes to the lungs, bone, liver and brain.

Clinical features

The most common symptom of renal carcinoma is painless haematuria. Other presenting features include backache, loin swelling, weight loss and low grade fever.

Investigations

The tumour may be palpable and will be well defined by radiological and ultrasonic investigations.

Therapeutic management

Renal cell carcinoma is treated by nephrectomy with or without ureterectomy.

Nursing intervention

Good patient–nurse relationships should be established to enable patients to express fears and anxieties. The patient's level of understanding should be assessed and appropriate information should be given. Adequate explanations about treatment should be given to ensure understanding and co-operation. Appropriate and adequate pain relief must be ensured. For nursing care following renal surgery see Nursing Care Plan 17.5.

Wilms' tumour (nephroblastoma)

This rare but usually very malignant tumour is one of the few that develops in children. Usually it is discovered in the first 3 years of life. It grows rapidly and gives rise to secondaries, especially in the lungs.

Clinical features

The child is noted to have a large abdomen and to be failing to thrive.

Therapeutic management

The prognosis for a child with a Wilm's tumour

has improved considerably and now there is a 90% survival rate. Treatment is by nephrectomy followed by combination chemotherapy. The parents of these children require considerable emotional support throughout the period of treatment.

BLADDER TUMOURS

Most cancers of the bladder originate from its epithelial lining. Bladder cancer is more common in men than in women and it generally affects the older age group (over sixties).

Aetiology

It appears that mutiple agents are responsible for the development of cancer of the bladder. The following are the most common associated factors:

- chemicals used in the manufacture of rubber, plastics, insecticides, cables and dyes
- cigarette smoking
- calculi
- chronic inflammation
- schistosomiasis.

The tumours develop in the epithelial lining of the bladder and often start as papillary growths. They may be benign to begin with and with treatment may remain so. Without treatment the tumours become malignant and invade by stages into the superficial muscle layer, the deep muscle and eventually into the surrounding tissues (Fig. 17.12).

Clinical features

The first evidence of bladder tumours is usually painless haematuria. Clot retention may develop. Some patients also have cystitis, frequency of micturition and dysuria.

Investigations

An intravenous urogram will exclude the presence of a renal tumour and show any ureteric obstruction.

Cystourethroscopy is used to visualize the tumour and to take biopsies. Computed tomography (CT scan) may be used for identification and staging of a bladder tumour. (For staging of bladder tumours see Table 17.1).

Therapeutic management

There is no single effective method of treatment. The

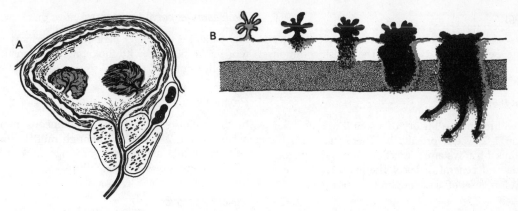

Fig. 17.12 Bladder tumours. (A) Pedunculated papillomata. (B) Stages of bladder tumours showing extension through the bladder wall and invasion of the neighbouring structures

---

Table 17.1 TNM staging of bladder tumours

Tis – Tumour in situ
T1 – Tumour invades subepithelial connective tissue
T2 – Tumour invades superficial muscle
T3 – Tumour invades deep muscle or perivesical fat
T4 – Tumour invades one or more of prostate,
     uterus, vagina, pelvic wall, abdominal wall.

---

treatment of choice depends on the characteristics of the tumour and whether or not bladder wall infiltration and local or distant metastases have occurred. Benign papillomas are treated by cystodiathermy. This generally has to be repeated at regular intervals as papillomas tend to recur. Non-invasive tumours can be treated with intravescical chemotherapy. Treatments for invasive tumours include transurethral resection, radiotherapy, systemic chemotherapy and cystectomy with urinary diversion.

INFLAMMATORY DISORDERS OF THE KIDNEYS

GLOMERULONEPHRITIS

Glomerulonephritis refers to a group of disorders associated with non-bacterial inflammation of the glomeruli of both kidneys. Inflammation is initiated by immune complex deposition or formation in the glomeruli. The best known antigen which can stimulate this reaction is the haemolytic streptococcus.

There are many different types of glomerulonephritis and they are are classified according to histological appearance. However, in **all** types the glomeruli are abnormal allowing leakage of protein. Proteinuria is therefore a constant feature of glomerulonephritis (Uldall 1988).

Altered physiology

Circulating antigen–antibody complexes become trapped in glomerular capillaries giving rise to:

- thickening of the glomerular filtration membrane
- inflammation and scarring
- increased glomerular capillary permeability
- leakage of red blood cells and proteins
- **haematuria** and **proteinuria**.

Clinical features

Glomerulonephritis presents either as **acute nephritic syndrome** or as **nephrotic syndrome** depending on the histological type.

In acute nephritic syndrome the patient complains of facial oedema and of passing small volumes of smoky-coloured urine containing small amounts of blood and protein (less than 3 g in 24 hours).

Nephrotic syndrome is typified by oedema, heavy proteinuria (more than 3 g in 24 hours) and hypoproteinaemia.

Acute proliferative glomerulonephritis

The incidence of acute glomerulonephritis has declined dramatically because of better nutrition, hygiene and use of antibiotics. Although the disease is commonest in childhood, it may occur throughout adult life.

Aetiology

The disease usually follows a throat infection after a latent period of 1–2 weeks. The most common causative organism is haemolytic streptococcus.

Clinical features

There will often be a history of a sore throat or other infection 1–2 weeks previously. There may also be symptoms of a systemic infection, such as pyrexia, anorexia and general malaise. The main features are the sudden onset of acute nephrotic syndrome.

Investigations

Urinalysis will reveal scanty amounts of cloudy urine which contain varying amounts of blood and protein.

A throat swab may confirm the presence of streptococcal infection.

Renal biopsy will confirm the diagnosis of glomerulonephritis and show the histological type.

Therapeutic management

Drug therapy   The original infection, if still present, will be treated with an appropriate antibiotic. Diuretics may be given to relieve oedema and antihypertensives may be required to control blood pressure.

Diet   This can be adjusted according to the patient's blood urea and electrolytes.

Fluid intake   It may be necessary to restrict fluid intake depending on the patient's urinary output.

Nursing strategies

The patient should be encouraged to rest in bed during the acute phase until the urine clears and blood urea and blood pressure return to within normal limits.

Adherence to a low protein, high carbohydrate diet is important in controlling uraemia and preventing tissue breakdown. Salt intake may also be restricted while oedematous or if there are any signs of congestive cardiac failure. Fluid intake is usually restricted to half a litre plus the equivalent of the volume of the previous day's urinary output. The nurse's role in the management of fluid intake and accurate fluid balance is therefore vital.

Daily weight will also help to assess the patients' fluid status. Any symptoms of renal failure should be recognized and treated promptly. Monitoring of temperature, pulse, respirations and blood pressure are important in the early recognition of complications.

Evaluation (expected outcomes)

The patient is no longer oedematous. Urinary output returns to normal with no abnormal constituents. Renal function and blood pressure are normal.

Prognosis

In the majority of patients spontaneous remission occurs within 2–3 weeks, although mild haematuria and proteinuria may persist for longer. About 5–10% of patients progress to renal failure.

Patient education

The nurse should explain to the patient the importance of follow-up urine and blood tests. He/she should also ensure that the patient can recognize the early signs of infection or renal failure and knows the importance of seeking medical help.

Minimal lesion glomerulonephritis and membranous glomerulonephritis

These two conditions are described together as initially they are clinically indistinguishable. Minimal lesion glomerulonephritis usually occurs in the 5–15-year-old age group while membranous glomerulonephritis more commonly occurs in those approaching middle age.

Clinical features

The main features are those of the nephrotic syndrome.

Investigations

See 'Nephrotic syndrome' below.

Therapeutic management

Minimal lesion glomerulonephritis responds well to steroid therapy. However, some cases will relapse when the steroids are discontinued, in which case cyclophosphamide can be prescribed (Anderton 1988). The prognosis of patients with membranous glomerulonephritis is less favourable and at present there is no form of drug treatment for this condition. One-third will recover spontaneously but the remainder will progress to chronic renal failure.

Nephrotic syndrome

Nephrotic syndrome is not a distinct disease but a

clinical picture brought about by **heavy proteinuria** due to damage to the glomerular capillary membrane.

Aetiology

Any condition that seriously damages the glomerular capillary membrane, such as chronic glomerulo-nephritis, diabetic nephropathy or connective tissue disorders, will cause nephrotic syndrome.

Altered physiology

The route leading to the altered physiology of oedema is given in Figure 17.13.

Clinical features

The patient will have marked oedema which increases gradually over a period of 2–3 weeks. There will also be heavy proteinuria (more than 3 g in 24 hours) which will lead to extensive depletion of body proteins, which in turn causes increased susceptibility to infection. The patient may also complain of malaise, lethargy and anorexia.

Investigations

Urinalysis will reveal reduced volumes of urine containing large amounts of protein (more than 3 g in 24 hours).

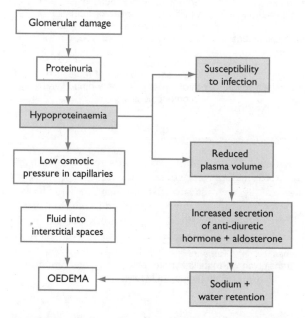

Fig. 17.13 Flow chart showing altered physiology leading to oedema

Therapeutic management

The cause of the nephrotic syndrome should be diagnosed and treated appropriately; for example, steroid therapy in minimal lesion glomerulonephritis. Oedema can be relieved by restricting sodium in the diet and by giving diuretics, for example frusemide. Amounts of protein and carbohydrate in the diet can be adjusted as required.

Nursing strategies

Assessment Monitoring of urinary output will show reduced volumes. General assessment of the patient will show marked generalized oedema. The oedematous areas are generally soft and readily pit on pressure.

Planning and implementing See Nursing Care Plan 17.3 for care of a patient with nephrotic syndrome.

Evaluation (expected outcomes)

The patient is no longer oedematous and shows no sign of proteinuria or infection. Urinary output and blood protein levels return to normal. The patient is free of complications.

IMPAIRED RENAL FUNCTION

ACUTE RENAL FAILURE

Acute renal failure can be defined as a sudden and severe reduction in renal function, which was previously apparently normal, causing retention of waste products of metabolism. It is usually reversible.

Epidemiology and aetiology

The causes of acute renal failure can be classified as prerenal, intrarenal or postrenal.

Prerenal causes are associated with diminished blood flow to the kidneys such as in haemorrhage or hypotension. Intrarenal causes are associated with damage to kidney tissue, for example glomerular disease. Postrenal causes are associated with urinary outflow obstruction (Table 17.2).

Altered physiology

Decreased renal perfusion, nephrotoxic injury and ischaemia can all lead to rapid deterioration of renal function causing fluid and electrolyte imbalance and retention of waste products of metabolism.

Nursing Care Plan 17.3   Care plan for a patient with the nephrotic syndrome

Problem	Goal	Nursing intervention	Rationale
1. Oliguria	Monitor urinary output and prevent overhydration	❐ Measure and record all urine passed ❐ Restrict intake of fluids according to urine output	Accurate assessment of output to allow calculation of volume of fluid permitted for next 24 hours Prevents overhydration
2. Heavy proteinuria	Prevent excessive protein loss	❐ Test urine daily for protein, blood and glucose ❐ Save continuous 24 hour urine collections ❐ Give high protein, low sodium diet	Monitors progress of disease Haematuria may indicate infection and/or further glomerular damage Glycosuria may indicate steroid induced diabetes Monitors amounts of protein being excreted High protein to replace loss, low sodium to lessen oedema
3. Oedema	To minimize oedema and prevent skin damage	❐ Bed rest if unwell, otherwise encourage mobility ❐ Care of skin and pressure areas ❐ Measure and record daily weight ❐ Measure and record lying/standing blood pressure ❐ Monitor pulse ❐ Measure daily girth ❐ Give diuretic therapy as prescribed	Reduces risk of venous thrombosis Oedematous tissue is fragile and very prone to damage More accurate assessment of fluid retention or loss Monitors hypertension due to renal disease or hypotension due to reduced circulating volume Assessment of cardiovascular competence To identify presence of ascites Assist in reduction of oedema
4. Infection risk	Prevent infection	❐ Monitor temperature Take regular skin and throat swabs Send regular urine specimens for culture	Serum immunoglobulin levels, which are essential for formation of antibodies, are low due to loss into urine
5. Thrombosis risk	Prevent venous thrombosis	❐ Encourage mobility Encourage leg exercises while in bed	Increased incidence of renal vein thrombosis pulmonary emboli and thrombophlebitis

Table 17.2   Causes of acute renal failure

Prerenal	Intrarenal	Postrenal
Surgical shock Severe dehydration Extensive burns Septicaemia Myocardial infarction Ante- or postpartum haemorrhage	Glomerular disease Nephrotoxic substances Incompatible blood transfusion	Calculi Tumours Prostatic hypertrophy Retroperitoneal fibrosis

Clinical features

These may be difficult to recognize, masked by symptoms of the primary acute condition.

Most patients with acute renal failure will become oliguric. However there are some who continue to pass 2–3 litres of urine daily in spite of having a decrease in renal function and increasing nitrogen retention. For those with diminished urinary output the clinical features in the oliguric phase are related to retention of fluid and electrolytes and uraemia.

Oliguric phase

1. *Oliguria*: urinary output diminishes to less than 500 ml per day. Sodium and water retention cause oedema and unless fluid intake is controlled pulmonary oedema and cardiac failure may result.

2. *Hyperkalaemia*: rapidly rising serum potassium is a serious threat to the cardiac muscle. In addition to not being eliminated by the kidneys, haemolysis and breakdown of tissue cells due to the primary condition increase levels of potassium in the blood.

3. *Uraemia*: blood urea levels generally rise rapidly as patients with acute renal failure tend to be in a highly catabolic state due to infection, fever and tissue destruction. Uraemia is characterized by nausea, vomiting, pruritis and hiccoughs. If untreated, lethargy, drowsiness and eventually coma may occur.

Diuretic phase There is usually an abrupt transition from the oliguric to diuretic phase. This is characterized by a high urinary output – more than 3 litres of urine per day is produced. However, kidney function has not yet recovered completely and the tubules are unable to concentrate urine. If fluid and electrolytes are not replaced at this stage, excessive loss of sodium and water can cause hypotension and muscle cramps. Excessive loss of potassium will cause cardiac arrhythmias. The uraemic symptoms will continue.

Recovery phase Improvement in renal function is gradual over 3–12 months. Urinary output decreases to normal, balancing intake. There may be some residual impairment, although for most patients full function is restored.

Investigations

1. Urinalysis of the small amounts of urine passed is helpful in diagnosing the cause of the renal failure; e.g. red cells and protein indicate glomerular disease.

2. Measurement of serum urea, creatinine and electrolytes will monitor the progress of renal function.

3. Ultrasound will show kidney size and may show the presence of calculi.

4. Retograde pyelography may be necessary if obstruction is suspected.

5. Renal biopsy is the only way of confirming a histopathological diagnosis.

Therapeutic management

Early diagnosis of the cause of the renal failure is essential for full recovery. Prompt treatment of the cause, for example restoration of fluid loss or relief of obstruction, is required. Uraemia should be minimized either by conservative methods or by dialysis.

Nursing strategies

Assessment An accurate record of fluid intake and output is essential. Frequent checking of vital signs is necessary to monitor cardiac function and fluid overload. Daily weight allows assessment of fluid loss or retention.

Planning and implementation The patient will still require care related to the primary disorder – haemorrhage, trauma or burns. If uraemia is being controlled by conservative methods the nurse must assist in the regulation of fluids and electrolytes. Tissue breakdown and hence rising blood urea and potassium are minimized by giving a high calorie intake at the same time as reducing protein. (Nursing Care Plan 17.4 gives care for a patient with acute renal failure.)

If uraemia needs to be controlled by dialysis to prevent further metabolic deterioration, arrangements should be made promptly.

Evaluation (expected outcomes)

Fluid and electrolyte balance is achieved and metabolic wastes are excreted. The patient is free from complications.

CHRONIC RENAL FAILURE

Chronic renal failure has an insidious onset and results from irreversible kidney damage.

Aetiology

- glomerulonephritis
- chronic pyelonephritis
- obstructive nephropathy
- polycycstic disease
- diabetes mellitus
- hypertension.

Nursing Care Plan 17.4 Care plan for management of a patient with acute renal failure

Problem	Goal	Nursing intervention	Rationale
1. Altered urinary elimination	To achieve fluid balance	❏ Measure and record accurate intake and output	Accurate assessment of output allows calculation of fluid permitted for next 24 hours
		❏ In oliguric phase restrict fluids to 500 ml and total of previous 24 hours output	Prevents overhydration
		❏ Observe for oedema	Assesses fluid balance
		❏ In diuretic phase increase fluid intake to compensate fluid loss	Prevents dehydration from excessive fluid loss
		❏ Monitor pulse and blood pressure	Assess cardiovascular status when over- or underhydrated
2. Electrolyte abnormalities	To achieve electrolyte balance	❏ In oliguric phase restrict salt in the diet	Kidneys are unable to excrete sodium
		❏ In diuretic phase give liberal amounts of salt in diet	To replace sodium being lost
		❏ Monitor serum potassium and if necessary restrict potassium in diet or give potassium supplements	In oliguric phase potassium not excreted by kidneys, therefore intake must be restricted. In diuretic phase excessive amounts may be lost in urine
		❏ Test urine specimens for abnormalities	Assesses progression of disease
		❏ Save 24 hour urine collections	Monitors electrolytes excreted over a 24 hour period
3. Retention of metabolic wastes	To minimize uraemia	❏ Give patient a low protein diet	Urea is a waste product of protein metabolism and is normally excreted via kidneys
		❏ Ensure high carbohydrate intake	Minimize utilization of patient's own body protein
4. Potential for infection	To minimize infection risk	❏ Nurse in a single room if possible	Minimize airborne and contact infection
		❏ Monitor temperature regularly	Early detection of infection
		❏ Send MSUs for culture and sensitivity	Monitor for urinary infection

Clinical features

Every system of the body can be affected (Box 17.1). Initially the patient passes large volumes of dilute urine (polyuria, nocturia) due to the kidneys' inability to concentrate urine. He/she may also complain of constantly feeling thirsty. Cramps and postural hypotension can also be problematical due to sodium depletion.

Tiredness, lethargy and breathlessness due to anaemia are often the first symptoms complained of by patients with chronic renal failure. Another common problem is anorexia, nausea and vomiting because of high levels of blood urea.

Skin changes which are typical of renal failure occur. These are pallor due to anaemia, yellowish discoloration due to retention of the pigment urochrome and pruritis because of retained urea, uric acid and calcium salts.

As kidney function deteriorates urinary output diminishes and in some patients stops completely (anuria). This leads to the problems of sodium and water retention, such as oedema, hypertension, pulmonary oedema, pericarditis and congestive cardiac failure.

Anaemia persists and many patients with end-stage renal failure have haemoglobin levels of 5–6 mmol/litre (normal 12–14 mmol/litre). Symptoms of uraemia worsen and blood potassium levels start to rise and, if not controlled, can lead to cardiac arrest.

Investigations

1. Blood urea and creatinine levels will be elevated and haemoglobin levels will be very low.

2. Radiology or ultrasound may show abnormal renal structure such as polycystic kidneys.

3. Renal biopsy may be carried out in the early

Box 17.1 Systemic manifestations of endstage chronic renal failure. (Adapted with permission from Read et al 1984, p. 276)

General
  Tiredness
  Irritability
Ocular
  Retinopathy
  Band keratopathy
  'Red eye'
Dermatological
  Pigmentation
  Pruritus
  Dry skin
  Purpura
Musculoskeletal
  Bone disease
  Weakness
  Myopathy
  Muscle cramp
  Restless legs
Endocrine
  Secondary hyperparathyroidism
Neurological
  Headache
  Parasthesia
  Convulsions
  Coma
Gastrointestinal
  Nausea
  Vomiting
  Anorexia
  Diarrhoea

GT haemorrhage
  Hiccough
Haematological
  Anaemia
  Susceptibility to infection
  Haemorrhagic tendency
Respiratory
  Dyspnoea and orthopnoea
  Pulmonary oedema
Cardiovascular
  Oedema
  Hypertension
  Pericarditis
  Ischaemic heart disease
Reproductive
  Impotence
  Subfertility
  Menstrual disturbances
Urinary
  Nocturia
  Enuresis
  Polyuria–oliguria
Metabolic
  Elevated urea
  Elevated creatinine
  Hyperuricaemia
  Hyperkalaemia
  Hyperphosphataemia
  Metabolic acidosis

---

stages of renal failure if glomerulonephritis is suspected.

Nursing strategies

Assessment Assessment should be made of the patient's fluid and electrolyte balance. Monitoring pulse, respirations, blood pressure and weight will reveal problems related to fluid retention and overload. Identify potential sources of imbalance and observe for early signs of complications, for example, infection.

Patient problems

- Altered fluid balance.
- Altered electrolyte balance.
- Altered nutritional status.
- Stress and anxiety related to lack of knowledge of condition and its treatment.

Planning and implementation The nurse's main role is to educate the patient regarding the regulation of fluids and electrolytes as well as the dietary management and the drugs required to control the uraemia.

Regulation of fluids and electrolytes Initially water and sodium are being lost in large quantities and must be replaced, therefore patients should be encouraged to take a high fluid intake and liberal amounts of salt in the diet.

Later, water and sodium are retained and therefore fluids must be restricted and so must dietary salt.

A low protein, high carbohydrate diet with electrolytes regulated as necessary will be required. The dietician should see the patient to give advice on the types of food to be taken and avoided. The lower the intake of protein the smaller the amount of nitrogenous waste. To minimize tissue breakdown a high calorie diet is essential.

Minimize psychological problems Depression is a common feature in patients with chronic renal failure. Not only does the patient feel generally unwell but he/she realizes that this is a chronic illness which will not disappear. Patients who are supported in the initial adaptation period can usually proceed to an appropriate level of acceptance. It is necessary for the family to be closely involved when teaching the patient about his illness and about future plans for the management of the chronic renal failure.

Evaluation (expected outcomes)

The patient maintains fluid balance, has improved electrolyte levels and demonstrates the ability to cope with the condition.

DIALYSIS

Dialysis is the process of removing waste products from the blood. It can be used in acute renal failure until spontaneous recovery occurs or in chronic renal failure to prolong life. Prior to the development of dialysis techniques, chronic renal failure meant inevitable death. For dialysis to take place it is necessary for blood from the patient to be brought into contact with dialysing fluid through a semipermeable membrane. Dialysis occurs by the natural physiological processes of diffusion and osmosis.

Peritoneal dialysis

The peritoneum is the largest semipermeable membrane in the body and has a rich blood supply. In peritoneal dialysis, dialysing fluid is inserted into the peritoneal cavity where it is in contact with the blood capillaries of the peritoneum (Fig. 17.14). Urea, creatinine, potassium and other toxic substances diffuse out of the capillaries into the dialysing fluid which is then drained away. Peritoneal dialysis can be used as a temporary measure in acute renal failure or as an alternative to haemodialysis in the management of chronic renal failure.

Methods of peritoneal dialysis

The two main methods of peritoneal dialysis are intermittent and continuous.

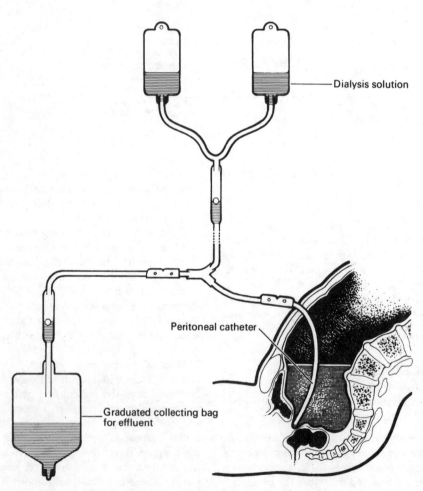

Dialysis solution

Peritoneal catheter

Graduated collecting bag for effluent

Fig. 17.14   Peritoneal dialysis

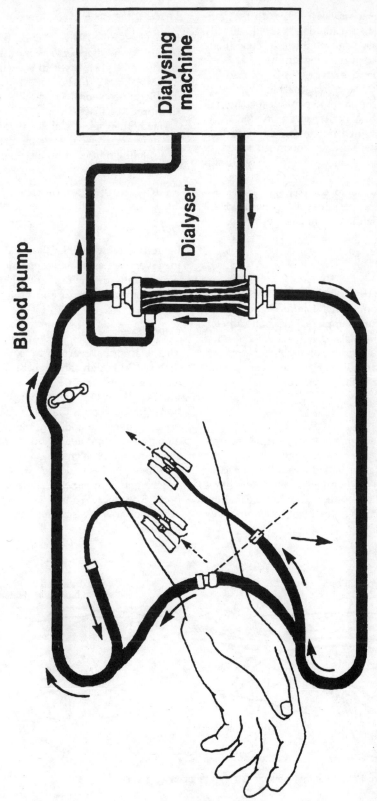

Fig. 17.15 Haemodialysis. Blood is removed from and returned to the patient in a continuous cycle. In the machine, blood is passed through fine, hollow fibres which are bathed in a flow of dialysate. Wastes diffuse from the blood into the dialysate.

Intermittent peritoneal dialysis Access to the peritoneal cavity is via a cannula inserted directly through the abdominal wall under local anaesthetic and held in place by a pursestring suture.

Intermittent peritoneal dialysis can be carried out manually or by automatic cycling machine.

Dialysing fluid is run into the peritoneal cavity via the cannula, left in the peritoneal cavity for 15–30 minutes and then drained out into a drainage bag. These dialysis cycles are usually continued for 24–48 hours at a time then repeated after 2–3 days if still required.

Continuous cycling peritoneal dialysis The automatic cycling machine performs the dialysis for 12 hours overnight while the patient is asleep.

Continuous ambulatory peritoneal dialysis (CAPD)

CAPD is an alternative to haemodialysis in the management of chronic renal failure. A permanent peritoneal catheter, for example a Tenckhoff catheter, has to be inserted. The dialysis cycles involve leaving dialysing fluid in the peritoneal cavity for approximately 4–6 hours and exchanges are carried out four times a day, every day of the week.

Haemodialysis

Haemodialysis uses a synthetic semipermeable membrane. Blood from the patient flows through the hollow fibres of the 'artificial kidney' and at the same time dialysing fluid is pumped around the fibres (Fig. 17.15). Haemodialysis depends upon the maintenance of adequate access to the bloodstream to allow blood flow to the dialyser.

Vascular access

It is necessary to have a good blood flow from the patient to the dialyser. The most usual method is an arteriovenous fistula which is created surgically in the forearm (Fig. 17.16). For emergency vascular access a double-lumen subclavian catheter or an arteriovenous shunt may be inserted.

Haemodialysis is usually required for 3–4 hours three times a week and can be carried out in hospital, in a satellite unit or at home.

Psychosocial problems of long-term dialysis

Dependence

Patients having regular hospital haemodialysis are in a very stressful and dependent position relying permanently on the skills of others. This can lead to resentment and aggression.

Depression

This is a normal reaction by patients having haemodialysis. Although they generally feel better than in end-stage renal failure, they soon realize that they must continue to adhere to dietary and fluid restrictions. Reliance on a dialysis machine means restrictions on life-style and may mean loss of earnings or employment. Impotence and loss of sexual drive may cause marital problems.

Nursing staff should be aware of these normal reactions and give patients and relatives help and support. The local Kidney Patients Association can also be of great assistance to many patients and their families.

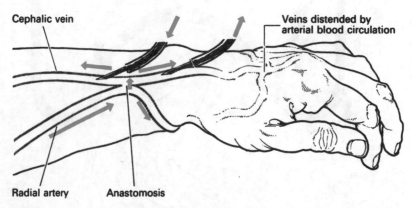

Fig. 17.16 Internal (subcutaneous) arteriovenous shunt

RENAL TRANSPLANTATION

Renal transplantation is now an accepted treatment for patients with end-stage renal failure. The kidney for transplantation may be taken from a living related donor (5–10%). The majority however are from cadeveric donors (Anderton 1988). Kidney donation is only considered after the patient has been declared brainstem dead (see Ch. 5) and the consent of relatives has been obtained. The donor and recipient must be ABO blood group and HLA tissue type compatible to reduce the risk of renal graft rejection.

For many patients with chronic renal failure a successful renal transplant means that their quality of life is greatly improved. However, for others the fear of rejection and loss of the kidney or dependence on immunosuppressive drugs and their side-effects are unacceptable.

Patients must be made aware of possible adverse effects as well as benefits before deciding to go on the waiting list for kidney transplantation. Rejection of a transplanted kidney means a return to dialysis treatment. Prior to transplantation the following procedures may be necessary:

1. Tissue typing to assess histocompatability.
2. Blood transfusion which induces beneficial immunological processes in the majority of recipients and thus better transplant survival.
3. Dialysis to ensure that the patient is in the best possible condition for surgery.

Transplant procedure

The donor kidney is sited in the right or left iliac fossa. Its renal artery is anastomosed to the patient's iliac artery and its renal vein is anastomosed to the iliac vein. The ureter is implanted into the bladder of the recipient via a submucosal tunnel, to prevent urinary reflux (Fig. 17.17).

Postoperative nursing strategies

Assessment   Fluid and electrolyte balance should be monitored as the transplanted kidney needs to be kept well perfused. The recipient should be observed for signs of rejection and any early signs of infection.

Planning and implementation

1. Maintenance of fluid balance   Central venous pressure is recorded to give accurate assessment of fluid status to prevent dehydration or fluid overload. The patient will have a urinary catheter in situ and urine output should be measured and recorded hourly. The amount of fluid given intravenously is adjusted according to CVP measurement and urinary output.

2. Prevention of infection   The kidney recipient is susceptible to infection because of the high doses of immunosuppressive drugs used in the initial postoperative period and also because of renal failure. Body temperature should be monitored for early signs of infection. The patient should be nursed in a single room if possible and strict asepsis should be maintained when carrying out wound care or any invasive procedures. Regular specimens of urine are taken for culture for the early detection of infection.

3. Prevention or early detection of rejection   Immunosuppressive drugs should be given as prescribed. The nurse must be alert for early signs of rejection which can occur as early as the second or third day postoperatively. There may be swelling or tenderness

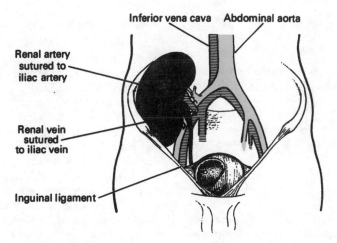

Fig. 17.17   Kidney transplant

Inferior vena cava   Abdominal aorta

Renal artery sutured to iliac artery

Renal vein sutured to iliac vein

Inguinal ligament

over the kidney. The patient may have a slight elevation of temperature and may complain of feeling generally unwell. Urinary output diminishes and serum creatinine and blood urea levels start to rise. Prompt antirejection treatment should be given as prescribed. High doses of steroids are usually given intravenously.

4. Psychological support The patient must be allowed to discuss anxieties. Nursing staff should be aware of the many stresses, such as fear of rejection, uncertain future, renewed independence and problems related to immunosuppressive drugs and give relevant information and support. The patient should be kept informed of progress and discharge planning should be discussed with the patient and his relatives.

Complications post transplantation

- Organ rejection.
- Viral, fungal and bacterial infections.
- Bone marrow suppression.

Patient education

It is important that patients are psychologically prepared for discharge from hospital. They must be made fully aware of their long-term treatment and be instructed how to recognize rejection.

Education on the importance of adhering to any dietary and fluid restriction is essential, as is the importance of taking immunosuppressive drugs as prescribed. The patient should be instructed to report to the doctor if any symptoms of rejection or infection develop. Advice should be given to avoid contact sports and the importance of follow-up care must be emphasized.

Evaluation (expected outcomes)

The patient will show no signs of rejection, will be free from infection and will have adapted to his/her new life-style.

FUNCTIONAL DISORDERS OF THE URINARY TRACT

ACUTE RETENTION OF URINE

Acute retention of urine is the inability to pass urine in spite of the desire to do so or being able to pass only very small amounts of urine with no relief.

Aetiology

Retention may be due to obstruction such as prostatic enlargement, but can occur after surgery, in acute illness and neurological disorders. Distension of the bladder causes back-pressure on the kidneys which can lead to renal damage and stasis of urine predisposes to infection.

Clinical features

The patient will complain of the inability to pass urine for several hours, suprapubic pain and will possibly appear shocked and anxious. A palpable bladder and distended lower abdomen will be found on examination.

Investigations

An intravenous urogram may be performed to check for obstructive uropathy. Renal function tests will be carried out in case of kidney damage. A midstream or catheter specimen of urine will be sent for culture and sensitivity in case of infection.

Therapeutic management

Most patients with acute urinary retention will require catheterization. Insertion of a suprapubic catheter may be the preferred treatment if retention is due to prostatic or urethral obstruction. However, patients with postoperative retention should be catheterized only as a last resort when other methods of encouraging micturition have failed.

Nursing strategies

Assessment The nurse should ascertain the patient's fluid intake and urinary output in the previous 12 hours. The patient should be assessed for degree of discomfort and his bladder palpated to assess level of distention.

Planning and implementation In postoperative retention the nurse should ensure privacy and assist the patient to the side of the bed if permitted. Running taps in the vicinity and lots of reassurance may help the patient to empty his bladder naturally. Giving adequate analgesia to relieve postoperative pain will also facilitate bladder emptying.

After catheterization ensure rest and reassurance. Analgesia may be required to make the patient more comfortable.

CHRONIC RETENTION OF URINE

In this condition the retention is incomplete. The patient will have a distended bladder with overflow incontinence or will be able to pass only small amounts of urine leaving large quantities in the bladder (residual urine). Urinary stagnation gives rise to infection in the urinary tract. The constant high pressures in the bladder cause changes in the bladder wall in which trabeculae and diverticulae form. In addition to increased bladder pressure, hydroureter and hydronephrosis may develop causing impaired renal function and eventual renal failure.

Therapeutic management

It is necessary for the patient to be catheterized and the catheter may need to be left in situ for several weeks until the blood urea and electrolytes return to within normal limits.

As soon as the patient's condition allows and when the investigations are complete, the underlying condition is treated.

INCONTINENCE OF URINE

Urinary incontinence is an extremely distressing problem and can occur at any age. In childhood, bedwetting (nocturnal enuresis) is often a problem and congenital abnormalities can result in incontinence. For adults urinary tract infections, weakened pelvic muscles and spinal cord injury are the main causes. In the elderly precipitating factors are the physiological changes of ageing, for example lack of bladder tone and loss of dexterity.

Aetiology

Urethral urinary incontinence is classified as being due to sphincter weakness, bladder instability, obstruction to outflow or congenital abnormality.

Types of incontinence

Enuresis is repeated involuntary urination especially at night in children who have reached the age when voluntary bladder control is possible. Factors thought to predispose to enuresis include emotional trauma, delayed development and hereditary factors.

Stress incontinence is due to sphincter weakness and occurs on coughing, straining or on exercising.

Stress incontinence in women is usually caused by overstretching of the pelvic floor muscles related to childbearing. Symptoms may improve with loss of weight, pelvic floor exercises and treatment for urinary tract infection. If these methods fail, surgery, for example anterior colporrhaphy or suprapubic repair (Marshall-Marchetti), is usually required.

Stress incontinence in men is usually caused by traumatic or surgical damage to the urethral sphincter, for example trauma from transurethral resection of the prostate or from a fractured pelvis. The only treatment is surgery, such as sling operations or perineal support, and this is not always successful.

Urge incontinence This is due to bladder instability. The sufferer recognizes the need to pass urine but is unable to reach the toilet in time. It can be caused by overactive detrusor muscle function or hypersensitivity of the bladder wall. The management of urge incontinence includes training to re-educate the bladder and the use of anticholinergic drugs (e.g. propantheline, emepronium bromide, Urispas) to decrease smooth muscle activity.

Overflow incontinence Outflow obstruction causes hypertrophy of the bladder muscle which eventually becomes atonic leading to overflow incontinence. Obstruction may be due to prostatic enlargement, constipation or pelvic tumour. The cause of the obstruction should be treated, followed by bladder training and possibly the use of parasympathomimetic agents (e.g. Ubretid) to help the bladder muscle regain normal tone.

Neurogenic bladder This bladder disturbance is due to a lack of nerve stimulation. There are two types: (1) spastic where there is an upper motor neurone lesion and the bladder behaves in a reflex fashion, and (2) flaccid where a lower motor neurone lesion enables the bladder to fill until greatly distended leading to overflow incontinence. Potential problems include recurrent urinary tract infections due to stasis of urine, urinary calculi, hydronephrosis and renal failure. The management of a neurogenic bladder is now usually by self-catheterization. Other methods of treatment include bladder training to avoid overdistension, parasympathomimetic drugs, surgical resection of bladder sphincters and urinary diversion.

Nursing strategies

Assessment The nurse should record the pattern of the patient's incontinence so that an appropriate plan for management can be made. Urine specimens are sent to bacteriology to identify any infection. Assessment is made of the skin for any excoriation.

The patient's dexterity is also assessed to ensure that clothing can be removed easily when visiting the toilet.

Planning and implementation Appropriate toilet facilities should be provided for individual needs. The nurse should assist the patient to plan realistic goals for bladder training. A good fluid intake should be ensured to prevent infection, but fluids are restricted after 6 p.m. to reduce incontinence overnight. Charting of urinary output and any episodes of incontinence is continued. Appropriate skin care is provided.

For patients with neurogenic bladders a teaching programme for self-catheterization may be required.

If surgery is required appropriate counselling and preparation are given. If all forms of treatment are unsuccessful, visits from a continence advisor and appropriate aids are arranged.

Evaluation The patient regains continence and has no skin excoriation. If this is not possible the patient's incontinence is managed in a manner which allows an acceptable quality of life.

SURGICAL MANAGEMENT OF URINARY TRACT DISORDERS

Renal surgery

Preoperative preparation

Increasingly the preliminary investigations are being carried out as an outpatient and patients are generally only admitted a day or two before operation for final tests and preparation. The general preparation for renal surgery is the same as for any patient having major abdominal surgery. Good preoperative preparation greatly reduces the patient's fears and anxieties and the risk of postoperative complications.

Postoperative nursing strategies

General postoperative care is the same as for any major abdominal operation. Particular attention must be paid to the prevention of complications, relief of pain and discomfort and the management of drainage tubes and catheters.

Assessment The patient should be monitored for respiratory and circulatory status, assessment is made of pain level and the effectiveness of pain control. Frequent checking of patency and adequacy of urinary drainage may be necessary. The wound dressing and wound drainage system are assessed regularly for early detection of excessive bleeding.

Actual potential patient problems
- Potential for shock and haemorrhage.
- Potential for respiratory complications.
- Potential for urinary complications.
- Potential for paralytic ileus.
- Pain and discomfort.
- Need for intravenous fluids.
- Impairment of skin integrity.
- Anxiety related to loss of kidney.

Planning and implementation See Nursing Care Plan 17.5 for a patient following renal surgery.

Evaluation (expected outcomes)

The patient's pain and discomfort are relieved and he/she remains free from complications throughout the postoperative period. The patient is able to discuss any anxieties and make plans for discharge, showing an awareness of follow-up care required.

Urinary diversion

There are times when it is necessary to divert the flow of urine away from the bladder to preserve renal function or alleviate incontinence. Urinary diversion is carried out primarily when a large or invasive tumour necessitates cystectomy. Other conditions requiring urinary diversion include birth defects (e.g. extrophy of the bladder) trauma (e.g. vesico-vaginal fistula) and neurogenic bladder.

There are various methods of urinary diversion:

1. *Nephrostomy tube insertion*: where a tube is inserted into the pelvis of the kidney to drain. This is mainly used as a short-term solution where there is ureteric blockage.

2. *Cutaneous ureterostomy*: the ureter is detached from the bladder and brought out through the abdominal wall to form an opening in the skin.

3. *Ureterosigmoidostomy*: the ureters are implanted into the sigmoid colon so that urine flows through the colon and is voided rectally.

4. *Ileal conduit*: a small loop of ileum is disconnected from the rest of the small bowel, retaining its mesentery and blood supply. Continuity of the small bowel is restored and the ureters are connected to the isolated ileal segment. One end of the ileal segment is brought out onto the skin surface as a stoma (Fig. 17.18). This is the method of urinary diversion that is used most frequently.

5. *Continent ileal urinary reserve (Koch pouch)*: the ureters are implanted into an isolated loop of ileum with a nipple-like one-way valve. A catheter is

Nursing Care Plan 17.5   Care plan for a patient following renal surgery

Problem	Goal	Nursing intervention	Rationale
1. Potential for shock and haemorrhage	Prevention or early detection of shock or haemorrhage	❑ Monitor and record pulse and blood pressure ❑ Observe colour and general condition of patient ❑ Check wound regularly ❑ Check wound drainage regularly	Early detection: shock or haemorrhage diagnosed from drop in blood pressure and increase in pulse rate Observing for signs of pallor or restlessness which could indicate shock or haemorrhage Observing for any visible signs of bleeding Observing for signs of excessive blood loss
2. Potential for respiratory complications	Prevention or early detection of respiration complications	❑ Monitor and record respiratory rate ❑ Encourage deep breathing exercises ❑ Prop up in bed using pillows and back rest for support	Observing for marked increase or decrease in respiratory rate To ensure full expansion of lungs Position to assist lung expansion
3. Potential for urinary complications	Prevention or early detection of urinary complications	❑ Measure and record urinary output ❑ Observe colour of urinary output ❑ Send regular MSUs for culture and sensitivity ❑ Ensure adequate fluid intake Urinary catheter may be in situ if accurate monitoring of remaining kidney required, hourly urine measure, ensure free drainage, ensure patency, catheter toilet	Monitors function of remaining kidney Observing for any abnormality Early detection of infection For adequate hydration of remaining kidney and to prevent infection
4. Potential for paralytic ileus		❑ Nil orally ❑ Commence fluids gradually when bowel sounds return Commence light diet when free fluids tolerated Full diet commenced when able	Initial paralytic ileus due to disturbance of retroperitoneal area Allows adequate peristalsis to become re-established
5. Pain and discomfort	To keep patient free from pain or discomfort	❑ Give analgesia regularly as prescribed Monitor patient for adequacy of pain control/amount and type of pain Help patient to turn regularly and make comfortable with pillows Plan analgesia to be given before physio or other procedures and before mobilization	Loin incision is painful
6. Need for intravenous fluids	To ensure adequate hydration	❑ Give i.v. fluids as prescribed Record amounts on fluid balance chart Check i.v. cannula site for any problems	Ensures adequate hydration of patient and remaining kidney To detect signs of inflammation, infiltration etc, and take appropriate action.

Nursing Care Plan 17.5 (*cont'd*)

Problem	Goal	Nursing intervention	Rationale
7. Impairment of skin integrity		❑ Check wound regularly for soakage Observe healing process Check wound drainage for patency, amount of drainage and type of drainage ❑ Maintain personal hygiene by daily bed bathing for first 2–3 days Encourage daily shower when drain removed ❑ Assist patient to turn regularly whilst in bed ❑ Encourage occasionally to turn towards side of operation with help of pillows	To detect excessive bleeding To evaluate progress of wound healing To prevent wound infection To assist wound drainage
8. Anxiety		❑ Allow patient to discuss any anxieties Give up to date information about progress Reassure over loss of kidney	Reduces anxiety levels and aids recovery

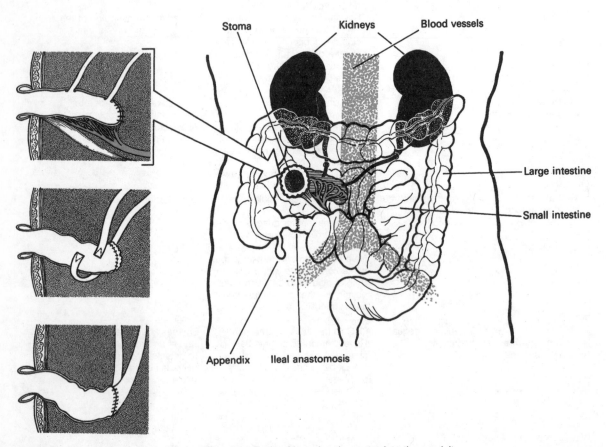

Fig. 17.18 Ileal conduit showing three different methods of inserting the ureter into the conduit

inserted to drain urine. This is the most recent development in urinary diversion.

Ileal conduit urinary diversion

Preoperative nursing strategies The general preparation is the same as for any major intestinal surgery. Explanation and counselling are necessary to ensure understanding of the nature of the operation. The patient should be encouraged to talk of any anxieties. The stoma is sited taking into account individual needs and life-style and a trial of the appropriate urostomy appliance should be given.

Preparation of the bowel for surgical intervention is necessary to minimize faecal stasis and reduce pathogenic bacterial flora.

Potential patient problems

- Wound infection.
- Leakage at anastamosis site.
- Paralytic ileus.
- Intestinal obstruction.
- Peritonitis.

Postoperative nursing strategies

Assessment General observation of the patient and monitoring of vital signs are the same as for any patient after intestinal surgery (see Ch. 15). The stoma is observed frequently for colour and size. Urinary output is measured and recorded and the patient monitored for signs and symptoms of potential complications.

Planning and implementation

1. *Management of stoma.* Frequent observation of the stoma colour and size is made to check for swelling and adequate blood supply. A clear two-piece drainable appliance is used to facilitate cleaning and observation of the stoma. The urinary output is measured and recorded to monitor for signs of impaired renal function. Care must be taken when changing the urostomy bag so that the ureteric stents, which are left in situ to allow healing without stenosis and narrowing of the ureters, are not dislodged.

2. *Management of fluids and nutrition.* The patient may have parenteral nutrition to ensure full nutritional requirements until oral feeding can recommence. Nil orally is permitted for approximately 5 days until bowel sounds return. An intravenous infusion, if properly managed, will ensure adequate hydration.

Patient education and psychological support The nurse must assist the patient to accept their altered body image. The sight of the stoma may be distasteful at first, so a gradual introduction needs to be given. The patient should be helped to plan realistic goals in the self-management of the stoma and frequent supervised practise at stoma care should be given. Visits from the stoma therapist who will be caring for the patient in the community should be arranged and reassurance given that discharge home will only be planned when the patient is able to look after the stoma competently.

DISORDERS OF THE MALE REPRODUCTIVE SYSTEM

STRUCTURE AND FUNCTION

The male reproductive system consists of paired testes, epididymis, vas deferens, common ejaculatory ducts, urethra, penis and scrotum. The accessory organs are the seminal vescicles, prostate gland and bulbourethral glands (Fig. 17.19).

The testis is made up of coiled seminiferous tubules in which spermatozoa are formed. These tubules drain posteriorly into a system of fine efferent ducts which pass into the epididymis and then to the vas deferens which passes upwards through the inguinal canal into the abdominal cavity behind the peritoneum. The course of the vas deferens then turns downwards towards the base of the bladder where a reservoir for testicular secretions, the seminal vesicle, branches off. The vas deferens continues as the ejaculatory duct which passes through the prostate gland to enter the urethra (Fig. 17.19).

INFECTIVE DISORDERS
Orchitis

Inflammation of the testis may complicate a viral infection such as mumps or rubella, or may result from an ascending infection, torsion of the testis or severe trauma. It causes sudden onset of acute testicular pain and swelling and may be accompanied by fever.

Therapeutic management

With conservative treatment of bed rest, scrotal support and analgesia the swelling will usually resolve within a few days. An antibiotic may be required for orchitis due to ascending infection.

Prostatitis

Inflammation of the prostate gland may result from

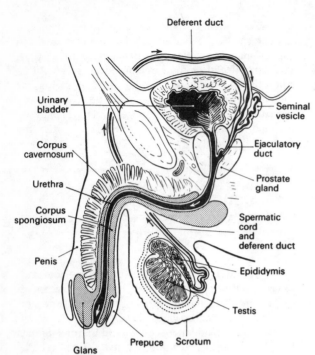

Fig. 17.19 Section of the male reproductive organs. Arrows show the structures through which spermatozoa pass. (Reproduced with permission from Wilson 1990, p. 241)

blood-borne infection or from bacteria ascending through the urethra.

Clinical features

Clinical features include fever and pain in the perineum, rectum, lower back and head of penis. These may be accompanied by urinary symptoms such as frequency, dysuria and haematuria.

Investigations

The diagnosis is mainly by rectal examination which reveals a very tender and swollen prostate, warm to the touch.

Therapeutic management

An appropriate antibiotic will be prescribed according to the organisms found on culture of prostatic fluid and urine specimens.

Nursing strategies

Encourage bed rest and assist with personal hygiene as required. Warm immersion baths may relieve discomfort. Monitor for signs of fever persisting and for signs of other complications. Given antibiotics, analgesics and antipyretics as prescribed when necessary.

NEOPLASTIC DISORDERS
Prostatic tumours

Cancer of the prostate is the most common cancer in men over the age of 65 years.

Aetiology

The precise aetiology of prostatic cancer remains unknown. However, associated factors include family history, diet, chemical exposure and viral infection.

Clinical features

Cancer of the prostate seldom gives rise to symptoms while in a curable stage. Often the symptoms are indistinguishable from those of benign prostatic hypertrophy, although some patients will present with back pain due to secondary deposits.

Therapeutic management

Prostatic cancer is potentially curable at an early stage, however the majority of patients present when the tumour has already spread. The management is therefore mainly palliative. Transurethral resection of the prostate may be performed to relieve urethral obstruction. Radiotherapy to the prostate may be used to prevent invasion of the rectum and also to metastases to treat bone pain. Prostatic cancers are androgen dependent, therefore suppression of androgen production can alleviate symptoms and retard the progress of the disease. Hormonal manipulation can be achieved by bilateral orchidectomy, oestrogen therapy or antiandrogens.

Testicular tumours

The aetiology of testicular tumours is unknown, although those with a history of undescended testes have an increased risk. They are the commonest cancer in men between the ages of 20 and 40. Sixty per cent of tumours are teratomas and 40% seminomas.

Clinical features

The onset is often gradual with an expanding palpable mass in the scrotum. Symptoms of metastatic spread include abdominal mass or pain and troublesome cough.

Therapeutic management

Combination chemotherapy has proved highly successful in the treatment of testicular tumours. The introduction of Cis-platinum has revolutionized the prognosis of testicular tumours – 90% can now be cured. This could improve further with early diagnosis and young men should be encouraged to carry out self-examination of the testes at regular intervals.

Tumours of the penis

Malignant tumours of the penis are uncommon. They are rare under the age of 45 years but thereafter the incidence increases with age. The tumour arises as a warty growth or ulcer on the glans penis usually hidden by the foreskin.

The first presenting symptoms may be pain, bleeding or a foul-smelling discharge.

Therapeutic management

For stage T1 and T2 tumours treatment is either by radiotherapy or partial amputation. More advanced tumours require radical amputation.

SURGERY TO THE MALE REPRODUCTIVE SYSTEM

Benign prostatic hypertrophy

Benign prostatic hypertrophy is a common problem in men over the age of 50. Enlargement of the prostate gland results in urinary output obstruction. This in turn can lead to infection, progressive hydronephrosis and eventual renal failure.

Aetiology

The aetiology is uncertain but may be related to endocrine changes associated with ageing.

Clinical features

The presenting features are dependent on the degree of bladder outlet obstruction. The initial problems are of difficulties in micturition, such as increasing urinary frequency, nocturia, poor stream, hesitancy and urgency. If these symptoms are ignored, increasing obstruction will result in incomplete emptying of the bladder with progressive distension. The patient then presents with chronic urinary retention perhaps accompanied by overflow incontinence and probably a degree of uraemia. Acute urinary retention may also be the presenting problem with the patient admitted as an emergency (see p. 604).

Investigations

Diagnosis of benign prostatic hypertrophy is generally made on history and rectal examination.

Urinalysis is performed and a specimen sent for microbiological examination.

A flow rate may also be requested, where the volume of urine passed per second is measured.

An intravenous urogram is used to reveal upper urinary tract damage due to obstruction. Blood tests are required to determine any deterioration in renal function. As most of the patients are elderly, a thorough assessment of their physical condition is required.

Therapeutic management

There are four routes available for removal of the prostate gland (Fig. 17.20).

Transurethral resection of the prostate is in most cases the operation of choice. However, if the gland is particularly large retropubic prostatectomy may be required. Transvesical prostatectomy is mostly used when there is co-existing bladder pathology which can be dealt with at the same time. Perineal prostatectomy is seldom used in this country, but is used in some centres in USA.

Transurethral resection of prostate

Potential patient problems

- Haemorrhage.
- Clot retention.
- Infection.
- Difficulty in re-establishing normal micturition.

Postoperative nursing strategies

The aim of postoperative management is to ensure free drainage of urine and the early detection of complications with prompt treatment. As the prostate gland is a very vascular organ haemorrhage is a potential problem.

The following measures should be taken:

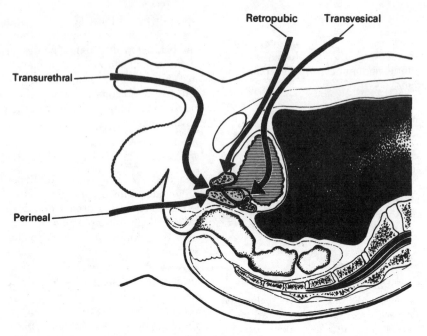

Fig. 17.20 Four routes for removal of prostate gland

1. *Monitor the patient for signs of shock and haemorrhage.* Vital signs are recorded frequently and the patient is observed for pallor and restlessness.

2. *Minimize the incidence of clot retention.* Continuous bladder irrigation may be in progress via a three-way catheter and the flow rate of irrigation fluid is adjusted according to the degree of haematuria. If the catheter lumen becomes blocked by clots the patient will complain of suprapubic pain and a desire to pass urine. Bladder lavage can be carried out adhering to a strict aseptic technique.

3. *Prevent urinary tract infection.* A closed urinary drainage system should be maintained. Ensure that the catheter can drain freely and check patency frequently. Catheter toilet should be carried out if the patient has any discharge at the urethral meatus or if the catheter has been 'by-passing'. A high fluid intake should be encouraged.

4. *Monitor fluid balance.* Fluid intake and amount of bladder drainage should be measured and recorded. The amounts of irrigation fluid used should be recorded and deducted from the amount of bladder drainage to ascertain urinary output.

5. *Minimize pain and discomfort.* As there is no skin incision with transurethral resection of the prostate, analgesia is not normally required. If pain or discomfort is felt, this is generally due to bladder spasm or a blocked catheter and should be treated appropriately.

Patient education

It should be explained to the patient to expect symptoms of urgency and frequency after catheter removal. Give reassurance that these will diminish. Pelvic floor exercises should be encouraged to help gain urinary control and the patient is advised to pass urine at regular intervals. Encourage the patient to continue to take a high fluid intake.

Torsion of testis

This is a surgical emergency. Torsion occurs if the testis can rotate freely within its capsule and may be due to congenital abnormality, undescended testes or trauma. Unrelieved strangulation causes vascular occlusion and ischaemic necrosis. The patient presents with acute scrotal pain, tenderness, swelling and nausea.

Surgical repair is required with fixation of the testis in the scrotum.

Hydrocele

This is a collection of watery fluid in the tunica vaginalis of the testicle. Hydrocele is caused by inadequate reabsorption of normally produced fluid and may be secondary to trauma, torsion, tumour or infection. Primary hydrocele can occur at any age without any obvious cause.

Therapeutic management

Most hydroceles, even when quite large, will usually reabsorb. If persistent surgical excision may be required. For poor risk patients periodic aspiration of hydrocele fluid will relieve discomfort.

Varicocele

This is a disorder of the blood vessels draining the testes. The veins from the testes are dilated causing enlargement of the spermatic cord in the upper part of the scrotum and in the groin. It may cause discomfort and an aching pain. In addition, the temperature of the testes is raised which may cause testicular dysfunction in the form of oligospermia.

Treatment

Usually no treatment is required. However, in cases of infertility and where discomfort is persistent ligation of the varicocele is required, but this is not always successful in increasing fertility.

Postoperative nursing strategies

Patients after ligation of hydrocele and excision of varicocele will require to wear a scrotal support to relieve discomfort. They may have a small wound drain and dressing in situ for 24 hours.

Vasectomy

Vasectomy involves division of the vas deferens and may be required where infections of the epididymis are recurrent. Bilateral vasectomy is the male sterilization procedure (see p. 624).

Postoperative nursing strategies

This surgery is usually carried out as an outpatient. The nurse's role is to give reassurance and advice before the patient is sent home. He should be advised to rest for 48 hours after surgery to prevent discomfort and a scrotal support should be worn. Reassurance is given that discoloration and swelling are quite normal and will gradually diminish. It is important that the patient understands the necessity of using contraceptives until two negative specimens, 1 month apart, have been given.

Day case surgery

Much of the minor surgery to the male reproductive and urological systems is carried out as day cases.

To ensure safety and effectiveness of day case surgery patients have to be carefully selected, taking into account the patient's age and home circumstances. The type of operation must have a low incidence of postoperative complications and the surgery must be of short duration. The nurse has a key role in assessing the patient, planning pre- and postoperative care and monitoring, instructing and evaluating the patient's progress.

Postoperative nursing assessment

The patient's vital signs should be stable, he/she should have no excessive pain, be fully orientated and have no complaints of dizziness. Before discharge home the nurse should ensure that the patient fully understands the postoperative instructions.

Advantages to patient

It is more pleasant and convenient for the patient and there is a lower incidence of postoperative complications. Children do not have to be separated from the family any longer than necessary and there is less disruption for mothers.

Advantages to NHS

Day case surgery is an efficient way to reduce hospital waiting lists. It is economical and releases ward beds for major cases.

Disadvantages

There is less time to assess and evaluate the patient and to establish patient–staff relationships. The patient has to cope at home with any complications. Accompanied transport is needed to take the patient home and the community nursing service workload may be increased.

DISORDERS OF THE FEMALE REPRODUCTIVE SYSTEM

STRUCTURE

The female reproductive tract is generally divided for descriptive purposes into internal organs and external organs.

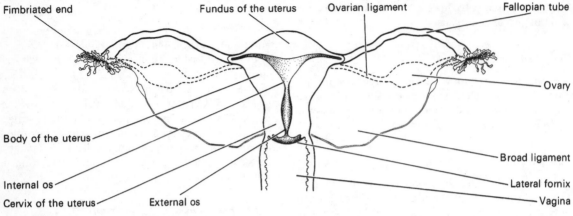

Fig. 17.21   Internal genitalia of the female

Internal organs

The internal organs consist of two ovaries, two fallopian or uterine tubes, uterus and vagina (Fig. 17.21).

The ovaries

The ovaries are the female sex glands which produce the hormones oestrogen and progesterone. They are approximately 3 cm long and 1.5 cm wide and lie in the peritoneal cavity on the back of the broad ligament near the fimbriated ends of the uterine tubes. During childbearing years the ovaries produce a mature ovum during each menstrual cycle (Fig. 17.23).

The uterine tubes

These are two thin muscular tubes which provide a passageway directly from the uterus into the peritoneal cavity. At the distal end of each tube are finger-like processes called **fimbriae**.

The uterus

The uterus is a hollow muscular pear-shaped organ measuring 7.5 cm × 5 cm × 2.5 cm. It lies almost at right angles to the vagina and bent over the urinary bladder (Fig. 17.22). Its lower end, the cervix, projects into the vagina for about half of its length. The opening of this part into the vagina is called the external os. The upper end of the cervix opens into the body of the uterus at the internal os.

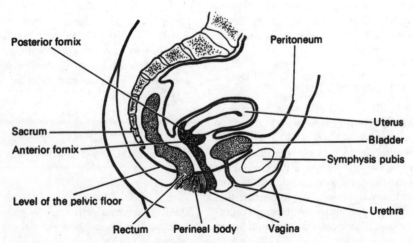

Fig. 17.22   Sagittal section of pelvis in the female

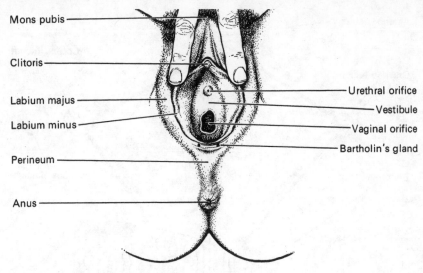

Fig. 17.23 External genitalia in the female

The uterus has an outer covering of peritoneum, a middle muscular layer (myometrium), and an inner lining of epithelium (endometrium), which alters in thickness during each menstrual cycle.

The uterine supports

The uterus is supported in the pelvic cavity by the surrounding organs, the muscles of the pelvic floor and ligaments, which are derived from folds of peritoneum and connective tissue.

The **broad ligaments** are formed by double folds of peritoneum on either side of the uterus. They hang down over the uterine tubes and are attached to the sides of the pelvis. They contain the round and ovarian ligaments.

The two **cardinal ligaments** are attached to the sides of the cervix and extend laterally to the walls of the pelvis.

The two **uterosacral ligaments** are attached to the posterior wall of the cervix and extend backwards, on either side of the rectum, to the sacrum. A deep depression between the vagina and rectum formed by peritoneum is known as the **pouch of Douglas**.

The vagina

The vagina is the link between the internal and external organs. It is a muscular canal which begins at the introitus, passes upwards and backwards and ends at the uterus. Its lining is arranged in rugae or folds allowing it to expand easily.

External organs

The external organs of the female reproductive tract are shown in Figure 17.23.

THE MENSTRUAL CYCLE

Menstruation and the events leading up to it are termed the menstrual cycle (Fig. 17.24) and are under the control of hormones.

The anterior pituitary gland secretes the follicle stimulating hormone (FSH) which stimulates a primordial follicle to grow and mature.

As the follicle develops it secretes oestrogen which eventually inhibits the secretion of FSH and stimulates the release of the luteinizing hormone (LH), also from the anterior pituitary. Oestrogen causes the endometrium to begin to thicken.

When it is sufficiently mature the follicle ruptures and releases an ovum which is then carried slowly along the uterine tube towards the cavity of the uterus. Ovulation has now taken place.

The remainder of the ruptured follicle develops into the corpus luteum which secretes progesterone. Progesterone prepares the breast and uterus for **gestation** and is only present in the circulation after ovulation, unlike oestrogen which is secreted throughout the cycle.

If the ovum is not fertilized, about 12 days after ovulation the corpus luteum degenerates and the secretion of progesterone and oestrogen ceases. Lack of progesterone causes the endometrium to break down giving rise to the menstrual flow which normally lasts from 3 to 5 days.

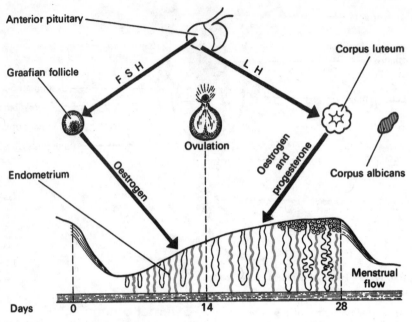

Fig. 17.24 The menstrual cycle

This entire process is under the control of the hypothalamus (Tortora 1989).

Menstrual disturbances

Amenorrhoea

Amenorrhoea or absence of menstruation may be primary or secondary.

Primary amenorrhoea

This is when a girl of 16–17 years of age has never menstruated. It may be due to congenital abnormality, imperforate hymen, anorexia nervosa or stress and needs to be investigated.

Secondary amenorrhoea

This occurs months or years after menstruation has begun and before the menopause. The main cause is pregnancy, however, endocrine, emotional or systemic disturbances (e.g. anorexia nervosa, diabetis mellitus) can also cause secondary amenorrhoea.

Some patients experience secondary amenorrhoea after stopping the contraceptive pill. The treatment depends on the cause.

Dysmenorrhoea

Dysmenorrhoea is pain experienced at the time of menstruation.

Primary dysmenorrhoea This is a spasmodic type of pain, usually occuring during the first 48 hours of a menstrual period.

Aetiology This remains uncertain but appears to be associated with excessive production of prostaglandins during breakdown of secretory endometrium causing muscular contractions. Their influence on smooth muscle may also cause nausea, vomiting, pallor and fainting (Tortora 1989).

Therapeutic management Usually the symptoms can be controlled with the use of mild analgesics and prostaglandin inhibitors such as aspirin and ponstan.

Regular exercise should be recommended and the woman advised to avoid constipation. A change in diet avoiding refined and processed food can help to relieve period pains. If the symptoms are not controlled the use of oral contraceptives may be successful.

Nursing strategies

1. *Assessment.* School nurses or occupational health nurses are most commonly involved in dealing with dysmenorrhoea. The degree and type of pain should be assessed. The nurse should ascertain whether the patient is menstruating, if these symptoms have oc-

curred before and if she is receiving any treatment from her doctor.

2. *Planning and implementation*. A sympathetic and understanding approach is essential. The patient is permitted to lie down with a blanket to keep her warm and a hot water bottle for local heat on the lower abdomen. Mild analgesia may be given if other medication has not been taken. Often symptoms are relieved in a short time allowing return to work. If this is a regular occurrence causing frequent loss of school or work time, it is the nurse's responsibilty to suggest that investigations are carried out by a gynaecologist.

3. *Evaluation*. The patient will have complete relief from symptoms and be able to continue with her normal daily routine.

Secondary dysmenorrhoea This usually occurs after several years with normal menstruation. It is a more constant type of pain which starts 2–3 days before the menstrual period and continues for several days thereafter. Secondary dysmenorrhoea is associated with endometriosis, inflammatory diseases and tumour. It is essential that these symptoms are investigated.

Menorrhagia

Menorrhagia is excessive bleeding at the time of the menstrual period. It may be due to hormonal disturbances, inflammatory diseases, fibroids or uterine carcinoma. Sometimes the cause cannot be found. As well as heavy bleeding the woman will usually complain of tiredness due to anaemia.

Therapeutic management Endometrial biopsy is necessary to eliminate organic disease, therefore a dilatation and curettage (D & C) is usually performed. If there is no organic cause treatments include the use of prostaglandin inhibitors, e.g. ponstan, or giving hormone therapy. Anaemia is treated with iron therapy. Surgical treatment, if required, usually means hysterectomy. However, a relatively new and minimally invasive procedure is now available as an effective alternative. Transcervical endometrial resection is carried out vaginally and the patient can be discharged after 24 hours.

Premenstrual syndrome (PMS)

PMS refers to a group of symptoms which occur regularly 1 week to 10 days prior to menstruation and diminish 1–2 days after it begins.

Clinical features Symptoms include any of the following:

1. Water retention, particularly breast swelling and abdominal distension.
2. Mood changes such as tension, irritability and depression.
3. Headaches or backache.
4. Dizziness, cold sweats and loss of concentration.

Therapeutic management No one form of treatment is consistently successful. Treatments are:

1. Medications, e.g. pyridoxone, progesterone, tranquillizers and diuretics.
2. Diet: restrict salt intake, increase potassium intake, increase fibre intake. Frequent small meals may help to keep blood glucose levels stable.
3. Counselling and self-help groups may be beneficial.

Menopause

The menopause usually occurs between the ages of 45 and 55 years and is characterized by the cessation of menstruation and of ovarian function. At this time a woman's reproductive function gradually diminishes.

Clinical features Many women will only notice a reduction in menstrual flow, which becomes irregular and finally ceases. However, for others there may be symptoms which are mainly related to oestrogen deprivation but may also be related to loss of fertility. Oestrogen decline may cause hot flushes, sweats, atrophic vaginitis and osteoporosis. Urinary frequency, headaches general aches and pains may be problematical. Often women notice feelings of irritability, anxiety and depression.

Therapeutic management For the small amount of women who have symptoms which are distressing, hormone replacement therapy will give relief.

Premature menopause

Ovarian function ceases before the age of 40. If oestrogen supplements are not given there is an increased risk of osteoporosis, fractures and heart disease.

Hormone replacement therapy (HRT) There has been a dramatic increase in the use of HRT in the last decade to relieve the unpleasant symptoms of the menopause, to protect bones against osteoporosis and to prevent ischeamic heart disease. Doses of HRT vary according to need and may be given orally, transdermally using patches, or subcutaneously by implant.

However, HRT can be accompanied by a number of undesirable side-effects. There is an increased risk of thromboembolism and possible increased risks of endometrial and breast cancers.

INTERRUPTIONS OF PREGNANCY

Abortion

Abortion is defined as the interruption of pregnancy before the 24th week of gestation, whether it occurs therapeutically or spontaneously.

Spontaneous abortion

Spontaneous abortion more commonly occurs about the 12th week of gestation, but may occur at any time before the 24th week of pregnancy. It is thought that more than half the abortions occuring spontaneously are caused by fetal malformation and the remainder caused by uterine fibroids, incompetent cervix or progesterone deficiency. Spontaneous abortion can be classified under the following headings:

1. *Threatened abortion.* There is some bleeding and pain but the cervix remains closed. With rest abortion may be prevented.

2. *Inevitable abortion.* There is strong, regular lower abdominal pain and vaginal bleeding with clots. On examination the external os is usually dilated which means that the pregnancy cannot continue.

3. *Incomplete abortion.* Expulsion of some products of conception occurs and there may be some heavy bleeding. Evacuation of the uterus is required.

4. *Habitual abortion.* This refers to three or more consecutive abortions and is usually due to cervical incompetence, uterine abnormality or chromosomal abnormality. In some cases the cause can be treated, for instance an incompetent cervix can be treated by inserting a Shirodkar suture.

Nursing strategies

Assessment Assessment of blood loss should be made and any clots passed vaginally should be saved. The degree and type of pain should be monitored. Observe closely for signs of shock.

Planning and implementation For patients with threatened abortion ensure bed rest until bleeding ceases. Mild sedation may be given as prescribed to ensure rest. If abortion is inevitable, prevent shock by maintaining circulatory blood volume. An intravenous infusion may be required. Analgesia is given when required. The patient is prepared for general anaesthetic for evacuation of retained products.

Evaluation In threatened abortion, pregnancy continues with no further bleeding. In inevitable abortion, the uterus contracts to its prepregnant state and the couple are then able to grieve for their lost child. Reassurance is given that future pregnancies need not necessarily be aborted.

Therapeutic abortion

The British abortion laws permit therapeutic abortion under certain conditions (Box 17.2). New regulations came into effect on 1 April 1991. The 1967 Abortion Act was amended in the following respects:

- 24 week time limit for abortions performed on existing grounds.
- New grounds for abortion: grave permanent injury to physical or mental health, no time limit.
- The following two existing grounds to be without time limit:
  — risk to the life of the pregnant woman
  — substantial risk that if the child was born it would suffer from such physical or mental abnormalities as to be seriously handicapped.

Before abortion can be performed legally agreement must be signed by two doctors. Therapeutic abortions may be carried out in the following ways:

1. suction termination of pregnancy
2. intra-amniotic administration of prostaglandins
3. hysterotomy.

Nursing strategies The nurse's role in care of the patient after termination of pregnancy is to monitor her general condition and to give psychological support and advice.

Box 17.2 Grounds for abortion under the Abortion Act of 1967

1. The continuance of the pregnancy would involve risk to the life of the pregnant woman greater than if the pregnancy were terminated
2. The continuance of the pregnancy would involve risk of injury to the physical or mental health of the pregnant woman greater than if the pregnancy were terminated
3. The continuance of the pregnancy would involve risk of injury to the physical or mental health of the existing children of the family greater than if the pregnancy were terminated
4. There is a substantial risk that if the child were born it would suffer from such physical or mental abnormalities as to be seriously handicapped
5. To save the life of the pregnant woman
6. To prevent grave permanent injury to the physical or mental health of the pregnant woman

Care of the patient after suction termination of pregnancy is related to care after general anaesthetic. Many patients experience some cramp-like pains after abortion and a mild analgesic may be required. Checks are made of vaginal blood loss and the patient monitored for a few hours. When the patient's general condition permits she will be discharged home. Intra-amniotic prostaglandins are used when the pregnancy is more than 12 weeks' gestation. The patient is monitored carefully during labour and subsequent abortion. All support and nursing care of a patient in labour is required.

Hysterotomy is generally carried out if the pregnancy is more than 16 weeks' gestation. Pre- and postoperative care is similar to that of caesarean section.

Ectopic pregnancy

Ectopic pregnancy occurs when the embedding and growth of the fertilized ovum occurs outside the uterine cavity. The most common site is in the uterine tube.

Aetiology

Predisposing factors include salpingitis, endometriosis and congenital abnormalities of uterine tubes.

Clinical features

The patient has had amenorrhoea for about 6 weeks and may have noticed some early signs of pregnancy. Small amounts of bleeding, usually less than that of a normal period, are common and the woman complains of cramp-like pains and abdominal tenderness.

Therapeutic management

This a surgical emergency. The patient may initially need to be treated for shock prior to laparotomy and salpingectomy.

Nursing strategies

Assesssment Monitor the amount of bleeding and assess the degree of pain and shock. As shock and haemorrhage are potential complications of ectopic pregnancy regular recording of vital signs and observation of the patient are essential.

Planning and implementation The patient may be shocked on admission and may require blood transfusion. Sedation and analgesia are given as prescribed when required and the patient prepared for emergency surgery. Reassurance and sympathy are required as the patient may be frightened and also grieving for the loss of the pregnancy.

Postoperative nursing

Patient problems

1. *Potential haemorrhage*: the patient's vital signs are monitored and vaginal loss checked at regular intervals.

2. *Pain and discomfort*: analgesia is given as prescribed. The degree of pain and adequacy of pain relief are monitored.

3. *Grief*: sympathy and support are given to assist the patient through the natural grieving process.

4. *Lack of knowledge about condition*: it is important that the patient understands what has happened and the prospects for future pregnancies.

Evaluation (expected outcomes) The patient is free from pain and discomfort and displays no signs of shock. She starts to show acceptance of the loss and an understanding of her condition.

INFECTIVE DISORDERS

Vaginal infections

Monilial vaginitis

Fungal infection of the vagina is caused by *Candida albicans*. This is commonly associated with pregnancy, diabetes mellitus, oral contraception and antibiotic therapy.

Clinical features The patient has a thick white creamy discharge which causes pruritis and vulval irritation. The vaginal walls are reddened and covered with white patches.

Therapeutic management Treatment is with Nystatin cream or cotrimazole vaginal pessaries. The patient's partner may also require treatment to prevent reinfection.

Trichomonas vaginitis This is a very common protozoan infection. It is mainly transmitted during sexual intercourse but can be acquired from infected articles, for example a speculum.

Clinical features The patient has a heavy greenish-yellow frothy discharge which causes vulval irritation, pruritis and excoriation. The vaginal mucosa is reddened and oedematous.

Therapeutic management Treatment is with oral administration of Flagyl (metronidazole). To prevent reinfection the woman's partner should be treated concurrently with Flagyl.

Atrophic vaginitis

This is due to hormonal changes after the menopause. The vagina loses its elasticity and becomes smooth and shiny.

Clinical features   The patient complains of burning in the vagina, dyspareunia and vulval pruritis.

Therapeutic management   Since this condition is due to oestrogen deprivation, treatment with oestrogen should resolve the problem but must be maintained. It may be preferable to use an oestrogen vaginal cream. Any infection present is also treated.

Pelvic inflammatory disease

This is an ascending pelvic infection causing endometritis or salpingitis. The commonest causative organisms are *Staphylococcus aureus* and *gonococcus*.

Clinical features

The patient has symptoms of a systemic infection which may be accompanied by nausea and vomiting and lower abdominal pain. There may also be a purulent vaginal discharge.

Nursing strategies

Assessment   A high vaginal swab is taken and the type of discharge should be ascertained. The patient's vital signs are monitored and assessment made of the degree of pain and discomfort. The vulval area is checked for redness and excoriation.

Patient problems

- pain and discomfort
- pruritis
- febrile illness.

Planning and implementation

Pain and discomfort are relieved by giving analgesia and sedation as prescribed.

To minimize pruritis frequent vulval toilet is helpful. Appropriate antibiotics are commenced. Nursing the patient in the semi-upright position will assist with pelvic drainage.

All care required during a febrile illness should be given (see Ch. 4). After the acute stage the woman is encouraged to shower rather than having an immersion bath and, if available, to use a bidet. She should be advised about the importance of handwashing to prevent reinfection and cross-infection.

Evaluation

The woman has no pain, pruritis is relieved and there is no discharge.

NEOPLASTIC DISORDERS

New growths of the genital tract may be benign or malignant. Benign growths are far more common than malignant.

Benign growths: fibroids

Fibroids are benign new growths arising from the muscle wall of the uterus. Symptoms are related to their position in the uterine wall (Table 17.3).

Table 17.3 Types of fibroid and symptoms resulting	
Type of fibroid	Symptoms
Submucous – lie beneath the endometrium	Menorrhagia
Intramural – grow within the wall of the uterus	Menorrhagia

Subserous – grow outwards into the peritoneal cavity; frequently multiple and if large cause pressure symptoms	a. Pressure symptoms, e.g.:
	  • frequency
	  • haemorrhoids
	  • varicose veins
	  • constipation
	b. Abdominal swelling

Pedunculated – some fibroids develop a pedicle or stalk which becomes twisted, i.e. torsion	Acute abdominal pain

Table 17.4 Staging of cervical cancer and treatment	
Staging of cervical cancer	Treatment
0 *Preinvasive intraepithelial carcinoma*	Colposcopy Cryocautery Diathermy Laser therapy
I *Limited to the cervix*	Intracavity irradiation Hysterectomy
II *Growth extends to upper two-thirds of vagina*	Wertheim's hysterectomy Intracavity irradiation
III *Involvement of parametrium to pelvic wall. Spread to lower one-third of vagina*	External radiotherapy Intracavity irradiation
IV *Metastases beyond pelvis or involvement of rectum and/or bladder*	Palliative treatment depends on presenting features

Therapeutic management

Small fibroids can be symptomless and no treatment is necessary. Larger fibroids, if causing distressing symptoms, will require surgery.

Myomectomy is the removal of fibroids from the uterine wall and is usually carried out in women who want to have children.

Hysterectomy is the recommended form of treatment for women who do not wish to have any more children.

Nursing strategies

See Nursing Care Plan 17.6 for a patient following hysterectomy.

Malignant growths

Cancer of the cervix

More than 2000 women in Britain die every year from cancer of the cervix.

Aetiology The risk of developing cervical cancer is closely related to sexual habits. Early age at first intercourse and multiple partners are high risk factors. The causes of the disease are not known but a sexually transmitted infection (possibly genital wart virus) is implicated. Smoking is thought to increase susceptibility and women of lower socioeconomic classes have a higher incidence of the disease.

Cervical screening The aim of screening is to detect early cancers while they are still small, have not spread and are easily removable. Cervical screen-

ing can detect precancerous lesions, the treatment of which results in virtually a 100% cure rate. Hence the importance of regular screening.

Therapeutic management Treatment of cervical cancer in relation to staging is given in Table 17.4.

Cancer of the uterus

Endometrial cancer causes about 1000 deaths in Britain per year.

Aetiology It typically occurs in the 50–65 years age group in obese, nulliparous women. It is often associated with diabetes mellitus and links are made with high levels of oestrogen.

Clinical features Postmenopausal bleeding is the most common feature, however any abnormal uterine bleeding must be investigated.

Therapeutic management Treatment of uterine cancer in relation to staging is given in Table 17.5.

Cancer of the ovary

Ovarian cancer is the fifth commonest cancer in women. The overall prognosis is poor and two-thirds of patients die from the disease, which is mainly due to its late diagnosis in the majority of patients.

Aetiology This is predominantly a disease of older, postmenopausal women. The rates are higher in nulliparous women, in those who are infertile and in those women who have had a relative with ovarian cancer.

Clinical features These are often vague and lead to delay in diagnosis. The commonest symptoms in-

Table 17.5 Staging of uterine cancer and treatment

Staging of uterine cancer	Treatment
I Confined to the body of the uterus	Total hysterectomy and bilateral salpingo-oophrectomy with or without radiotherapy
II Extended to the cervix	Wertheim's hysterectomy
III Extended to other organs in the pelvis	Pelvic radiotherapy
IV Further extension to bladder or rectum and distant spread	Palliative radiotherapy Palliative surgery if required

clude abdominal swelling, pain, vaginal bleeding and weight loss.

Therapeutic management Treatment of ovarian cancer in relation to staging is given in Table 17.6.

Cancer of the vulva

This is comparatively rare.

Aetiology This is most common in elderly women and is usually preceded by vulval dystrophy. The tumour appears as a small hard painless ulcer on the labia, which if untreated will eventually spread to involve the whole of the vulva and inguinal and femoral glands.

Therapeutic management If the condition can be identified in the non-invasive stage laser treatment may be given. Otherwise the treatment is surgical. Radical vulvectomy is mutilating surgery and healing after operation is slow.

Radical vulvectomy
Postoperative nursing strategies
1. *Assessment.* General observation of the patient and monitoring of vital signs are important for early detection of shock and haemorrhage. Assessment of the degree of pain and discomfort and adequacy of pain relief is essential. Regular checks of wound dressings and drains are made for excessive bleeding or leakage.
2. *Patient problems.*
   a. potential for shock
   b. pain and discomfort
   c. potential for wound infection
   d. impaired skin integrity
   e. potential for thrombosis
   f. altered body image.

Planning and implementation Monitoring of vital signs and patient's condition is continued. Comfort and pain relief are promoted by giving appropriate analgesia as prescribed and the patient is positioned carefully to relieve tension on sutures. A bed cradle is generally used to protect the wound from the weight of the bed clothes and sometimes a pillow under the patient's knees will give support and relieve pressure on the wound.

To prevent wound infection and facilitate wound healing it is necessary to ensure adequate drainage and compression of tissues. Redivac drains are generally used and it is important to ensure that suction is maintained. A pressure dressing is usually necessary to prevent accumulation of lymph and serum. It is usually more comfortable to keep perineal dressings in place with a T-binder. Prophylactic antibiotics are given intravenously to prevent wound infection. A urethral catheter is normally in situ to prevent wound contamination with urine. Although it is necessary to position the patient to ensure comfort and healing of the wound, it is also important to ensure that pressure areas remain intact.

Table 17.6 Staging of ovarian cancer, treatment and 5-year survival

Staging of ovarian cancer	Treatment	5-year survival
I Growth limited to ovaries	Hysterectomy and bilateral salpingo-oophrectomy	60–70%
II Growth limited to the pelvis	Chemotherapy	40–45%
III Growth extending to abdominal cavity	Chemotherapy	17%
IV Distant metastases	Chemotherapy	5%

As thrombosis is a potential problem the patient will wear antiembolitic stockings and be encouraged to do leg exercises whilst in bed. Early mobilization is essential.

Recovery from such mutilating surgery is slow and breakdown of wounds is not uncommon, necessitating skin grafting in some cases. Assisting the patient to readjust to her altered body image is an important role for the nurse (see Ch. 15).

Evaluation (expected outcomes) The patient has no pain and discomfort from wounds is diminishing daily. There is no wound breakdown or infection and no other postoperative complications are reported. The patient shows knowledge of the discharge plan and is coming to terms with her altered body image.

INFERTILITY

Infertility is the state in which a couple who desire conception are unable to achieve it.

Infertility may be either primary, when the woman has never conceived, or secondary, when there has been at least one confirmed pregnancy whether or not it has gone to term.

Infertility in the female is commonly caused either by some factor preventing the spermatozoa from having free passage to the uterine tubes where the ovum is fertilized or by the woman failing to ovulate so there is no ovum to be fertilized. The most common reason for male infertility is the inability to produce sperm or the production of very few sperm.

Initially the couple are seen by the GP but are usually referred to an infertility clinic. A thorough investigation is carried out to exclude ovarian factors, tubal factors, cervical factors, uterine factors and seminal factors.

The nurse's role is to explain the investigations, discuss the causes and possible treatments for infertility and to give support and encouragement throughout.

Therapeutic management

In some cases after investigation the cause of the problem has not still not been found. Advice is therefore given about improving the chances of contraception. Re-investigation can be carried out after 12–18 months of unprotected intercourse.

If the women is not ovulating hormone therapy is given to induce ovulation. Surgery is aimed at restoring function in both the male and female by correcting any anomalies or malformations.

Artificial insemination techniques can be used when male infertility is the problem. Approximately 65% of women successfully conceive in this way.

With in vitro fertilization techniques, eggs are taken from the woman or a donor and are then mixed with sperm in the laboratory. If fertilization is successful then one or more is replaced in the uterus. These treatments are, however, costly and success rates are low.

CONTRACEPTION

The nurse can discuss with the client the type and adequacy of contraception required. A sympathetic approach with a full explanation of the advantages and disadvantages of the various methods should be given. If assisting a client to make a choice, age and any relevant medical history should be taken into account. The chosen method should be explained thoroughly and appropriate literature given to the client to take home.

Types of contraception

Natural methods

'**Safe period**' The lifespans of spermatozoa and ova are short and fertilization occurs near the time that the ovum is released. This method is based on calculating the time of ovulation and avoiding intercourse during the fertile period, that is for approximately 10 days. The remaining days of the cycle are termed the 'safe period'.

Coitus interruptus This method of withdrawal before ejaculation is better than no contraception but has a high failure rate, usually because withdrawal is too late. However, this is the only method accepted by some cultures.

Mechanical methods

Vaginal diaphragm This is a dome of fine latex or plastic. It fits across the upper vagina to provide a barrier preventing the ejaculated spermatozoa from reaching the cervix. It is made in various shapes and sizes and every woman using it is individually fitted.

Male condom This is placed over the penis and acts as a barrier to the spermatozoa entering the vagina. As a method of contraception it is fairly reliable if used properly. The use of condoms is recommended to prevent the spread of AIDS, gonorrhoea, trichomonal vaginitis and other sexually transmitted diseases. It may also give some protection against development of cervical neoplasia.

Female condom This is a new form of barrier contraception with a polyurethane sac lining the vagina. Its acceptability and efficiency have yet to be assessed.

Intrauterine devices (IUDs)

IUDs are simply foreign bodies in the uterus. There mode is not fully understood but they set up an inflammatory response in the endometrium. They come in a variety of shapes and are made of inert radio-opaque plastic and must be fitted into the uterus by a skilled practitioner. Threads are attached to them so that the woman can check that the IUD is in place. They have a moderately reliable contraceptive effect.

Oral contraceptives

1. The combined oestrogen and progesterone pill is used by more than 25% of women in the UK for contraception and is very reliable if used correctly. It is most suitable for young women who are healthy and non-smoking.

2. Progesterone-only pills contain a small amount of progesterone and have to be taken regularly at the same time each day. They are used when oestrogen is contraindicated and are effective if taken regularly.

Depot medroxyprogesterone acetate (Depot-Provera)

This is given by intramuscular injection every 12 weeks. It is a very effective contraceptive, particularly for those who cannot manage to take oral contraceptives regularly.

Postcoital contraception

The aim is to prevent implantation if fertilization occurs and must be given within 72 hours of unprotected intercourse.

Sterilization

Male sterilization Vasectomy is performed by removing a short length of each vas deferens. It is easier to perform than female sterilization and has fewer complications. Reversal of vasectomy is very difficult. Microsurgical techniques can be used (vasovasostomy) but success cannot be guaranteed and therefore vasectomy must be considered as permanent. (For nursing management after surgery see p. 613.)

Female sterilization This is effective immediately. It involves a general anaesthetic and a short stay in hospital. The uterine tubes can be occluded by the application of clips or rings or by diathermy under laparoscopic vision. Clips cause the least damage to the tubes and allow the best chance of reversal.

SURGICAL MANAGEMENT OF DISORDERS OF THE FEMALE REPRODUCTIVE SYSTEM

For a summary of gynaecological surgery see Table 17.7.

Hysterectomy

Hysterectomy is the surgical removal of the uterus. For possible indications and types of hysterectomy see Table 17.8.

Postoperative nursing strategies

Assessment General observation of the patient and monitoring of vital signs are the same as for any patient after abdominal surgery (see Ch. 4). The wound and any drains are checked frequently for excessive blood loss. Vaginal loss is also checked regularly. The patient is assessed for degree of pain and adequacy of pain control and urinary output is monitored.

Patient problems

- Potential for shock and haemorrhage.
- Pain and discomfort.
- Potential urinary problems.
- Potential infection.
- Potential thrombosis.

Planning and implementation See Nursing Care Plan 17.6 for care for a patient following hysterectomy.

Patient education

1. If salpingo-oophorectomy has been performed in women of child-bearing age it produces surgical menopause. The nurse should explain to the patient the importance of hormone replacement therapy.

2. Advise patient to rest as much as possible initially on discharge and to resume only light household tasks during the first month after operation in order to avoid putting any strain on abdominal muscles.

3. Explain that tiredness and depression are common after hysterectomy but will not last so they should not feel discouraged. Advise against heavy lifting for at least 6 weeks and suggest that driving a car is delayed for 3–4 weeks as this may cause lower abdominal discomfort. Advise that the resumption of

Table 17.7 Gynaecological surgery

Operation	Indications	Specific nursing strategies	Potential complications
D & C Dilatation of cervix and curetting of endometrium	Diagnostic: to establish cause of abnormal bleeding, e.g. menorrhagia, intermenstrual bleeding Therapeutic: to evacuate uterus, e.g. termination of pregnancy, evacuation of retained products of conception to correct dysfunctional bleeding or dysmenorrhoea	Observe for signs of haemorrhage	Haemorrhage Infection Perforation of uterus Laceration of cervix
Laparoscopy	Diagnostic: infertility or pelvic pain Therapeutic: tubal occlusion (sterilization)	Analgesia may be required for pain Encourage mobilization to disperse CO_2 gas	Haemorrhage from vessel damage Perforation of bowel
Total hysterectomy – removal of uterus	Dysfunctional uterine bleeding, cancer of uterus, fibroids in patients who do not want children	Observe for haemorrhage Monitor urinary output Give appropriate analgesia Encourage early mobilization Monitor for signs of infection Ensure patient is wearing antiembolitic stockings	Haemorrhage Urinary retention Urinary tract infection Wound infection Thrombosis
Total hysterectomy and bilateral salpingo-oophorectomy – removal of uterus, fallopian tubes and ovaries	Endometriosis Malignancy	As for total hysterectomy	In premenopausal women will cause sudden, severe menopausal symptoms unless hormone replacements are given
Wertheim's hysterectomy – removal of uterus, fallopian tubes, ovaries, upper third of vagina and lymph nodes in groin	Cancer of cervix or endometrium	Patient should be carefully monitored as this is extensive surgery, otherwise as for total hysterectomy Psychological support	Leg oedema Damage to adjacent organs Shock and haemorrhage Urinary retention Paralytic ileus Thrombosis
Vaginal hysterectomy – vaginal removal of the uterus	Fibroids Uterovaginal prolapse	Monitor urinary output Catheter care if patient has urethral catheter Perineal care	Haemorrhage Wound infection Urinary tract infection Thrombosis
Trans-cervical endometrial resection – resection of the endometrium via vaginal route (alternative to hysterectomy)	Dysfunctional uterine bleeding	Check PV loss Check urinary output	Perforation of uterus Electrolyte imbalance
Radical vulvectomy – removal of surface tissue of vulva and lymph glands in groin	Malignancy of vulva	Appropriate analgesia Position to ensure comfort Care of urethral or suprapubic catheter Ensure drainage and compression of tissues Prevent infection and promote wound healing Psychological support	Shock Thrombosis, embolism Chronic oedema of legs Wound infection Delay in healing

Table 17.7 (*cont'd*)

Operation	Indications	Specific nursing strategies	Potential complications
Anterior/posterior colporrhaphy – repair of anterior/posterior vaginal wall prolapse	Cystocele Rectocele	Care of urethral catheter If no catheter monitor urinary output to keep bladder pressure low Vulval and perineal care	Urinary complications Thrombosis
Manchester repair – repair of uterine prolapse, amputation of cervix, anterior and posterior colpoperineorrhaphy	Uterovaginal prolapse	As for anterior/posterior colporraphy	Urinary complications Thrombosis
Marshall–Marchetti suprapubic urethrovesical suspension	Stress incontinence	Monitor urinary output Appropriate analgesia Early mobilization Observe for signs of haemorrhage or infection	Urinary complications Haematoma

Table 17.8   Types of hysterectomy and indications

Types of hysterectomy	Indications
Total abdominal hysterectomy	Menorrhagia Dysfunctional uterine bleeding Fibroids
Total abdominal hysterectomy and bilateral salpingo-oophrectomy	Endometriosis Chronic pelvic infection Menorrhagia Malignancy
Wertheim's hysterectomy	Stage I and II cancer of cervix Cancer of body of uterus
Subtotal hysterectomy	Usually in technical difficulties Only justifiable if total hysterectomy is not feasible
Vaginal hysterectomy	Uterine prolapse Procidentia

sexual intercourse should wait until after follow-up examination.

4. Stress the importance of attending for follow-up appointment and advise patient to see her GP if she has any abnormal bleeding or vaginal discharge before then.

Evaluation (expected outcomes)

The patient has no pain from the operation and dis-comfort is becoming less each day. She is able to pass urine without difficulty and reports no complications. She shows knowledge and understanding of discharge advice.

Uterovaginal prolapse

Uterovaginal prolapse occurs as a result of weakening or damage to the supporting structures of the pelvic organs. This allows the uterus to prolapse into or

Nursing Care Plan 17.6 Care plan for a patient after hysterectomy

Problem	Goal	Nursing intervention	Rationale
1. Potential for shock and haemorrhage	Prevention or early detection of shock and haemorrhage	❒ Monitor pulse and blood pressure Observe patient for signs of shock Check wound dressing regularly If there is a wound drain check amount and type of drainage regularly Check PV loss regularly	Haemorrhage may occur within 24 hours The nurse should observe for signs of internal as well as external bleeding Haemorrhage is more common after vaginal hysterectomy
2. Pain and discomfort	Relief of pain and discomfort	❒ Give appropriate analgesia as prescribed Restrict oral fluids and food until peristalsis resumes Ensure adequate hydration with intravenous fluids Encourage mobility Give antiemetics as prescribed when required	Patient will have pain related to the surgical procedure but will also often have pain and discomfort from abdominal distention. This is due to partial stasis of the gut preventing gaseous escape per rectum
3. Potential urinary problems	To minimize urinary disturbances	❒ Measure and record urinary output May require catheterisation if unable to pass urine or unable to empty bladder completely If catheter in situ regularly measure and record urine volumes	Urinary difficulties are common due to proximity of surgical site to the bladder Oedema or nerve trauma may cause temporary bladder atomy Distended bladder may pull on newly sutured pelvic tissues causing discomfort and possible haemotoma
4. Potential infection	To minimize risk or early detection of infection	❒ Monitor temperature Take regular urine specimens for culture Check for PV loss at regular intervals Check wound for signs of inflammation or for any abnormal discharge	Wound infection and urinary tract infection are the most common infections after hysterectomy
5. Potential thrombosis	Prevention of thromboembolitic complications	❒ Ensure that patient has antiembolitic stockings Encourage leg exercise Encourage early mobilization	Thrombosis is a common complication after gynaecological surgery This may be due to the site of surgery, with its interruption to pelvic venous return

through the vagina. As the uterus prolapses traction causes the vagina to prolapse which in turn causes the bladder and rectum to herniate into it. Vaginal wall prolapse can occur without uterine descent.

Aetiology

Factors which predispose to uterovaginal prolapse are multiparity and overstretching during childbirth. Also the decline in muscle tone and atrophy of reproductive organs due to lack of oestrogen after the menopause.

Uterine prolapse

Uterine prolapse is classified into degrees according to the descent of the uterus:

1st degree: the uterus has descended slightly but the cervix is still inside the vagina (Fig. 17.25).

2nd degree: the cervix appears outside the vagina.

3rd degree (Procidentia): the uterus is completely outside the vagina (Fig. 17.26).

Vaginal wall prolapse

This is the descent of vaginal walls due to weakness

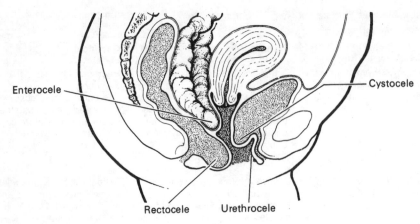

Fig. 17.25 Prolapse of the uterus

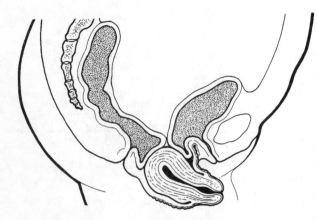

Fig. 17.26 Uterovaginal prolapse (procidentia)

in their supporting structures. It will also cause descent and herniation of adjacent organs.

There are two types of vaginal prolapse:

- Cystocele: prolapse of bladder and anterior vaginal wall (Fig. 17.25).
- Rectocele: prolapse of rectum and posterior vaginal wall (Fig. 17.25).

Clinical features

The patient may complain of fullness in the vagina or the feeling of 'something coming down'. There may be a dragging ache, worsening with prolonged standing or coughing. Often urinary symptoms are problematical with urinary frequency, stress incontinence or incomplete emptying leading to urinary tract infection. Bowel symptoms such as constipation or inability to empty the rectum completely may also occur.

Therapeutic management

Pelvic floor exercises may be sufficient to tighten the muscles of the pelvic floor and relieve symptoms. In postmenopausal women oestrogen therapy may be helpful. The use of a ring pessary can help to relieve symptoms in younger women who wish to have more children or in the elderly who are unfit for or refuse surgery.

Surgery is usually required and the operation will depend on the type and degree of prolapse. Operations include:

- vaginal hysterectomy
- Manchester repair
- anterior colporrhaphy
- posterior colporrhaphy
- perineorrhaphy.

Nursing strategies

Assessment General observation of the patient and monitoring of vital signs are important in the immediate postoperative period. The patient is checked regularly for degree of pain or discomfort and adequacy of pain control.

Patient problems

- Potential for urinary complications.
- Pain and discomfort.
- Impairment of perineal skin integrity.
- Potential for infection.
- Potential for thrombosis.

Planning and implementation Most patients will have a urethral or suprapubic catheter to prevent bladder distension. Those patients with no catheter should be encouraged to empty their bladder every

3–4 hours to keep bladder pressure low. If difficulty is experienced in voiding a catheter will have to be inserted. Accurate assessment of intake and output should be made. A high fluid intake should be encouraged while the catheter is in situ to help reduce the incidence of urinary tract infection.

Analgesia is given when required as prescribed to ensure patient comfort. Sitting may be uncomfortable so other positions should be encouraged. Cleanliness of the vulval and perineal area is important to prevent secondary infection of sutures. Regular vulval toilet should be given until the patient is ambulant. When ambulant encourage daily baths and use of the bidet after visits to toilet. Encourage a high fibre diet and give aperients if necessary to avoid straining on defaecation.

Thrombosis is a potential complication, therefore early mobilization is essential, however, tightness of perineal sutures may make walking uncomfortable so mobilization may have to be gradual.

For early detection of infection temperature is monitored and vaginal loss checked regularly.

Evaluation (expected outcomes)

The patient has no pain or discomfort. She is able to pass urine without difficulty and has no post-operative complications.

Patient education

The patient is advised to rest as much as possible after discharge and very gradually resume normal activity over a 3 month period. Emphasize the importance of permanently avoiding any heavy lifting as this could cause further damage. Advise to refrain from sexual intercourse until after the 6 week check-up to ensure that healing has taken place.

BREAST

The breast plays an important part in a woman's body image. Some women pay large sums of money for surgical operations that either enlarge their breasts, make them smaller or improve their shape. It follows that removal of a diseased breast will have a profound psychological effect upon a woman.

Anatomy and physiology

The anatomy of the breast is illustrated in Figure 17.27. It is important to note that blood and lymphatic supplies to the breast are liberal; this is of particular

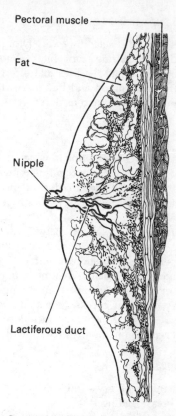

Fig. 17.27 Section showing breast in resting phase

significance in relation to some disorders and their treatment.

Blood supply is via the mammary branches of the axillary, internal thoracic and intercostal arteries.

Venous drainage takes place through veins following similar routes to those of the arteries.

Lymphatic drainage is through vessels distributed all over the breast which drain mainly into the axillary lymph nodes.

The breasts develop at puberty under the influence of the ovarian hormones to which they continue to respond throughout reproductive life. Each menstrual cycle therefore brings changes within the breast, premenstrually there is an increase in blood supply and in growth of glandular tissue, which gives rise to the discomfort experienced by many women. The slightly nodular feel of the breasts at this time is also regarded as physiologically normal. The breasts resume a resting phase after menstruation (Fig. 17.27). The cyclic changes continue throughout reproductive life unless pregnancy intervenes, but cease at the menopause with the decline in the production of the ovarian hormones.

Disorders of the breast

The breasts may be affected by a variety of pathological conditions including congenital abnormalities, infections, tumours and diseases that affect the skin. By far the most common and important disorder is cancer, which is, therefore, considered in more detail.

Fibrocystic disease

Aetiology   This is a condition in which there is dysfunction of the breast, it is not an inflammatory state. The cyclic changes that occur during menstruation due to stimulation of the breast by oestrogen become abnormal.

Clinical features   The cyclic changes cause part or all of the breast to become fibrous or cystic and the patient experiences pain and discomfort.

Therapeutic management   Treatment may involve aspiration or excision. The nurse must emphasize the importance of regular checks, as patients with fibrocystic disease have an increased incidence of malignancy and self-examination is very difficult.

Acute mastitis

This is an inflammatory condition generally associated with breast feeding.

Clinical features   The woman complains of pain and tenderness in the affected breast. There may be signs of systemic infection. The infection may be blood borne or introduced through a fissured nipple.

Therapeutic management   Early diagnosis and antibiotic therapy have greatly reduced the possibility of abscess formation and in most cases breast feeding may be continued once the local symptoms have cleared up.

Benign tumours of the breast

Aetiology   Fibroadenomas occur as encapsulated lumps, commonly in the breasts of young women.

Therapeutic management   They are usually removed, although they will not grow very large, because a benign tumour may undergo malignant changes. The usual investigations will be carried out to confirm that it is indeed benign (see Ch. 4).

Malignant tumours of the breast

Each year in the UK 24 000 women are newly diagnosed with breast cancer and 15 000 women die from the disease. Breast cancer is by far the most common type of cancer in women.

Aetiology   It seems highly probably that hormones, particularly oestrogen, play an important role in the development of breast cancer. Risk factors include increasing age, late childbearing and family history (first degree relative).

Clinical features (Fig. 17.28)   The earliest symptom is a painless lump or thickening in the breast. Alteration in the shape of the breast or retraction of the nipple suggest that the tumour has begun to infiltrate locally. Dimpling of the skin, which is said to look like the peel of an orange (*peau d'orange*), indicates that the small lymphatics beneath the dermis have become blocked. Ulceration through the skin is a late feature.

Malignant tumours spread by the lymphatics and the bloodstream. Metastases will be found in the

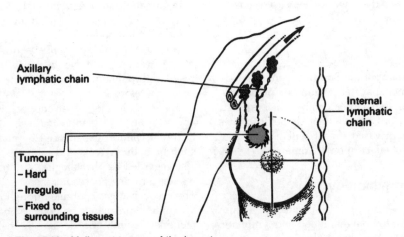

Axillary lymphatic chain

Internal lymphatic chain

Tumour
- Hard
- Irregular
- Fixed to surrounding tissues

Fig. 17.28   Malignant tumour of the breast

lymph nodes of the axilla on the affected side initially and later elsewhere (Baum 1988).

Investigations

Breast examination Breast examination involves inspection and palpation to detect abnormalities.

Self-examination of the breast The earlier breast cancer is diagnosed the better are the survival rates. Women should therefore be encouraged to examine their own breasts visually noting any asymmetry and by palpation (Fig. 17.29).

Mammography Mammography (X-ray) is used to detect lesions which may or may not be palpable and is diagnostically very accurate. Other imaging techniques such as thermography and ultrasonography are not as reliable.

Screening Breast cancer incidence rises sharply with increase in age. Age is the only risk factor of sufficient significance to influence screening policy. Accordingly mammography is being offered to all women aged 50–64 years and repeated at 3 yearly intervals.

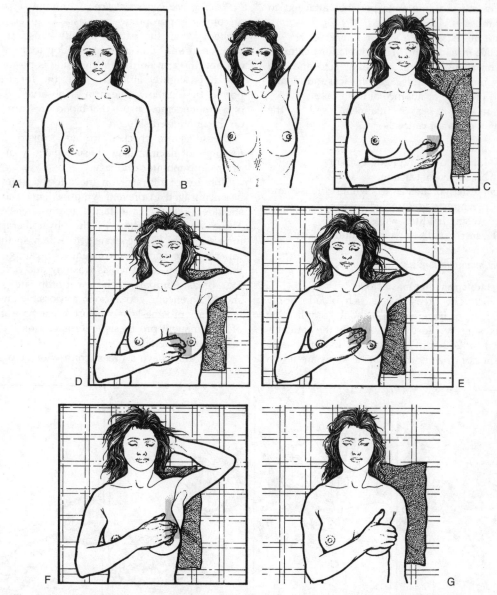

Fig. 17.29 (A), (B) Breast inspection by looking into a mirror. (C)–(G) Self-examination by palpation

Aspiration cytology This procedure can be carried out as an outpatient. After injection of local anaesthetic, a fine bore needle is inserted into the site to be sampled and the tissue aspirated into a syringe (Fig. 17.30).

Open biopsy This is carried out under general anaesthetic. A specimen of tissue is sent to the laboratory for frozen section.

Staging of tumour

I   Small moveable tumour confined to breast.

II Spread to lymph nodes.

III Locally advanced tumour possibly attached to chest muscles.

IV Distant metastases.

Therapeutic management The criteria for treatment depends on many factors, including size and site of tumour, menstrual status, age, physical and mental health and presence or absence of metastases.

There are four types of treatment used in the management of breast cancer.

1. *Surgery*: mastectomy
          lumpectomy and node excision
          breast reconstruction.
2. *Radiation*: external beam to whole breast and lymph nodes sealed local radiotherapy using irridium wires.
3. *Chemotherapy*: usually a combination of drugs is used.
4. *Hormone manipulation*: e.g. tamoxifen.

Nursing strategies after mastectomy

Assessment The breast has a rich blood supply therefore haemorrhage is a potential complication after breast surgery. Close observation of the patient is maintained for 24 hours after surgery to detect early signs of shock or haemorrhage. Vital signs are monitored frequently and wound dressings checked at regular intervals for bleeding. The amount and colour of any wound drainage in the Redivac drain is noted. The affected arm is checked frequently for oedema.

Patient problems

- Pain and discomfort.
- Impaired mobility of affected arm.
- Impaired skin integrity.
- Altered self-image.
- Potential for lymphoedema.

Planning and implementation To minimize pain and discomfort appropriate analgesia is given as prescribed. When the patient is fully conscious she is positioned in a semi-upright position to assist drainage and the arm on the affected side is positioned so that it is slightly abducted with the forearm supported by a pillow. The arm is observed for signs of lymphoedema. Ensure that blood pressure is taken on the unaffected side.

Dressings are checked for any constriction and for signs of haemorrhage. Ensure patency of wound drains and monitor drainage.

Mobility of the arm on the affected side should be encouraged to prevent lymphoedema and frozen shoulder. Exercises are started gently after 24 hours. These are usually done by the physiotherapist but nurses should be encouraged to watch so that they can reinforce correct movements. Encourage use of the arm in self-care such as washing and hair brushing. Breast support with an appropriate soft bra should be encouraged as soon as possible and a soft temporary prosthesis may be used. The type and style of a permanent prosthesis will depend on individual needs and preferences.

Many units have a breast counsellor who will see

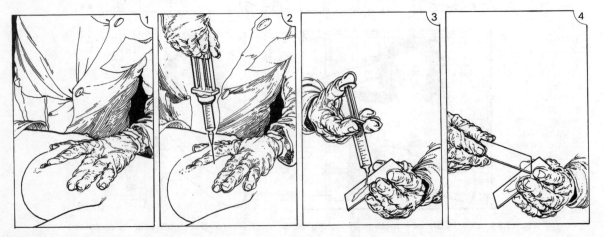

Fig. 17.30 Procedure for aspiration cytology

the patient before and after surgery. Education and support of the patient are of paramount importance for good physical and psychological recovery following mastectomy. The patient must be allowed to discuss her fears and anxieties and be assisted in coming to terms with her altered body image (see Ch. 15). The patient's husband or partner should be prepared for a supportive role.

Patient education Encourage the patient to continue exercises after discharge and advise on skin care a round incision site and how to recognize signs of infection. Following mastectomy there is inevitably a feeling of deep personal loss and the time required to adjust to the situation varies considerably. Local self-help groups or the Mastectomy Association should be recommended as sources of continued support.

Further information
BACUP
121/123 Charterhouse Street
London EC1M 6AA
Cancer Information Service (from London): 071 608 1661
Freeline (from outside London): 0800 181199
Counselling Service (London based): 071 696 9000

Offers medical and non-medical information and support to patients, their families and friends. Publications include: *Understanding Cancer of the Breast, Understanding Secondary Breast Cancer, Understanding, Radiotherapy* and a *Tamoxifen factsheet.*

Breast Cancer Care
15/19 Britten Street, London SW3 3TZ
Help and Information Line: 071 867 1103
Administration: 071 867 8275

Suite 2/8, 65 Bath Street, Glasgow G2 2BX
Tel: 041 353 1050

9 Castle Terrace, Edinburgh EH1 2DP
Tel: 031 221 0407
Also Freeline 0500 245 345

Charity Registration Number: 271078

Suggested assignments

DISCUSSION TOPICS
1. Incontinence is a taboo subject. How can sufferers be helped to cope with this socially unacceptable problem?
2. The impact of renal disease and the necessity of regular dialysis can put patients and families under considerable anxiety and stress. Discuss the nurse's role in helping them cope.
3. Are nurses equipped to meet the emotional needs of women after miscarriage? Discuss.

ETHICAL ISSUES
1. In spite of an ever increasing demand for kidneys for transplantation the number of transplant operations carried out each year is fairly static. Should an 'OPT-OUT' organ donor card system be introduced instead of the 'OPT-IN' system used at present?
2. Evidence shows that increased screening could decrease the number of deaths from breast cancer. In the current financial climate should extra money be made available for breast screening?
3. Is it right that money is being spent on in vitro fertilization so that single women can have children? Discuss.

REFERENCES AND FURTHER READING

Anderton J L A, Thomson D 1988 Nephrology: colour aids. Churchill Livingstone, Edinburgh
Asscher A W, Moffat D B 1983 Nephro-urology. Heinemann Medical Books, London
Baum M 1988 Breast cancer: the facts. Oxford University Press, Oxford
Bullock N, Sibley G, Whitaker R 1989 Essential urology. Churchill Livingstone, Edinburgh
Daugirdas J T, Ing T S 1988 Handbook of dialysis. Little, Brown and Co, Boston
Fream W C 1979 Notes on gynaecological nursing. Churchill Livingstone, Edinburgh
Garrey M M, Govan A D T, Hodge C, Callander R 1978 Gynaecology illustrated, 2nd edn. Churchill Livingstone, Edinburgh

Genitourinary problems (Nurse Review) 1986 Springhouse Corporation,
Kilmartin A 1990 Understanding cystitis. Pan Books, London
Lerner J, Khan Z 1982 Manual of urologic nursing. CV Mosby, London
Lin D T, Lachelin G C 1989 Practical gynaecology. Butterworths, London
Mandelstam D 1977 Incontinence. Heinemann Health Books, London
Pfeiffer C H, Mulliken J B 1984 Caring for the patient with breast cancer. Reston Publishing Co, Virginia
Read A E et al 1984 Modern medicine, 3rd edn. Churchill Livingstone, Edinburgh
Renal and urologic disorders (Nurses Clinical Library) 1984

Springhouse Corporation, 1111 Bethlehem Pike, Springhouse PA

Ross & Wilson Anatomy and physiology, 5th edn. Churchill Livingstone, Edinburgh

Shorthouse M A, Brush M G 1981 Gynaecology in nursing practice. Baillière Tindall, London

Smith E K M 1987 Renal disease: a conceptual approach. Churchill Livingstone, Edinburgh

Tortora G J, Anagnostakos N P 1990 Principles of anatomy and physiology, 5th edn. Harper and Row, New York

Uldall R 1988 Renal nursing, 3rd edn. Blackwell Scientific Publications, Oxford

Whitworth J A, Lawrence J R 1987 Textbook of renal disease. Churchill Livingstone, Edinburgh

Wood R F M 1983 Renal transplantation: a clinical handbook. Baillière Tindall, London

Glossary

Abduction: movement of a limb away from the midline of the body.

'Acting out': the resolution of inner conflicts through anti-social or aggressive behaviour.

Acuity: sharpness of perception, for example, visual acuity.

Adduction: movement of a limb towards the midline of the body.

Amputation: traumatic or surgical removal of all or part of a limb.

Anorexic: having no appetite.

Anti-social personality: see personality disorder.

Arthrography: injection of contrast medium into a joint which is then gently inflated with carbon dioxide. Allows joint structures to be examined.

Arthroscopy: examination of a joint (usually the knee) carried out under general anaesthetic. An arthroscope is introduced into the joint to allow direct observation of the internal structure of the joint.

Articulating cartilage: hyaline cartilage which covers the epiphyses of bones in a synovial joint. It is continuous with the periosteum.

Articulation: a joint, contact between bones or cartilage and bones.

At risk: state of vulnerability to a particular health problem as a result of hereditary factors, health practices or family environment.

Atrophy: a decrease in size of cells, tissues, or parts of the body.

Balanced traction: uses a pulley and weight system to provide a pull against the counter traction which is the patient's body weight. It can be achieved using skin extensions or skeletal traction. Used to maintain alignment of fractures.

Base movement: begins with relaxation of the knees and the movement of a foot either forwards or in the direction of a possible fall. This movement reduces postural stiffening and widens the base area to allow balance to be maintained during handling and moving operations.

Behaviour therapy: a psychological treatment aimed at changing observable symptoms.

Benign tumour: non-malignant growth.

Biopsy: surgical removal of a very small piece of tissue which is sent for laboratory examination to aid diagnosis.

Calcitonin: hormone, which is necessary for bone growth and development produced by the thyroid gland.

Cancellous bone: latticework type of bone found in the epiphyses of long bones. Also known as spongy bone. Found in large quantities in short and flat bones. Red marrow is commonly found within cancellous bone.

Cellular immunity: specially sensitised T cells attach to antigens (foreign material) and destroy them.

Chronic illness: an illness that is long lasting and usually irreversible.

Classical conditioning: reflexive responses are attached to new stimuli by pairing the new stimuli with existing stimuli that naturally elicit the response.

Cognitive: adjective, referring to the processes of thinking, perception and reasoning.

Cognitive dissonance: a state of disequilibrium which occurs when a person's beliefs or values are inconsistent with their behaviour.

Compact bone: dense bone found in the shaft of long bones and in thin layers covering cancellous bone.

Congenital: being present at or from birth, usually referring to disease or deformity.

Contractility: ability of cells to shorten or draw together. Muscle fibres (cells) have a high degree of contractility.

Contracture: irreversible shortening of a muscle due to fibrosis or diminished blood supply. Can occur in both lower and upper limbs, causing deformity and loss of function.

Corticosteroids: hormones secreted by the adrenal cortex, for example hydrocortisone. These can be produced synthetically and have powerful anti-inflammatory properties.

Corticotrophin: a hormone secreted by the anterior pituitary gland which stimulates the adrenal cortex to produce corticosteroids. It can be given by injection if it is not produced in sufficient quantities.

Crepitus (bony): the grating sound when two ends of a fractured bone rub together.

Counselling: a process through which one person helps another by purposeful conversation in an understanding atmosphere.

Crisis intervention: action taken to minimise disruption in an actual or potential emergency.

Culture: the norms and values of a society, learned by the members of that society during socialisation; includes language and convention.

Debilitated: weakened, usually as a result of disease or injury.

Delusion: a false belief held in spite of reasoning to the contrary.

Depression: a low mood state.

Diaphysis: shaft of a long bone.

Elasticity: the ability of tissue to return to its original shape following extension or contraction.

Embolus: a clot or other substance brought by the blood from another vessel and forced into a smaller one, thus obstructing the circulation.

Empathy: the ability to be sensitive to another individual's feelings and to communicate this understanding to that individual.

Endosteum: the membrane that lines the medullary cavity of bones.

Epidemiology: the study of patterns of disease in human populations.

Epiphysis: the end of a long bone.

Ethnic: refers to a group in society who share cultural values and/or physical characteristics.

Ethnic minority: a group of people who share cultural and racial factors but who constitute a minority within a larger social group.

Euthanasia: ending the life of a person suffering from a terminal disease, or assisting them to end their own life.

Excitability: the ability of muscle tissue to receive and respond to stimuli.

Extensibility: the ability of muscle tissue to stretch when pulled.

External fixation: a method of immobilising a fracture from the outside of the affected limb. Usually involves the insertion of pins through the bone above and below the fracture which is then held in place by a clamp.

External splintage: Immobilisation of a fracture with a plaster cast. Usually used in stable fractures.

Exudate: discharge from cells or blood vessels.

Fixed traction: application of a pulling force to a limb; does not involve a pulley and weights system.

Flexion: a movement resulting in the decrease of an angle between two bones.

Fracture: a break in the continuity of bone.

Galactose: soluble sugar which is derived from lactose.

Glycoprotein: a protein with sugar groups attached.

Growth hormone: a hormone that stimulates the growth of tissues, produced by the anterior pituitary gland.

Fear appeals: efforts to change attitudes to health by arousing fear to induce the motivation to change behaviour.

Grief: a response to bereavement involving a feeling of hollowness and sometimes marked preoccupation with the dead person. The bereaved person may experience feelings of guilt and express hostility towards others. Symptoms may also include restlessness, inability to concentrate, and other psychological and physical problems. Similar emotional responses may arise following other losses such as divorce, examination failure.

Haematoma: a tumour or swelling filled with blood.

Haemopoiesis: formation of blood cells.

Haemorrhage: bleeding; the escape of blood from blood vessels.

Halitosis: offensive smelling breath.

Hallucination: a false perception in the absence of external stimuli.

Health beliefs: beliefs about the relationship between particular health practices and health outcomes.

Holistic care: an approach to health care which treats the individual as a whole person in relation to his or her environment.

Hormone: a substance produced by endocrine tissue which enters the blood stream and affects the activity of a target cell.

Humoral immunity: the component of immunity where B cells develop into plasma cells that produce antibodies.

Hypertension: high blood pressure.

Hypertrophy: an excessive enlargement or overgrowth of tissue without cell division, increasing the size of an organ as a result of an increased amount of work required of cells.

Hypnotics: a group of drugs which have sleep-inducing properties.

Internal fixation: surgical procedure during which wires, nails or screws are used to hold a fracture securely.

Ischaemia: inadequate or deficient blood supply to some part of the body.

Lacrimation: production of tears by the lacrimal glands.

Libido: sex drive.

Ligament: connective tissue that attaches bone to bone.

Living will: a will prepared by a person with a terminal illness, requesting that life-sustaining procedures should not be used in the event that their ability to make this decision is lost.

Macrophage: phagocytic cell which is derived from a monocyte; can be wandering or fixed.

Macule: small, flat blemish or discolouration of the skin, for example, a freckle.

Malignant: invasive form of cancer which becomes worse and can result in death.

Mania: elevated mood state.

Medical model: a model of health which proposes that health is the absence of disease in a person's body and that restoring a person to health is a matter of curing the disease. This model of health contrasts with the principles underlying holistic care.

Medullary cavity: the space in the diaphysis of long bones which usually contains yellow marrow.

Microbes: a minute living organism which can cause disease.

Mobility: the ability to move. Not purely concerned with walking.

Mourning: the social expression of grief, including culturally-specific funeral rituals and associated behaviour.

Morbidity rate: the number of people affected by a disease within a stated number of the population.

Mortality (death) rate: the number of deaths per year in a stated number of people (commonly a thousand) in a particular country or region, usually in relation to specific causes.

Muscle: may be skeletal, cardiac or smooth; tissue which is specialised for contraction to produce voluntary or involuntary movement.

Muscle spasm: a spasmodic contraction of one of many muscles; cramp.

Muscle tone: a sustained, partial contraction of portions of a muscle.

Myocardial infarction: gross necrosis of myocardial (heart muscle) tissue, due to interrupted blood supply. Also called a 'heart attack'.

Narcotics: group of drugs including opium and morphine.

Necrosis: death of a localised group of cells as a result of injury or disease.

Neoplasm: new growth of tissue which may be benign or malignant.

Neuromuscular: combined effects of the nervous and muscular systems.

Neurovascular checks: observations of circulation, sensation and movement in limbs.

Neurotransmitter: one of a group of chemicals by which nerve cells communicate with each other or with muscle cells.

Nystagmus: involuntary, rhythmic movement of the eyes. Movements may be vertical, horizontal or rotational.

Osteoarthrosis: a degenerative disease in which there is destruction of the articular cartilage. Often begins in the larger, weight-bearing joints.

Osteoblast: bone-forming cell.

Osteoclast: bone-destroying cell.

Osteogenic: the ability to form new bone during growth or repair.

Osteomalacia: a deficiency of vitamin D in adults which causes demineralization and softening of bones; see rickets.

Osteoporosis: a condition resulting from decreased levels of oestrogens, particularly in postmenopausal women. Bone mass is decreased and there is an increased risk of fracture.

Papule: a small, palpable elevation of the skin, for example, a pimple.

Parasuicide: intentional, non-fatal, self-injury or attempted suicide. The intention is not normally to commit suicide but rather to elicit help in resolving a life crisis.

Parathormone: hormone secreted by the parathyroid gland; necessary for bone growth and development.

Passive moments: movements of patients' limbs and joints which are carried out by the nurse on behalf of the patient who cannot perform the movement unaided.

Patient education: informing patients about their condition, its treatment, and methods of coping with the disorder and the limitations it imposes upon them.

Periosteum: tough outer fibrous layer which covers bone; contains osteoblasts and is essential for bone growth, repair and nutrition.

Personality disorder: deeply ingrained maladaptive behaviour patterns which endure most of adult life.

Petechial rash: small spots due to an effusion of blood under the skin.

Photophobia: sensitivity to light.

Physical restraint: a strategy of physical control of aggressive or violent behaviour whereby minimal force is applied in such a way as to obtain the desired results without causing harm.

Polydipsia: excessive fluid consumption usually arising from abnormal thirst.

Polyuria: frequent passing of urine.

Poultice: a local application used to improve circulation and relieve pain, for example, kaolin.

Preprandial: before a meal.

Presbycusis: a sensorineural hearing loss affecting mainly higher notes; associated with ageing.

Prone: lying face downwards.

Proprioception: awareness of the body's position, movement or balance.

Psychiatric emergency: acute mental health problems which require urgent attention from psychiatric services.

Psychoanalysis: a theory of human behaviour and a method of treatment. Psychoanalysis helps people become aware of unconscious thoughts and feelings, many of which, it is thought, have their roots in childhood.

Psychomotor retardation: slowing of thoughts and movements; sometimes present in severe depression.

Psychopathy: a personality disorder which results in abnormally aggressive, insensitive or irresponsible behaviour.

Psychotherapy: a form of treatment which uses verbal exchanges and the establishment of trust to help resolve problems and change behaviour.

Quality of life: the degree to which a person is able to maximise his or her physical, psychological, and social functioning; an important indicator of recovery from or adjustment to chronic illness.

Red marrow: marrow found in the epiphyses of long bones and in short and flat bones. Haemopoiesis occurs in red marrow.

Regression: a defence mechanism whereby the person goes back to earlier, more childlike behaviour.

Rickets: Vitamin D deficiency in children leading to demineralisation and softening of bones.

Rheumatoid disease: painful inflammatory condition affecting all connective tissue; commonly affects synovial joints.

Rubella: German measles.

Skeletal traction: insertion of a pin through a bone to which weights are attached in order to achieve a pull on a muscle or fracture. (See Balanced Traction.)

Skin extensions: application of bandages or elastoplast to a limb to which weights are then attached in order to produce traction. (See Balanced Traction.)

Sleep apnoea: multiple and transient cessations in respiration during sleep. May be associated with snoring.

Sociopathy: see psychopathy.

Stenosis: an abnormal narrowing or constriction of a duct or opening.

Still's disease: a form of rheumatoid arthritis in children.

Subluxation: partial dislocation of a joint.

Suicide: deliberate self-harm with a fatal outcome.

Supine: lying face up.

Synovial fluid: fluid secreted by the synovial membrane which lubricates joints and nourishes articular cartilage.

Synovial joint: a freely movable (diarthrotic) joint in which there is a joint space between the two articulating bones.

Tendon: fibrous connective tissue which attaches muscle to bone.

Thalidomide: a proprietary hypnotic drug which was prescribed as a sedative. It was withdrawn because it caused pregnant women for whom it was prescribed to give birth to children with abnormal or missing limbs.

Thrombolytic agent: chemical substance injected into the body to dissolve blood clots and restore circulation.

Thrombus: a clot formed in an unbroken vessel, usually a vein.

Top heavy movement: the knees are kept in extension and the body is bent forwards from the hip. The centre of gravity is moved forward creating stiffening in the lower limbs, back and shoulders. The amount of postural stiffening is often disproportionate to the activity being carried out.

Traction: the act of pulling or drawing; used to realign fractured bones or overcome muscle spasm.

Tranquillizer: medication prescribed to calm.

Vitamin D: vitamin synthesized by the action of sunlight on the skin. Necessary for the absorption of calcium into the blood stream from the gastrointestinal tract.

Yellow marrow: marrow found within the medullary cavity of adult long bones. Has the capacity to revert to red marrow in the presence of disease.

Index

Page numbers in **bold** type refer to main discussions of a subject; those in *italics* refer to figures, tables or application boxes.